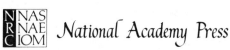

National Academy Press

The National Academy Press was created by the National Academy of
Sciences to publish the reports issued by the Academy and by the
National Academy of Engineering, the Institute of Medicine, and the
National Research Council, all operating under the charter granted to
the National Academy of Sciences by the Congress of the United States.

Mammalian Models for Research on Aging

Committee on Animal Models for Research on Aging
Institute of Laboratory Animal Resources
Division of Biological Sciences
Assembly of Life Sciences

NATIONAL ACADEMY PRESS
Washington, D.C.   1981

The primary support for this publication was provided by Contract No. N01-AG-7-2118, National Institutes of Health, National Institute of Aging.

LIBRARY OF CONGRESS CATALOGING IN PUBLICATION DATA

National Research Council. Committee on Animal Models
    for Research on Aging.
    Mammalian models for research on aging.

    1. Aging--Animal models. 2. Mammals--Age.
I. Title.
QP86.N38   1980   612'.67'0724   80-24383
ISBN 0-309-03094-3

Available from

NATIONAL ACADEMY PRESS
2101 Constitution Avenue, N.W.
Washington, D.C. 20418

Printed in the United States of America

Preface

In December 1976, the National Institute on Aging (NIA)
sponsored a workshop (Belmont House, Elkridge, Maryland)
at which the use of numerous vertebrate species for research on aging was reviewed. The participants generally
agreed that an intensive evaluation of selected species as
models of human aging was needed and that the NIA should

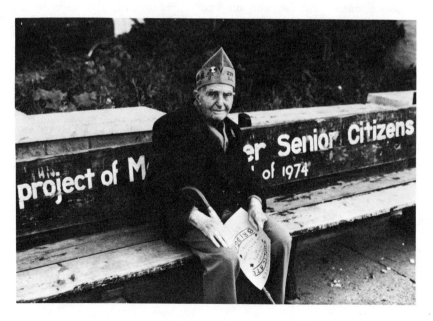

"The goal of biomedical research on aging is to prolong
the useful and active lives of the elderly and to raise
the quality of their lives" (NIA, 1977).

actively promote awareness in the scientific community of significant issues related to animal studies in aging. Subsequently, the National Academy of Sciences was asked to undertake such a study, which was then carried out by the Institute of Laboratory Animal Resources (ILAR) Committee on Animal Models for Research on Aging.

Old animals are expensive and often available in limited numbers for research. It is, therefore, essential to define carefully the goals and strategies of research on aging, and so to plan the research as to derive maximum benefit from the animals that are used. This report is intended to aid investigators in selecting animals and to highlight issues that bear on the relevance and appropriateness of various species as models of human aging.

In preparing this report, the Committee has benefited greatly from the whole-hearted participation of a broad range of scientific and clinical specialists (listed in the following pages) who provided the critical review of widely scattered information and helped to compile it as reflected here. The Committee is grateful, also, to the staff of the Institute of Laboratory Animal Resources for administrative and clerical support, especially to Dorothy D. Greenhouse, who served as Staff Officer.

COMMITTEE ON ANIMAL MODELS
FOR RESEARCH ON AGING

Bennett J. Cohen, Unit for Laboratory Animal Medicine, University of Michigan Medical School, Ann Arbor, Michigan (Chairman)
Richard C. Adelman, Temple University Institute on Aging, Philadelphia, Pennsylvania
Douglas M. Bowden, School of Medicine and Washington Regional Primate Research Center, University of Washington, Seattle, Washington
Carel F. Hollander, Institute for Experimental Gerontology TNO, Rijswijk, The Netherlands
Leah M. Lowenstein, School of Medicine, Boston University, Boston, Massachusetts
Takashi Makinodan, VA Wadsworth Hospital Center, Los Angeles, California
Roger McClellan, Lovelace Inhalation Toxicology Research Institute, Albuquerque, New Mexico
Henryk M. Wisniewski, New York State Institute for Basic Research in Mental Retardation, Staten Island, New York
John Aronson, The Wistar Institute, Philadelphia, Pennsylvania (Invited Contributor)
Vincent J. Cristofalo, The Wistar Institute, Philadelphia, Pennsylvania (Invited Contributor)

SUBCOMMITTEE ON CARNIVORES

Roger McClellan, Lovelace Inhalation Toxicology Research Institute, Albuquerque, New Mexico (Chairman)
Henry J. Baker, Jr., Department of Comparative Medicine, University of Alabama at Birmingham, Birmingham, Alabama
Robert W. Bull, Department of Medicine, Michigan State University, East Lansing, Michigan
Harold W. Casey, Department of Pathology, Armed Forces Institute of Pathology, Washington, D.C.
Webster S.S. Jee, Radiobiology Laboratory, University of Utah, Salt Lake City, Utah
Joe L. Mauderly, Lovelace Inhalation Toxicology Research Institute, Albuquerque, New Mexico
Robert Lee Pyle, Mississippi State University, Mississippi State, Mississippi
Stephen A. Benjamin, College of Veterinary Medicine and Biomedical Sciences, Colorado State University, Fort Collins, Colorado (Invited Contributor)

James Boulay, Collaborative Radiological Health Laboratory, College of Veterinary Medicine and Biomedical Sciences, Colorado State University, Fort Collins, Colorado (Invited Contributor)

Betsy Byrne, Collaborative Radiological Health Laboratory, College of Veterinary Medicine and Biomedical Sciences, Colorado State University, Fort Collins, Colorado (Invited Contributor)

Donald N. Kitchen, Collaborative Radiological Health Laboratory, College of Veterinary Medicine and Biomedical Sciences, Colorado State University, Fort Collins, Colorado (Invited Contributor)

Claire M. Lathers, Department of Pharmacology, Medical College of Pennsylvania, Philadelphia, Pennsylvania (Invited Contributor)

Hamilton Redman, Lovelace Inhalation Toxicology Research Institute, Albuquerque, New Mexico (Invited Contributor)

SUBCOMMITTEE ON LAGOMORPHS AND RODENTS
OTHER THAN RATS AND MICE

Carel F. Hollander, Institute for Experimental Gerontology TNO, Rijswijk, The Netherlands (Chairman)

Joe D. Burek, Dow Chemical Company, Midland, Michigan

Richard R. Fox, The Jackson Laboratory, Bar Harbor, Maine

Alan L. Kraus, University of Rochester Medical Center, Rochester, New York

George A. Sacher, Division of Biological and Medical Research, Argonne National Laboratory, Argonne, Illinois

Albert L. Vincent, Department of Comprehensive Medicine, College of Medicine, University of South Florida, Tampa, Florida

SUBCOMMITTEE ON MICE

Takashi Makinodan, VA Wadsworth Hospital Center, Los Angeles, California (Chairman)

Harold H. Draper, Department of Nutrition, College of Biological Sciences, University of Guelph, Guelph, Ontario, Canada

James F. Florini, Department of Biology, Syracuse University, Syracuse, New York

David Harrison, The Jackson Laboratory, Bar Harbor, Maine

Howard J. Hoffmann, Biometry Branch, National Institute of Child Health and Human Development, National Institutes of Health, Bethesda, Maryland

J. Michael Holland, Biology Division, Oak Ridge National Laboratory, Oak Ridge, Tennessee

C. K. Hsu, Division of Comparative Medicine, Georgetown University Medical Center, Washington, D.C.

Richard L. Sprott, The Jackson Laboratory, Bar Harbor, Maine

Henk H. Solleveld, Institute for Experimental Gerontology TNO, Rijswijk, The Netherlands (Invited Contributor)

SUBCOMMITTEE ON NONHUMAN PRIMATES

Douglas M. Bowden, School of Medicine and Washington Regional Primate Research Center, University of Washington, Seattle, Washington (Chairman)

Irwin S. Bernstein, Yerkes Field Facility, Lawrenceville, Georgia

Thomas B. Clarkson, Department of Comparative Medicine, Bowman Gray School of Medicine, Wake Forest University, Winston-Salem, North Carolina

Donna Cohen, Department of Psychiatry and Behavioral Sciences, University of Washington, Seattle, Washington

Andrew G. Hendrickx, California Primate Research Center, University of California, Davis, California

Robert W. Prichard, Department of Pathology, Bowman Gray School of Medicine, Wake Forest University, Winston-Salem, North Carolina

Peter S. Rodman, Department of Anthropology, University of California, Davis, California

William H. Stone, Laboratory of Genetics, University of Wisconsin, Madison, Wisconsin

Henryk M. Wisniewski, New York State Institute for Basic Research in Mental Retardation, Staten Island, New York

SUBCOMMITTEE ON RATS

Richard C. Adelman, Temple University Institute on Aging, Philadelphia, Pennsylvania (Chairman)

Miriam R. Anver, Unit for Laboratory Animal Medicine, University of Michigan, Ann Arbor, Michigan

Merrill F. Elias, Department of Psychology, University of Maine at Orono, Orono, Maine

Philip W. Landfield, Department of Physiology and Pharma-
cology, Bowman Gray School of Medicine, Wake Forest
University, Winston-Salem, North Carolina
Edward J. Masoro, Department of Physiology, University of
Texas Health Science Center, San Antonio, Texas
Joseph Meites, Department of Physiology, Michigan State
University, East Lansing, Michigan
Jay Roberts, Department of Pharmacology, Medical College
of Pennsylvania, Philadelphia, Pennsylvania
Paula B. Goldberg, Department of Pharmacology, Medical
College of Pennsylvania, Philadelphia, Pennsylvania
(Invited Contributor)

STAFF OFFICER

Dorothy D. Greenhouse

Participants

In compiling its report, the Committee on Animal Models for Research on Aging organized two workshops to prepare the section entitled "Comparative Models of Selected Problems of the Human Elderly." The first workshop was held May 6-7, 1979, in Winston-Salem, North Carolina; the second was held May 17-18, 1979, in Davis, California. The participants were:

NERVOUS SYSTEM AND BEHAVIOR

Philip W. Landfield, Department of Physiology and Pharmacology, Bowman Gray School of Medicine, Wake Forest University, Winston-Salem, North Carolina (<u>Chairman</u>)

Henry J. Baker, Department of Comparative Medicine, University of Alabama at Birmingham, Birmingham, Alabama

Douglas M. Bowden, School of Medicine and Washington Regional Primate Research Center, University of Washington, Seattle, Washington

Donna Cohen, Department of Psychiatry and Behavioral Sciences, University of Washington, Seattle, Washington

Peter S. Rodman, Department of Anthropology, University of California, Davis, California

James Severson, Andrus Gerontology Center, University of Southern California, Los Angeles, California

Henryk M. Wisniewski, New York State Institute for Basic Research in Mental Retardation, Staten Island, New York

VISUAL SYSTEM

Richard R. Fox, The Jackson Laboratory, Bar Harbor, Maine (<u>Chairman</u>)

Roy W. Bellhorn, Department of Ophthalmology, Albert Einstein College of Medicine, Montefiore Hospital and Medical Center, Bronx, New York

Kirk N. Gelatt, Department of Special Clinical Science, University of Florida, Gainesville, Florida

Robert L. Peiffer, Jr., Department of Ophthalmology, School of Medicine, The University of North Carolina at Chapel Hill, Chapel Hill, North Carolina

W. Keith O'Steen, Department of Anatomy, Bowman Gray School of Medicine, Wake Forest University, Winston-Salem, North Carolina

AUDITORY SYSTEM

Robert Lee Pyle, Mississippi State University, Mississippi State, Mississippi (<u>Chairman</u>)

James McCormick, Department of Surgery, Bowman Gray School of Medicine, Wake Forest University, Winston-Salem, North Carolina

Muriel Ross, Department of Anatomy, University of Michigan, Ann Arbor, Michigan

SKELETAL SYSTEM

Webster S.S. Jee, Radiobiology Laboratory, University of Utah, Salt Lake City, Utah (<u>Chairman</u>)

Douglas M. Bowden, School of Medicine and Washington Regional Primate Research Center, University of Washington, Seattle, Washington

Harold H. Draper, Department of Nutrition, College of Biological Science, University of Guelph, Guelph, Ontario, Canada

Carel F. Hollander, Institute for Experimental Gerontology TNO, Rijswijk, The Netherlands

Dike Kalu, Department of Physiology, University of Texas, San Antonio, Texas

Roy C. Page, Center for Research in Oral Biology, University of Washington, Seattle, Washington

RESPIRATORY SYSTEM

Joe L. Mauderly, Lovelace Inhalation Toxicology Research Institute, Albuquerque, New Mexico (<u>Chairman</u>)

Fletcher F. Hahn, Lovelace Inhalation Toxicology Research
Institute, Albuquerque, New Mexico
C. J. Martin, Institute of Respiratory Physiology, Virginia Mason Research Center, Seattle, Washington
Conrad Richter, Oak Ridge Associated University, Oak
Ridge, Tennessee

CARDIOVASCULAR SYSTEM

Thomas B. Clarkson, Department of Comparative Medicine,
Bowman Gray School of Medicine, Wake Forest University,
Winston-Salem, North Carolina (Chairman)
Merrill F. Elias, Department of Psychology, University of
Maine at Orono, Orono, Maine
Richard R. Fox, The Jackson Laboratory, Bar Harbor, Maine
David Lehr, Department of Pharmacology, New York Medical
College, Valhalla, New York
Robert W. Prichard, Department of Pathology, Bowman Gray
School of Medicine, Wake Forest University, Winston-
Salem, North Carolina
Robert Lee Pyle, Mississippi State University, Mississippi
State, Mississippi
Jay Roberts, Department of Pharmacology, Medical College
of Pennsylvania, Philadelphia, Pennsylvania

ENDOCRINE SYSTEM

Richard L. Sprott, The Jackson Laboratory, Bar Harbor,
Maine (Chairman)
Richard C. Adelman, Temple University, Institute on Aging,
Philadelphia, Pennsylvania
Thomas B. Clarkson, Department of Comparative Medicine,
Bowman Gray School of Medicine, Wake Forest University,
Winston-Salem, North Carolina
Robert L. Harris, Department of Comparative Medicine,
Bowman Gray School of Medicine, Wake Forest University,
Winston-Salem, North Carolina
C. Max Lang, Department of Comparative Medicine, College
of Medicine, Pennsylvania State University, Hershey,
Pennsylvania
Robert W. Prichard, Department of Pathology, Bowman Gray
School of Medicine, Wake Forest University, Winston-
Salem, North Carolina
Albert L. Vincent, Department of Comprehensive Medicine,
University of South Florida, Tampa, Florida

OBESITY

Edward J. Masoro, Department of Physiology, University of
Texas, San Antonio, Texas (Chairman)
Robert L. Harris, Department of Comparative Medicine, Bow-
man Gray School of Medicine, Wake Forest University,
Winston-Salem, North Carolina
Richard L. Sprott, The Jackson Laboratory, Bar Harbor,
Maine
Albert L. Vincent, Department of Comprehensive Medicine,
College of Medicine, University of South Florida,
Tampa, Florida

REPRODUCTIVE SYSTEM

Andrew G. Hendrickx, California Primate Center, University
of California, Davis, California (Chairman)
Michael Adams, Department of Comparative Medicine, Bowman
Gray School of Medicine, Wake Forest University,
Winston-Salem, North Carolina
Gordon C. Blaha, Department of Anatomy, University of Cin-
cinnati, Cincinnati, Ohio
Harold W. Casey, Department of Veterinary Pathology,
Armed Forces Institute of Pathology, Washington, D.C.
Caleb Finch, Andrus Gerontology Center, University of
Southern California, Los Angeles, California
Joseph Meites, Department of Physiology, Michigan State
University, East Lansing, Michigan
David R. Meldrum, Department of Obstetrics and Gynecology,
UCLA Medical Center, Los Angeles, California
Sydney A. Shain, Southwest Foundation for Research and
Education, San Antonio, Texas

STAFF OFFICER

Dorothy D. Greenhouse

Contents

Introduction

The primary focus of this report is the relevance and appropriateness of selected mammals as models of human aging. Animal experimentation provides a scientifically valid and ethical approach to the development of new knowledge and contributes to human and animal welfare. In this sense, the scientific and moral justification for using animals in research on aging is the same as for other areas of biomedical significance. Legal, ethical, and practical constraints limit the extent to which human subjects can be used in research on aging. Moreover, an understanding of human aging requires basic research on relevant biological principles and phenomena (NIA, 1977). Man is not an appropriate subject for much of this type of research. Accordingly, utilization of many biological systems and animal species is necessary to study the scientific questions that are relevant to human aging.

SCOPE OF THE REPORT

Animals have three broad roles in research on aging. They may serve as:

- models for studying biological mechanisms and normative aspects of aging, such as reproductive senescence and physiological decline in various other organ systems;
- models for research on the pathology of aging, i.e., effects and interactions of environment and genetics on disease and longevity; and
- sources of cells, tissues, organs, and fluids for in vitro studies in the above-mentioned areas.

These roles are elaborated upon in the following sections.

DEFINITION AND CRITERIA OF RELEVANCE AND APPROPRIATENESS OF ANIMAL MODELS OF AGING

It is difficult to use man as an experimental subject for most areas of human aging because of the practical problems in conducting longitudinal investigations that span human life and because of legal and ethical constraints on human experimentation. Accordingly, animals are used as surrogates. Information that is developed through research in different animals provides a basis for scientific judgments about extrapolation of data from animals to man.

Up to now, convenience has been the most important criterion in choosing animal models for research on aging. It has become necessary to examine the relevance and appropriateness of particular species for studies on aging. Such examination is needed because of the high cost and complexity of rearing and maintaining old animals, their limited availability, and the complex nature of the scientific questions that investigators in this area often must ask.

The term "relevance" refers to the comparability of a phenomenon being studied in an animal to that in the human aged. "Appropriateness" refers to the complex of other factors that make a given species the best for studying a particular phenomenon. In selecting animals, emphasis should be placed on their utility for resolving scientific questions that are particularly applicable to the problems of human aging. Thus, for the purposes of this report, Wessler's (1976) useful definition of an animal model is rephrased as follows: an animal model of aging is a living organism on which a normative biological or behavioral aspect of aging can be studied, or on which a spontaneous or induced age-related pathological process can be investigated, and in which the phenomenon in one or more respects resembles the same phenomenon in man.

Numerous practical and scientific considerations must be taken into account in determining the relevance and appropriateness of a particular animal for research on aging. The basic criteria for selecting animals include the following:

● Comparability of a phenomenon to that in man: Where the same phenomenon can be shown to occur in an animal as in man, its relevance as a model is enhanced. Lack of comparability, however, does not necessarily preclude its use for research on aging, since the study of alternative mechanisms sometimes can provide useful insights into human aging.

● Life span of the animal: The phenomenon of interest, such as a physiological mechanism, a metabolic process, or a disease entity should become manifest in a shorter time period than in man to facilitate its study.

● The frequency of occurrence of the phenomenon: This is particularly important where multiple observations are required to obtain statistically valid data, while using the minimum number of animals to meet the experimental objective(s).

● The genetic homogeneity or heterogeneity of the animal: This is particularly important where genetics and environment interact to affect aging or where predisposition to age-associated disease may be influenced by genetic factors.

● Availability of background data about the animal: Knowledge of past use of an animal, of increased variability among individuals with age, and of age-associated diseases or lesions can enhance the usefulness of a particular animal for research on aging.

● Unique anatomical, physiological, or behavioral attributes: The characterization of age-associated changes may reveal specific attributes that can influence the choice of animal for particular areas of investigation.

● Availability of techniques to permit research at adequate levels of sophistication: The availability of good research methods may sometimes dictate the choice of animal. In planning studies on aging, investigators should take into account that state of the art with respect to the specificity of research techniques for particular animals.

● Supply of animals: Adequate numbers of animals obviously must be available for study. Strategies must be developed to assure the availability of aged primates and of other animals that are difficult to rear or obtain for research on aging.

● Cost factors: Acquisition, rearing, care, and feeding of aged animals are costly matters. Strategies are needed to ensure efficient use of aged animals, such as by grouping or pooling of experiments where possible. Where the criteria of relevance and appropriateness can be met, the least costly animal obviously should be selected.

● Convenience factors: Behavioral attributes of the animal with respect to tractability and ease of handling can influence decisions on its choice. The size of the animals, the ease and availability of housing them, and the ease of controlling environmental variables also are important considerations in selecting animals for research on aging.

These criteria are discussed selectively in greater detail in the following sections.

CATEGORIES OF RESEARCH ON AGING

The term "research on aging" has no single, universally ac-cepted definition and often is a source of semantic confu-sion. Some of the confusion can be avoided by characteriz-ing the areas of scientific investigation on aging. Studies of aging tend to fall into one of two broad categories of research--biology of aging or pathology of aging (Figure 1). The two differ considerably in methodology, experi-mental strategy, and perspectives on the relationship be-tween aging and disease.

Categories of Aging Research   Areas of Investigation

	Predictors of longevity
Biology of Aging	Age-associated changes
	Changes that predispose to disease
Pathology of Aging	Individual genetic pre-disposition to disease
	Diseases of cumulative epigenetic etiology

FIGURE 1 Categories of research on aging.

Research on the biology of aging generally is based on the premise that aging and death are normal processes--part of a physiological continuum in which aging is a step in the development of the normal life span. Research on the pathology of aging tends to be based on the premise that aging is a disease. Thus, a change in any characteristic of the organism from the optimal state of the mature adult is pathological by definition; aging, disease, and death are part of a continuum involving progressively more severe limitation of adaptability.

A few of the broad areas of investigation in the biology and pathology of aging that may involve the use of animal models are listed in Figure 1. To identify characteristics that correlate with or account for species differences in longevity, biological studies of aging may involve the examination of closely related species whose maximal life spans vary greatly, or large numbers of a particular species may be studied to identify characteristics that change in close correlation with chronological age. A subset of the changes may predispose to disease in old age, but that usually is not the major focus of interest in studies on the biology of aging. It is more important to compare, analyze, or manipulate relationships among a wide variety of characteristics across a variety of species, genera, and phylogenetic orders, to understand more completely the mechanisms of aging in a broad biological sense.

Most research on the pathology of aging is aimed at understanding human diseases that have their peak incidence in old age. The strategy in selecting animal models is to search for pathological conditions that resemble diseases of the human elderly in one aspect or another. Of all the changes that occur with increasing chronological age, the ones of greatest relevance for studies of the pathology of aging are those that predispose to disease. Such changes seldom are the only factors that account for the development of specific diseases in the elderly. This means that in studying the changes, questions may be raised that have little to do with biological aging per se, but which bear importantly on the ultimate expression of disease in the aged. For example, a genetic predisposition to disease, present from birth, may require the evaluation of very young subjects to characterize its development and ultimate expression in the aged. Diseases of cumulative epigenetic etiology that have their peak incidence in the elderly may provide a focus of investigation at various life stages. Such diseases may become manifest clinically only after many years of cumulative exposure to infectious agents, environmental pollutants, or other toxic agents; thus, only individuals beyond a given age show them.

The categorization of research on aging into biological and pathological "spheres of interest" does not imply that one or the other approach is better or more relevant to solving problems and diseases of the human aged. What is known now or may be discovered in the future about aging and disease is certain to derive from a better understanding of aging as approached from the perspectives of "biology" and "pathology." The purpose of this discussion is to highlight these equally legitimate approaches to research on aging. Failure to recognize the semantic implications could inhibit constructive collaboration among workers in the biology and pathology of aging in an important area of overlap in their respective areas of interest--viz, that of changes associated with increasing age that predispose to disease (Figure 1). Effective communication among scientists approaching research from each perspective is essential to an eventual understanding of aging and disease in man.

An Agenda for Action
(Recommendations)

The primary goals of biomedical and behavioral research on aging are to improve the quality of life for the aged, guide development of effective health care services for the aged, and generate understanding of aging processes (NIA, 1977; Panel on Biomedical Research, 1978). These goals imply a lengthy research agenda whose implementation is of the utmost importance to human health. Advisory panels of the National Institute on Aging (NIA) have proposed a research program of national scope on the basic biology of aging and the relationship of aging to disease. The program requires the use of a broad range of animal species for investigating many of the fundamental scientific questions relevant to aging. In essence, animal research has been recognized as an essential component of a national plan toward understanding human aging (NIA, 1977; Panel on Biomedical Research, 1978).

We present here a brief discussion of the need to develop a research agenda on animal models as part of the national research plan on aging. This is followed by a series of recommendations for providing animals and other resources that are essential to implement the research agenda during the coming decade. This section is the conclusion of the report. It is placed at the beginning, rather than the end, to provide, with the introduction, a concise overview of the major issues and needs related to animal research on aging.

RESEARCH AGENDA ON ANIMAL MODELS OF AGING

The relevance and appropriateness of animals as models of human aging are based on the criteria outlined on pages 2-4. The validity of the criteria obviously depends on

the base of knowledge and experience from which they were
derived. While much is known about aging in animals, as
this report indicates, vast areas of ignorance remain, even
in relation to the most commonly used species. For example,
the natural life span of rabbits, guinea pigs, cats, and
most primates is not well established under defined laboratory conditions. This poses difficulties in assessing age-
associated functional decline in these species. There are
wide gaps in knowledge about the pathological changes that
accompany aging of many inbred and outbred rats and mice.
There is a dearth of information about the most suitable
nutritional regimens for aging rodents and other species
(B. J. Cohen, 1979). This is an important problem because
the incidence of certain age-associated lesions can be influenced by the animals' diet, and the lesions themselves
can influence the outcome of gerontological research projects. The relation to age of amyloidosis in certain mouse
strains, and the role of altered immune function in its
pathogenesis, is not clearly understood. How respiratory
control mechanisms and pulmonary reflexes are altered as
dogs age has not been well defined. Much remains to be
learned about the comparability of age-associated lesions
and diseases in animals and man. This is of great importance in defining models of specific diseases of the elderly. Similarly, much information is needed to assess
the applicability of patterns of biological and behavioral
aging in various animal species to human aging. The interactions of environment and genetics require study to determine their impact on animal aging. Knowledge of these interactions is important in differentiating lesions of aging
from lesions that result from cumulative exposure over many
years to exogenous factors. Finally, much baseline information is needed on physiological and pathological processes and alterations that may predispose to diseases or
to the loss of adaptive functions in old animals. From
these examples, it is evident that additional research is
needed to establish the relevance and appropriateness of
particular species as models of human aging.

Many areas of animal research should be encouraged, including systematic searches for models of diseases of the
human elderly and basic biological investigations on underlying mechanisms of aging. The normative and the pathological changes that occur with aging in animals should be
studied in continuing efforts to identify the precise contribution of age-related changes to disease. The interaction of nutrition and aging should be investigated in many
animal species to define the kinds of influence exerted

by dietary factors on longevity and diseases of old age.
Immunosenescence, neurosenescence, and cellular senescence
as mediators of aging in animals merit continuing intensive
study. Pharmacokinetic studies in animals should be broadened to develop better test systems for evaluating drug responses in elderly patients. These are but a few examples
of research areas that belong on the research agenda on
animal models of aging. Many others can be found elsewhere
in this report.

SUPPLY AND AVAILABILITY OF ANIMALS FOR RESEARCH ON AGING

Background

An adequate supply of well-characterized animals is an absolute requirement for research on aging. The maintenance
of animals throughout their life span under defined laboratory conditions is costly. Accordingly, a decision to rear
a particular genus, species, breed, stock, or strain to old
age for research must be based on well-documented requirements and on established expertise in rearing and maintaining the animals. There is a related need to examine the
possible availability of certain types of old animals from
public and community sources. At present, an adequate supply of old animals for research on aging is not assured.
Specific planning and action are necessary to remedy this
problem.

Several years ago, the NIA contracted with commercial
rodent breeders to rear outbred and inbred rats and mice
to 2 years of age and older under rigidly controlled conditions of environment and husbandry and to make these animals available to NIA grantees for research use. As a
result, several rodent strains and stocks have become
available in modest numbers, and additional strains are
in production for future use. This approach has been in-
strumental in enabling interested investigators to participate in research on aging, because it has not been feasible for most investigators to rear the animals they need
to old age. However, there are at least two important
limitations to this approach--availability is limited to
NIA grantees or researchers with NIA-approved pilot projects, and commercial rearing precludes research access to
animals during the first two-thirds of their life span,
thus limiting longitudinal and programmatic research on
the animals from birth to senescence. Accordingly, additional measures are needed to ensure an adequate supply

of old rats and mice, as well as adequate research settings where life-term studies relevant to human aging can be conducted.

With respect to rabbits and rodents other than rats and mice, such as hamsters, gerbils, mastomys, guinea pigs, and peromyscus, there is no mechanism at present to encourage the rearing of these species to old age. None of these species currently is available in significant numbers from commercial sources as old animals. Limited numbers of mastomys, peromyscus, hamsters, and gerbils are being maintained into old age in a few institutional colonies in the United States and abroad. Availability of the animals, however, is limited to only a small number of investigators, and there are no mechanisms for expanding development of these colonies for research on aging. The same situation applies to dogs, cats, and nonhuman primates, with the additional complication that the long life span of these species makes it especially costly to rear them specifically for research on aging. Strategies are needed to assure availability of long-lived species that are different from those that are appropriate for shorter-lived species.

Categorization of Animal Colonies

The recommendations on pages 16-19 concern the modification or expansion of existing animal colonies and the selective development of new colonies for research on aging. The colonies can be categorized by the terms dedicated, shared, and model-convergence. These terms require elaboration before presenting the specific recommendations on animal supply and availability.

Dedicated colonies serve research on aging as a primary mission. This implies their location at institutions having strong intramural programs for multidisciplinary characterization of biological and behavioral aging. Dedicated colonies consist of sufficient numbers of animals at all life stages to permit intensive characterization of the animals and study of aging by longitudinal, cross-sectional, and cross-sequential methods. Sufficient numbers are needed to accumulate life-table statistics for the species, especially for species whose longevity has not been well documented under defined laboratory conditions. Colony records include the genealogical information necessary to manage colony breeding and to analyze experimental results. Experimental data from long-term studies on colony animals

should be stored in a central computer file to assure ease
of retrieval and analysis.

Shared colonies serve more than one research field,
with the costs of maintaining the animals to be apportioned
among the agencies that fund research in these fields. Under this concept, for example, the NIA might contribute to
the support of animals originally maintained for purposes
of production or research in areas other than aging. In
this way, animals in the middle of their life span approaching the end of their reproductively active years, or no
longer useful for the research purposes for which they
were selected originally, could be continued in the colonies, to assure their availability for research on aging.
They could be screened for distribution to dedicated or
model-convergence colonies or studied on-site by resident
or visiting investigators when removal from the colony is
not necessary. It is implicit that adequate genealogical
records and case histories be maintained to assure the
availability of information on genetics, previous illnesses
or injuries, and reproductive events. Where wild-caught
animals are part of the colony, such as is likely in the
case of nonhuman primates, it is expected that the age of
each animal would be determined upon entry by dental analysis, radiographic analysis of long bones, or other suitable techniques. Presumably, for colony-born animals, the
precise age always would be known.

Model-convergence colonies consist of groups of animals
having particular age-related diseases that are relevant
to human aging and that have been assembled in order to
study those diseases. Development of such colonies requires a strategy for defining the diseases most urgently
in need of animal models and for identifying affected animals in existing research colonies and from other potential sources (e.g., zoos, veterinary hospitals, private
owners). A single institution having the relevant expertise might serve as the model-convergence center for one
or several diseases, based on established criteria and
capabilities for identifying and concentrating the models.
In addition to making animals available for study on-site,
the model-convergence concept implies that biological materials from affected animals and, occasionally, the animals themselves could be made available to investigators
at other institutions. Access to colony animals by visiting scientists at the host institution also is implicit
in the concept of the model-convergence colony.

Recommendations

Dedicated colonies of appropriate strains and stocks of rats and mice should be developed for research on aging and to complement and supplement commercial rearing of these animals to old age.
These research colonies should be located regionally at universities or other research institutions that are committed to biomedical research on aging and that have the expertise to rear and maintain old animals and use them wisely in research. The colonies should be established with disease-free animals and maintained under barrier conditions with appropriate monitoring to assure their continuing freedom from infectious diseases. Colony size and production, and selection of stocks and strains to be maintained, should be based on national and regional assessments of need. They should include animals at all life stages. Multiple use of animals from the colonies, consistent with humane standards, should be fostered by coordinated planning of research among individual investigators. Finally, the colonies should be organized to bank tissues, cells, and fluids for supply and exchange (see pages 17-18).

Colonies of rodents that differ in longevity from common laboratory strains of rats and mice, or which have other attributes especially suitable for research on aging, should be expanded or established to increase their availability for comparative research on biological gerontology.
Significant contributions to understanding the fundamental mechanisms of aging could result from identification of the factors (biochemical, physiological, behavioral, genetic) that account for differences in longevity among closely related species. The life span of peromyscus (the white-footed mouse; Peromyscus leucopus), for example, is 2.5 times that of the laboratory mouse (Mus musculus). Comparative study of these species would appear to have great potential value for biological gerontology. Obviously, species to be compared must be thoroughly defined with respect to maintenance, diet, risk of infectious disease, and age-associated lesions or diseases. Other rodent species (e.g., mastomys, gerbils, hamsters) also have particular value that may justify expansion of existing colonies. The guiding criteria for evaluating proposals for dedicated colonies of such species should include the scientific merit of the proposed use, the commitment of the host institution to research on aging, and the expertise of the staff in rearing and maintaining the animals.

The NIA should review its contract programs for the
rearing of rodents to old age in commercial breeding laboratories and should develop a projection of need for old
rats, mice, and other rodents through 1990.

The review should be undertaken to assess the adequacy
of current arrangements for production of old rodents, as
well as to project future requirements. The possibility of
sharing the contract costs of commercial rearing among the
NIA and other granting agencies that have an interest in
the supply of old animals for research should be explored.
There should be a selective expansion of contract rearing
programs as the need can be documented and justified.

Defined populations of rabbits should be reared to old
age at one or more multidisciplinary facilities having the
capability to maintain a disease-free colony, utilize the
animals in research on aging, and provide aged animals for
research use.

The potential utility of the rabbit for research on aging has been discussed (pages 170-179). Inbred and genetically defined rabbits of good quality are available in
limited numbers. They should serve as foundation animals
in developing research colonies. At least one large and
one small inbred strain should be reared to permit comparisons of the effect of size on longevity within the
species, as well as comparison with the longevity of small
rodents, carnivores, and nonhuman primates.

Existing colonies of dogs and cats should be expanded
and utilized to yield aged animals with defined backgrounds.

Dogs and cats of known age and background are needed
for research in many areas that are relevant to aging
(pages 180-242). Only a few such animals are available
now. One approach to increasing the supply for research
on aging is to expand existing research colonies of dogs
and cats by application of the shared colony concept. At
present, there are severe limitations on the extent to
which the old animals in these colonies can be used for
studies on aging, because they are serving primarily as
controls for other areas of research. Expansion of these
colonies would provide animals for a broader range of
studies on aging at relatively modest cost, compared with
the cost of establishing entirely new dedicated colonies.
The baseline information in existing colonies of dogs and
cats should be made available, as it is especially valuable
to an expanded program of research on aging involving these

animals. By using the shared-colony approach, additional information could be generated efficiently.

The use of companion animals for research on aging should be expanded, while simultaneously improving baseline actuarial data on these animals.
In the United States, dogs and cats kept as pets represent the largest number of animals that are allowed to live out their natural life span. Although accidental death is common among dogs and cats, many live much longer than a decade. Many are examined, vaccinated, and treated by veterinarians throughout their lives and, thus, have relatively complete medical records. A large number of animals receive care at veterinary schools, where excellent records on the animals' histories are maintained. The opportunity exists to observe these animals over their life span and, with appropriate authorization, to utilize their medical records for research on aging. In addition, by establishing appropriate collaborative arrangements, protocols can be developed to identify animals with diseases that are relevant to human aging. These animals could serve as research subjects locally or, in some instances, they could be sent to model-convergence centers for study. The development of improved systems for the actuarial analysis of life-table data should accompany increased use of companion animals for research on aging.

Existing nonhuman primate colonies should be utilized and expanded to yield aged animals with defined backgrounds.
The National Primate Plan (Interagency Primate Steering Committee, 1980) has established both general and specific guidelines on nonhuman primate utilization in research. In addition, special considerations that apply to the use of nonhuman primates in research on aging have been discussed in this volume (pages 243-278). Conservative use of nonhuman primates and careful selection of the species to be studied are among the major concerns that have been addressed. There is an urgent need to increase the availability and efficiency of using old nonhuman primates for research on aging. Dedicated colonies of at least one Old World and one New World species should be developed to determine similarities and differences between biological aging in primates compared to shorter-lived species more distantly related to the human. Shared and model-convergence colonies should be developed for the study of disease problems of the human elderly. All of these approaches should be utilized in adapting existing primate

colonies for participation in research on aging. An additional approach, especially pertinent to nonhuman primates, is that of utilizing animals in field-station colonies. Field stations are permanent sites where natural groups of animals living under free-ranging conditions can be studied to derive information that cannot be obtained in captive populations. Field-station colonies are necessary for studying biological and behavioral aging under natural conditions and in providing data essential for evaluating results of studies on laboratory-maintained nonhuman primates.

RESOURCES FOR ANIMAL RESEARCH ON AGING: FACILITIES,
SERVICES, PERSONNEL

Background

In addition to the need for old animals, there are unmet needs for other research resources. These needs must be addressed to promote good research on aging and to attract additional numbers of scientists into this field. The recommendations that follow relate to some of these resource needs, such as specialized research laboratories, diagnostic laboratories, facilities for maintaining aged and aging animals, banks for animal tissues and cells, computer-based record systems for colony records and experimental data, and training resources of various kinds. Some of these resources already exist in many scientific institutions, and although they are not being used invariably in support of research on aging, they could be mobilized readily. The approach recommended here is that of cost-sharing for support of resources that can serve several research areas. Gerontological research in animals spans the scientific disciplines. Often it is conducted in conjunction with research in related fields, providing opportunities for fruitful scientific collaboration and exchange. In such settings, investigators can share the use of costly animals, research supplies, equipment, facilities, and other resources. This approach should be encouraged. Gerontological research can best be served by coordinated development of resource programs and animal colonies in multidisciplinary scientific institutions committed to research on aging.

Recommendations

The National Institutes of Health (NIH) should develop mechanisms for supporting institutional research resources that
promote shared use of the resources for the mutual benefit
of the research fields they serve.
    A number of agencies within the NIH, such as the Divi-
sion of Research Resources (DRR), National Heart, Blood,
and Lung Institute (NHBLI), National Cancer Institute (NCI),
and NIA, support institutional animal resources of various
kinds. It is appropriate for these agencies to assess current programs and determine how best they can coordinate
their efforts in relation to their programmatic interests.
With proper coordination, additional resources can be made
available for aging and other fields of research at relatively modest cost.

    Institutional or regional laboratories having special-
ized research capabilities in aging should be developed,
together with the animal colonies that provide the experimental material for the research.
    Resource laboratories capable of defining a broad range
of age-associated changes in animals are needed for adequate characterization of biological aging in different
species. Laboratories that have access to model-convergence
colonies and special capabilities and interest in screening
for and identifying animal models of diseases of the human
elderly should be designated. Other laboratories are needed
to develop batteries of measures on biological aging of
nonhuman primates, dogs, and other species to be used in
screening for potential subjects in particular age groups.
Research laboratories capable of applying genetic-monitor-
ing techniques to characterize interactions of aging, environmental influences, and disease represent another area
of need. These are a few examples of the specialized research laboratories that should be expanded or established.

    Institutional or regional laboratories should be main-
tained for the diagnosis of infectious diseases and for
monitoring the quality of animals used in research on aging.
    Diagnostic laboratories are an absolute requirement for
disease prevention and assurance of high-quality animals.
There are at least 15 such laboratories in scientific institutions that are supported by the DRR, NIH. There are
also pathology sections at each of the seven NIH-supported
Primate Research Centers. Many of these laboratories could
serve also as diagnostic resources for research programs on

aging, on an institutional or regional basis. In some instances, the diagnostic laboratory staff could collaborate with scientists involved in specific areas of research to identify animals with age-related diseases. The laboratories also could collaborate in research by characterizing pathological changes in aging animals or by performing necropsies, clinical chemistry tests, or hematologic evaluations on aged animals as a professional service.

A program should be developed for renovation or construction of facilities to accommodate aged animals being maintained in dedicated, shared, or model-convergence colonies and to provide necessary cage equipment.
It is envisioned that many of the specialized colonies for aging research would be extensions of existing colonies; thus, renovation or construction of animal facilities need not necessarily be extensive. Any application for renovation or construction of animal facilities should be based on a meritorious research plan for utilizing the animals.

Banks of animal tissues, cells, and body fluids for research on aging should be maintained and made accessible to the scientific community on a continuing basis.
Many more investigators could participate in research on aging if tissues, cells, or body fluids derived from animals at various ages were more widely available. For cell-culture research, a first priority is to utilize cells from rodent species such as rats, mice, and peromyscus. It also is important to develop cell-culture systems from larger animals, such as nonhuman primates, including at least two with widely different life spans. The advantages of using species larger and longer-lived than the rodents are that their cells are relatively long-lived in culture, large amounts of material can be obtained from a given animal, and the cells have a lower propensity to transform than do rodent cells. For research that does not require live animals, the advantages of being able to obtain specific tissues or fluids from well-characterized, high-quality animals are obvious. Tissue banks can readily be developed in conjunction with dedicated colonies of all species. A decision to establish a bank should be based on a careful assessment of need and on the expertise available to develop this resource. Once a bank is established, the availability of tissues should be announced periodically. Development of a publication comparable to that of the Primate Supply Information Clearinghouse,

University of Washington, Seattle, would provide a mechanism for announcements of this kind, as well as for the exchange of information on availability of aged animals for research.

The development of computer-based record systems on aging animals should be strongly encouraged.

Adequate records must be kept on all animals maintained in dedicated, shared, and model-convergence colonies. The data base must include experimental data, as well as colony statistics such as husbandry records, medical histories, and genealogical information. This is necessary because it is probable that such colonies are likely to be maintained for many years, and the data must be kept in a form that is readily retrievable to the many investigators who need it.

To some extent, existing animal record programs can be utilized in the interest of research on aging. For example, many veterinary schools in the United States operate jointly a computerized clinical record system on dogs and cats. The ILAR Committee on Laboratory Animal Records (1979c) has issued recommendations for the managers of nonhuman primate colonies on a common record system that will make it possible for information to be shared among institutions and to be used for the management of captive, self-sustaining primate populations and for national planning of nonhuman primate resources. It would be extremely valuable to have longevity data and other relevant information on aging for companion animals generated from these systems or to have actuarial techniques incorporated to aid in identifying animals with age-associated diseases comparable to diseases of the human aged.

The NIA should continue to sponsor the training of scientists in research on aging.

A fundamental need in research on aging is for well-trained, motivated investigators in all disciplinary areas relevant to aging. The NIA should maintain continuing surveillance of areas where specialists are in short supply. For example, currently there is a well-recognized shortage of human and veterinary pathologists, especially those with training and experience in the pathology of aging. Similarly, there is a need for additional numbers of specialists in laboratory animal medicine with special expertise in aging. It may well be that existing laboratory animal medicine training programs could be augmented to accommodate veterinarians having a special interest in aging.

Biologists and other scientists have been very vocal in expressing interest in workshops and short courses dealing with pathology, clinical aspects of disease, and husbandry of aging animals. Such courses should be offered on a continuing basis and should include workshops designed specifically for technical personnel in gerontological research programs. A similar need exists for short courses on human age-associated diseases for veterinary pathologists to aid them in identifying animal models of these diseases.

Major Animal Groups for Research on Aging

There are features of aging that probably are unique to human populations. Other features of aging undoubtedly are expressed similarly or identically both in humans and experimental animals. The intent of this report is not to characterize selected animal models in encyclopedic detail. Rather, representative characteristics of selected mammals are presented to illustrate the advantages and limitations of using them as models. Certain animals already are well characterized under defined genetic and environmental conditions with respect to mortality, disease profiles, physiological capabilities, similarities to and differences from age-associated changes in humans, and underlying mechanisms that account for age-associated changes. Thus, the report is designed to aid investigators in selecting or avoiding an animal for research on aging based on specific attributes rather than on convenience alone.

The animals considered in this report are mice, rats, certain other rodents, rabbits, cats, dogs, and nonhuman primates. Other animals are mentioned, but the emphasis is on those listed. These are not the only appropriate models for research on aging; they have been selected for initial review because, presently, they are used most widely or are most likely to be used in studies on aging.

Rodents and Lagomorphs

INTRODUCTION

The comparative study of aging in rodents and lagomorphs is
becoming increasingly important in research on the basic
biology of longevity and aging and the relationship between
aging and disease. The order Rodentia is the largest order
of mammals, containing about 350 genera, and far exceeding
all other orders in numbers of species and individuals.
Adult body weights range from less than 10 g to about 50 kg
(Ellerman, 1940-1949; Simpson, 1945; Walker, 1975a).

The taxonomic tree shown in Figure 2 embodies the accepted classification of Rodentia (Simpson, 1945) and includes all genera now widely used as laboratory models,
plus several genera that are beginning to be used in research or that have good research potential. All but one
of the widely used laboratory rodent species, the cavy or
guinea pig (Cavia porcellus), belong to the large superfamily Muroidea, with its two major families, Muridae and
Cricetidae. The Muridae is an Old World family, but three
species, the laboratory (house) mouse (Mus musculus), the
Norway (laboratory) rat (Rattus norvegicus), and the roof
rat (Rattus rattus rattus), were distributed worldwide by
explorers and colonists during the sixteenth century. The
laboratory mouse and the Norway rat are widely used in research on aging; mastomys [Praomys (Mastomys) natalensis]
is finding growing use for its high susceptibility to age-
related diseases.

Two Old World representatives of the family Cricetidae
that have become widely used in the laboratory are the hamster (Mesocricetus or Cricetulus) and the gerbil (Meriones).
Several New World cricetids, particularly the deer mice
(Peromyscus) and the cotton rat (Sigmodon), are coming into
use as laboratory animals.

-23-

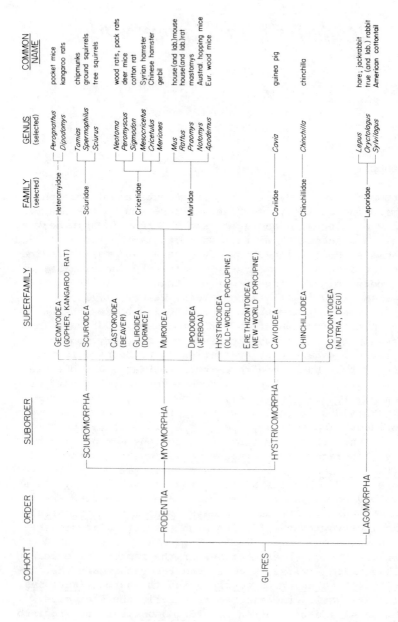

FIGURE 2 Classification of selected rodents and lagomorphs. Diagram courtesy of G. A. Sacher, Argonne National Laboratory, Argonne, Illinois.

The laboratory mouse, Norway rat, hamster, gerbil, and mastomys are all short-lived animals, none of them attaining ages much beyond 4 years; however, Peromyscus may live as long as 8 years. The availability of both short- and long-lived species is an advantage in research on aging because it enables the study of the biological basis for longevity by comparison of the genetic, biochemical, and physiological mechanisms in these species.

The South American rodents of the suborder Hystricomorpha are represented in laboratories only by the cavy or guinea pig (Cavia porcellus). This taxon has specialized toward a reproductive pattern characterized by small litters and long gestation times. Several small hystricomorph rodents, such as the degu (Octodon degus) and tuco-tuco (Ctenomys spp.), are well suited for laboratory use (Weir, 1974).

The laboratory rabbit (Oryctolagus cuniculus) and other rabbits, hares, and pikas were originally classified as members of the order Rodentia. However, for some time they have been classified in the separate order Lagomorpha, because they have six incisor teeth, rather than four, as the rodents have. The Lagomorpha and the Rodentia form the cohort Glires (Figure 2). The order Lagomorpha is comprised of two major families, Ochotonidae (pika) and Leporidae (rabbits and hares), with many genera and species native to all parts of the world. The laboratory rabbit (Oryctolagus cuniculus) is the only member of the order having widespread laboratory usage (Fox, 1974; 1975), and it is becoming increasingly important in research on the basic biology of aging and on the relationship between aging and disease. This is particularly evident by publications in the European literature. The development of inbred strains has provided additional benefit for research.

MICE

In this section the use of the mouse as a prospective animal model for research on aging at the population, individual, and cellular levels is reviewed. Small size, short life span, adaptability, and high fertility are important characteristics of the mouse that make it attractive for population and individual studies. The paramount advantage, however, is its relative tolerance to intensive inbreeding, a trait that has permitted the establishment of a variety of inbred strains in which interaction between and within genetic loci, and between genetic and environmental forces,

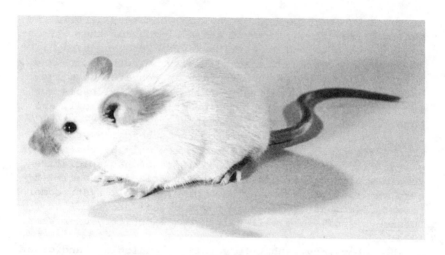

The laboratory mouse, <u>Mus</u> <u>musculus</u>, BALB/c strain. Photograph courtesy of The Jackson Laboratory, Bar Harbor, Maine.

can be evaluated systematically. Thus, over 500 different inbred strains are now available, many with unique advantages; e.g., strains that are either highly susceptible or highly resistant to diseases observed in humans. The mouse has its disadvantages though, as do all animal models. For example, tissue mass in an individual animal may be too small to analyze biochemically. However, recent advances in radioimmunoassays and similar micro procedures now make it possible to do accurate analyses on very small samples.

Types of Genetic Stocks Available

Nine population types of genetically defined mice are potentially useful in research on aging: inbred strains, F_1 hybrids, other crosses (e.g., F_2, four-way, and diallel), specific mutations, congenic lines, recombinant inbred strains, selected lines, "random-bred" lines, and wild stocks. Individuals of similar genotypes should not always be expected to show similar patterns of age-dependent change since patterns of genetic-environmental interactions vary. Genetic contributions to aging processes can be understood only with the use of genetically defined subjects. However, the use of strain comparisons as a

basic technique in research on aging has certain limitations. The demonstration of strain differences is a relatively simple matter, but it is difficult to interpret
these differences without additional genetic manipulation.
If several strains and F_1 hybrids are compared, the investigator is less likely to be misled by characteristics
unique to a single genotype.

Inbred Strains

An inbred strain, as defined by the Committee on Standardized Genetic Nomenclature for Mice (Staats, 1976), is the
product of 20 or more consecutive generations of brother x
sister matings. Parent x offspring matings may be used to
replace brother x sister matings. When consecutive parent
x offspring matings are used, the mating must always be to
the most recent generation parent. Bailey (1978) recently
has pointed out that when gene linkage is taken into account, inbreeding should not be considered complete until
after at least 40 generations of brother x sister matings.

The variety and availability of inbred strains, together
with their convenient and variable life spans (1 to 3 years
depending upon the strain), have made them valuable tools
in research on aging. By using animals of one strain, it
is possible to produce and study many individuals with the
same genotype, as alike as identical twins. Once their
characteristics are known, they can be reproduced repeatedly, but not necessarily indefinitely. Most inbred
strains have mean life spans in excess of 20 months.

Cross-strain surveys, involving the same kinds of observations on mice of different inbred strains, are useful for determining whether genetic variation in the expression of particular characters exists and for locating
especially favorable animal material for studying specific
phenomena. Strain comparisons make it possible to formu-
late hypotheses that can be tested, and lead to a genetic
analysis of physiological or behavioral factors of interest.

Virtually all inbred strains are adapted to the laboratory environment. However, most have been developed for
particular research purposes (e.g., the study of particular
disease entities) and, therefore, may not be suitable for
research on aging. Adaptation to the laboratory environment may be a problem during the development of a strain
or during the introduction of a captured population to the
laboratory. It is easy to "select" such a population for

laboratory suitability and inadvertently restrict the gene pool in the process.

Substrains

When a group of inbred mice is separated from the parent strain, it may come to differ genetically, even if it is maintained by brother x sister breeding. Bailey (1978) has concluded that much substrain variability results from separation before inbreeding is complete (i.e., before 40 generations). Therefore, substrain designations are given to inbred strains when:

  • animals that have been maintained by brother x sister mating for 8 to 19 generations are separated into different groups and continue to be inbred in the same laboratory without intercrossing for an additional 12 generations,
  • animals from the parent strain are transferred to another investigator, or
  • genetic differences become established (Staats, 1976).

In order to assure comparable results, investigators should use the same substrain as others engaged in similar work and should designate the animal properly so that it is clear to others which substrain is used (Lyon, 1978). Rules for designating substrains are given by Staats (1976).

F_1 Hybrids

To analyze patterns of genetic control, crosses between animals of differentially affected genotypes must be used. The first stage in any such analysis is typically a cross between two inbred strains to produce the genetically uniform F_1 hybrid that is heterozygous at all loci where the parental strains differ. F_1 hybrid mice have additional uses in research on aging. Each of the two parental inbred strains inevitably is homozygous for certain age-limiting genes, and many of the deleterious alleles carried in one parental strain will not be found in the other. As a result, the F_1 hybrid mouse usually has many more positive factors yielding vigor, disease resistance, and increased longevity. The mean life span of F_1 hybrid mice is almost always as long as that of the longer-lived parental strain, and sometimes the F_1 hybrid life span greatly exceeds that of either parental strain, especially when neither parent is long-lived (see pages 43-50).

F_2, Four-Way, and Diallel Crosses

F_2, four-way,[1] and diallel[2] crosses are second generation "stocks" derived from crosses between four parental inbred strains. Because these crosses are "special" stocks, used primarily to test very specific genetic hypotheses, such mice are rarely, if ever, available, except from an investigator engaged in such testing. Their primary utility in research on aging is to provide replicable populations of genetically heterogeneous subjects. These are all populations in which genetic segregation is occurring, but in which the gene pool can be reproduced by reconstituting the cross from the appropriate progenitor genotypes. For most purposes, these genetically controlled heterogeneous populations are preferable to the so-called "random-bred" and "wild type" populations, which cannot be reproduced (see below).

Mutations

Analyses of the action of single normal versus mutant genes may provide specific information on aging processes. Many mutant alleles severely limit total life span, and comparisons between affected mice homozygous for a particular recessive mutant gene and their normal littermates may be

---

[1] A four-way cross is derived from a mating between the F_1 hybrid strains A and B and the F_1 hybrid of strains C and D.
[2] A diallel cross is an array of all possible matings of three or more strains as shown below:

		Strain			
		A	B	C	D
Strain	A	AAF_1	BAF_1	CAF_1	DAF_1
	B	ABF_1	BBF_1	CBF_1	DBF_1
	C	ACF_1	BCF_1	CCF_1	DCF_1
	D	ADF_1	BDF_1	CDF_1	DDF_1

quite productive. This is particularly true if the mutation (or series of mutations) is of interest to other disciplines as well (e.g., neurological mutants and the
"obesity" mutations), since these mutations are likely to
be widely studied and reasonably well characterized. Mutant genes used in this manner can be viewed as "natural
lesions" that permit the study of rather specific morphological or biochemical alterations in otherwise healthy,
untreated animals. More than 500 different mutant stocks
are available from commercial sources and from the laboratories of individual investigators.

Congenic Lines

Many mutations are so pronounced that the effects due to
variation of genetic expression in animals with heterogeneous genetic background (genetic noise) may be negligible (e.g., most neurological mutants). However, genetic
noise is a serious problem with certain mutants systematically tested on different backgrounds (e.g., mutations resulting in obesity). The background problem can be avoided
by the use of congenic lines that are created by making
single gene substitutions against a common genetic background. This occurs spontaneously in the case of a new
mutation within an inbred strain, but can be created by
repeated backcrosses of mutant animals to a strain of interest. For example, the mutations, obese (ob), which
first occurred in the C57BL/6J strain, and diabetes, (db),
which first occurred in the C57BL/Ks strain, show a pattern
of decreased plasma insulin and degeneration of the islets
of Langerhans when maintained on a C57BL/Ks background and
a pattern of sustained high plasma insulin and hypertrophy
of islets of Langerhans when maintained on a C57BL/6J background. Direct comparison of the effects of the mutations,
without interaction with other background genes, was not
possible until the two mutations were placed on a common
background strain (C57BL/6J) in separate congenic lines.

Recombinant Inbred Strains (RIS)

A recently developed breeding technique promises to do much
to alleviate the problem of distinguishing between environmental and genetic influences on aging. Crosses are made
between two inbred strains known to show genetic differences
in some characteristics of interest (Figure 3). Following

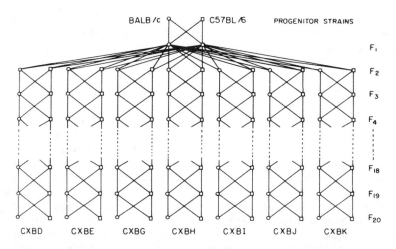

FIGURE 3 Recombinant inbred strains. A series of recom-
binant-inbred strains derived from a cross of two highly
inbred progenitor strains (BALB/c and C57BL/6 strains).
After the cross, inbreeding continues, although independently, for each new strain in the series. Circles represent females, squares represent males, and line segments
represent gametic pathways. Source: Bailey, 1979.

the production of an F_2 generation from this interstrain
cross, 20 or more different brother-sister pairs of F_2 individuals are mated, and offspring from each such pair are
used to start a new recombinant inbred strain (RIS) (Bailey,
1978). Some of these lines may die out during the course
of inbreeding, but all that survive through 20 successive
generations (6-8 years) of brother-sister inbreeding will
constitute new homozygous inbred strains.

In these new strains, the allele carried at each of the
genetic loci, by which the original parental lines differed,
must be identical with that in one or the other of those
lines. Thus, a new homozygous combination of these genes
carried by the two strains has been produced and can be
replicated indefinitely simply by continuing brother-sister
inbreeding. If a particular behavior or aging pattern,
for example, is controlled by alleles at one specific genetic locus, then half of any family of RIS will exhibit
the pattern of one of the original parental strains and the
other half will exhibit the pattern of the second original
parental strain. Finding an exact copy of a parental

characteristic in several of the RIS is very good evidence
that the characteristic is controlled by alleles at a
single genetic locus.

Selected Lines

Selected lines commonly are used in the analysis of quantitative traits (e.g., maze learning ability, aggression),
but have not been used much in research on aging, except
for the work of J. W. Elias et al. (1975) on selection for
high and low blood pressure. Genetic selection (usually
by repeated matings of the population extremes) is a time-
consuming and expensive technique. Its use in aging increases the time and expense involved. Therefore, such
a technique is likely to be more attractive when evidence
for a particular aging correlate cannot be obtained by
using currently available genetic stocks.

Random-Bred Populations

Random-bred populations are commonly believed to offer the
advantage of genetic heterogeneity in a somewhat uniform
population (e.g., albino Swiss mice). In fact, these populations are rarely truly random-bred. Instead, they are
the product of unintentional, undirected selection for
docility, fertility, rapid weight gain, and other characteristics that make them easy to raise and handle and,
therefore, economically attractive. A systematic method
for "random mating" has been discussed by Poiley (1960).
While the genetic heterogeneity could be advantageous in
some studies, the gene pool in a truly random-bred population cannot be reconstituted in further generations. Over
a few generations, this might cause genetic differences between groups of young and old animals in addition to the
age-related differences. In most situations, the progeny
of an 8- or 10-way cross of unrelated inbred strains will
produce a greater degree of genetic heterogeneity with the
advantage of replicability of the gene pool.

Wild Stocks

Wild stocks often are suggested as potentially useful for
research on aging, since it is assumed that they are "more
natural" than laboratory strains. What is meant by "more

natural" usually is not specified and is more an an article
of faith than the result of investigation. On the other
hand, it is probably true (and some evidence does exist)
that in the process of adapting wild progenitor stocks to
laboratory environments some genes are lost (e.g., those
that produce extreme jumpiness, shock reactions to testing procedures, or reduce fertility in a cage environment).
The use of wild stocks in an aging context could reveal
the effects of such genes as long as the gene pool is continually replenished by matings with captured animals.

Biological Characteristics

Because of the large variety of random-bred, inbred, hybrid, and mutant mice available for research, it has been
necessary for us to limit the scope of this discussion.
Emphasis will be placed on six inbred strains of mice:
A, BALB/c, CBA, C3H, C57BL/6, and DBA/2, and three hybrids
of these strains: B6C3F1 (C57BL/6 x C3H), B6DF1 (C57BL/6
x DBA/2), and CB6F1 (BALB/c x C57BL/6). These strains and
hybrids were chosen because they are genetically defined,
young animals are available commercially, and they are relatively easy to breed and maintain. Substrain relationships
for these six inbred strains have been summarized (Bailey,
1978). Investigators planning to use aged mice may have to
produce them themselves because aged mice of these strains
and hybrids are not available commercially and the few colonies of aged mice that exist can seldom provide more than
the needs of one or two investigators.

These strains and hybrids have been commonly used in the
past for research on aging; thus, their patterns of longevity and pathological change are somewhat understood.
They die from a variety of causes, none have an unusually
short life span, and each differs from the others. The
origin and history of these mice have been reviewed by
Bailey (1978), and their characteristics have been described by Staats (1976).

The selection of these strains and hybrids should not be
construed to mean that these are the only mice of value in
research on aging. Indeed, many useful models will be
found in less frequently utilized strains.

Ease of Breeding

The researcher frequently has the choice of breeding his own mice or purchasing them from commercial sources. The danger that damaging microorganisms and parasites may be introduced from a commercial supplier is a strong argument for laboratory breeding, but the danger can be minimized by limiting purchases to a reliable supplier(s). In addition, newly received mice should be quarantined and tested before being introduced into the aging colony. Successful long-term control of parasites and pathogens demands the application of painstaking precautions in receiving and handling shipments of new mice.

If the researcher needs a steady supply of mice of both sexes at frequent intervals, such as monthly, laboratory breeding may well prove easier and less costly than commercial procurement. Production must be sufficient to provide adequate numbers of 2- to 3-year-old mice. When large numbers of mice of a single sex are needed at infrequent intervals, purchase from a commercial supplier may be more appropriate.

Breeding performance depends on the interactions between genetics and environment. Many commonly used inbred strains tend to breed well (Table 1) and are inexpensive to produce. F_1 hybrid and outbred mice often are even easier to produce. However, to meet the requirements of particular experiments on aging, there may be a need for certain strains that do not breed well and that are more costly to produce.

Table 1 gives breeding performances for 14 inbred strains of mice (Heiniger and Dorey, 1980). The genetic relationships of various substrains have been discussed by Bailey (1978). Before weaning, all abnormal and sickly mice are culled and are not counted in determining the percentage of productive mated pairs and the number of offspring weaned per pair. The Jackson Laboratory makes detailed records for a large number of inbred strains accessible to qualified scientists who would like to study breeding performances.

Age-Related Functional Changes

Many different parameters are altered with age in mammals. Similarities and differences between animals of various genotypes and different species are interesting in themselves. Age-associated changes also may be useful in developing "assays" of aging. Correlations can be evaluated

TABLE 1   Reproductive Performance of Selected Inbred
Strains of JAX Mice[a]

Strain	Breeding Period (weeks)[b]	Pairs in Sample		Weaned of Those Born[d]	No. Pups Weaned per Productive Pair	
		No.	% Productive[c]		Mean	SE[c]
A/HeJ	26	240	58	79	9.4	± 0.6
A/J	26	240	69	82	14.3	± 0.7
BALB/cByJ	30	122	98	94	31.3	± 0.7
BALB/cJ	30	240	65	88	14.4	± 0.6
CBA/CaJ	26	167	96	94	19.8	± 0.6
CBA/H-T6J	26	157	84	89	16.8	± 0.6
CBA/J	26	240	95	78	13.8	± 0.5
C3H/HeJ	26	240	94	83	13.6	± 0.6
C3HeB/FeJ	26	240	95	90	23.7	± 0.7
C57BL/KsJ	30	217	90	93	25.8	± 0.5
C57BL/6J	30	240	85	87	21.1	± 0.6
C57BL/10J	26	194	87	85	12.3	± 0.5
DBA/1J	30	241	91	77	15.8	± 0.4
DBA/2J	26	240	92	87	13.8	± 0.5

[a]These data were collected between April 1976 and June 1977
(Heiniger and Dorey, 1980). These records are offered as
examples of breeding performance of inbred strains that
were maintained under clean conventional conditions at The
Jackson Laboratory, outlined in the husbandry section of
The Handbook of Genetically Standardized JAX Mice, third
edition (Heiniger and Dorey, 1980). Mice were fed pasteurized food and acidified water. The diets were formulated
for balanced nutrition and good breeding performance, not
to provide maximum longevity. Cages and bottles were
sterilized with detergent and hot water; bedding and other
materials were autoclaved with steam. Cages were changed
once each week; new births were recorded and weanling mice
removed at that time. All mouse cages were filtered, and
mouse rooms had sufficient positive air pressure for at
least 15 air changes per hour. People who worked with the
mice made liberal use of disinfectants to keep all mouse
room facilities clean. Most rooms were maintained at 21
to 25°C with 30 to 50 percent relative humidity, although
a few rooms had only heating facilities and occasionally
exceeded upper temperature and humidity levels in July
and August.

TABLE 1 (continued)

Mouse rooms were very strictly quarantined from contact with microorganisms. No biological materials were allowed to enter The Jackson Laboratory until they had been approved by the Animal Health Department. Live mice and unsterilized animal products were imported as infrequently as possible, and then only after painstaking testing. People who had been in contact with laboratory animals within the past 10 days were not allowed to come in contact with mice.

[b]The number of weeks between pairing and retirement is given under "Breeding Period (weeks)." Times in ages are accurate to $\pm$ 0.5 week. All mice are paired when they are weaned at 4 weeks of age, except the C3H/HeJ and C3HeB/FeJ strains, which are paired at 3 weeks of age.

[c]A pair is scored as productive if at least a single litter (one or more pups) is born before the retirement date.

[d]Before weaning all abnormal or sickly animals are culled and are not counted as pups weaned.

among biochemical, physiological, and behavioral changes and life span, and the effects of procedures to alter the rate of aging can be tested. However, susceptibility to many diseases increases with age; thus, functional changes may be caused by disease, entirely apart from aging.

Biochemical Changes

Few biochemical studies of aging mice have been done. For example, the changes in enzyme levels observed in mice (Florini, 1975) represent a very small part of the total literature on age-related changes in enzyme levels (P. D. Wilson, 1973). The reason is that although many inbred strains of mice are available, and although the mouse is easy to breed and has a short life span, it is difficult to obtain adequate sample mass from a single animal. Accordingly, studies on age-related changes for which extensive fractionation procedures or large initial samples are required have usually involved rats. Mice have been used more frequently when having genetically defined animals is essential or for experiments in which small sample mass is adequate. Thus, in general, larger organs,

such as the liver, have received more attention than
smaller organs, such as the pituitary.

Tissue and Organ Composition   The only components of tissues and organs that have been studied to any extent in
mice are the DNA and protein content. The DNA and protein
content of brain, liver, heart, and kidney remain relatively stable postadolescence (Beauchene et al., 1967;
Zorzoli and Li, 1967; Franks et al., 1974; Leto et al.,
1976); however, there can be changes in specific proteins.
This is reflected in age-related changes in levels of enzyme activity in the mouse, changes that are complex and
often confusing (P. D. Wilson, 1973) because they can be
due to qualitative and/or quantitative changes in the enzyme. For example, there is an alteration in the molecular structure of certain enzymes (Gershon and Gershon,
1973); however, this alteration need not occur in every
cell (Yagil, 1976). It should be recognized that organs
consist of parenchyma and stroma and that each may contribute in different ways to enzyme changes (Knook and
Sleyster, 1976).

Gene Replication and Expression   The effect of aging on
the synthesis and function of nucleic acids and proteins
has been investigated to some extent. Analysis of chromatin composition of the liver, kidney, and brain of C57BL/
Icrf mice reveals no gross change with age (B. T. Hill,
1976). The accessibility of DNA in isolated chromatin to
deoxyribonuclease digestion also remains unaltered with
age (Hill and Whelan, 1978). Very interesting results have
been reported by Paffenholz (1978) in his study on the relationship between aging and DNA repair of fibroblasts cultured from three inbred strains with different life spans.
Finally, although Hoffman and McCoy (1974) have reported
only minimal difference in nucleoside composition of liver
tRNA between young adult and aged C57BL/6 mice, Frazer and
Yang (1972) have shown differences in the aminoacylation
capacity of liver and brain tRNA between young adult and
aged BC3F1 (C57BL x C3H) mice.
     Various age-related protein metabolic changes have been
detected. For example, a decrease in the rate of protein
synthesis has been detected in isolated muscle ribosomes
(Britton and Sherman, 1975) and in liver microsomes (Mainwaring, 1969; Hrachovec, 1971). Other age-related changes
in protein metabolism, including posttranslational modification of proteins, have been reviewed (Florini and Sorrentino, 1976; Rothstein, 1977).

Adaptive Responses Delays in various adaptive responses
similar to those characterized in rats by Adelman (1975)
have been reported in C57BL/6J mice. For example, Finch
et al. (1969) found an age-related decrease in the induction of liver tyrosine aminotransferase following exposure
to cold, and Florini et al. (1973) observed that induction
of cardiac hypertrophy by thyroxine injection was substantially delayed in 26-month-old (compared to 8-month-old)
animals. On the other hand, Baird et al. (1974) found no
age-related decrease in the rate or extent of induction of
liver catalase by clofibrate (α- p -chloropenoxyisobutyrate)
in this strain of mice.

Hormonal Changes Age-related changes in the level and activity of a number of hormones have been reported. Eleftheriou and Lucas (1974) have found that plasma testosterone
levels do not change significantly between 2 and 28 months
of age in male DBA/2 or C57BL/6 mice. Eleftheriou (1975)
also noted that protein-bound iodine (PBI) and the PBI response to thyrotrophic hormone (TSH) decrease progressively
from 2 to 30 months of age in both strains of mice, with a
significantly greater decrease in DBA/2 mice. Age-related
reduction in the rate of catecholamine metabolism has been
observed by Finch (1973a) in C57BL/6 mouse brain, and Gosden
(1976) has found that a decrease in estradiol uptake by
the pituitary, but not the uterus, hypothalamus, cerebrum,
or serum, of aging CBA/H-T6 mouse.

The numbers and activities of receptors for several hormones also have been studied (see review by Roth and Adelman, 1975). A decrease in the number of estrogen receptors
with age has been detected in the uterus of C57BL/6 mice
(Nelson et al., 1976a). However, no change has been detected in the number of corticosterone receptors in the
brain of C57BL/6 mice (Nelson et al., 1976b) and of insulin
and growth hormone receptors in the liver of C57BL/6 mice
(Sorrentino and Florini, 1976).

An area of growing interest is the hypothalamic-pituitary
interactions and related neurotransmitters that play essential roles in the brain and in the interactions between
the nervous and endocrine systems. Mice of the C57BL/6J
strain have been used in demonstrating decreased brain
dopamine and norepinephrine turnover under conditions in
which there was little or no change in the levels of these
compounds, serotonin, or of the enzymes dopa decarboxylase,
acetylcholine esterase, glutamic dehydrogenase, and others;
this area recently has been reviewed by Finch (1977), who
concluded that, "many phenomena of aging that may ultimately

be traced to neuroendocrine and autonomic loci cannot be seriously evaluated until a great deal more information is available."

Hormones or enzymes associated with reproductive processes have been studied in female and male mice because of widespread interest in age-related losses in fertility and/ or sexual function (Bronson and Des Jardins, 1977; Parkening et al., 1978). These losses usually occur relatively early in the life span, before the onset of age-related decline in other systems.

Physiological Changes

Many age-related physiological changes have been measured in mice; only a few will be reviewed here. Emphasis will be placed on tests that can be repeated on individuals. Mice are useful in physiological testing, because large numbers can be maintained and studied longitudinally more conveniently and inexpensively than larger mammals; in addition, their life spans are short enough to make longitudinal studies practical. Proper husbandry minimizes environmental variability, and inbred strains or F_1 hybrids can be used to control genetic variability.

Transplantation Studies The relationship between age and function can be studied in certain cell lines by transplanting cells from old mice into young mice of the same inbred strain. For example, studies suggest that hemopoietic stem cells from old and young donors function equally well when transplanted into young hosts. This observation indicates that the loss of hemopoietic function in the aging individual is due to the environment of the stem cell (Harrison, 1979). Inbred strains are particularly useful because individuals of the same strain are genetically identical, eliminating the problem of rejection. Congenic lines are valuable because they carry genetic markers that make it possible to identify cell lines. In addition, certain mutants, such as the mutant anemias, are useful not only in identifying cell lines, but also in testing cell function (Harrison, 1978, 1979).

Changes in Immune Response Age-related changes in immune responses in mice have been extensively studied and reviewed (Walford, 1969; Good and Yunis, 1974; Adler, 1975; Makinodan, 1978). Recently, Kay (1978a) has compared age-related changes in several different immunological tests

using mice of eight genotypes; demonstrating concurrently
the great effect of Sendai virus infection on the immune
response of apparently healthy mice. In general, responses dependent on thymus-derived cells (T cells) show
the largest decline with age. The thymus itself is most
active before puberty, losing active tissue mass progressively thereafter. Large age-related declines occur in
the following immune responses:

● The T cell-dependent antibody response declines due
to a decrease in the number of spleen cells forming the
antibody in response to sheep erythrocyte stimulation
(Makinodan and Peterson, 1962; Price and Makinodan, 1972).
● There is a decline in the ability of T cells to syn-
thesize DNA in response to mitogenic stimulation as measured by incorporation of tritiated thymidine by spleen
cells (Hori et al., 1973; Mathies et al., 1973).

Other immune responses, such as T cell-mediated cytotoxicity, skin graft rejection time, and response to bacterial
lipopolysaccharides, show mixed results--declining in some
studies, remaining unchanged in others. The conflicting
results are probably due to differences in techniques,
mouse genotypes, age ranges used, and the health status
of the mice.

Although most tests of immune response can be done without harming the mouse, they are not repeatable because subsequent tests are affected by those done previously. If
the mouse is immunized against a particular antigen, subsequent responses to that antigen will be greatly improved.
It can often have an adjuvant effect as well, increasing
subsequent responses to additional antigens; therefore,
in vitro testing is preferred. Cells are collected for
testing immune response in vitro either from the circulating blood or from excised spleens and lymph nodes. Only
the former tests are repeatable in the same mouse. Astle
and Harrison (1976) and Horneffer and Weksler (1976) have
used the circulating blood method, but have not shown significant age-related changes. Neither group compared old
and young individuals.

Changes in Response to Stress   Many age-related physiological changes are not obvious until the animal is stressed.
Some examples of this are age-related declines in the
ability of:

- C57BL/6J female mice to produce erythrocytes follow-
ing severe bleeding (Harrison, 1975);
- C57BL/6J mice, CBA/HT6J mice, and their F_1 hybrids
to concentrate urine following exposure to dry food, but
no water for 24 to 48 hours (Burich, 1975; D. E. Harrison,
The Jackson Laboratory, Bar Harbor, Maine, Unpublished);
- C57BL/6J female mice to conserve calcium (Draper,
1964); and
- C57BL/6J male mice to consume oxygen maximally (D. E.
Harrison, The Jackson Laboratory, Bar Harbor, Maine,
Unpublished).

Minimum Oxygen Consumption An age-related reduction in the
amount of oxygen consumed per gram of metabolically active
mass in anesthetized C57BL/6J male mice, maintained at a
constant body temperature, has been observed by D. E. Harrison (The Jackson Laboratory, Bar Harbor, Maine, Unpublished)
using the method of Denckla (1974). Similar results have
been reported by Pettegrew and Ewing (1971), although their
data are more variable, probably because they did not control anesthesia or body temperature and calculated their
results on the basis of body weight, rather than on metabolically active mass.

Proliferative Capacity of Submandibular Glands The proliferative capacity of submandibular glands, measured by
incorporation of tritiated thymidine in response to the
beta-adrenergic agonist, isoproterenol, declines linearly
by about 300 percent between 2 and 18 months of age in male
BALB/c mice (Piantanelli et al., 1978). Similar changes
in rats have been reported by Adelman et al. (1972).

Electroencephalography Age-related changes in sleep time
and in rapid eye movement (REM) sleep are found in both
DBA/2J and C57BL/6J male mice (Eleftheriou et al., 1975).
The declines are much more rapid in DBA/2J mice.

Reproductive Performance Female reproductive performance
has been reviewed by Finch (1978b). Distinct declines can
be detected in the decidual response of the uterus to transplanted ova or to certain irritations by 10 months of age
in C57BL/6J virgin females. Male A/CRe mice have been reported to show rapid reproductive aging (Beatty and Mukherjee, 1963), as judged by the increase in abnormal sperma-
tozoa of 300-day-old as compared with 80- to 100-day-old
mice.

Hair Regrowth Capacity   The regrowth of hair after plucking declines with age in the CBA strain (Horton and Whiteley, 1969), but not in the C57BL/6J strain (Finch, 1973b). This discrepancy may result from strain differences or from differences in health status. Finch (1973b) has found that unhealthy aged mice have slower rates of hair regrowth than healthy aged mice.

Blood Pressure   The blood pressures of 4 inbred strains and 12 F_1 hybrids have been shown to decline from about 4 to 20 months of age (Weibust and Schlager, 1968). Associated with this decline is an increase in variability of the level of cholesterol in the blood.

Collagen Breaking Time   The aging of collagen has been tested in mice of 13 different genotypes by removing individual tail tendon fibers and measuring fiber breaking times in a solution of concentrated urea (Harrison and Archer, 1978). Breaking times increase nearly linearly from approximately 30 to 500 days of age, and thereafter increase exponentially.

Bone Thickness   The cortical thickness of long bones decreases with age in $B6D2F_1$ female mice. The cortices of 18-month-old mice are only about 50 percent as thick as those of 6-month-old mice. An additional 20 percent decrease in thickness occurs by 30 months of age (Rao and Draper, 1969).

Changes in Behavior

Mice probably are not mature behaviorally until 4 to 6 months of age. Accordingly, studies on aging using 2- to 3-month-old subjects to determine baseline behavior levels have nothing to say about senescence. Most behavior measures that have a large activity or motor component decline with advancing age, simple learning measures usually do not, and complex learning tasks produce conflicting results. Cross-sectional studies that use one immature (2 to 4 months) and one older group of subjects are a waste of time and effort. A life span developmental approach in combination with cross-sectional studies probably is best, but it is beyond the resources of some investigators. If a cross-sectional approach must be used by itself, then at least four age groups should be included: one immature (2 to 4 months), two mature (6 to 12 months

and 18 to 24 months), and one senile (30 to 36 months).
The use of genetically defined subjects can greatly increase the precision of studies on aging if more than one
genotype is used in combination with a life span developmental approach. Some behavioral characteristics of the
strains and hybrids emphasized in this report are presented in Table 2.

Aggression is a problem with male mice of particular
strains (e.g., DBA/2J, BALB/cJ, AKR/J, and C57BL/6J). The
problem can be avoided (except for BALB/cJ mice) by keeping cage groups intact from weaning through the rest of
the life span. However, unpublished observations at The
Jackson Laboratory suggest that "stress-inducing" test procedures in older mice of these genotypes may significantly
increase aggression levels. To avoid loss of subjects in
such a situation, isolation may be the only appropriate
housing arrangement.

Life Span[1]

The wealth of previously collected survival data for the
mouse provides the investigator with many published reports
in which genetic and environmental effects on life span
have been documented. There is an abundance of information
on survival characteristics from several inbred colonies of
mice used as controls for aging or age-related experiments.
The survival data reported below pertain to cohorts in
which two inbred parental strains and an F_1 hybrid cross
between the two parental strains were set aside contempo-
raneously and housed in the same environment.

In contrast, survival information on inbred strains or
randomly bred stocks of rats is usually limited to a single
strain or stock, and available usually for either the male
or female only. The previous use of hybrid rat crosses
derived from two inbred rat strains has been practically
nonexistent (Hoffman, 1979). For the mouse, however, there
are studies in which even the F_2, F_3, and/or backcross

---

[1]For uniformity, information on life span in rodents is
presented in months. Data from the literature given in
days or weeks have been converted to months by using the
following formulas:
- life span in months = life span in days x 12/365.
- life span in months = life span in weeks x 12/52.

TABLE 2 Behavioral Characteristics of Selected Inbred Strains of Mice and F_1 Hybrids[a]

Strain or Hybrid	Alcohol Preference[b]	Tasters of PTC[c]	Aggression Level	Emotionality	Activity	Learning	Mating[d]	Vision
A	PA		low	high	low	slow		normal
BALB/c			high	high	low	moderate		normal
CBA			low	moderate	moderate			abnormal
C3H	PA		moderate	moderate	low	rapid		abnormal
C57BL/6	PA	+	low	moderate	high	rapid	RI; RE	normal
DBA/2	AA	+	moderate	moderate	moderate	rapid	SI; RE	normal
B6C3F1								normal
B6D2F1	IA		moderate				SI; RE	normal
CB6F1						rapid		normal

[a]The characteristics described in this table have been reviewed by Sprott (1975).
[b]PA prefers alcohol
   IA intermediate alcohol preference
   AA alcohol avoidance
[c]PTC phenylthiocarbonate
[d]RI rapid intromission
   RE rapid ejaculation
   SI slow intromission

populations have been characterized in survival studies (Grahn, 1972; Goodrick, 1975).

Figures 4-6 illustrate standard survival distributions obtained from three different life span studies. In each study, two parental strains and the F_1 hybrid were set aside for the collection of normative survival and pathology data. The data in Figure 4 are derived from cohorts of mice bred and maintained at the Charles River Breeding Laboratories, Wilmington, Massachusetts, under contract to the National Institute on Aging, National Institutes of Health, Bethesda, Maryland. Survival data were collected only for male mice of the two parental strains, BALB/cNNia and C57BL/6NNia, and the F_1 hybrid cross (BALB/cNNia female x C57BL/6NNia male). Each of these three cohorts contained 270 male mice, weaned at 1 month of age and set aside in alternating groups of 30 and 60 animals each month from December 1972 through May 1973.

The survival distributions shown in Figure 5 are based on cohorts of mice set aside to collect baseline information that was needed for several related studies of the processes of aging conducted at The Jackson Laboratory, Bar Harbor, Maine (D. E. Harrison and D. D. Myers, Unpublished). Survival distributions for both male and female

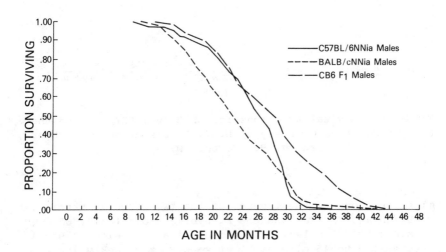

FIGURE 4 Survival functions for male BALB/c, C57BL/6, and the F_1 hybrid. Diagram courtesy of H. J. Hoffman, National Institute of Child Health and Human Development, Bethesda, Maryland.

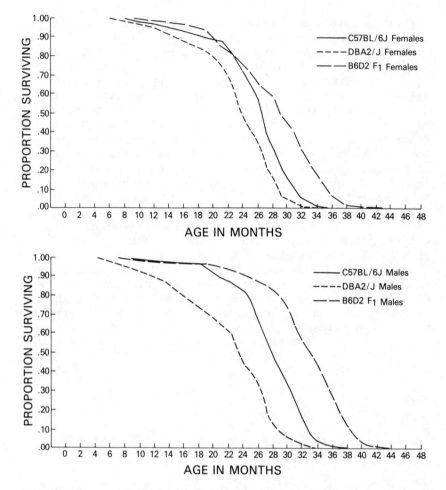

FIGURE 5   Survival functions for C57BL/6J, DBA/2J, and the
F_1 hybrid.   Data Courtesy of D. E. Harrison and D. D. Myers,
The Jackson Laboratory, Bar Harbor, Maine.

mice are shown in the figure for the two parental strains,
C57BL/6J and DBA/2J, and the F_1 hybrid cross (C57BL/6J
female x DBA/2J male).   These mice were set aside in small
batches (10 to 15 mice each) at weekly or biweekly intervals throughout 1974.   A total of 195 mice of each sex
and strain were set aside.   However, approximately 40 percent of each cohort were preselected for serial sacrifice

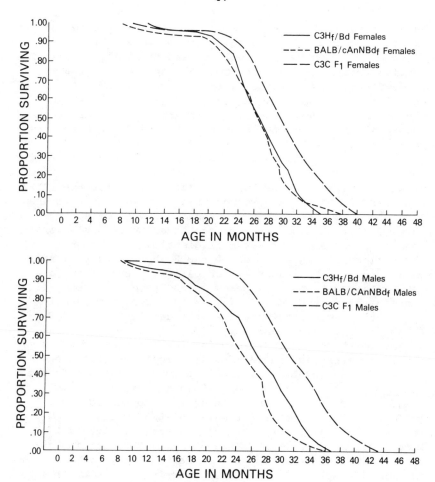

FIGURE 6   Survival functions for BALB/c, C3H, and the F₁ hybrid.   Data courtesy of J. M. Holland, Oak Ridge National Laboratory, Oak Ridge, Tennessee.

at specific ages that ranged from 1 through 3 years of age. The remaining 60 percent of these cohorts were undisturbed. These latter animals were used in calculating the survival functions shown in Figure 5.

   Figure 6 illustrates additional survival data that were obtained at Oak Ridge National Laboratory, Oak Ridge, Tennessee.   The data for these mice were acquired as control information for comparison with mice of the same inbred strains receiving 300 R doses at 5 to 6 weeks of age of whole body X-irradiation (Holland and Mitchell, 1976). The survival distributions for both male and female mice are shown for the two parental strains, $C3H_f/Bd$ and BALB/ $cAnNBd_f$, and the F_1 hybrid cross ($C3H_f/Bd$ female x BALB/ $cAnNBd_f$ male). The number of mice set aside ranged from 139 to 170 for these sex-specific cohorts. These cohorts were set aside between 1968 and 1970.

Survival distributions for four of the six principal mouse strains are illustrated in Figures 4-6. Also, survival distributions for two separate sublines of the BALB/c and C57BL/6 strains are represented in these three figures. In spite of the fact that these data were obtained from three different experimental locations, there are several common features of the survival distributions shown in all three figures. In every case, the F_1 hybrid has a longer median survival age than either parent. Several authors have referred to this tendency of an increased average life span in the F_1 hybrid and have applied the term "hybrid vigor" to describe the phenomenon (Russell, 1966; G. S. Smith et al., 1973; Goodrick, 1975).

The relative median life spans for these selected parental strains also reflect earlier reports. Based on Figure 4, the C57BL/6 strain has a longer median life span (26.2 months) than the BALB/c (22.3 months). Goodrick (1975) reported mean longevity of 21.3 months for male BALB/cJ and 27.2 months for male C57BL/6J mice. G. S. Smith et al. (1973) reported a mean survival age of 27.2 months for male C57BL/10J mice. The C57BL/6 strain has been shown repeatedly in various settings to have a longer median life span than the BALB/c strain. Although this statement holds true for the data shown in Figure 4, if the median or mean life span is compared between the BALB/c and C57BL/6 mice, there is no apparent difference in survival of the longest lived one-sixth of either mouse population. In fact, 1 of the 270 original BALB/cNNia mice lived longer (1239 days) than any 1 of the 270 C57BL/6NNia mice originally set aside.

Figure 5 confirms that the C57BL/6 strain also has a longer median life span (26.8 months) compared to the DBA/2 strain (23.7 months). Myers (1978) reviewed the literature on life span and aging in the mouse and showed that for the majority of studies in which both the C57BL/6 and DBA/2 strains were included, the C57BL/6 has the longer mean life span. The data published by Storer (1978) provide an exception to the general observation. However, the data in

that report were collected in the early 1960s when the
C57BL/6J strain had a much shorter mean life span (19.7-
21.4 months) than is typical of later data (Kunstyr and
Leuenberger, 1975). A recent study by Les (1979) found a
mean life span of 31.2 months for the C57BL/6J strain at
The Jackson Laboratory, Bar Harbor, Maine. His study confirms the same pattern for the relative survival distributions of the C57BL/6J and the DBA/2J strains as the data
shown in Figure 4.

Comparing the top and bottom panels in Figures 5 and 6,
it is apparent that male F_1 hybrid mice have a longer median life span than do female F_1 hybrid mice. Also, one
of the parental strains, the C57BL/6, shows a similar tendency for males to survive longer than females. On the
other hand, the C3H and DBA/2 males and females have nearly
identical life spans, while the BALB/c males show a shorter
life span than the females. Thus, only in the longest
lived mice (the F_1 hybrids and the C57BL/6) is a male
advantage in median life span observed.

The survival distributions in Figure 6 indicate that
for females, the C3H and BALB/c strains are almost indistinguishable in life span characteristics. The male BALB/c
strain has a shorter mean life span, however, than does
the male C3H strain (Festing and Blackmore, 1971; Storer,
1978; and Les, 1979). Ebbesen (1972) has reported that
when BALB/c males are isolated in individual cages, longer
mean life spans can be expected. This can be attributed
to the prevention of fighting. Since behavioral and other
differences have been reported between the BALB/cJ and the
BALB/cN substrains (Ciaranello et al., 1974), the mean life
span of the male BALB/c may be somewhat different for individual substrains. Bailey (1978) has provided an argument based on the genealogical tree of substrain differentiation in the BALB/c strain that can account for the
observed differences between substrains.

The two principal strains for which no survival data
have been presented, the A and CBA strains, generally have
been found to have survival distributions similar to the
BALB/c, C3H, and DBA/2 strains (G. S. Smith et al., 1973;
Goodrick, 1975; Myers, 1978). Blankwater (1978) has recently reported survival distributions for the CBA strain
and summarized the age-related pathology. She found that
the median survival of both male and female CBA mice was
about 28.6 months for animals maintained at the Institute
for Experimental Gerontology TNO, Rijswijk, The Netherlands. Of the six principal mouse strains, only the

C57BL/6 appears consistently to have a longer mean life
span than any of the other strains.

Factors Affecting Life Span

Nutrition

Although the requirements of mice for specific nutrients
have not been as extensively investigated as those of rats,
satisfactory growth, maintenance, reproduction, and lactation have been reported in mice fed a number of natural-
ingredient and purified diets. In formulating such diets,
it is necessary to allow for variations in nutrient requirements arising from differences in growth rate, body
weight, and litter size among the large number of genetic
strains used in research. There are physiological characteristics of mice that limit extrapolation of nutritional
information from other species of laboratory animals such
as the rat. For example, the nutrient requirements for
lactation in the mouse are relatively more stringent than
in the rat, because the mouse achieves a higher proportion
of its adult weight during the suckling period.

A further consideration in formulating diets for animals
used in research on aging is that diets that promote maximum growth are not necessarily those that support maximum
life span. In fact, caloric restriction is the most effective means known of increasing longevity in the mouse
and rat (Ross, 1978). As for most other species, the nutrient requirements of the mouse during the postreproductive period of the life span are the least understood.

Nutrient Requirements Estimates of the dietary concentrations of nutrients required for growth and reproduction of
mice have been published by the Board on Agriculture and
Renewable Resources (BARR) (1978c). The requirements for
these essential nutrients for which data are not available
(chloride, sodium, and selenium) probably can be estimated
reliably from the requirements of rats (BARR, 1978c).
There is evidence that certain additional trace elements
(molybdenum, nickel, vanadium, silicon, tin) may be required in the diet of laboratory animals; however, it appears likely that sufficient amounts are present in natural-
ingredient diets, as well as in purified diets that are not
formulated to be low in these elements. The evidence for
the essentiality of fluoride is still controversial.

No estimates are available on the optimal concentrations of carbohydrate and fat (BARR, 1978c). Most mouse diets contain about 5 percent fat and 5 percent fiber. It should be noted that a higher fat content will lead to reduction in food intake arising from the greater caloric density of the diet and, hence, to a reduced intake of essential nutrients. Additionally, no recommendations are given as to the most desirable proportions of complex and simple carbohydrates.

Natural-Ingredient Diets   A committee of the American Institute of Nutrition has recommended that the open-formula diet formulated by Knapka et al. (1974) be adopted as a standard reference mouse diet (BARR, 1978c). This diet provides all known essential nutrients in excess of their estimated requirements and has been shown to support reproductive performance in three strains of mice equivalent to that obtained by feeding a leading commercial closed-formula ration. This formula is used in most conventional mouse colonies in the National Institutes of Health. Quality control can be assured by issuing ingredient standards based on data published by the Subcommittee on Feed Composition (1969) and by requiring that production facilities comply with sanitation standards of the National Institutes of Health Standard No. 1 (NIH, 1964). Meat-packing products such as meat and bone meal are not included in this formula because of the danger of bacterial contamination. Data on longevity of mice fed this diet have not been reported.

Purified Diets   It is generally necessary to employ purified diets when control of the intake of specific nutrients is required. The American Institute of Nutrition has developed a purified diet that has been found satisfactory for growth and reproduction of mice and rats during the first year of life (BARR, 1978c). The diet contains sucrose as the main carbohydrate source and, thus, may be cariogenic.

The Institute of Laboratory Animal Resources (ILAR) Committee on Laboratory Animal Diets (1978c) has stressed the importance of reporting the details of diets used in animal experimentation. It is particularly important to identify explicitly the forms of nutrients used in purified diets (e.g., dl-α-tocopheryl acetate rather than vitamin E). The trade name and source of major nutrients should be given, and the specific details of diet composition should be reported.

Control of Experimental Diet Ingredients   The importance of
maintaining adequate control of diet ingredients, particularly in long-term studies such as those frequently required in research on aging, has been emphasized (ILAR,
1978c). Fluctuations in diet composition may result in
subtle changes in intestinal microflora, enzyme activity,
and tissue composition, which may complicate the comparison of results obtained in different laboratories.

Deterioration of diet ingredients during storage, particularly at high temperatures, often is an important experimental variable, especially in purified diets. Among
the most labile nutrients are vitamin A, which should always be used in a stabilized form, and vitamin E, which
should be used in an esterified form such as the acetate.
To allow for losses during storage, it is recommended
(ILAR, 1978c) that vitamins be included at 2 to 3 times
the estimated requirement. Similar allowances should be
made for losses incurred during pasteurization of diets
for conventionally housed animals. Large excesses, however, should be avoided. Vitamin C and p-aminobenzoic
acid are not required by mice and should not be added
to purified diets. Minerals (with the exception of calcium and phosphorus) should be provided at 1.5 times the
estimated requirements to allow for variations among
strains and individual animals.

Care should be taken to use up-to-date vitamin and mineral mixes that reflect recent knowledge of the requirements for these nutrients. A fresh supply of a natural-
ingredient stock diet should be fed to a control group of
animals as a check on the ability of purified diets to
promote maximal growth. Since the ingredients in commercial stock diets are subject to change, use of a standard
open-formula reference stock diet is recommended. A standard formula not only gives assurance of nutritional adequacy, but also minimizes complications arising from the
presence of toxicants, plant hormones, etc., in some natural materials. If possible, an investigator should establish a diet quality-assurance program by routinely sub-
jecting each new lot of animal feed to the Salmonella
mutagenesis test or any other rapid assay for demonstration of potentially reactive electrophiles.

Investigators should be aware that any substitution of
one ingredient for another that alters the caloric density
of the diet (for example, fat for carbohydrate) will alter
food intake and thereby the intake of all ingredients.
Animals tend to adjust their eating habits to maintain
constant energy intake rather than constant food intake.

Therefore, substitutions of calorigenic ingredients should be made on an isocaloric basis. This precaution is particularly relevant when the long-term effects of a minor ingredient, such as a suspected carcinogen, are being investigated as a function of the fat, carbohydrate, or protein content of the diet. Natural-ingredient diets should not be used to test the effects of supplements that constitute more than 10 percent of the diet (ILAR, 1978c).

Coprophagy in mice results in the ingestion of significant quantities of some vitamins that are produced by microbial synthesis in the gut. Indeed, it is difficult to produce deficiencies of folic acid, biotin, and vitamin K without the use of an antibacterial agent. While coprophagy generally represents an uncontrollable variable in the nutrition of conventionally reared mice, it is probably not a significant problem except in studies in which control over the intake of certain vitamins is required. It is a more serious complication, however, in studies on the effect of drugs and other nonnutrients on aging, since they may be recycled in fecal material.

Water restriction has an important influence on food consumption, and unrestricted access to water ordinarily should be provided. Tap water from different sources varies significantly in its content of calcium, magnesium, and fluoride, and in some studies it may be necessary to provide distilled or deionized water. When an automatic watering system is not available, sanitized or sterilized water bottles should be used.

Diet Additives Investigators should be aware that commercial natural ingredient diets frequently contain additives that are intended to maintain the nutritional quality of the diet during storage. For example, the synthetic lipid antioxidants, butylated hydroxyanisole, and butylated hydroxytoluene, are designed to inhibit the oxidation of fats and oils in the diet and the co-oxidation of other lipids such as β-carotene and vitamin A. These compounds have been tested for safety in life-cycle studies and should not constitute a risk to the interpretation of the results of most experiments. They may represent a complication, however, in studies on such subjects as the effect of saturated versus unsaturated fats or of natural antioxidants on life span or the incidence of cancer.

Diet Contaminants Natural ingredient diets are subject to contamination with pesticide and herbicide residues arising from the use of these chemicals in agriculture. However, the concentrations of these substances are normally far below the "no effect level," and they do not appear to constitute a significant hazard in biological experiments on laboratory animals. The same conclusion has been drawn with respect to traces of nitrosamines in laboratory animal diets (Lijinsky, 1978). The usual precautions should be taken against heavy metal contamination from mixing equipment and from industrial pollutants such as polychlorinated biphenyls.

Natural feed ingredients may contain mycotoxins and other toxicants of plant or microbial origin. Maximum allowable concentrations of these substances have been suggested (ILAR, 1976b).

In long-term feeding studies, it is desirable to obtain sufficient supplies of diet ingredients to last throughout the experiment. This precaution provides assurance against fluctuations in the levels of contaminants in the diet as well as in nutrient composition, during the course of the study. Of course special precautions must be taken for storage of labile diet ingredients (BARR, 1978c).

Diets for Germfree Mice Germfree and gnotobiotic mice require higher levels of some B vitamins in the diet because of losses during diet treatment and the unavailability of vitamins normally produced by the intestinal microflora. They may also require a dietary source of inositol (BARR, 1978c). Losses during autoclaving are greater in purified diets, being particularly severe in the case of thiamine, vitamin B_6, and pantothenic acid. Prior addition of water substantially reduces the destruction of vitamins during autoclaving. Commercial diets suitable for autoclaving are offered by several suppliers, and some of these diets have been found to sustain normal growth and reproduction in mice over several generations. Satisfactory, chemically defined liquid diets also have been developed for both germfree and conventionally reared mice. γ-irradiation is an acceptable means of sterilization, provided precautions are taken against overexposure, which may cause lipid oxidation, protein damage, and destruction of vitamins (BARR, 1978c).

Germfree mice are susceptible to cecal distention with accompanying growth depression and impaired reproductive performance. Although the cause of this problem is obscure, diet modifications have been suggested that are designed to minimize any effect of nutrition (Wostmann, 1975).

Diet and Longevity The relationship between nutrition and aging recently has been reviewed by Barrows and Kokkonen (1977). It is apparent that the intake of total diet, as well as that of certain specific nutrients, may affect the life span of mice and other species. In evaluating the effect of nonnutritional agents on the life span, it is therefore important to monitor their influence on food consumption and to employ, if necessary, an appropriate method of controlled feeding.

Moderate diet restriction during growth or adult life has been shown to increase the life span of several strains of mice. Although this effect is most conspicuous with respect to energy, in strains susceptible to the early development of autoimmune disease, such as the DBA/2, moderate protein restriction appears to increase longevity by interfering with disease expression (Fernandes et al., 1976). Protein restriction (e.g., 6 percent) also results in maintenance of cell-mediated and humoral immunity functions that usually decline with age in the autoimmunity-susceptible NZB strain (Fernandes et al., 1976). Likewise, diet restriction has been found to extend the developmental and maximum age of immunocompetence in mice of the longer-lived C57BL/6J strain (Gerbase-DeLima et al., 1975). In this strain, reduction of food intake also increases longevity and oxygen consumption and decreases rectal temperature. A dramatic demonstration of the effect of diet restriction on the life span has been presented by the genetically obese (ob/ob) mouse, which survives to at least the age of its nonobese siblings when obesity is prevented by food intake regulation (Lane and Dickie, 1958).

In some studies, it is not possible to differentiate between the effects of protein restriction and the effects of consequent energy restriction. However, restricted feeding of a balanced diet increases the life span of mice; this effect is most evident in animals in which growth retardation is induced by restricting food intake during early life. Nevertheless, Stuchlikova et al. (1975) have observed that longevity in mice is enhanced by diet restriction after 1 year of age, though not as much as by restricting the diet prior to this age.

A high proportion of fat relative to carbohydrate in the diet increases the incidence of obesity and decreases the life span of mice. This effect is apparent even when

energy consumption is equated. Obesity is generally more
severe in mice fed purified diets (which usually have a
higher caloric density) than in mice fed natural ingredient diets. The fatty acid composition of the mesenteric
adipose tissue of B6D2Fl mice fed a stock diet throughout
adult life has been observed to shift toward a higher
proportion of saturated and monoenoic fatty acids and
a lower proportion of linoleic acid (Draper et al., 1970).

Pasteurization of normal pelleted diets has been shown
to increase the life span of 3 of the 10 inbred strains at
The Jackson Laboratory (Heiniger and Dorey, 1980). It is
clear that different diets are required to produce the
maximum longevity in various strains of mice. What is
needed now is a study to determine which commercially
available diet is best suited for each commonly used
strain for purposes of research on aging, rather than
for production purposes. Studies of three such diets are
currently being conducted at The Jackson Laboratory, but
it will be 3 or 4 years before the results are available.

Diet and the Diseases of Aging   Diet restrictions that increase the life span must delay the onset of some diseases
of aging. Prominent among these are cancer, cardiovascular
disease, diabetes, and other pathological correlates of obesity. Diet restriction, sufficient to maintain adult body
weight, has been reported to prevent diabetes and sustain
sensitivity to insulin in the Wellesley mouse (a hybrid of
the C3H and I strains) (Cahill et al., 1967). High energy
intake is associated with obesity, hyperglycemia, and a
rise in serum immunoreactive insulin. Progressive, diet-
related atheromatous disease has been documented in the
C57BL/6J strain when it is fed a diet high in saturated
fat and cholesterol (Thompson, 1969).

Diet restriction reduces the incidence of some forms of
cancer in mice, including spontaneous mammary carcinoma in
the C3H strain and leukemia in the AKR strain (Barrows and
Kokkonen, 1977). Diets high in fat increase the incidence
of skin and mammary tumors (Carroll, 1975). In studies on
the relationship of dietary fat, carcinogenesis, and survival, an increase in the intake of polyunsaturated fatty
acids entails an increased requirement for the lipid anti-
oxidant vitamin E. Restricting the intake of vitamin E
increases the rate of accumulation of lipofuscin pigments
("age pigments") in the tissues of mice (Csallany, et
al., 1977). These pigments are believed to arise from
the peroxidation of polyunsaturated fatty acids in cell
membranes.

The finding that restricted feeding enhances immunocompetence in aging C57BL/6J mice (Gerbase-DeLima et al., 1975), as well as in short-lived strains that are susceptible to autoimmune disease (Fernandes et al., 1976), suggests that nutrition may have a general influence on mortality caused by such diseases. It appears, however, that there may be strain differences in this regard. Stoltzner (1976) found no effect of protein restriction on immunocompetence in BALB/c mice.

Like man and other vertebrate species, mice are susceptible to aging bone loss with corresponding decrements in breaking strength (Krishnarao and Draper, 1969). Aging bone loss is enhanced by feeding diets that are either low in calcium or high in phosphate (Shah et al., 1967). Restriction of physical activity during confinement is probably a contributing factor.

Husbandry

If observations made in aging mice are to be interpreted, interrelated, and reproduced, the environment must be well controlled. The standards of environmental control required for maintaining mice in reproducible, healthful conditions throughout their lives are at least as high as those required for breeding. Thus, animal colonies adequate for maintaining mice to old age also will be adequate for breeding them. In addition, if observations are to be affected minimally by intercurrent infectious disease, it follows that husbandry procedures must be designed to prevent or limit these factors. A thorough discussion of husbandry practices is beyond the scope of this presentation. Fortunately, several recent reports are available that provide excellent surveys of the subject (ILAR, 1976c; 1977; 1978a). There is no optimal set of procedures that will, in all cases and in all strains, guarantee maximum longevity. A laboratory environment is a compromise between research needs and convenience of colony management.

Husbandry is both an art and a science, more empirical than quantitative, and constrained more by economics and expediency than any other single parameter. The ultimate test of any arbitrary set of procedures and recommendations is how successfully they satisfy the requirements for maintenance of a stable, minimally stressful environment.

Other Factors

A variety of additional factors are believed to affect
life span, but very little solid experimental evidence
exists that could be used to confirm or deny these beliefs.
These factors include housing (cage size, airflow, cleanliness, temperature, and cage bedding); cage density;
early environmental enrichment; isolation; lighting; and
handling. Chino et al. (1971) investigated the effects
of "clean versus dirty" cages and found no significant
differences in the mean life span of BC3F1 mice in two
environments. Finkel and Scribner (1955) have found no
survival differences in metal versus plastic cages that
could not be accounted for by an acute infection outbreak
in one group; however, cage size and density also differed.
   Mills (1945), in a study of temperature (13°, 24°, or
33.5°C) effects on the longevity of DBA and C3H mice, has
reported longer life spans in mice raised in a "hot"
environment, and has concluded that the effect is probably
due to reduced food intake and slower growth. Grad and
Kral (1957) have found young (4-7 months) female C57BL/6J
mice to be significantly more resistant to cold stress
than old (16-21 months) female C57BL/6J mice. Gradual ac-
climatization to low temperature reduces, but does not
eliminate, the excess mortality of the older mice.
   Cage density, early environmental enrichment, isolation,
lighting, and handling are occasionally referred to as possible factors in increased longevity in nutritional or behavioral studies. No agreement exists on the effects of
these factors, and indeed they may be strain and/or sex
specific (especially isolation and handling).

Infectious Diseases

The susceptibility of a host to infection and disease increases with advancing age. This is a manifestation of
the aging process presumably due to factors such as the
decline in immune system response, physiological condition,
metabolism, and organ function. There are at least 70 infectious diseases in mice, induced by pathogenic bacteria,
viruses, mycoplasma, fungi, and parasites (ILAR, 1971;
G. S. Smith, et al., 1973; Crispens, 1975), that should
not be present in research animals at any time throughout
experimentation, especially for studies on aging.
   Strain differences in sensitivity to pathogens do exist, and sensitivity may change drastically with age.

Unpublished experience at The Jackson Laboratory suggests
a dramatic increase in susceptibility to pinworms in
DBA/2J mice 24 months of age or older. Parker et al.
(1978) have reported greater sensitivity to Sendai virus
infection in A/J, A/HeJ, C3H/Bi, DBA/1J, DBA/2J, 129/J,
129/ReJ, and nude mice than in C57BL/6J, RF/J, and SJL/J
strains. Greater susceptibility to ectromelia infection
has also been demonstrated in A, C3H, and DBA/1 than in
AKR, BALB/c, and C57BL/6 strains.

Infectious diseases influence age-related changes and
life span through a complex series of mechanisms. Pathogens infect and proliferate in animals, resulting in subtle
or inapparent, long- or short-term changes in organ function, metabolism, physiological state, morphology, enzyme
levels, and the immune system, even though animals appear
clinically "healthy," and these changes may affect experimental results. With recent advancements in laboratory
animal medicine and technology, it now is feasible to
prevent or control infectious diseases and maintain animals free from pathogens.

The effects of infectious diseases on age-related
changes in mice have not been explored extensively. Although the longevity of animal species and the functional
period of tissues are genetically predetermined, infectious
diseases undoubtedly alter biological processes in infected
animals and, thus, reduce life span, hasten tissue death,
cause cellular impairment, and increase the incidence of
other diseases (autoimmune disease or neoplasia). Unfortunately, many early studies, as well as some current
studies on aging, do not give the microbiological status
or define the health quality of experimental animals. This
may account for the variation in life span of identical
mouse strains that exists between laboratories (Myers,
1978). Examples of some adverse effects of unspecified
infectious diseases of rodents for gerontology research
are briefly cited by B. J. Cohen (1968). Improvements
in disease control and other environmental factors have
remarkably increased the life span of several inbred
strains of mice (B. J. Cohen, 1968). If data from different laboratories are to be comparable, specific information on the presence or absence of at least the common
mouse pathogens, including Sendai virus, mouse hepatitis
virus, pneumonia virus of mice, reovirus 3, mouse encephalomyelitis virus, lactic dehydrogenase virus, Salmonella typhimurium, Pasturella, Bordetella bronchiseptica,
Streptococcus pneumoniae, Mycoplasma pulmonis, pinworms
(Syphacia and Aspicularis), Hexamita, Giardia, and

Trichomonas, in animals must be provided even when the
terms "conventional," "barrier-maintained," "specific
pathogen-free (SPF)," or "germfree" are used in reporting.
This is necessary because, in many instances, the health
status of conventional and barrier-maintained animals is
essentially the same due to a breakdown in animal facility
management. In view of these considerations, it is im-
perative to properly characterize and define the health
status of animals used for long-term gerontological research and to maintain them in a barrier facility under
optimal environmental conditions throughout the
investigation.

At least 17 viruses cause infections in mice of all
ages: lymphocytic choriomeningitis virus, mouse hepatitis
virus (including lethal intestinal virus of infant mice--
LIVIM), mouse adenovirus, cytomegalo-virus, pneumonia
virus of mice, Sendai virus, polyoma virus, minute virus
of mice, H-1 virus, mouse encephalomyelitis virus, mouse
encephalomyocarditis virus, ectromelia, reovirus 3, mouse
rotavirus (epizootic diarrhea of infant mice--EDIM), lactic
dehydrogenase virus, and thymic virus. Many of them cause
long-term and subclinical infections in normal mice and
perpetuate in the colony. Morbidity and mortality become
evident when the immune response of animals is altered due
to aging, stress, experimental manipulation, immunosuppres-
sion, poor nutrition, etc. The biology and pathogenesis
of these viruses are reviewed by G. S. Smith et al. (1973),
Parker et al. (1978), and Riley et al. (1978).

It has been postulated that chronic viral infections
are associated with the aging process (Oldstone and Dixon,
1974). Lymphocytic choriomeningitis virus (LCM), like
other slow virus infections, is involved in the pathogenesis of chronic lesions of aging such as glomerulonephritis
and autoimmune diseases resulting in progressive, degenerative changes (Gajdusek, 1972; Lewis, 1974; Oldstone and
Dixon, 1974). LCM significantly depresses the T cell-
related immune responsiveness in old mice (Doherty, 1977).

The chronic infection by reovirus 3 causes runting,
amyloidosis, liver necrosis, damage to or change in the
lymphoid system, and an increase in the incidence and
early onset of lymphoma (Stanley and Keast, 1967; Stanley,
1974). Reovirus 3 also induces diabetes mellitus by de-
stroying pancreatic β cells (Onodera et al., 1978). Mouse
encephalomyocarditis virus (M-variant) also infects pancreatic β cells and produces a diabetes-like syndrome in
certain strains of mice (Notkins, 1978).

Lactic dehydrogenase virus (LDV) is extremely common in mice and mouse cell lines. It causes persistent asymptomatic infections and accelerates the high incidence of autoimmune-related lesions such as glomerulonephritis due to the deposition of circulating virus-antibody complex in the kidney (Morrison and Wright, 1977). LDV infection is known to induce significantly elevated levels of corticosterone and many enzymes, such as lactate dehydrogenase, isocitric dehydrogenase, malic dehydrogenase, glutamic oxalacetic transaminase, phosphohexase isomerase, and glutathione reductase (Riley et al., 1978). Other biomedical complications induced by LDV are reviewed by Riley et al. (1978).

Sendai virus is an important and common pathogen in rodents. The infection is very contagious and persists in animal colonies. Recently, Parker et al. (1978) have reported that as many as 80 percent of commercial mouse colonies in the United States are infected by Sendai as evidenced by the presence of antibodies. Sendai causes clinical symptoms and pathological changes in immunologically depressed or deficient old mice and immature mice. Kay (1978a,b) has studied the long-term sequelae of an outbreak of Sendai infection in mice for gerontological studies. Its adverse effects on aging mice include a decrease in body weight, an increase in fragility and decrease in proliferative capabilities of T and B cells, a reduction in T cell function, and an increase in susceptibility to autoimmune disease.

Mouse hepatitis virus (MHV) infection affects mice of all ages. It causes severe clinical signs and high mortality in athymic mice and immunologically immature or suppressed mice. Pathological changes are found in the liver, brain, intestine, and lymphoid tissues. MHV infection induces an elevation of the levels of serum glutamic-oxalacetic transaminase (SGOT), serum glutamic-pyruvic transaminase (SGPT), and phosphoglucomutase. It also inhibits microsomal enzyme function and depresses the function of the reticuloendothelial system.

Bacterial infections caused by a number of species still constitute a major disease problem in conventionally reared mouse colonies. Bacterial infections may have synergistic effects with other viral, mycoplasmal, or parasitic infections, inducing diseases and pathological changes in mice. No longitudinal studies have been conducted to define the long-term effects of bacterial diseases on the age-related changes at cellular or whole animal levels.

Some species of parasitic infection, such as pinworms and Spironucleus (Hexamita) are still common in conventional mice purchased from many animal vendors. These parasites usually cause no clinical signs. For example Innes et al. (1962) have reported a 50 percent incidence of occult encephalitozoonoses due to Encephalitozoon (Nosema) cuniculi in the brains of mice from a "disease-free" colony. The infection rate increases with age and induces a nonsuppurative, meningo-encephalitis with no apparent effect on the life span of the mice. However, if the environment of the animals or of their parasites is altered, a breakdown in the balance of the host-parasite relationship could occur, which may have adverse effects on the hosts. As with bacterial infections, no information is available on the effects of subclinical parasitic infestation on the life span, tissue and cellular function, or metabolic status in mice. For example, the effect of intestinal parasites, such as pinworms or Spironucleus (Hexamita), on the aging of intestinal tissue is unknown.

Spontaneously Occurring Diseases

General Considerations The likelihood that lesions will be present in tissues from aged animals should always be taken into account. That is, the cellular, architectural, and functional characteristics of these tissues may depart significantly from the norm, and any data obtained may be more indicative of a particular pathological state than organ- or tissue-specific senescence. Steps must be taken to limit this potential problem, or at least recognize when it occurs. The first requirement is to become thoroughly familiar with the gross and, if possible, microscopic characteristics of the tissue. Second, it is necessary to develop explicit gross, microscopic, and, if possible, functional criteria for normality, with appropriate allowances for natural, time-dependent changes. If inexperienced persons are primarily responsible for collecting and processing tissues, it is even more important to adhere to an explicit set of descriptive criteria that are designed to exclude pathological tissues from the data set. In preparing these criteria, the advice and assistance of a qualified pathologist should always be sought, but if these services are unavailable, there are a few approaches that will at least minimize this source of potential bias. The investigator can prepare color photographs that bracket the normal range of color, shape,

and texture of the organ under whatever set of conditions
prevail. When departures are observed, they can be excluded from the analysis or handled separately. In addition to general macroscopic examination, useful insight
can be obtained by weighing the tissue and referencing
the individual organ weight to an average obtained from
all animals of the same strain, sex, and approximate age.
A general impression then can be obtained concerning
whether the particular specimen falls within a predetermined range.

This approach will exclude only the most abnormal tissues from the study set and provides little or no guarantee that some degree of pathological change is not present
in the remaining samples. It would be extremely helpful
if there were a systematic survey of disease incidence
in various tissues that are frequently of interest to
the experimental gerontologist based upon the commonly
used inbred strains of mice. However, there are many difficulties, some technical, some practical, and others biological, why such a survey does not exist. First and
foremost, there are very few populations of mice, of known
genetic constitution, that have been followed sufficiently
long or in which a high percentage of the mice have received an adequate histopathological evaluation. Most of
the reports in the published literature, especially those
prior to 1970, present spontaneous disease data in terms
of crude incidence that may be reproducible for only a
single strain under a single set of conditions (environment, infectious disease burden, and diet). However,
these data seldom can be extrapolated, since crude incidence is highly dependent upon the underlying mortality
distribution of the study sample. Since the overall mortality rate reflects the summation of all lethal genetic-
environmental interactions, it is not surprising that from
experiment to experiment or from laboratory to laboratory,
it should prove to be a variable dimension.

Strain-Specific Chronic Disease   No survey of spontaneous
disease literature can do justice to the vast amount of
information available on the mouse. Fortunately, much of
this information has been summarized in the Biology of the
Laboratory Mouse (Green, 1966), and for many of the less
commonly untilized strains, it is the only source of information. The descriptions of pathological states commonly
observed in various strains can be found in monographs em-
phasizing the spontaneous pathology of laboratory animals
(Ribelin and McCoy, 1965; Benirschke et al., 1978).

The incidence of various neoplasms in mice is summarized
in Table 3. Many well known characteristics are reflected.
Even more impressive is the variation among mice of the
same strain, often greater in magnitude than that observed
between strains. By far the most prevalent of the pathological conditions observed in aged mice of all strains
are the lympho- and myeloproliferative diseases. In certain strains (AKR, RFM), leukemia and lymphoma are the
principal causes of death. However, in the longer-lived
strains chosen for emphasis in this chapter, the combined
incidence of lethal lymphoproliferative diseases rarely
exceeds 20 percent prior to 2 years of age.

The so-called retroviruses or oncornaviruses contribute
to the pathogenesis of these diseases. Considerable data
exist concerning strain differences in susceptibility and
host genetic factors that control virus expression (Pincus,
1980). Retroviruses are capable of causing an extensive
variety of pathological tissue changes that could alter
interpretation of biochemical data obtained from whole organ extracts. In addition to lymphoid and hematopoietic
tissue involvement, there is also frequent involvement of
the liver, gonads, adrenals, and perivascular regions of
a variety of other tissues. As a precaution, it would be
wise to determine the spleen weight of all aged mice used
in studies of cellular and molecular aging. If the spleen
weight is positively correlated with the parameter of interest, disseminated lymphoreticular disease may have contributed to the differences observed.

The importance and popularity of neoplasia as a disease
entity often overshadow less spectacular, but potentially
no less relevant, disease states that also occur with some
frequency in aging mice. Table 4 lists the scanty amount
of data found on these "nonneoplastic" disease states in
inbred strains. About all that can be said, on the basis
of these data, is that degenerative diseases are observed,
especially in the last 10-20 percent of survivors, and the
possible contribution of these diseases to mortality is
rarely addressed.

There are several things that can be done to facilitate
a more critical comparison of disease incidence among inbred strains. The primary objective must be determination
of age-specific mortality rates caused by specific pathological states. To do this, animals should be housed under
conditions that preclude early infectious disease mortality
(not necessarily in a "barrier"); they must be examined at
least daily, especially after 18 months, to remove dead and
moribund mice; investigators must resist the temptation to

kill sick mice on Friday afternoons; and all mice (auto-
lyzed or otherwise) should be necropsied and all gross observations recorded on a standard form, such as shown in
Figure 7. Tissues that are impossible to adequately evaluate visually should be routinely processed for microscopic
examination. This includes decalcification and sectioning
the skull at several levels to examine the cranial vasculature, tongue, eyes, Harderian glands, and pituitary. When-
ever individual organs or portions of the animal cannot be
evaluated either as a result of cannibalism or autolysis,
the missing tissues should be noted on the necropsy record.
When the data are subsequently analyzed, these animals can
be excluded from the analysis of those diseases for which
diagnosis depends upon examination of the missing tissue.

There are several approaches that, if systematically
applied, could reduce some of the uncertainty in the interpretation of disease surveys based upon aged animals, including mice. The experimentalist should consult a bio-
metrician for suggestions of how best to adjust the
incidence data for overall mortality. Once this is done
other investigators can more readily compare data. Several
approaches are available, and each has its advantages and
limitations (Upton et al., 1960; Lindop and Rotblat, 1961;
Ullrich et al., 1977; Turnbull and Mitchell, 1978).

There remains the difficult problem of drawing conclusions from survival experiments concerning the relative
contribution of individual pathological states to overall
mortality. This implies that it is of interest to identify
those processes most directly responsible for mortality in
specific individuals. The basic reason for the study is
frequently to identify the effects of an exposure to toxic
materials, environmental manipulation, mutant gene, or
altered nutrition. In this analysis, it must be kept in
mind that not all occurrences of single disease are equally
lethal in all individuals and that different diseases tend
to vary greatly in their potential lethality in a particular strain or under a particular set of conditions.

Statistical analysis of necropsy information obtained
from animals permitted to die naturally requires the discussion of a term known as "competing risk." Under the
competing risk concept, different diseases are viewed as
"competing" with one another for the life of the animal.
In a stochastically aging population, the observation of
a disease process is conditional upon death of the animal,
and since death is not an entirely random sample of the
population (not all diseases are contributing equally),

TABLE 3   Percent Incidence of Tissue or Site Specific Neoplasms in Aged Inbred Mice

Strain	Reference	Sex	Number Autopsied[a]	Breeding Status	Environment[c]	Total Neoplasms	Lymphoreticular Tissue	Muscle and Connective Tissue
1. BALB/cAnNBdf	Cosgrove et al., 1978	F	331	V	BR	94%	67	nd[h]
2. BALB/cAnNCr	Peters, 1972	F	2065	B	C	nc[e]	23	2
3. BALB/cAnHPi	G. S. Smith, 1971	M&F	67	B	GF	43	8	nd
4. BALB/cAnNCr	Madison et al., 1968	M&F	2088[d]	V	C	20	10	.0004
5. BALB/cLacf	Festing and Blackmore, 1971	M&F	21	B	BR	2-32	0-17	nd
6. C3H/HeBdf	Holland et al., 1978	M	58	V	GF	67	7	4
		F	74	V	GF	93	10	25
7. C3H/HeLacf	Festing and Blackmore, 1971	M&F	131	B	BR	48-67[f,g]	0-4	nd
8. C57BL/Icrfa[t]	Rowlatt, et al., 1976	M	497	B&V	C	40	16	1
		F	293	B&V	C	50	19	1
9. C57BL/10ScSn	G. S. Smith et al., 1973	M	30	V	C	33	31	0
		F	21	V	C	31	29	0
10. CBA/Lacf	Festing and Blackmore, 1971	M&F	21	B	B	14-57	0-17	nd
11. CBA/J	G. S. Smith et al., 1973	M	17	V	C	29	6	0
		F	28	V	C	54	15	3
12. DBA/2Lacf	Festing and Blackmore, 1971	M&F	30	B	BR	20-56	0-17	nd
13. DBA/2J	G. S. Smith et al., 1973	M	31	V	C	15	10	3
		F	29	V	C	49	12	0
14. A/Lacf	Festing and Blackmore, 1971	M&F	30	B	BR	6-35	10-43	nd

[a] Unless otherwise noted, the disease observations were based upon mice dead or killed moribund.
[b] V = virgin; B = breeder.
[c] BR = barrier-reared; C = conventional; GF = germfree.
[d] Mice killed at 18 months of age, sexes not distinguished in the analysis.

it is necessary to distinguish lethal from nonlethal occurrences. This will enable one to approximate the true population frequencies of disease, especially those of low overall lethality. Additional examples of their application can be found elsewhere (Hoel and Walburg, 1972; Holland et al., 1977).

TABLE 3 (continued)

Strain	Vascular	Liver	Lung	Mammary	Pituitary	Adrenal Cortex	Adrenal Medulla	Testis and Ovary	Uterus	GI Tract	Bone	Harderian Gland
1.	5	nd[h]	32	13	8	29	nd[h]	8	3	4	nd[h]	11
2.	2	.01	17	5	nd	4	nd	3	nd	nd	.002	.02
3.	6	3	21	3	nd	3	nd	1.5	nd	nd	nd	nd
4.	.0009	.006	16	.0004	nd	1	.0004	.004	.0004	nd	nd	.0004
5.	nd	0-17	2-32	0-17	nd	nd	nd	nd	nd	nd	nd	nd
6.	4	40	9	0	nd	0	4	0	-	0	1	4
	2	11	6	6	nd	1	2	60	2	1	3	12
7.	nd	9-23	2-10	21-36	nd	nd	nd	nd	nd	nd	nd	nd
8.	.004	10	6	-	nd	nd	0	nd	-	7	0	1
	2	11	8	.003	nd	nd	.003	6	.01	11	.003	.01
9.	nd	3	0	0	nd	nd	nd	nd	nd	0	nd	nd
		0	3	0						3		
10.	nd	1-26	0-17	3-37	nd	nd	nd	nd	nd	nd	nd	nd
11.	nd	24	0	0	nd	nd	nd	nd	nd	0	nd	nd
		0	0	33						0		
12.	nd	6-35	1-23	0-11	nd	nd	nd	nd	nd	nd	nd	nd
13.	nd	2	0	0	nd	nd	nd	nd	nd	0	nd	nd
		0	0	31						2		
14.	nd	0-12	4-31	0-12	nd	nd	nd	nd	nd	nd	nd	nd

[e]These entries could not be calculated from the data as reported.
[f]The calculated 95 percent confidence that the true incidence lies between these limits.
[g]Total neoplasms, not including tumors of lymphoreticular tissue.
[h]Category not used by author; therefore, the incidence could not be determined.

TABLE 4   Percent Incidence of Various Nonneoplastic Disorders in Aged Inbred Mice

Strain	Reference	Sex	Number Autopsied[a]	Breeding Status[b]	Environment	Hepatitis
1. BALB/cAnNBdf	Cosgrove, et al., 1978	F	331	V	BR	4
2. BALB/cAnNCr	Madison et al., 1968	M&F	2088[d]	V	C	5
3. BALB/cLacf	Festing and Blackmore, 1971	M&F	21	B	BR	(0-17)[f,g]
4. C57BL/6Lacf	Festing and Blackmore, 1971	M&F	13	B	BR	(0-26)
5. A/Lacf	Festing and Blackmore, 1971	M&F	30	B	BR	(15-50)
6. C3H/HeLacf	Festing and Blackmore, 1971	M&F	131	B	BR	(0-3)
7. DBA/2Lacf	Festing and Blackmore, 1971	M&F	30	B	BR	(0-11)
8. CBA/Lacf	Festing and Blackmore, 1971	M&F	21	B	BR	(0-17)
9. C3H/HeBdf	Holland et al., 1978	M F	67 93	V V	GF	-
10. C57BL/Icrfa_t	Rowlatt et al., 1976	M&F	43[e]	B&V	C	46

[a]Unless otherwise noted, the disease observations were based upon mice dead or killed moribund.
[b]V = virgin; B = breeder.
[c]BR = barrier-reared; C = conventional; GF = germfree.
[d]Killed at 18 months of age.
[e]Based on number of mice autopsied at 30 months of age. 20 male and 23 female mice were pooled for the incidence calculation.
[f]Infections were pooled without specifying location. A range is given that reflects the upper and lower 95 percent confidence limits.
[g]If the range includes 0, this indicates that no occurrences of the disease were observed.
[h]The author did not include this diagnostic category.
[i]Data for both ovarian and uterine cysts. Sexes were pooled, so the actual incidence is lower than that reported.
[j]Data based upon female autopsies only.

TABLE 4 (<u>continued</u>)

Strain	Nephritis	Pneumonia	Cardiac Calcinosis	Ovarian Cysts	Amyloidosis	Arterio-sclerosis	Polyarteritus	Glomerulo-sclerosis	Hemorrhage/Thrombosis
1.	nd[h]	nd	21	8	1	8	4	74	24
2.	nd	11	8	nd	nd	nd	0.4	nd	0.1
3.			2-3	0-17[i]	nd	nd	nd	nd	0-17
4.			0-2	0-26	nd	nd	nd	nd	0-26
5.			0-1	0-12	nd	nd	nd	nd	0-12
6.			8-2	13-26	nd	nd	nd	nd	0-7
7.			0-1	0-17	nd	nd	nd	nd	4-31
8.			1-2	3-37	nd	nd	nd	nd	3-37
9			nd	nd	nd	nd	nd	6	3
10.	nd	51	nd	17[j]	37	nd	nd	28	nd

ANIMAL NECROPSY RECORD Prosector______________

UCN-8062
(3 10-78)

Experiment No. _ _ _ _ _ _ Birth date _ _ _ _ _ _ Sex F, M.

Histology No. _ _ _ _ _ _ Death date _ _ _ _ _ _ Strain _________.

Cage No. _ _ _ Treatment __________. Dose __________.

Animal No. _ _ Start date __________. Stop date __________.

Body wt.____. Disposition: Dead, Sick, Moribund, Accidental, Sacrifice.

Organ wts.: lung___, liver___, spleen___, kidney___, ___.
heart___, testis/ovary___, ___, brain___.

General condition: Healthy, debilitated, emaciated, obese, other______.

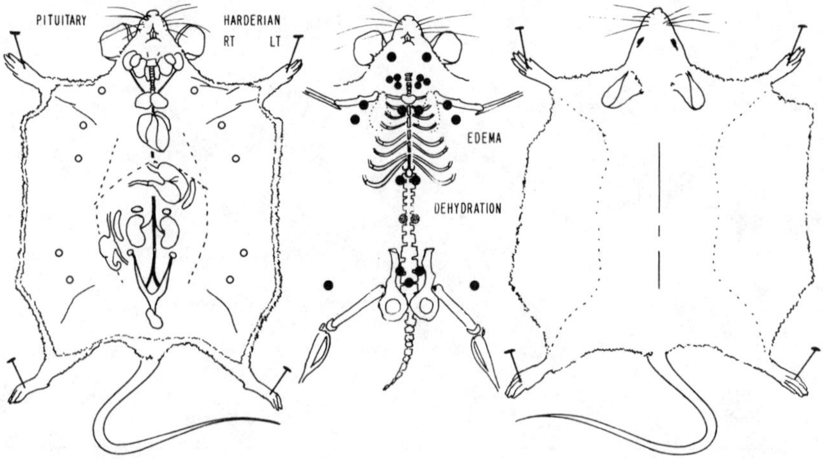

HYDROTHORAX
CLEAR
MILKY
BLOODY

ASCITES
CLEAR
MILKY
BLOODY

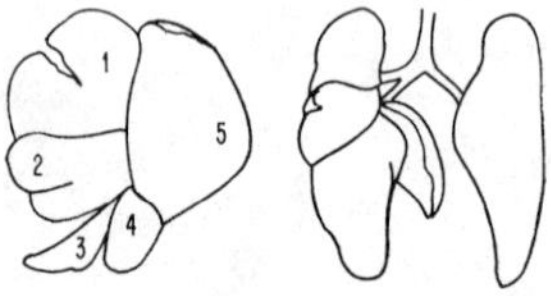

COMMENT

FIGURE 7 Animal Necropsy Record. Figure courtesy of J. M. Holland, Oak Ridge National Laboratory, Oak Ridge, Tennessee.

Systems Examination

A. <u>Integumentary</u> - 1 hair, 2 skin, 3 external ear r, l, 4 nails, 5 subcutis,
6 breast, 7 gingiva, 8 oral cavity

    Gross -   Micro. -   Codes -

B. <u>Musculoskelatal</u> - 1 skelatal muscle, 2 diaphragm, 3 sternum, 4 joints,
5 fore limb, r, l, 6 rear limb r, l, 7 pelvis, 8 spine,
9 cranium, 10 ribs, 11 tail

    Gross -   Micro. -   Codes -

C. <u>Lymphohemopoetic</u> - 1 superficial lymphnodes, 2 deep lymphnodes, 3 Peyer's patches,
4 spleen, 5 bone marrow, 6 thymus

    Gross -   Micro. -   Codes -

D. <u>Cardiopulmonary</u> - 1 heart, 2 blood vessels, 3 lung, 4 trachea/larynx, 5 pleura,
6 sinus/nares

    Gross -   Micro. -   Codes -

E. <u>Gastrointestinal</u> - 1 esophagus, 2 forestomach, 3 glandular stomach, 4 small intestine,
5 colon, 6 cecum, 7 rectum, 8 salivary glands, 9 liver,
10 gall bladder, 11 exocrine pancreas, 12 omentum/mesentery,
13 peritoneum

    Gross -   Micro. -   Codes -

F. <u>Genitourinary</u> - 1 kidney r, l, 2 ureter, 3 uretus, 4 bladder, 5 urethra,
6 testis/ovary r, l, 7 seminal vesicles/uterus,
8 prostate/cervix, 9 prepace/vagina, 10 accessory glands

    Gross -   Micro. -   Codes -

G. <u>Sensory</u> - 1 brain, 2 spinal cord, 3 mininges, 4 eye r, l, 5 peripheral nerves,
6 spinal ganglia, 7 cranial nerves, 8 middle ear

    Gross -   Micro. -   Codes -

H. <u>Endocrine</u> - 1 pituitary, 2 harderian r, l, 3 thyroid, 4 islets of langerhans
5 adrenal r, l, 6 paraganglia

    Gross -   Micro. -   Codes -

FIGURE 7 (<u>continued</u>)

Adaptation of Germfree Mice to Conventional Environments

It is advisable for scientists in gerontological research to use "clean conventional" rodents, meaning that they are derived either from a germfree colony or from an SPF colony and maintained within a closed colony system. This will help prevent contamination of the colony with infectious diseases that may obscure the results of an experiment or affect longevity adversely.

The effects of introducing germfree mice into a conventional environment have been studied by a number of investigators. Reyniers and Sacksteder (1958) have found that each genotype responded somewhat differently, and within each genotype, the survival rate was age-dependent. Germfree C3H mice seemed unusually sensitive to contamination when brought out of the germfree system; less than 15 percent survived 48 hours after exposure. In marked contrast was the 80 percent survival rate for germfree Swiss mice brought into a conventional environment. The survival times of male and female C3H mice were not significantly different, but only mice over 1 month of age survived. Outzen and Pilgrim (1967) showed that the death rate of germfree C3H/Pi mice introduced into a conventional colony was highest during the first month after exposure, but in contrast to the work of Reyniers and Sacksteder (1958), showed that the death rate was dependent on both age and sex, being higher in males and in mice over 6 months of age. This higher death rate in older mice was also found by Outzen (1969), when he exposed germfree mice to Salmonella typhimurium and Salmonella newport.

Gordon et al. (1966) compared the longevity of germfree and conventional colonies of Swiss-Webster mice derived from the same parental stock. The ancestors of the conventional animals were germfree mice that, soon after formation of the original nucleus, were removed from the isolators and adapted to conventional quarters. It was not reported whether this change was attended by deaths. The germfree mice showed a higher mean survival age than the conventional animals (Table 5).

Walburg and Cosgrove (1967) have compared the mean survival age of germfree, barrier-maintained, and conventional random-bred ICR mice. The data for their germfree and conventional animals indicate no significant difference in the mean survival age of these mice under the different microbial conditions (Table 5).

Wostmann (1968) concluded from his data that the life span of germfree mice (most likely a Swiss-Webster stock) is at least as long as that of comparable conventional animals. In fact (see Table 5), his data indicate that there is a clear-cut difference in the 50 percent survival and maximum ages between the germfree and conventional mice.

Less data of this type are available for species other than mice. Germfree rats, removed from isolators to conventional conditions, have been reported to show severe inflammation of lymph nodes, but no mortality (Reyniers and Sacksteder, 1958; Gordon and Wostmann, 1959). Germfree guinea pigs reportedly die within 2-10 days after removal from the isolator, due to Clostridium perfringens type E infection (Madden et al., 1970).

Based on experiences such as those mentioned above, the Radiobiological Institute, Institute for Experimental Gerontology and the Primate Center (REP Institutes) of the Organization for Health Research TNO, The Netherlands, adopted a new procedure for conventionalization of germfree animals in the late 1960s. It was known that mice colonized with known anaerobic intestinal flora showed colonization resistance (CR) when subsequently exposed to gram-negative organisms. Offspring of germfree mice, contaminated with the intestinal flora of a conventional mouse that had been treated with antibiotics, also showed colonization resistance, and these mice were called CRF mice (van der Waaij and Sturm, 1968; van der Waaij et al., 1971; Wensinck and Russeler-van Embden, 1971), since it appeared that this flora constituted a colonization resistance factor (CRF).

The REP Institutes have established an SPF colony of animals to provide large numbers of rats and mice in common use to all the Institutes. This SPF colony originally was established by transferring pregnant, germfree mice and rats to an isolator in which they were exposed to CRF flora for 14 days. The animals were then moved to the SPF unit where they served as foster mothers for cesarean-derived young from conventional animals. Such animals from this colony as are to be used for experimental purposes are transferred to a clean, conventional environment (Hollander, 1976; Solleveld, 1978; Hollander, 1979).

A possible alternative to this procedure is to contaminate germfree animals with CRF flora and then transfer them directly to a conventional environment. Although there are no deaths when this procedure is used, the animals exposed to CRF flora are housed under the same rigid conditions (in isolators) as germfree animals, which is a limiting factor in the production of large numbers of

TABLE 5 Fifty Percent Survival and Mean and Maximum Survival Ages of Different Mouse Strains Under Germfree and Conventional Conditions

	Age in Months												
	50% Survival[a]				Mean Survival[a]				Maximum Survival				
	Male		Female		Male		Female		Male		Female		
Mouse Strain	GF[b]	C[b]	GF	C	GF	C	GF	C	GF	C	GF	C	Reference
Swiss-Webster	25	15	23	17	24	16	23	17	37	27	33	28	Gordon et al., 1966
ICR	19	20	18	15	19	18	18	18	31	31	25	28	Walburg and Cosgrove, 1967
Swiss-Webster?	25	16	23	17					36	26	33	28	Wostmann, 1968

[a]Modified from original data
[b]GF = germfree
C = conventional

animals for experimental purposes. Therefore, the above-
described procedure is preferred.

RATS

More information is available concerning aging in rats
than for any other species with the possible exception of
man. This reflects the relatively short life span, ease
of handling, convenient size, and moderate maintenance
cost of rats compared to other animals. These attributes,
combined with age-associated physiological and pathological changes that are similar to those of humans, make rats
useful animals for research on aging. The stocks and
strains that have been characterized under well-defined
environmental and genetic conditions with respect to age-
associated changes are primarily the inbred Fischer 344
(F344) and outbred Sprague-Dawley®[1](SD) rats, and to a
lesser extent, the outbred Long Evans (LE) and Wistar
(WI) rats. The principles of genetics and husbandry are
essentially the same as those discussed in the section on
mice. The following discussion focuses on the specific
life span properties of these stocks and strains, the
ways in which life span is affected by environment, and
the use of rats as animal models for studying the biology
and pathology of aging. There is no attempt to be encyclopedic or to focus research in specific directions.
Instead, illustrative examples, with appropriate references, are used to alert prospective investigators to
potential values and pitfalls of using rats in research
on aging.

Reliably Characterized Stocks and Strains

Mortality Statistics

The survival characteristics of rat stocks and stains are
dependent on environmental conditions, as well as genetic
factors. Differences in diet, population density, microbiological status, etc., may have a profound effect on
mortality statistics. The reported life spans for F344,
SD, LE, and WI rats are presented in Table 6. Differences

---

[1]Sprague-Dawley® is a registered trademark of Harlan Indus-
tries, Inc., Indianapolis, Indiana.

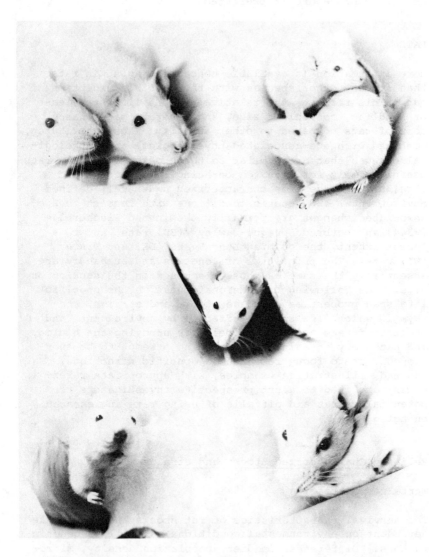

The laboratory rat, Rattus norvegicus. Photograph courtesy of Mr. James Young, Temple University Institute on
Aging, Philadelphia, Pennsylvania.

TABLE 6 Reported Life Spans of Ad Libitum-Fed F344 and SD Rats

Stock or Strain	Sex[a]	Microbio-logical Status[b]	Housing (no./cage)	Length of Life (months)			Reference
				Mean	Median	Maximum	
F344	M	BR	5 until 6 mo; 3 thereafter		29	35	Coleman et al., 1977
	M	BR	1	23.1	23.4	31.7	Masoro, 1980
	M	C	3	21.1	21.7	39.2	Chesky and Rockstein, 1976
	M	BR	4-5		27.5		Sass et al., 1975
	F	BR	4-5		26.5		Sass et al., 1975
SD	M	C	1		23.2		Nolen, 1972
	F	C	1		24.9		Nolen, 1972
	M		1	24.0		35.2	Ross, 1961
	M	C	8-9		25.2		Lesser et al., 1973
	M	C	8-9		25.3		Lesser et al., 1973

TABLE 6 (continued)

Stock or Strain	Sex[a]	Microbiological Status[b]	Housing (no./cage)	Length of Life (months)			Reference
				Mean	Median	Maximum	
SD	M	--			26.4		Simms, 1967
	M	--	1	19.3			Leveille, 1972
	F	--			27.5		Shellabarger et al., 1974
	M	BR	5-7		30	40	Adelman et al., 1978
LE	M	C	--		19-24	30-36	Riegle et al., 1977
	M				27.5		Kozma et al., 1973
	F				28		Kozma et al., 1973
WI (inbred)	M	BR	2	21.2			Festing and Blackmore, 1971
	F	BR	2	24.6			Festing and Blackmore, 1971

	Sex[a]	Condition[b]				Reference
WI (outbred)	M	BR	2	24.0		Festing and Blackmore, 1971
	F	BR	2	25.7		Festing and Blackmore, 1971
	M/F	C	--		25.5	Paget and Lemon, 1965
	M/F	BR	--		29.0	Paget and Lemon, 1965
	M	C	8		23.7	Schlettwein-Gsell, 1970
	F	C	8		26.7	Schlettwein-Gsell, 1970
	M	C			18.3	Stuchlikova et al., 1975

[a] M = male, F = female.
[b] C = conventional, BR = barrier maintained.

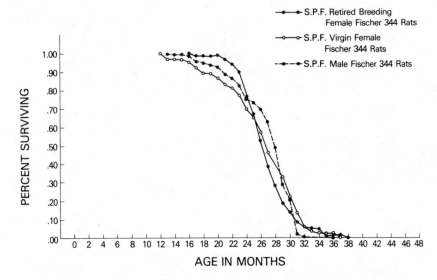

FIGURE 8   Survival curves for specific pathogen free (SPF)
F344 rats.   Source: Hoffman, 1979.

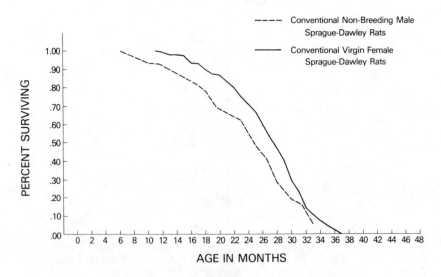

FIGURE 9   Survival curves for SD rats.   Source: Hoffman,
1979.

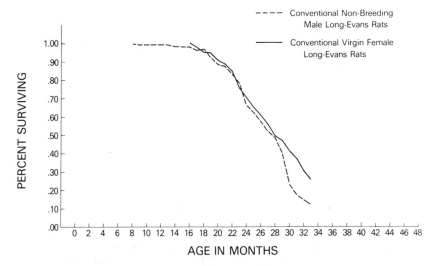

FIGURE 10   Survival curves for LE rats.   Source: Hoffman, 1979.

in life span may be due to variation in microbiological or breeding status or to other environmental factors. Figures 8-10 present survival curves for F344, SD, and LE rats. Further information on the longevity of WI and WI-derived, and on the Brown Norway (BN) and BN-derived, stocks can be found in a recent monograph by Burek (1978).

Growth Patterns

F344 Strain   As with mortality statistics, growth patterns of rats are influenced by environment. The data in Figure 11 describe the growth pattern of male F344 rats main-tained at the University of Texas Health Science Center, San Antonio, Texas, in a barrier facility, fed ad libitum (Masoro, In press). There is a rapid increase in body mass during the first 8 months of life, followed by a less rapid, linear increase until 16 months of age, with a very slow further increase until peak weight is reached at 20 months. After 20 months, there is a significant decrease in body mass. Lean body mass increases through much of the life span, but declines after 95 percent of the life span has been achieved. Adipose tissue mass

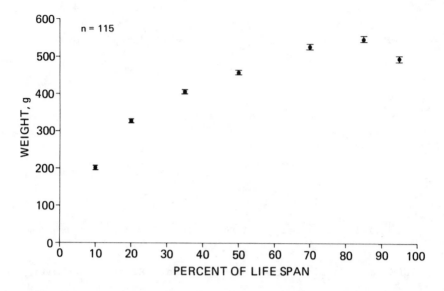

FIGURE 11 Changes in body weight of F344 rats. Changes in body weight are recorded throughout the life span for 115 F344 rats fed ad libitum. Mean length of life is 702 ± 10 days. Source: Masoro, 1980, by permission of the author and editor, Beech Hill Enterprises, Inc.

increases during the first two-thirds of the life span and usually declines thereafter.

Data made available by the Charles River Breeding La-boratories, Wilmington, Massachusetts (Unpublished), on 15 male F344 rats indicate a similar growth pattern, but because such a small number of rats are reported, it is difficult to know precisely at what age the peak weight for a large population might occur, or if mean body weight between 15 and 25 months of age remains nearly constant. The greatest mean weight observed for this small population occurs at 18 months of age. There are appreciable differences in the absolute value of the mean weights between the Charles River and the San Antonio populations (Table 7). Chesky and Rockstein (1976) have reported that the weights of 572 male F344 rats increase throughout their life span to a maximum mean weight of 346 ± 33 g.

SD Stock The data in Figure 12 describe the growth pat-tern reported by Berg (1960) for SD rats. The males

TABLE 7 Mean Weights of Male F344 Rats (g)

Mean at:	Charles River Study[a] (n=15)	San Antonio Study[b] (n=115)
2 mo. of age	150	173
4 mo. of age	276	310
Maximum weight attained	454	569

[a]Data from the Charles River Breeding Laboratories, Wilmington, Massachusetts, Unpublished.
[b]Data from Masoro, 1980.

reach a maximum weight of approximately 450 g by 18 months of age; female rats reach a maximum weight of approximately 280 g by 24 months of age. Ross (1969) states that male SD rats increase in body weight until 18 months of age, reaching about 600 g, a weight that is maintained until after 24 months of age. Nolen (1972) reports that ad libitum fed male and female SD rats increase in body weight until 24 months of age, at which time the average weight of the males is 880 g and that of the females is 600 g. Lesser et al. (1973) have found that a maximum weight of 750 g is reached by SD male rats in conventional facilities by approximately 24 months of age. Lean body mass does not decline with advancing age until the onset of severe disease. Adelman et al. (1978) report that barrier-maintained, male SD rats continue to increase in weight until 24 months of age; their weight at this time is around 700 g.

Other Stocks Riegle et al. (1977) have reported that 4-month-old, ad libitum fed LE male rats have a mean weight of 416 $\pm$ 10 g and 26-month-old rats have a mean weight of 570 $\pm$ 17 g. Leathem and Albrecht (1974) have found that the weight of LE males increases markedly throughout the first year of life, with only a small additional increase until 18 months of age, when the weight is about 540 g. Information on changes in body weight with respect to age of WI- and BN-derived rats is discussed by Burek (1978).

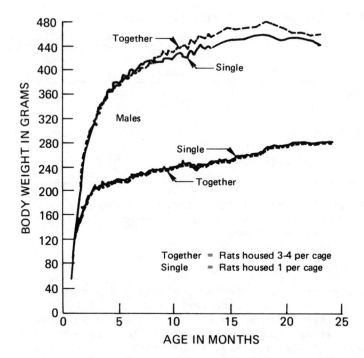

FIGURE 12   Changes in body weight of SD rats.
Changes in body weight are recorded throughout
the life span for SD rats fed ad libitum.   n = 25
for each group.   Source: Berg, 1960.

Spontaneous Diseases

The spectrum of age-associated lesions in rats can be influenced by both genetic factors and environment.   However,
regardless of stock or strain, the most consistent nonneoplastic, age-associated lesions are chronic renal disease,
polyarteritis nodosa, myocardial degeneration, skeletal
muscle degeneration, and radiculoneuropathy.   There are
numerous other lesions in most organ systems.   Aging rats
also develop benign and malignant neoplasms that may be
multiple.   The most common rat tumors are pituitary and
mammary neoplasms (Cohen and Anver, 1976; Anver and Cohen,
1979).

   Berg's (1967) paper remains the definitive study of
age-associated, nonneoplastic lesions of the SD rat.

Anver and Cohen (1979) have more recently reviewed age-associated, nonneoplastic lesions in a variety of stocks and strains. Coleman et al. (1977) have characterized age-associated lesions in virgin male F344 rats. The pathology of aging BN/Bi, WAG/Rij, and (WAG x BN)F$_1$ rats has been described in detail by Burek (1978). Altman and Goodman (1979) have reviewed neoplasms in various stocks and strains. The histopathology of rat tumors has been described by Tursov (1973, 1976).

Numerous age-associated lesions can produce marked clinical and experimental effects. Advanced renal disease and malignant neoplasms, in addition to being life-threatening, result in alterations of biochemical, hematological, and other parameters. Benign mammary tumors may become large and ulcerated, which may necessitate surgical removal or euthanasia of rats for humane reasons. Neoplasms of endocrine glands, such as the adrenal cortex and medulla, pituitary, pancreatic islets, and thyroid C cells, can secrete active hormones that markedly alter homeostasis. Nerve degeneration in the central nervous system is reflected by alterations in peripheral nerve and organ function. Therefore, unlike their younger counterparts in which homeostatic mechanisms are optimal, old rats have deficiencies or derangements of many systems. These abnormalities must be recognized and accounted for when experimental results are interpreted.

Renal Disease Chronic renal disease is the most significant cause of morbidity and mortality in many rat stocks and strains. According to Gray (1977), renal disease has its greatest prevalence in populations of male rats more than 12 months of age and, hence, is a major complication of using rats in gerontologic research. Female rats also develop renal disease, but onset is later, prevalence lower, and lesions often less extensive. Sequelae of chronic renal disease are proteinuria, changes in serum proteins, hypercholesterolemia, hypertension, decreased glomerular filtration rate, azotemia, elevated serum creatinine, secondary renal hyperparathyroidism, fibrous osteodystrophy, ascites, hydrothorax, polydypsia, polyuria, and eventually, death. The most severe sequelae of renal disease occur in rats older than 24 months (Berg, 1967; Gray, 1977; Anver and Cohen, 1979).

Progressive renal disease occurs in SD (Foley et al., 1964; Berg, 1967; Cohen et al., 1978), F344 (Coleman et al., 1977), WI (Hirokawa, 1975), and many other rat stocks (Anver and Cohen, 1979). The disease is essentially

identical in all of these stocks, and maximum prevalence
may reach 60-100 percent. Mild or focal kidney lesions
not leading to clinical disease have been described in
WAG/Rij (WI-derived) and BN/Bi in the Netherlands (Burek,
1978) and Osborne-Mendel (OM) and Buffalo (BUF) rats at
the National Cancer Institute (Snell, 1967). The history,
morphology, and theories concerning pathogenesis and etiology of rat renal disease have been extensively reviewed
by Gray (1977).

Cardiovascular Lesions Myocardial degeneration, atrophy,
and fibrosis occur in stocks of barrier-reared and conventional, but not germfree, rats (Pollard and Kajima, 1970;
Anver and Cohen, 1979). In SD rats, prevalence is higher
and onset earlier in males than females. Onset of the
lesion in males is usually after 12 months of age. Maximum prevalence in both sexes can be as high as 60-80 percent (Berg, 1967). In the F344 rat, myocardial lesions
appear to be secondary to an inflammatory lesion of rats
less than 4-6 months of age, chronic interstitial myocar-
ditis. Prevalence of myocardial lesions in aged male
F344 rats is comparable to that in SD animals (Coleman
et al., 1977; Cohen et al., 1978), and the lesions are
generally not life-threatening.
    Polyarteritis nodosa (PAN) is an inflammatory lesion
of muscular arteries, principally in the pancreas, mesen-
tery, and testicle. Inflammation may be acute or chronic
with sequelae of thrombosis, infarction of tissue supplied by the affected artery, and/or hemorrhage due to
rupture of aneurysms (Anver and Cohen, 1979). The reported prevalence of PAN in the SD rat varies. Berg
(1967) has found a prevalence of 60 percent in SD males
at 29.6 months (900 days); Yang (1965) reports 14-17
percent in both sexes at an average age of 23 months
(699 days). The prevalence of PAN is greater in outbred
SD than in inbred F344 virgin males (Coleman et al.,
1977) and in more intensively bred than in seldom-bred
or virgin animals (Wexler, 1970).

Radiculoneuropathy Spinal cord and nerve root degeneration have a late onset. In SD rats, the lesions are most
extensive in animals over 24 months of age; prevalence
ranges from 75 to 96 percent. A study by Berg et al.,
(1962) describes lesions that develop earlier in males
(mean age, 16.4 months) than in females (mean age, 23
months). Gilmore (1972), on the other hand, has not observed a sex difference.

Clinical motor disfunction, posterior paresis, posterior paralysis and atrophy, and degeneration of skeletal muscles of the hind quarters have been correlated with nerve root lesions of demyelination, axonal degeneration, and malacia (Burek et al., 1976). Other investigators (Berg et al., 1962; Gilmore, 1972) maintain that CNS lesions are clinically silent and unrelated to skeletal muscle changes. The prevalence of radiculoneuropathy in F344 rats is not known. The condition has been seen in strains other than SD as reviewed by Anver and Cohen (1979).

Skeletal Muscle Degeneration and Atrophy This condition, which affects the muscles of the hind quarters, has an onset time similar to that of radiculoneuropathy (approximately 24 months). Microscopically, muscle fiber diameter decreases; there is sarcolemmal nuclear proliferation; and, in the later stages, there is degeneration and fragmentation of the sarcoplasm and eventual loss of the myofiber (van Steenis and Kroes, 1971). This condition has been described in SD rats (Berg et al., 1962) and associated with clinical signs in other strains (van Steenis and Kroes, 1971). Muscle lesions are not a problem in F344 rats.

Neoplasia Neoplasms in rats can be derived from all germ layers; mixed tumors, such as mammary fibroadenoma and nephroblastoma, are not uncommon. There appears to be minimal difference between barrier-reared and conventional animals in tumor development (Paget and Lemon, 1965), provided conventional animals do not die of intercurrent disease at an early age. Cancer also appears in germfree rats, although incidences vary (Pollard and Kajima, 1970; Sacksteder, 1976). Other than renal disease, neoplasia often is the main reason that rats older than 24 months are presented for necropsy (Paget and Lemon, 1965; Boorman and Hollander, 1973)

Almost the entire spectrum of rat neoplasia has been described in SD (Davis et al., 1956; Thompson et al., 1961; Durbin et al., 1966; Schardein et al., 1968, Cohen et al., 1978) and F344 rats (Jacobs and Huseby, 1967; Sacksteder, 1976; Sass et al., 1975; Coleman et al., 1977). Although many tumors are similar, prevalence between outbred SD and inbred F344 animals varies as discussed by Cohen et al. (1978). For example, mononuclear cell leukemias and testicular interstitial cell tumors are more common in F344 rats, while SD animals have a

greater prevalence of adrenal and pancreatic endocrine
neoplasms. SD and F344 animals have a similar prevalence
of pituitary tumors. Sacksteder (1976) reports a lower
prevalence of "solid tumors" in germfree F344 males as
compared to conventional animals. Certain tumors of the
endocrine glands may produce physiological alterations
due to hormone secretion, e.g., pancreatic islet cell
tumors (insulin), pituitary chromophobe adenomas (prolactin), and medullary thyroid tumors (calcitonin).

Availability

Outbred SF, LE, and WI and inbred F344 rats are available
as young animals or as retired breeders (9-12 months old)
from a variety of commercial sources in the United States.
These animals may be reared under conventional or barrier
systems, and investigators should determine the microbiological status of their animals prior to experimental use.
A very limited number of commercial suppliers sell aged
(18- to 24-month-old) SD, F344, and LE rats. The breeding
and microbiological status of these rats varies. In addition, a number of stocks and strains of aged rats are kept
in individual investigator colonies at various institutions throughout the United States and in Europe. Acquisition of such rats must be negotiated on an individual
basis.

Aged rats from the National Institute on Aging (NIA)
are available to NIA grantees, and under special circumstances, to investigators wishing to do pilot projects.
To obtain these rats, application should be made to:
Chief, Biophysiology and Pathobiology Aging Program, Biomedical Research and Clinical Medicine, National Institute
on Aging, Building 31, Room 5C35, National Institutes of
Health, Bethesda, MD 20205.

Information concerning suppliers of aged rats may be
obtained from the Institute of Laboratory Animal Resources, National Academy of Sciences, 2101 Constitution
Avenue, N.W., Washington, D.C. 20418.

Factors Affecting Stock Characteristics

Infectious Diseases

Mycoplasmosis Murine respiratory mycoplasmosis, a chronic
disease caused by the highly contagious Mycoplasma pulmonis, is the most common and devastating infectious disease
of rats. It can involve any portion of the respiratory
tract from the nares to the lungs and may also extend to
the tympanic bulla via the eustachian tube. In addition,
there is a genital (uterine) form of mycoplasmosis. At
the end stages of the disease, chronic suppurative inflammatory lesions are seen in the upper respiratory tract,
eustachian tube, and middle and inner ears (Kohn, 1971;
Lindsey et al., 1971, 1978). Environmental ammonia from
urine and feces contributes to the pathogenesis of lower
respiratory infections, leading to the development of bron-
chiectasis, chronic pulmonary abscesses, and pneumonia
(Broderson et al., 1976). Antibiotic therapy may amelior-
ate clinical signs but will not eliminate the infection in
sick animals or in asymptomatic carriers.

Mycoplasmosis is the disease that most complicates the
use of rats in gerontologic research (Lindsey et al.,
1971), and because it significantly shortens life span
(Paget and Lemon, 1965; Cohen, 1968; Lindsey et al., 1971;
Burek and Hollander, 1980) it is considered the most
serious problem in chronic rodent studies (NCI, 1973).

Other Infections Many other pathogenic organisms can produce clinical disease with variable morbidity and mortality. An animal may be asymptomatic, when not under an
experimental stress such as irradiation or immunosuppres-
sion, even though it carries such organisms as Corynebacterium kutscheri (pneumonia), Bacillus piliformis (necro-
tizing hepatitis and enteritis), Pseudomonas aeruginosa
(otitis media, otitis interna, abscesses, and meningitis),
and the unclassified Pneumocystis carinii (pneumonia). All
but the latter are bacterial pathogens (Flynn, 1963; Giddens et al., 1968; Jonas et al., 1970, ILAR, 1971). Infectious diseases and parasites and their effects on the rat
host have been reviewed in a number of publications (Cotchin and Roe, 1967; ILAR, 1971; Flynn, 1973; Baker et al.,
1979).

Prevention of Infectious Disease The practices of cesar-
ian derivation, barrier rearing, and barrier maintenance
of rat stocks have done much to eliminate mycoplasmosis

(Weisbroth, 1972) and to keep rats free of other agents
as well. It is more difficult to exclude viruses than
bacteria or parasites from barrier systems. Many rats
that are barrier reared and maintained have serologic
evidence of virus infection, most commonly, Sendai virus,
rat coronavirus, and PVM (pneumonia virus of mice) (Coleman et al., 1977; Burek, 1978). These infections are
transient or subclinical and have no overt effects on
life span.

Nutrition

The mortality statistics of rats and the age of onset of
disease can be greatly modified by nutritional influences
(Barrows and Roeder, 1977; B. J. Cohen, 1979). These influences include the total caloric intake, the amounts of
carbohydrate and protein consumed, and the temporal pattern of intake.

F344 Rats   A study on male rats carried out at the University of Texas Health Science Center at San Antonio (Yu et
al., In press) has revealed a 23.4-month (711-day) median
length of life for ad libitum-fed rats and a 34.4-month
(1046-day) median life span for rats fed the same diet at
60 percent ad libitum intake. The major diseases in these
rats are chronic nephropathy and testicular interstitial
cell tumors. The occurrence of both types of lesion is
much later in food-restricted rats.
    Nutrition may also account for the differences in mor-
tality and body weights between the male F344 rats fed ad
libitum at the Charles River Breeding Laboratories, Wilmington, Massachusetts (median length of life 29 months;
mean maximum body weight 454 g) (Coleman et al., 1977)
and those transferred from Charles River at 4 weeks of
age to San Antonio (median length of life 23.4 months;
mean maximum body weight 569 g). All aspects of the
maintenance are the same in these two studies (temperature, barrier facility, acidified drinking water, etc.),
except for the number of rats housed per cage and the
nature of the diet. Charles River animals are housed
5 per cage until 6 months of age and 3 per cage thereafter; San Antonio animals are housed 1 per cage throughout their life span. Charles River rats are fed the
Charles River 4RF Rat-Mouse Diet, which is a pasteurized
diet containing a minimum of 26 percent protein and 5
percent fat and a maximum of 5 percent fiber. San Antonio
rats are fed a nonpasteurized, semisynthetic diet composed

of 21 percent casein (vitamin-free), 15 percent sucrose, 10 percent corn oil, 3 percent Solka-Floc, 46.65 percent dextrin, 0.15 percent DL-methionine, 2 percent Ralston-Purina vitamin mix, 0.2 percent choline chloride, and 5 percent Ralston-Purina salt mix. Although further work is necessary to establish unequivocally whether the life span differences relate to the number of rats per cage or to the diet, the work of Berg (1960) and Berg and Simms (1960) on SD rats indicates that the number of rats per cage probably is not the important factor.

SD Rats   Berg and Simms (1960) have reported that restricting the food intake of male SD rats to 67 or 54 percent of the ad libitum intake markedly extends longevity. In addition, the rats on restricted food intake have a much lower incidence of cardiac, renal, and vascular lesions at 26.3 months (800 days) of age than rats fed ad libitum. Nolen (1972) has studied the effects of food restriction in both male and female SD rats (Table 8). The food-restricted rats have a longer life span and the onset of various diseases appears later in life. In a study restricting the access to food each day to a single, 2-hour period, male SD rats consumed 75 to 80 percent of the amount eaten by ad libitum-fed rats (Leveille, 1972). The mean length of life of the rats with limited access to food was 22.6 months (688 days), compared to 19.3 months (587 days) for the rats fed ad libitum.

Ross and his colleagues have reported on the effects of various, lifelong dietary regimens upon the life span of male SD rats. Restriction of intake has a life-extending effect. Restricting the intake of the protein component only (in diets allotted on an isocaloric basis) has little effect on life span, while restricting intake of carbohydrates, with simultaneous restriction of caloric intake, does enhance life expectancy (Ross, 1961). Restricting the intake both of protein and carbohydrates, with simultaneous restriction of caloric intake, enhances life expectancy to the greatest degree.

In another study (Ross and Bras, 1973), the life expectancy of male SD rats increases as the percent protein in an ad libitum-fed diet increases from 10 to 51 percent. Restriction of intake, in addition to variation of the protein content, also increases the length of life. The influence of the level of protein intake on the risk of incurring spontaneous tumors depends on the tissue of origin and the type and malignancy of the tumor. There

TABLE 8   Effect of Food Restriction Regimens on Life Span of SD Rats[a]

Group	Diet Regimen	Mean Survival Time for Males in Months (days)	Mean Survival Time for Females in Months (days)
1	ad libitum	23.2 (706)	24.9 (756)
2	80% ad libitum postweaning	28.1 (856)	28.7 (872)
3	60% ad libitum postweaning	30.4 (924)	28.7 (872)
4	ad libitum for 12 weeks post-weaning: 80% ad libitum thereafter	26.3 (801)	28.6 (871)
5	ad libitum for 12 weeks post-weaning; 60% ad libitum thereafter	30.5 (927)	31.0 (943)
6	80% ad libitum for 12 weeks postweaning; ad libitum thereafter	23.8 (723)	25.9 (788)
7	60% ad libitum for 12 weeks postweaning; ad libitum thereafter	25.7 (782)	26.5 (805)

[a]From Nolen, 1972.

is a remarkable reduction in the age-associated progression of renal lesions in male SD rats when intake of protein, carbohydrate, or calories is restricted, the greatest effect occurring when carbohydrate intake is restricted, regardless of the level of protein intake (Bras and Ross, 1964). This reduction in renal lesions is directly correlated with the life-prolonging effects of the diets.

In a freedom-of-choice mode of feeding, the protein content of the diet that a rat elects to consume early in life correlates highly with longevity (Ross and Bras, 1975; Ross et al., 1976). When the same choices are made after midlife, the amount of protein the rat consumes is inversely correlated with life span.

Other Stocks   WI rats have also been used for studies on nutrition and aging (Barrows and Roeder, 1965; Barrows and Kokkonen, 1975; Stuchlikova et al., 1975). LE rats have not been extensively used for studies in this area; however, the work of Segall and Timiras (1975) on tryptophan-deficiency suggests that these rats are suitable models.

The Rat as a Model for Human Nutrition and Aging   To study the effects of nutrition on the biology of aging, it is desirable that no single disease be a dominant factor in the life and death of animals of the stock under study, because nutritional manipulation may exert its effects by influencing the disease process rather than aging per se. For example, renal lesions are a dominant factor in many aging rat stocks, a major disadvantage of using these animals in nutrition studies. In addition, the rat should grow during the first 20 to 25 percent of its life span, after which lean body mass should decline slowly with increasing age. No rat stock currently available has this characteristic. Further, there should be no marked differences in body mass between rats of the same age, fed identical diets ad libitum. Unfortunately, both F344 and SD rats show large differences in body weight among individuals of the same age in the same environment (R. C. Adelman, Temple University, Institute on Aging, Philadelphia, Unpublished; Masoro, In press).

Marked adiposity, unless being specifically studied, should not be present in stocks being used for the study of nutrition and aging. The F344 male rat is relatively lean, with a mean fat content of 14.8 (range 8.2 to 18.2) percent at 20 months of age (Masoro, In press). The SD rat, on the other hand, tends to become obese in old age,

with a mean fat content of 24 (range 13.2 to 30.2) percent
at 24 months of age (Lesser et al., 1973).

Other Environmental Factors

A rat's macro- and microenvironment can influence its
physiological, biochemical, and behavioral status, and
this influence is even more pronounced when rats are held
for long periods of time. Experimental data in gerontological research will be more uniform if the temperature,
humidity, room noise level, ventilation (both in the room
and within the cage), and light duration and intensity
are controlled. For example, toxicity patterns of drugs
may be affected by cage temperature, the lowest toxicity
occurring at thermal neutrality (Weihe, 1973). Light
levels of 50- to 100-foot candles at the cage level cause
retinal degeneration that becomes more severe with age
(O'Steen et al., 1974). Details of the effects of these
factors on rats and the optimal methods of control have
been well reviewed (ILAR, 1976c; Lindsey et al., 1978).
   Other environmental factors can produce great variability in studies on drug metabolism, drug response, and organ function even in reliably characterized stocks and
strains. Examples of such factors are types of bedding
used, cleanliness of the environment, and concentration
of chemicals in the animal environment. Hepatic microsomal enzyme activity can be increased by aromatic hydro-
carbons in cedar bedding or chlorinated-hydrocarbon in-
secticides used to control vermin in animal rooms, whereas
ammonia generated from urine and feces in unchanged pans
can inhibit hepatic microsomal activity (as well as
exacerbating mycoplasmosis). Failure to control these
environmental factors can make experimental results difficult to interpret within or between laboratories even
if a genetically uniform rat is used (Vessell et al.,
1976).

Housing   Rats are gregarious animals and live in colonies
under natural conditions (Lorenz, 1963). Many physiological and behavioral responses in this species are influenced by whether rats are individually or group-housed
in the laboratory. There are variations in plasma cortisol levels, immune responsiveness, temperament, and life
expectancy between rats housed in isolation, small groups,
or large, crowded groups. It is, therefore, important
to specify the type of housing used when reporting

experimental results with rat subjects. Although it is difficult to generalize about such a wide range of parameters, rats housed in small groups seem to come closer to the physiological norm than animals that are crowded or kept in isolation (Lindsey, et al., 1978).

During life span studies, a certain percentage of rats will be lost due to death and autolysis or cannibalism before an adequate necropsy can be performed. They represent a complication of group-housing that leads to loss of valuable data in gerontological research (Burek and Hollander, 1980).

Sex Sex differences in longevity of certain rat stocks have been observed. For example, it is generally accepted that female SD rats have a longer life expectancy than males (Simms, 1967; Wexler, 1970; Hoffman, 1979). Barrier-reared WI-origin rats (Alderly Park Strain 1) show little difference in longevity between virgin males and females except for a prolongation of life of those females surviving to the 85th percentile of life span (Paget and Lemon, 1965; Hoffman, 1979). Other studies on WI-derived animals (WAG/Rij) show that virgin males have a significantly shorter life expectancy than virgin females (Burek, 1978). Among F344 rats, the male is not at a survival disadvantage relative to the female until after 30 months of age (Hoffman, 1979). LE males and females have a similar median survival age, but females survive longer after the 50 percent mortality age is reached (Hoffman, 1979). Mortality statistics of laboratory rats have been reviewed extensively by Hoffman (1979).

Brain Aging

A major control problem in using rats for research on brain aging is that of infectious and/or advanced disease processes. Disease may be manifested in widespread brain deterioration in aging rats, thereby suggesting that such widespread changes are normal concomitants of aging. In fact, when healthy, aged rats (barrier-maintained) are studied, there appear, at least in some cases, to be only limited and highly specific alterations in brain function, even in animals approaching the age of median longevity for the stock (e.g., Landfield et al., 1978b). Since early and discrete changes with aging are of interest in analyzing etiological phenomena, avoiding the extensive brain deterioration associated with systemic disease may

be of considerable importance. However, since methods
for controlling against infectious disease (e.g., use of
barrier-protected colonies, pathology and bacteriology
analyses) have already been described at some length,
they will not be considered again here. Only those methodological problems that are specific to research on the
aging brain will be reviewed below.

Neurochemical Research

Two major control problems particularly relevant to the
large majority of neurochemical studies of aging rat
brains are:

● the established loss of neural elements (cells,
synapses, fibers) and
● altered brain composition, in particular, the increase in glial elements (see Table 9).

If a change in the concentration of a neuronal component (e.g., receptor, transmitter, etc.) in a whole brain
or in brain regions is found, there may be some confusion
as to whether this change reflects an altered level of
metabolism or synthesis within individual neurons, or
whether it simply indicates an overall loss of neuronal
elements (e.g., synapses). Our increased understanding
of brain aging may depend upon the interpretation given
to the results. Expressing these changes per mg of DNA
or protein is not as useful as it is in neurochemical
studies on nonaging brains, since synaptic loss may
cause undetectable changes in overall weight and since
the increase in glial cells and their size affects DNA
and protein. Additionally, observed changes in brain
chemistry or metabolism may not reflect altered functions within individual neurons, but may instead reflect
the increased ratio of glial-to-neuronal elements. Independent chemical or morphological measures of the relative
composition of the brain tissue under study (e.g., synaptic or cell volume counts, measurements of glial marker
enzymes, etc.), or the fractionation of neural and glial
elements, are of some use in controlling for these difficult problems, but require major research efforts in
themselves.

A major problem in studying the distribution or uptake
of metabolic precursors administered to aging animals may
be the reported age-dependent decline of extracellular

brain space (e.g., Bondareff and Narotzky, 1972), which
may arise from astroglial hypertrophy (e.g., Landfield
et al., 1977, 1978a; Lindsey et al., 1979). Further,
altered vascular and blood-brain barrier factors can substantially affect precursor distribution and uptake
(Appel, 1974).

Neuromorphological Research

Several major considerations relevant to most neuromorphological studies of the aging brain are:

● age-related changes in the volume and size of neural
elements (Table 9) and
● differences in the susceptibility of aging tissue
to artifacts of preparation and/or staining procedures
(Table 9). By comparing two methods (e.g., electron
microscopy and specialized light microscopic staining)
that employ substantially different preparation procedures, many, but not all, of these problems can be
controlled.

Studies counting the density of cells or synapses must
take into account the possibility of greater shrinkage or
swelling of aged tissue. Age-dependent size differences
in brain elements may affect the numbers obtained when
using selected slides. Abercrombie's (1946) correction
for nuclear size differences is sometimes employed in
studies of cell counts using tissue from animals of
different ages (e.g., Brizzee et al., 1968; Ling and Le-
Blond, 1973). Independent measures of structure, volume,
or area are also particularly important in density counts
(cf., Brody, 1976; Brody and Vijayashankar, 1977; Geinisman et al., 1977; Landfield et al., 1979).

Neurophysiological Research

Although neurophysiological studies of the aging rat
brain have not been as common as morphological or chemical studies, some specific control problems are:

● the loss of cells or synapses;
● altered intra- or extracellular ionic concentrations arising from endocrine, kidney, or vascular diseases; and

TABLE 9 Brain Changes During Aging

Age Change	F344	SD	LE	WI and Others
Nerve cell loss	Reduced density of hippocampal pyramidal cells (Ordy and Brizzee, 1977; Landfield et al., 1977) No loss in dentate gyrus (Geinisman et al., 1977)	Reduced density in neocortex, by 18 mo. (Brizzee, 1973)	No major loss in neocortex (Brizzee et al., 1968)	
Brain volume changes	Tendency to increased hippocampal depth (Lindsey et al., 1979) No change in depth of dentate gyrus (Geinisman et al., 1977)		Decrease in neocortical depth, increase in hippocampal depth (Diamond et al., 1975)	
Neuronal size-- cytoplasmic changes	Reduced hippocampal nuclear size (P.W. Landfield, Department of Physiology and Pharmacology, Bowman Gray School of Medicine, Winston-Salem, North Carolina, Unpublished)	Decreased perikaryal volume in cortex (Feldman, 1976) Decreased perikaryar size in auditory cortex (Vaughan, 1977)		Reduced nuclear volume in hypothalamic cells (Lin et al., 1976) WI--Dispersed endoplasmic reticulum (Hasan and Glees, 1973)

Increased size of olfactory bulb mitral cells (Hinds and McNelly, 1977)

Lipofuscin accumulation

Progressive accumulation in hippocampal pyramids, particularly at base of apical dendrites (Landfield et al., 1978c)

WI--Extensive in Purkinje, hippocampal and cortical cells; low in cerebellar granule cells (Reichel et al., 1968)

Holtzman--Progressive accumulation in cortical neurons, particularly at base of apical dendrites (Brizzee et al., 1969)

Neurofibrillary tangles and amyloidosis--not yet reported in any rat strain or stock

TABLE 9 (continued)

Age Change	F344	SD	LE	WI and Others
Synaptic deterioration	Decreased synaptic terminals and dendritic volume in dentate gyrus (Geinisman et al., 1977, 1978a) Apparent degenerating terminals and synaptic elements in hippocampus (Landfield, 1978; Landfield et al., 1978c) Reduced synaptic vesicles in hippocampus (Landfield et al., 1979)	Apparent phagocytosis of axon terminals by microglia in cortex (Vaughan and Peters, 1974b)	Dendritic atrophy and loss of spines in cortex (Feldman, 1976) Dendritic atrophy and loss of spines in olfactory bulb (Hinds and McNelly, 1977) Dendritic atrophy and loss of spines in auditory cortex (Vaughan, 1977)	Degenerating terminals in motor nerve (Fujisawa, 1976) WI--Reduced density of axodendritic synapses in hippocampus; increased dendrodendritic synapses--qualitative observations (Hasan and Glees, 1973).
Neuroglial cells	Hypertrophy but not increased numbers of astrocytes in hippocampus and caudate nucleus, mild hypertrophy in neocortex (Landfield, et al.,	No increase in astrocyte numbers or size in cortex; increased filaments and inclusions (Vaughan and Peters, 1974b)	Increased glial-to-neuronal ratios in cortex (Brizzee et al., 1968)	WI--Increased oligodendrocyte satellitosis in hippocampus; glial inclusions; no change in astrocytes--qualitative obser-

1977, 1978a,c; Lindsey et al., 1979; Geinisman et al., 1978b)

Increased filaments and inclusions in astrocytes; increased numbers of microglia in hippocampus (Landfield, 1978; Landfield et al., 1978c)

Increased glial-to-neuronal ratios in cortex (Brizzee, 1973)

Increased inclusions and numbers of microglia in cortex; transformation "gitter" cells; increased oligodendrocyte satellitosis; but no increase in numbers (Vaughan and Peters, 1974b)

vations (Hasan and Glees, 1973)

Neurotransmitters, related enzymes and receptors

Reduced cAMP response to norepinephrine (NE) in cortical slices (Berg and Zimmerman, 1975)

Reduced density of β-adrenergic receptors in pineal, neostriatum and cerebellum (Greenberg and Weiss, 1978)

Decreased cAMP in neostriatum and cerebellum (Walker and Boas-Walker, 1973; Puri and Volicer, 1977)

Reduced hypothalamic content of catecholamines (Miller and Riegle, 1975)

Decreased spinal cord ChAT activity (Timiras, 1972)

Decreased glutamate, glycine, and taurine in spinal cord, but not in cortex (Timiras et al., 1973)

WI--Reduced catecholamine levels and metabolism in caudate nucleus and hypothalamus (Simpkins et al., 1977)

WI--Reduced levels of striatal dopamine (DA) and DA receptors (Joseph et al., 1978)

TABLE 9 (continued)

Age change	F344	SD	LE	WI and others
				WI--Reduced cAMP response to NE in cerebellar slices (Schmidt and Thornberry, 1978)
				Decreased AChe in forebrain (Hollander and Barrows, 1968); in cerebral cortex (Moudgil and Kanungo, 1973)
				WI--Possibly impaired preoptic dopamine functions (Clemens and Bennett, 1977)
				WI--Reduced tyrosine hydroxylases ChAT and AChE in neostriatum (McGeer et al., 1971)

| Neurochemistry (macromolecules, lipids) | Lipids stable with age, myelin increases (Rouser et al., 1972; Norton and Poduslo, 1973) | Decreased neuronal concentrations of RNA (Wulff et al., 1963)
No brain changes in DNA, RNA, protein, or Na-K ATPase (Hollander and Barrows, 1968)
Decreased thermal lability of brain DNA-protein complex (Zs-Nagy and Zs-Nagy, 1975)
Reduced uptake of labeled amino acids by neural tissues (Jakoubek et al., 1968; Ford and Rhines, 1969) |

TABLE 9 (continued)

Age Change	F344	SE	LE	WI and Others
Cerebral metabolism	Cerebral blood flow normal at rest, but reduced adaptability when challenged (Haining et al., 1970)	Reduced oxidative metabolism of glucose in cortical slices; reduced activity of some mitochondrial enzymes (Patel, 1977) Altered oxidative metabolism when demand is high (Sylvia and Rosenthal, 1979)		Reduced oxygen consumption by brain homogenates (Peng et al., 1977)
Neuro-physiology	Impaired monosynaptic potentiation in hippocampus during repetitive stimulation, in vivo and in vitro; many other responses, including antidromic, are normal (Landfield and Lynch, 1977; Landfield et al., 1978b; Landfield, 1979)	No reduction of conduction velocity or refractory period in sciatic nerve (Birren and Wall, 1956) Reduced long-term potentiation and field potential amplitude in dentate gyrus (Barnes, 1979)		Reduced frequency of spontaneous release of transmitter quanta at neuromuscular junction (Vyskocil and Guttmann, 1972) Increased spinal synaptic delay; reduced conduction velocity in efferent, but not afferent, nerves (Wayner and Emmers, 1958)

• possible differential responses of aged brain tissue
to anesthetics (during acute experiments), either because
of changes in liver, adipose tissue, or neuronal sensitivity or the distribution and uptake factors noted above.

It is particularly important to monitor and control
body temperature during acute neurophysiological experiments employing anesthesia (e.g., Landfield, In press).
The regulation of body temperature is generally impaired
in aging mammals (Finch et al., 1969), and the animal
cannot compensate for the drop in temperature often accompanying anesthesia. Brain temperature is of course an
important factor in controlling neural activity.

Comparison of in vitro and in vivo neurophysiological
preparations (e.g., Landfield and Lynch, 1977; Landfield
et al., 1978b) is useful in dealing with many of these
problems. In vitro the extracellular ionic environment
can be held relatively constant and the use of anesthesia
can be avoided. In vivo preparations of the same system
are also necessary to guard against increased susceptibility of aged neural tissue to damage from in vitro
techniques, as well as against results specific to in
vitro preparations.

The loss of brain cells or synapses may be a major
factor in the interpretation of many neurophysiological
results (e.g., reduced amplitudes of evoked field potentials, EEG amplitudes, altered thresholds, etc.). It is
important to determine whether a physiological change reflects altered dynamics of individual cell function or
whether it is simply an indicant of cell or synaptic
loss. To compensate for effects due to cell loss, it is
often possible to adopt an experimental design in which
the animal is employed as its own control. In many cases,
single cell recording can provide direct solutions to
these problems (for a review see Landfield, In press).

Comparison of Human and Rat Brain Aging Patterns

Changes in the rat brain with age resemble those in the
human brain in several respects, including the presence
of apparent deterioration of both pre- and postsynaptic
elements, reactive glial changes, and probable decrements
in the size of some neurons. The topography of deterioration is similar in both species, affecting particularly
the hippocampus, neocortex, caudate nucleus, and catecholaminergic brain stem nuclei (Brody, 1976; Tomlinson and

Henderson, 1976; Ball, 1978). There is also a pattern of lipofuscin accumulation and a loss of neocortical granule cells in humans (Brody, 1973), which are consistent with observations in rats (Table 9).

Neurochemically, there appears to be an age-related change in macromolecular synthesis in both humans and rats, but data are sparse and technical problems considerable (Appel, 1974). Preliminary evidence suggests that there also may be an analogous shift in brain fatty acid composition (Rouser et al., 1972; Horrocks et al., 1975) and alterations in cerebral metabolism (Obrist, 1972; Toole and Sulkin, 1974). This latter effect, however, is far more notable in humans with senile dementia (Ingvar et al., 1975).

Unlike the human (Tomlinson and Henderson, 1976; Ball, 1978), the rat apparently does not show granulovacuolar degeneration of hippocampal neurons, extracellular amyloid, or neurofibrillary tangles (Table 9). Lack of these phenomena does not seem to seriously impair the usefulness of the rat as a model, however, since amyloid and neurofibrillary tangles do not appear to be critical to the etiology of synaptic deterioration and glial reactivity in humans and nonhuman primates (Wisniewski and Terry, 1973, 1976). Large clusters of degenerating neurites (e.g., human plaques) have not yet been observed ultrastructurally in rats, although clusters of reactive astroglia in synaptic terminal fields have been observed (Landfield et al., 1977, 1978a; Lindsey et al., 1979). Age-related changes in myelin also appear dissimilar, and the question of whether there is a decrease in the brain weight of rats is still unclear.

The amplitude of large, scalp-recorded electrical waves (EEG, EPs) declines with age in humans, particularly in humans with senile dementia (Obrist, 1972; Feinberg et al., 1967; Thompson et al., 1978). Although EEG age changes in rats have not been extensively studied, synaptic deficits in the brain neurophysiology of aging rats have been noted during repetitive stimulation at frequency ranges similar to EEG rhythms (Table 9). Such stimulation elicits synchronized patterns of unit firing which are partly analogous to the single cell firing patterns seen during rhythmic EEG activity.

Conclusions

Several rat stocks appear to exhibit patterns of brain
aging that are qualitatively similar, in many fundamental
aspects, to human and to general mammalian patterns of
age-related synaptic, glial, lipofuscin, and nerve cell
changes. The present data indicate that F344, SD, LE,
and possibly other rat stocks may provide reasonable
models for the study of cell loss, glial changes, altered
synaptic elements, macromolecular and oxidative metabolic
alterations, and nuclear changes.

There also are areas in which the rat does not appear
to serve as a good model for brain aging in humans. For
example, myelin and certain specific patterns of degenerative changes that occur in the human brain during the
aging process do not seem to occur in the rat. Nonetheless, the general similarity between patterns of brain
changes seen in the rat and other mammalian species, suggests that the rat is a good model for the study of the
basic, underlying principles governing aging of the mammalian brain.

Cardiovascular Aging

Information is presented here on age-related structural,
physiological, and biochemical changes characteristic of
the cardiovascular system of rats and humans. Additionally, the suitability of rats as models for the study of
aging of the cardiovascular system is evaluated. The
literature cited in many instances represents original
work. However, recent reviews are also cited that bring
together much information and place in proper perspective
what is known and not known about cardiovascular aging.
Data have been retabulated for ease of comparison, and
information has been subdivided, where possible, on the
basis of rat stock and sex. No specific distinction has
been made between characteristics of "normal" aging and
diseases of old age since, in some instances, the diseases
may be considered a consequence of aging (e.g., increased
incidence of cardiac arrhythmias).

Several parameters of cardiovascular structure and
function have been characterized in both rats and humans,
and sufficient parallel information exists to show that,
particularly for cardiovascular function, the effects of
increasing age appear to be similar in both species.

Generally, decreases in heart rate, cardiac output, and contractility; increases in blood pressure; and altered cardiac electrical activity with increasing age have been observed in humans and in F344, SD, and WI rats. Studies have not been done using LE rats. The majority of work in the rat has been done using males; however, since in most human studies sex is not specified, there is not sufficient information to allow a comparison to be made by sex.

Structurally, the heart and vasculature of the rat undergo some age-related changes that are similar to, and others that are different from, changes in the human heart (Table 10). For example, left ventricular wall thickness increases both in humans and in rats (WI), whereas heart size decreases in humans and increases in rats (F344). Studies on fine structure are not sufficiently parallel for comparison. A comparison of age-related physiological changes is presented in Table 11.

Age-related changes in biochemical processes of rat cardiac tissue are summarized in Table 12. These data are difficult to evaluate because of differences in experimental approach and in data expression. On the whole, however, it can be seen that there is an age-related increase in protein content and metabolic enzyme activity during growth and maturation (e.g., myoglobin content and glucose phosphate isomerase activity in SD rats), whereas collagen content and lipid metabolism increase through senescence (e.g., microsomal cytochrome C reductase in SD rats). Such changes are consistent with some of the structural changes observed in rats (e.g., increased connective tissue in SD rats) and in humans (e.g., increased pericardial elastic fibers).

Biochemical parameters for humans have not been included in this study because of the vastness of the human literature and because the variation in experimental approaches to studying the rat would make adequate comparisons extremely difficult.

Advantages and Disadvantages of the Rat Model

Overall, rats appear to be good models of age-related changes in human cardiovascular physiology. The differences between F344, SD, and WI rats, particularly with respect to cardiac function, are minor and appear to be due to differences in experimental design rather than to some basic cellular mechanism. Since virgin F344, WI,

and SD rats generally do not develop arterio-athero-
sclerotic lesions spontaneously, whereas breeder rats do
(Table 10), the latter may be more suitable models for
studies of the interaction between age and such lesions
on cardiovascular function. In addition, spontaneously
hypertensive rats (SHR) or other rats on appropriate diets
may be more suitable for studies on hypertension and
arteriosclerosis.

Reproductive Aging

The rat and mouse have been the two most widely used models in the study of reproductive senescence. Some of the
salient features exhibited by aging female rats as they
come to the end of their reproductive life are as follows
(Huang and Meites, 1975; Meites et al., 1978). Between
8 and 15 months of life, irregularities first appear in
the estrous cycles, characterized by lengthening of the
cycle from 4 or 5 days to 6, 7, or more days, with prolonged periods of estrus or diestrus. Next there is a
constant estrous syndrome, characterized by the presence
of both cystic and well developed follicles, no corpora
lutea, and estrogen secretion similar to that of the
cycling rat. This constant estrous syndrome may last
for many months, and appears in the majority of aging
female rats. Prolonged pseudopregnancies of irregular
length (10 to 30 days or more in duration) usually follow, and many corpora lutea in the ovaries activity secrete high levels of progesterone. In rats 2 to 3 years
of age, the ovaries often become atrophic and the uterus
appears infantile. These anestrous rats secrete very
little estrogen or progesterone and many have pituitary
tumors.

The hypothalamo-pituitary system of aging female (and
male) rats shows a reduced capacity to secrete gonadotropins (LH and FSH) and an increased capacity to secrete
prolactin (Huang et al., 1976a; Meites et al., 1978).
Associated with these changes in pituitary function is a
decrease in hypothalamic catecholamines, an increase in
serotonin turnover, and a reduction in release of hypothalamic LHRH to the pituitary. Thus, the changes in
hypothalamo-pituitary function in aging female rats appear to be primarily responsible for the failure of the
ovaries to function normally (Meites et al., 1976, 1978).
Estrous cycles have been reinitiated in old female rats
by appropriate treatment with drugs acting on the central

Table 10 A Comparison of Age-Related Changes in Cardiovascular Structure of Humans and Rats

Structure	Human Data	Reference	Rat Data	References
Heart size or mass	Size of heart decreases; thickness of ventricular walls increases	Harris, 1975; Lakatta, 1978	F344--increased heart mass, but no change in ratio of heart mass to total body mass	Roberts and Goldberg, 1975
			WI--increase in heart mass and in ratio of left ventricular mass to total body mass;	Lakatta, 1978
			WI--left ventricular wall thickness increases or shows no change; left ventricular volume increases	Weisfeldt, 1975
Endocardium	Thickened whitish patches appear	Harris, 1975		
Heart valves	Become thickened and more rigid	Harris, 1975		
Other heart changes	Pericardial elastic fibers increase	Harris, 1975	SD--increase in myocardial lipofuscin pigmentation, connective tissue, and golgi structures; mitochondria accumulate in small, dense foci; vesicles and intercalated discs become dilated; myofibrils become irregular.	Tomanek and Karlsson, 1973

Vasculature	Progressive deterioration of intima and muscle wall	Timiras, 1972; Blumenthal, 1975	WI--increase in connective tissue;	Landowne and Stanley, 1960;
			WI--increase in mitochondrial rows between myofilaments; lysosomes associate and coalesce with mitochondria; increase in lipid droplets	Travis and Travis, 1972
	Small vessels decrease in number, become gnarled and tortuous	Landowne and Stanley, 1960	Unspecified--increase in small mitochondria;	Edington and Cosmas, 1972
			Unspecified--mitochondrial number decreases, but individual volume increases	Levkova and Trunov, 1970
			F344--males rarely show vascular lesions	Coleman et al., 1977
			SD, WI, LE, and Holtzman-- breeders develop more arteriosclerotic lesions than virgins regardless of sex	Wexler, 1964

Table 10 (continued)

Structure	Human Data	Reference	Rat Data	References
	Increased colla-gen/elastic ratio, calci-fication of media	Harris, 1975	WI--thickening of aortic intima and accumulation of debris within arterial wall	Laver-Rudich et al., 1978

TABLE 11 A Comparison of Age-Related Changes in Cardiovascular Function of Humans and Rats

Function	Human Data	Reference	Rat Data	Reference
Heart rate	Decreases from adult to old age; Fluctuates throughout life	Brandfonbrener et al., 1955; Montoye et al., 1971	F344--decreases in vivo (unanesthetized, re-strained males) and in vitro; pacemaker rates decrease in vitro. SD--decreases during rest and exercise in males between 1-18 mo. WI--increases in vivo in unanesthetized males 12-24 mo. WI--decreases in vivo in anesthetized, open-chest males 6-24 mo	Roberts and Goldberg, 1976; Goldberg, 1978; Goldberg and Roberts, 1978; Tomanek, 1970; Rothbaum et al., 1973; Lee et al., 1972
Cardiac output	Decreases from adult to old age	Brandfonbrener et al., 1955	WI--decreases in un-anesthetized males; WI--increases in anes-thetized, open-chest males	Rothbaum et al., 1973; Lee et al., 1972

TABLE 11 (continued)

Function	Human Data	Reference	Rat Data	Reference
Electrical activity	Increased duration of P-R interval, QRS complex, and S-T segment	Cheraskin and Ringsdorf, 1971; Golden and Golden, 1974; Shah et al., 1968; Sprague, 1954	F344--decreased amplitude, duration, overshoot, and plateau duration of action potential	Roberts and Goldberg, 1976; Goldberg, 1978; Goldberg and Roberts, 1978
	Increased incidence of arrhythmias	Golden and Golden, 1974	F344--atrial Na^+ increases, atrial K^+ decreases; atrial and vetricular Ca^{++} increases	Goldberg et al., 1975; Kendrick et al., 1978
			SD--cardiac muscle Na^+, K^+, Ca^{++}, Mg^{++}, and Cl^- decrease in females 1-35 mo	Mori and Duruisseau, 1960
Blood pressure	Increased systolic and diastolic pressures; increased peripheral resistance	Harris, 1975; Landowne and Stanley, 1960; Master and Lasser, 1961; Master et al., 1958	SD--decreases in unanesthetized males between 2 and 6 mo	Frangipane and Aporti, 1969
			WI--decreases in unanesthetized males between 12 and 24 mo	Rothbaum et al., 1973
			WI--increases in anesthetized males between 6 and 24 mo	Lee et al., 1972

		WI--increased in anesthetized rats between 1 and 13 mo	Vizek and Albrecht, 1973
Blood flow	Regional blood flow decreases to a lesser extent to brain and heart than to viscera and muscles	WI--aortic flow decreases	Lee et al., 1972; Rothbaum et al., 1973; Vizek and Albrecht, 1973
			Bender, 1965
Mechanical properties	Left ventricular work decreased	F344--contractility of isolated ventricular tissue decreases in male	Roberts and Goldberg, 1976; Goldberg, 1978; Goldberg and Roberts, 1978
		SD--ventricular mechanical properties decrease between 1 and 10 mo	Heller and Whitehorn, 1972
	(Harris, 1975)	WI--ventricular contractility decreases in vitro between 12 and 24 mo	Shreiner et al., 1969; Weisfeldt et al., 1971

TABLE 11 (continued)

Function	Human Data	Reference	Rat Data	Reference
Other functions	Cardiac reserve and response to stress decreases	Harris, 1975		
	Preejection period increases	Montoye et al., 1971		
	Ventricular ejection time increases	Willems et al., 1970		

TABLE 12   Age-Related Biochemical Changes of Rat Cardiac
Tissue

F344 (males, 1-28 mo)
ADP-stimulated mitochondrial respiration and ATP production decrease (Chen et al., 1972).
Dopa decarboxylase and monoamine oxidase activities increase; catechol-o-methyl transferase activity shows no
change (Thompson et al., 1974).
Na-K stimulated ATPase activity decreases (Kendrick et
al., 1978).
Norepinephrine uptake decreases (Thompson et al., 1974).
Catecholamine content decreases (Roberts and Goldberg,
1976).
Serotonin shows no change; histamine increases (Thompson
et al., 1974).

SD (males and females, 1 day-28 mo)
Glycogen phosphorylase, fructose diphosphate aldolase,
glucose phosphate isomerase, and succinate oxidase ac-
tivities are increased (Burleigh and Schimke, 1969).
Microsomal NADH cytochrome C reductase and -hydroxybuty-
rate dehydrogenase activities are increased (Grinna and
Barber, 1972).
Monoamine oxidase activity is increased (Horita, 1968).
Hexokinase activity is decreased (Burleigh and Schimke,
1969).
Lactic dehydrogenase activity is decreased (Porter et al.,
1971).
Myoglobin increases (Burleigh and Schimke, 1969).
Microsomal and mitochondrial phospholipids remain un-
changed (Grinna and Barber, 1972).
Phosphatidyl inositol, palmitate, and stearate decrease
(Glende and Cornatzer, 1966).
Proteolipid N-terminal and C-terminal amino acids present
(Whikehart and Lees, 1973).

WI (males and females, 1 day-27 mo)
Monoamine oxidase activity is increased (Callingham and
Della Corte, 1972).
NADH cytochrome C reductase activity is increased (Call-
ingham and Laverty, 1973).
Succinate dehydrogenase activity is increased (Rebel and
Stegmann, 1973).
Lactic dehydrogenase activity is decreased (Singh and
Kanungo, 1968).

TABLE 12 (continued)

Cytoplasmic malate dehydrogenase and mitochondrial malate
dehydrogenase activities are decreased (Singh, 1973).
Guanyl cyclase, c-GMP phosphodiesterase and adenylate
cyclase, and c-AMP phosphodiesterase activities are decreased (Williams and Thompson, 1973).
No change in mitochondrial oxidative phosphorylation (Gold
et al., 1968).
Collagen increases (von Knorring, 1970)
Protein decreases (Singh and Kanungo, 1968).

Holtzman (female, age unspecified)
Glutamine and tuarine increase, threonine and glycine decrease (Kuttner and Lorincz, 1969).

---

nervous system (CNS) (Quadri et al., 1973; Huang et al.,
1976b), and ovulation has been induced by electrical stimulation of the preoptic area of the hypothalamus (Clemens
et al., 1969; Clemens and Bennett, 1977).

Advantages of the Rat as a Model for Reproductive Aging

The endocrinology and neuroendocrinology of rats have been
more widely investigated than in any other species, with
the possible exception of humans. The estrous cycle of
the rat has many features in common with the menstrual
cycle of women. In both species the same hypothalamic decapeptide, LHRH, controls release of LH and FSH by the
pituitary. LH and FSH in rats and humans have similar
actions on the ovaries in producing development and growth
of follicles, ovulation, formation of corpora lutea, and
in the male, control of spermatogenesis and secretion of
testosterone by the testes. The negative and positive
feedback actions of the ovarian hormones, estrogen and
progesterone, on secretion of gonadotropins is similar in
both species, as are the effects of estrogen, progesterone, and testosterone on the reproductive tracts and on
other tissues.

There are several major differences between the cycles of female rats and women. The cycle is shorter in the rat than in women, and there is no bleeding (although there is desquamation of the epithelial lining in the uterus and vagina). In women there is no behavioral phenomenon comparable to "heat" seen in rats during the estrous phase of the cycle. In addition, the hormone, prolactin, is important for maintaining progesterone secretion by the corpora lutea of rats, whereas it appears to be of relatively minor importance in maintaining progesterone secretion by the ovaries of humans. However, there is recent evidence that prolactin may promote progesterone secretion by the corpus luteum of women under in vitro conditions. The positive feedback of estrogen (or estrogen and progesterone) on LH release that occurs normally prior to ovulation was first demonstrated in the rat and has since been confirmed in primates and other mammals. In addition, the negative feedback by estrogen and progesterone on LH and FSH secretion appears to be similar in rats and humans.

The irregular cycles exhibited by female rats approaching the end of their fertility period resemble the irregular menstrual cycles of women during the 2 or 3 years premenopause. In both species, there is a tendency for follicular cysts to develop during this period, and ovulations become fewer. Both species may show a reduction in progesterone and estrogen secretion.

Another advantage of the female rat is that it remains polyestrous during the entire year under good laboratory conditions, has a short estrous cycle (4-6 days duration) and pregnancy (about 21 days), and comes into puberty (begins cycling) at about 35 to 40 days of age. Regular estrous cycles usually cease at 10 to 15 months of age, well before termination of life, and in this respect are similar to loss of reproductive cycles of women. Both male rats and men exhibit a more gradual decline in reproductive function, continuing to produce sperm and testosterone into old age.

Some stocks of rats probably are more suitable for studies on reproductive senescence than others. The LE rat appears to be superior to either the SD or WI stock (J. Meites, Department of Physiology, Michigan State University, East Lansing, Unpublished). All three stocks appear to be similar in their manifestations of reproductive decline, but the SD rat appears more susceptible to respiratory and other diseases and develops a much higher incidence of spontaneous mammary tumors than LE rats.

Both male and female WI rats develop large fat deposits
during aging that may influence their reproductive
functions.

The male rat appears to be a very good model for studies on reproductive aging in men. The fundamental controls by the hypothalamus, pituitary, and testes appear
to be similar in the male rat and human. The decline in
reproductive function is more gradual than in the female
and can continue, although at a reduced rate, into advanced age. In both species, there is a gradual decline
in testosterone production and spermatogenesis. There is
also a reduced hypothalamic capacity to respond to stimuli
that normally elicit release of LHRH (Riegle and Meites,
1976), perhaps due to a decrease in hypothalamic catecholamines and an increase in serotonin (Simpkins et al.,
1976). The aging male rat also shows a decrease in blood
LH and FSH levels (Bruni et al., 1977), and an increase
in blood prolactin values (Riegle and Meites, 1976).
Preliminary observations indicate that these changes are
potentially reversible and that male reproductive functions may be enhanced and extended by appropriate neuroendocrine treatments (J. Meites, Department of Physiology,
Michigan State University, East Lansing, Unpublished).
Similar possibilities may exist for the aging human male.

Disadvantages of the Rat as a Model of Reproductive Aging

The biggest difference between the aging female rat and
the postmenopausal woman is that the ovaries of the rat
appear to be capable of normal or near normal function
throughout their life span, whereas the ovaries of women
are not. Even the atrophic, seemingly nonfunctional
ovaries, with their few tiny follicles, seen in the oldest female rats (24 months or older) can be made to function normally or near normally under appropriate gonadotropic stimulation (Meites et al., 1978). When these
ovaries are transplanted into young ovariectomized rats,
they increase in size, show development of follicles, and
ovulate and form corpora lutea. Although the secretion
of serum gonadotropins and ovarian steroids tends to be
low, the ovaries in old female rats remain responsive and
can be activated by the use of appropriate central acting
drugs (L-dopa, ipronmiazid, etc.), hormones (LHRH, estrogen, progesterone, ACTH), or environmental stimuli (diet,
stress, etc.). On the other hand, the ovaries of postmenopausal women become fibrotic, lose their follicles,

and become essentially unresponsive to gonadotropic hormone stimulation, even though secretion of gonadotropins
is high. Thus, the fundamental causes for the loss of
reproductive cycles in aging women and female rats are
not the same. By contrast, reproductive decline in men
has many features in common with that in male rats.

Biochemical Adaptations

One feature that in part characterizes all aging populations is the altered ability to adapt to environmental
challenges. However, interpretation of underlying mechanisms may be complicated by the simultaneous expression
of other chronic, nongerontological characteristics of specific animal models. The following paragraphs illustrate:

● two examples of adaptive response to the stress of
starvation in SD rats;
● the manner in which responsiveness changes as these
rats age from 2 to at least 24 months;
● the difficulty in distinguishing between manifestations of aging and the continuous increase in body weight
that also characterizes SD rats between 2 and 24 months
of age; and
● two experimental approaches that have been designed
to resolve the issue (Britton et al., 1975; Adelman et
al., 1978).

When 2-month-old male SD rats from the colony maintained for R. C. Adelman at the Charles River Breeding
Laboratories are subjected to the stress of starvation,
activity of the liver enzyme, tyrosine aminotransferase,
increases more than 100 percent within 2 days. Similarly, circulating levels of corticosterone (the adrenal
glucocorticoid hormone whose adaptive secretion into the
circulation is necessary for the hepatic enzyme adaptation to occur) also are increased several fold. Both the
enzyme and hormone adaptations occur to a markedly diminished extent as the rat population ages.
The temptation to characterize these changes in responsiveness as age-associated phenomena must be tempered by
an evaluation of the life span profile of body weight for
SD rats. Under the specific conditions utilized for maintenance of this rat colony, body weight is approximately
150-175 g at 2 months, approximately 500 g by 12 months,
and approximately 700 g by 24 months of age. The older

and much larger rats may not recognize short-term starvation as very much of a stress; hence, there could be little need to secrete corticosterone and no mechanism to elicit an adaptive increase in hepatic tyrosine aminotransferase activity.

One experimental approach to resolution of this difficulty entails assessment of alternative physiological manifestations of starvation. Apparently, the older SD rats do recognize and respond to the absence of food. Liver and body weights and the serum concentration of glucose decrease significantly at 2, 12, and 24 months of age, although the decrease is more notable in the youngest rats. Serum levels of free fatty acids similarly increase at all three ages.

A second experimental approach to resolution of this issue entails assessment of the capabilities for the enzyme and hormone adaptations in experimental animal models that exhibit a broad spectrum of growth patterns during aging. The male COBS®CDF®F344/Crl[1] rats and C57BL/6NNia mice (from the NIA colonies maintained at the Charles River Breeding Laboratories) and Crl:COBS®CD® (SD)[1] rats used in this experiment are cesarian-derived and barrier-maintained under virtually identical environmental conditions throughout their life span. They are housed 5-7 per cage and fed a defined diet ad libitum until 2 years of age. The body weight of the SD rats increases continuously between 2 and 24 months of age, while that of the F344 rats increases to a lesser extent until 12 months of age and then remains constant until at least 24 months of age. Body weight remains constant beyond sexual maturity in the C57BL/6 mice. When responsiveness to starvation is expressed as adaptive increases in the activity of hepatic tyrosine aminotransferase or in the circulating level of corticosterone, aging exerts the identical effects in F344 and SD rats and C57BL/6 mice. Therefore, the progressive change in regulation of corticosterone levels and hepatic tyrosine aminotransferase activity represents a manifestation of aging rather than a consequence of species- or strain-specific differences in life span profiles of change in body weight.

---

[1]COBS®, CDF®, and CD® are registered trademarks of the Charles River Breeding Laboratories, Wilmington, Massachusetts.

Behavior and Aging

In the following review, an experiment is defined as a
study on aging if it includes a minimum of two age
groups, one of which is at least 10 months (300 days)
old. This is not a satisfactory definition, but more
stringent criteria would severely limit the discussion.
Reviews of the literature on aging and various aspects
of behavior in the rat have been written by Botwinick
(1959), Jerome (1959), Jakubczak (1973), Elias and Elias
(1975, 1977), and Arenberg and Robertson-Tchabo (1977).
A review by Elias (1979) is particularly relevant to the
aging rat. The following sections provide selected examples of studies with F344, SD, and LE rats.

Escape/Avoidance Learning

The ability of a rat to perform in active and passive
avoidance tests decreases in very old age, but when a
broad range of ages representing the whole life span is
investigated, curvilinear relationships are sometimes observed, with the youngest and oldest animals showing the
poorest performance (Elias, 1979). The specific nature
of the results depends on the strain or stock employed,
the nature of the response to be learned, and the interval between trials (Elias and Elias, 1975, 1977; Arenberg
and Robertson-Tchabo, 1977; Elias, 1979). What are sometimes interpreted as differences in learning ability may
reflect age-related differences in motivation to perform,
shock threshold, and/or attention to relevant stimuli
(Birren and Kay, 1958; Doty and Dalman, 1969; Paré, 1969;
Bengelloun et al., 1977; McNamara et al., 1977; Gordon
et al., 1978; Elias, 1979).
 Generally, studies with F344 rats indicate that age-
related deficiencies in memory are exaggerated when the
length of time that the rat is required to retain material
is increased (Gold and McGaugh, 1975). Some recent studies indicate that synaptic potentiation in the hippocampus
may be related to inferior memory in old F344 rats (Landfield and Lynch, 1977; Landfield et al., 1978b).

Discrimination Learning

Because of their greater visual acuity relative to albino
rats, LE rats have been chosen most frequently for studies

of pattern discrimination learning. Regardless of stock, age differences in discrimination learning are rarely obtained when the test consists of only two choices, unless the task involves a reversal learning paradigm (Birren, 1962; Kay and Sime, 1962; Botwinick et al., 1963).

Bar-Press Studies

Studies to determine age-related differences in bar-press tests have been unsuccessful in showing these differences about as often as they have been successful (Jakubczak, 1973; Arenberg and Robertson-Tchabo, 1977; Elias, 1979). SD rats will bar-press for milk and food rewards and to turn off a light. Bar-press differences where shock is used as the incentive may reveal age differences that are related to shock threshold rather than to learning ability (Elias, 1979). In any discriminated bar-press study using aged animals, the question may be raised as to what extent poor learning performance is related to impaired ability to perform and other variables unrelated to learning ability per se (Elias and Elias, 1977; Elias, 1979).

Reaction Time and Speed of Response

Age differences in swimming and response times may be related to differences in sensory thresholds or to an increased tendency for old animals to fatigue more quickly (Birren, 1955; Elias, 1979). Some of the variables that may be associated with a decreased response have been investigated. The monosynaptic reflex has been studied in 18 male and 5 female hooded rats, 3.8, 9.7, 14.6, and 27.2 months of age (Wayner and Emmers, 1958). Mean synaptic delays for the flexor hallucis longus monosynaptic reflex decrease with advancing age. Afferent condition velocity is approximately the same for young and old animals, but ventral root conduction velocity decreases from 64.2 m/sec in young animals to 43.7 m/s in old animals.

Motivation and Incentive

There have been many indices of hunger motivation used in studies on aging. The best index appears to be weight loss relative to predeprivation weight (Elias and Elias, 1977; Elias, 1979). In recent studies it has been suggested that, while regulation of caloric intake remains constant over a significant segment of the life span of SD rats (3.5 to 26.2 months of age), it is influenced by the "sensory and hedonic" aspects of the diet (Jakubczak, 1977).

The incentive value of cold stress has been examined using a bar-press task (Jakubczak, 1966). SD rats (7, 12, and 28 months old) serving as controls or subjected to cold stress show equal heat loss and perform equally well in lever pressing to turn on a heat source. This relationship may not hold for all temperatures or for all stocks of rats.

Activity, Exploratory Behavior, and Emotionality

A decrease in activity from late to old age is a frequently replicated finding for rats (Elias and Elias, 1975; Elias et al., 1975; Elias, 1979), but data with regard to emotionality are considerably less consistent. The problem lies with the use of defecation scores that may not be particularly valid (Collins, 1966; Bindra and Thompson, 1953) or sensitive (Hunt and Otis, 1953) measures of response to fear stimuli. One solution is to use multiple behavioral indices of emotionality (Werboff and Havlena, 1962), or better yet, to use hormonal indices of physiological response to stress (Elias and Elias, 1975; Elias and Redgate, 1975). Differences in results for various studies of wheel-running activity are related to the strain or stock of rat used (Elias, 1979) and the time sample (Jones et al., 1953). Wheel running itself influences the amount of food and water consumed; thus, it is difficult to explore the relationship between food and water deprivation and activity when using the activity wheel (Elias, 1979).

Stress and Early Experience

Environmental enrichment or stressors influence behavior of aging rodents (Arenberg and Robertson-Tchabo, 1977; Elias and Elias, 1977). For example, it has been shown that irradiation for 7 days postpartum accentuates the effects of aging on brain weight, ataxia, tremor, defecation, and activity in the open field test (Wallace and

Altman, 1970; Wallace et al., 1972). Studies such as
these relating to early treatment and experience have important implications for rearing and handling of animals
and in making the decision of whether to obtain animals
from outside sources or rear them in the home colony.
Under no circumstances should these variables be con-
founded with age-related variables.

Sexual Behavior

Studies of sexual behavior have been reviewed by Jakubczak
(1967) and Elias and Elias (1975), among others. Particularly interesting work has been done by Finch and Girgis
(1974).

Aging and Drug Action

Pharmacological effects in aging animals may be modified
by genetic factors, environmental and nutritional status,
age-specific biological and pathological characteristics,
mean survival time, and life expectancy (NIA and NIGMS,
1978). Specifically, these factors may cause differences
in absorption, binding, metabolism, and excretion of a
drug (Bender, 1964, 1967; Bender et al., 1970; Goldberg
and Roberts, 1976; Richey and Bender, 1977). The relationship of drug effects and aging has been studied most
commonly using the SD, WI, and F344 rats. The LE stock,
with the exception of endocrine studies, seldom has been
used in pharmacological or toxicological studies. Other
stocks and strains also are used infrequently (see Tuttle,
1966; Baird et al., 1975; Kelly, 1978) and will not be
considered here. Only those studies that address stock
identification, sex, and husbandry will be included, since
it is well known that these parameters significantly affect drug action.
   Perhaps the most striking difference in drug action
with age occurs in the pharmacokinetic aspects. These
differences are common to all stocks. Tables 13, 14, and
15 indicate age-related changes in drug action from the
perspectives of pharmacokinetic parameters, species and
stock differences, and dose-response relationships,
respectively.

TABLE 13   Changes with Age That May Affect Pharmacokinetic
Parameters of Drug Action

Property	Direction of Change with Age	Effect
Metabolism by the liver	Decrease	Prolonged half-life Failure to convert agent to active form of drug
Induction of microsomal enzymes	Variable	Variation in rate of metabolism of drug
Body-water (extracellular compartments)	Decrease	Drug distribution in body fluids
Binding to plasma proteins	Reduced	Increased concentration of free drug
Ratio lean to fat body weight	Decrease	Drug distribution changes
Ratio of organ weight to body weight	Variable	Sequestration of drug in a particular organ, change in organ sensitivity to drug
pH of body fluids	Variable	Drug distribution
Gastrointestinal motility	Decrease	Delayed absortion

TABLE 14 Relationship Between Species, Stock, and Drug Action as a Function of Age

Drug	Response	Effect of Age	Specie	Stock	Reference
Atropine	Anticholinergic	Increased sensitivity	Dog		Lasagna, 1956
		Decreased sensitivity	Rabbit		Lasagna, 1956
		Increased sensitivity	Rat		Lasagna, 1956
		No effect	Guinea pig		Farner and Verzar, 1961
	Effect on heart rate	Decrease	Human		Bender, 1964
Morphine	Analgesic	More sensitive at either end of age spectrum	Rat		Bender, 1964
		Decrease in older animals	Mice		Spratto and Dorio, 1978
Carbon monoxide	Poisoning	Increased susceptibility	Rabbit		Lasagna, 1956
		No change	Guinea pig		Lasagna, 1956
		Increased susceptibility	Rat		Lasagna, 1956
Phenobarbital	Induction of liver microsomal enzymes	Decrease	Rat	WI	Baird et al., 1975
		No change	Rat	CFN	Baird et al., 1975

Substance	Effect	Result	Species	Strain	Reference
Methylcho-lanthrene	Increase in hepatic demethylase	Decrease in the adult	Rat		Schwartz, 1971
	Renin release	Increase	Rat	SHR and SD	Aoi and Weinberger, 1976
		No change	Rat	WI Kyoto	Aoi and Weinberger, 1976
Hexobarbital	Sleep time	Increase with age	Rat	SD	Baird et al., 1975
			Rat	CFN	Baird et al., 1975
Barbiturates	Sedative effect	Increase	Human		Bender, 1964
N-nitroso-methylurea	Tumor induction	Increase	Rat	SD	Chan et al., 1977
	Synthesis of brain neurotransmitters	Small increase	Rat	F344	Chan et al., 1977
		Changes depend on area and enzyme	Rat	F344	Reis et al., 1977
		No change	Mouse	CB6F1	Reis et al., 1977
	Enzymes involved in synthesis of adrenal gland neurotransmitters	Increase	Rat	F344	Reis et al., 1977
		Increase	Mouse	CB6F1	Reis et al., 1977

TABLE 15 Dose-Response Relationship in Various Strains

Drug	Response	Effect of Age	Stock	Sex	Remarks	Reference
Codeine	Toxicity	No change	WI	M		Bender, 1964; Braunlich, 1966
Morphine	Toxicity	Decrease	WI	M		Bender, 1964; Braunlich, 1966
	Analgesic	Increase	SD	M		Spratto and Dorio, 1978
Neurohypophyseal hormones	Life span	Increase	WI	M		Friedman et al., 1965
Cortisol	Life span	Increase	WI	M		Friedman et al., 1965
	Rate of H_2O turnover	Reduced	WI	M		Friedman et al., 1965
Epinephrine	Lipolysis	Decrease	SD	M		Hruza, 1973
	Blood pressure	Increase	SD	M	Due to decreased metabolism	Hruza, 1973
Epinephrine	Lipolysis	Decrease	WI	M		Jelinkova et al., 1970
Norepinephrine	Lipolysis	Decrease	WI	M		Jelinkova et al., 1970
Theophylline	Inhibition of phosphodiesterase	Decrease	WI	M		Jelinkova et al., 1970

Substance	Effect	Response	Strain	Sex	Comments	Reference
ACTH, theophylline, norepinephrine	Lipolysis of isolated fat cells	Decrease	Holtzman	M		Nakano et al., 1971
Chloral hydrate	Sleeping time	Increase	F344	M		Mende and Viamonte, 1967
Camphor	Convulsions	No effect	F344	M	Due to increased variations in older groups	Mende and Viamonte, 1967
Amphetamine	Convulsions	Decrease	NI[a]	NI[a]		Farner and Verzar, 1961
Amphetamine	Body temperature and weight; motor activity	Increase	WI	M		Ziem et al., 1970
Hexobarbital, phenobarbital	Duration of hypnotic effect	Increase	WI	M/F		Kato and Takanaka, 1968
OMPA	Toxicity (cholinesterase inhibition)	Decrease	WI	M	Due to decreased liver function	Kato and Takanaka, 1968
Anticonvulsants	ED_{50}	Decrease	SD	M		Petty and Karler, 1965
Acetylcholine	Synthesis in atria	Decrease	NI[a]	NI[a]		Verkratsky, 1970

TABLE 15 (continued)

Drug	Response	Effect of Age	Stock	Sex	Remarks	Reference
Procaine	Life span	No change	WI	M/F		Verzar, 1959
Procaine (gerovital H_3)	Life span	Increase	WI	M/F	Effect seen only in male	Aslan et al., 1965
Alcohol	LD_{50}	Decrease	WI	M		Wiberg et al., 1970
Catecholamines	Contractility	Decrease	WI	M		Lakatta et al., 1975 Limas, 1975
Dopamine, apomorphine	Stimulation of adenylate cyclase activity (brain)	Decrease	SD	M		Govoni et al., 1977
Epinephrine	Effect on adenylate	Increase	WI	M/F		Kalish et al., 1977
Glucagon	Cyclase activity (liver)	Increase	WI	F	Age not a factor in males	Kalish et al., 1977

[a]NI = not indicated.

GERBILS

The Mongolian gerbil (dark-clawed gerbil, black gerbil,
or more correctly, jird), Meriones unguiculatus (Milne-
Edwards, 1867), is placed within the subfamily Gerbillinae, family Cricetidae, superfamily Muroidea (Figure 2).
The gerbil's noteworthy relatives occupy the genera Ger-
billus, Tatera, and Desmodillus.
     The gerbil was originally found in "la Mongolie Chi-
noise," possibly a reference to what is now Saratsi,
Northwest Shansi, China (Allen, 1940). Few observers have
studied the gerbil in its natural habitat. It is described as a social, burrowing rodent, excavating communal
galleries in high desert and and semidesert areas. Multiple tunnels, each about 4 m in length, converge upon
a central nest chamber lined with the chewed leaves of
grasses, sedges, buckwheat, and millet (Loskota, 1974).
Allen (1940) states that seeds are stored in the burrow
prior to the hibernation period. According to Tanimoto
(1943), the jird is active on the surface both by day
and night, but neither hibernates nor aestivates.
     In 1935, Dr. C. Kasuga captured 20 pairs of wild Mongo-
lian gerbils in the basin of the Amur River in Eastern
Mongolia and sent them to the Kitasato Institute in Japan.
Some were transferred, in 1949, by Miss Michiko Nomura to
Japan's Central Institute for Experimental Animals. Dr.
V. Schwentker, Tumblebrook Farm, Westbrook, Massachusetts,
obtained several animals from the Central Institute in
1954. These animals are the original source of all Mongolian gerbils in the United States.

General Characteristics

The gerbil is small and sandy brown with a light ventrum.
It weighs 85-100 g at 2 years of age (Kramer, 1964). Combined head and body length is 13-14 cm; tail length is
only slightly shorter than body length. A small tuft of
hairs is present at the tip of the tail. The hind legs
are moderately enlarged and the brain case is broadened
posteriorly with enlargement of the mastoids and tympanic
bullae (Rich, 1968). Gerbil hematology has been studied
by Ruhren (1965), Mays (1969), and Dillon and Glomski
(1975); embryonic and fetal hematopoiesis has been reviewed by Smith and Glomski (1977). The diploid number
of chromosomes is 44. Of the 42 autosomes, 32 are metacentric or submetacentric and 10 are acrocentric (Pakes,

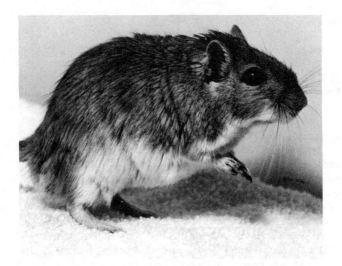

The Mongolian gerbil, _Meriones unguiculatus._
Photograph courtesy of Mr. Max Lent, University
of California at Los Angeles, Los Angeles,
California.

1969; Cohen, 1970; Leonard and Deknudt, 1970; Majumdar and
Solomon, 1970; Weiss _et al._, 1970).

Life Span

The mean survival time is 25.4 months (maximum, 48.0
months) for males and 32.1 months (maximum, 48.2 months)
for females (Troup _et al._, 1969). The authors note that
the mean survival time for males is biased by an epizootic
of acute pneumonia that occurred between 11.5 and 23
months (Figure 13). Longer mean survival times (35 $\pm$
7.8 months for males and 37.8 $\pm$ 7.7 months for females),
but similar maximum life spans (48.3 months for males,
47.8 months for females), have been reported (Arrington
_et al._, 1973).

Husbandry

The following procedures are generally accepted for rearing gerbils. Standard laboratory cages, suitable for rats

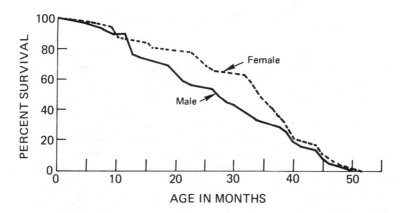

FIGURE 13 Survival curves of 35 male and 33 female
Mongolian gerbils. Modified from Troup et al., 1969.

or Syrian hamsters, may be used. A breeder pair requires
at least 929 cm^2 and mature animals should be allowed
232 cm^2 each. Gerbils may be kept on pine sawdust or
wood shavings, but the addition of absorbent is desirable.
Generally, fecal pellets are dry and soiling by urine is
minimal. Environmental conditions are not critical, but
the following are recommended: 21-22°C room temperature,
less than 50 percent relative humidity, and a 10- to 12-
hour photoperiod (Schwentker, 1968; Robinson, 1975).
Gerbils are docile and generally do not bite unless
provoked.

The nutrient requirements and maximal growth rates of
the gerbil are unknown. Available information has been
reviewed recently (BARR, 1978c). Gerbils thrive on standard pelleted laboratory chows as long as drinking water
is provided ad libitum (Schwentker, 1968, McManus, 1972).
Under natural conditions, the gerbil, a semidesert rodent,
can maintain hydration from metabolic water alone. Acceptable supplementary foods are mixed grain seeds, let-
tuce, carrots, cabbage, and apples. Sunflower seeds are
the food of choice for motivation tests; however, the
gerbil develops a high serum lipidemia, traced to sunflower seeds in the diet, that may prevent meaningful
hemoglobin determination in older animals (Ruhren, 1965).

A semipurified casein-glucose diet suitable for gerbils
has been developed by Zeman (1967).

Ease of Breeding

In the laboratory, gerbils are monogamous; older females
that have lost their mates usually will not accept another. Aggressive behavior leading to substantial mortality
may develop when sexually mature animals are first paired
(Marston and Chang, 1965; Norris and Adams, 1972a,b).
When mature males are transferred to a cage with a multiparous female or vice versa, mortality may reach 10 percent and usually involves the introduced animal. This
loss is greatly reduced when pairing occurs in a clean,
"neutral" box. Best results are obtained when animals
are paired at 6-12 weeks of age and not separated
thereafter.

Gerbils are less prolific than some other rodents; however, careful selection for long reproductive life, large
litter size, and, most importantly, for maternal capacity
to wean, will promote good reproductivity (Marston and
Chang, 1965). The greatest single cause of mortality in
gerbils is maternal neglect or agalactia. Twenty percent
of newborns fail to survive to weaning (Norris and Adams,
1972b). Ovarian cysts are common in gerbils older than
1 year. This condition is associated with reduced litter
size and premature infertility (Norris and Adams, 1972c).

Genetic Stocks Available

The Mongolian gerbils in the United States represent the
progeny of only nine animals and may be highly inbred
(Schwentker, 1963). There are apparently only a few histocompatibility genes; thus, tumor homografts and possibly heterografts are not rejected (Handler et al., 1966).
In parabiotic gerbils, major antigenic differences between
partners result in separation or death (Levine and Hoenig,
1972). Effects of genetic homogeneity are also evident
in peculiarities of territorial behavior (Thiessen et al.,
1971).

Four strains of syngeneic gerbils have recently been
developed by D. G. Robinson, Jr., Tumblebrook Farm, Inc.,
West Brookfield, Massachusetts. Strain 532 or MON/Tum
strain has been inbred for more than 26 generations.
Karavodin and Ash (1977a) have developed a semimicro mixed

lymphocyte culture and have found a weak allogeneic response with cells from Uclp:(MON) stock gerbils responding to stimulating cells from MON/Tum strain gerbils; the reverse has not been seen. The authors have demonstrated histocompatibility within strains and have found only weak histoincompatibilities between strains. Work with lymphoid graft-versus-host reactions has confirmed these conclusions (Karavodin and Ash, 1977b).

A mutation to acromelanic albinism (C^h) has been reported by R. Robinson (1973), and gerbils with a full black coat (except for a white patch on the throat) have been described by Cramlet et al. (1974). A selectively bred, seizure-sensitive strain (WJL/Uc) has been described by Loskota et al. (1974).

Germfree gerbils have been raised to maturity in limited numbers, but thus far have failed to reproduce. A small colony of animals with a known, limited microflora has been established, however (Wostmann et al., 1978).

Factors Affecting Life Span

Infectious Diseases

Major, life-threatening infectious diseases of gerbils include Tyzzer's disease, salmonellosis, and acute pneumonia. Tyzzer's disease of the liver is a major cause of gerbil mortality, killing up to 75 percent of young gerbils (Carter et al., 1969; Port et al., 1970; Vincent et al., 1975). High mortality due to Salmonella enteritidis has been noted (Olson and Shields, 1977); the severity of the disease is possibly related to the stress of Hymenolepis nana infection and to shipping shortly after weaning. Gerbils also are susceptible to alopecia or generalized dermatitis associated with Staphylococcus aureus (Peckham et al., 1974).

Acute pneumonia in gerbils with bronchial changes and significant mortality has been reported (Troup et al., 1969; Vincent et al., 1975). Males appear more susceptible than females. The etiology has not been demonstrated, but a viral agent has been postulated (Vincent et al., 1975).

Parasites in the gerbil are largely nonpathogenic and not restrictive in most laboratory investigations. Naturally occurring helminths (Wightman et al., 1978), protozoa (Loew, 1968; Vincent et al., 1975), and mites

(Schwarzbrott et al., 1974) have been reported. The presence of Tryophagus castellani in the feces probably reflects contamination of feed grain and is a potential cause of allergic dermatitis in the colony. Najarian's observation (1961) of Hemobartonella within gerbil erthyrocytes has not been substantiated by subsequent workers (Ruhren, 1965; Smith et al., 1976).

Spontaneously Occurring Diseases

Spontaneously occurring lesions occurring in gerbils are listed in Table 16. The incidence of tumors in the gerbil has been calculated by various authors as 8.4 to 24 percent (Benitz and Kramer, 1965; Leathers and Bullock, 1975;

TABLE 16 Neoplastic and Nonneoplastic Lesions of the Gerbil (Meriones unguiculatus)[a]

Neoplastic Lesions	Nonneoplastic Lesions
Malignant melanoma	Pancreatic islet cell
Malignant blue nevus	hypertrophy
Pigmented nevus	Pancreatic cell degeneration
Amelanotic melanoblastoma	Hydropic degeneration of
Squamous cell carcinoma	pancreatic islets
Pancreatic islet cell	Fatty change of liver
adenoma	Atypical nuclear change
Uterine and ovarian	of liver
leiomyoma	Arteriosclerosis
Ovarian dysgerminoma	Chronic interstitial
	nephritis
Uterine carcinoma	Glomerular hyperplasia and
Plasmacytoma	sclerosis
Prostatic adenoma	Follicular cysts
	Periodontal syndrome

[a]From reviews and case reports of Benitz and Kramer (1965), Troup et al. (1969), Cramlet et al. (1974), Shumaker et al. (1974), Leathers and Bullock (1975), Vincent et al. (1975), and Vincent and Ash (1978).

Troup et al., 1969). The mean age at death of tumor-
bearing gerbils is 52.3 months (Leathers and Bullock,
1975).

Spontaneous arteriosclerosis, evidence of steroid diabetes, and other metabolic derangements that develop in
breeder gerbils are highly reminiscent of a similar "syndrome" in breeder rats. It is ascribed to "over-activity
of the hypothalamic-pituitary-adrenal-gonadal axis in connection with the reproduction effort" (Wexler et al.,
1971). Arterial connective tissue derangements, including
ground substance alterations, elastolytic degeneration,
or calcification, are found in the majority of male and
female breeders; little demonstrable lipid is present in
these lesions. Serum CPK, triglycerides, free fatty
acids, cholesterol, glucose, BUN, and cortisol levels all
are greatly elevated.

The gerbil has been tentatively recommended as a model
of experimental diabetes. (See section entitled "Comparative Models for Problems of the Human Elderly.")

After approximately 6 months on a standard diet, the
gerbil may show a slowly developing periodontal syndrome.
Progressive accumulation of plaque, calcareous deposits,
round cell infiltration, and resorption of supporting tissues may be followed by multiple root fractures and ce-
mental tears (Moskow et al., 1968). Spontaneous exfolia-
tion of the third molar sometimes occurs. In short-term
trials, standard laboratory chow produces somewhat fewer
soft and calcified tissue lesions than mixed grains (Gupta
and Shaw, 1960).

An increase in relative spleen weights with advanced
age (ninth and tenth decile of survivorship), coupled with
an apparent substantial increase in serum gamma globulin
in 28-month-old gerbils (Dellenback and Ringle, 1963), is
not inconsistent with a heightened autoimmunity in advanced age (Troup et al., 1969).

Research Use

Techniques for Use

Experimental procedures (not specifically for research on
aging) suitable for gerbils and other rodents have been
reviewed by Schuchman (1974). Pentobarbital sodium solution (60 mg/ml) is a satisfactory anesthetic given at
0.01 ml/10 g body weight, not exceeding a total dose of

0.1 ml (Allanson, 1970). Intravenous injections and withdrawal of blood samples are easily accomplished at the
orbital sinus; injection of the tail vein is not practical. A technique of thymectomy of newborn, 17- and 34-
day-old gerbils has been reported by Benten et al. (1977).

Use in Research on Aging

Research areas related to aging for which the gerbil may
be a useful model are: cholesterol metabolism, maturity-
onset diabetes mellitus, various infectious and degenerative diseases, and some forms of neoplasia. A unique
aspect of the gerbil's cholesterol metabolism is that
the formation of steroid hormones is probably its most
important pathway of cholesterol metabolism, while in
other animals, bile acids comprise the major pathway (Roscoe and Fahrenback, 1962). This difference may reflect
the gerbil's need to retain salts and water. Feeding diets rich in fats or cholesterol uniformly elevates serum
cholesterol, but unlike other animals, atheromatous lesions do not result. Cholesterol gallstones form when the
diet is supplemented with cholic acid and cholesterol (van
der Linden and Bergman, 1977). As in man, bile acids are
cholic and chendeoxycholic acids; in this respect, the
gerbil is perhaps a better candidate for the study of
cholesterol metabolism than is the rat (Wostmann et al.,
1978).

GUINEA PIGS

Cavia porcellus (Linnaeus) is the scientific name of the
common laboratory guinea pig or cavy. It is classified
taxonomically in the order Rodentia, suborder Hystricomorpha (Figure 2), which includes the chinchillas, porcu-
pines, and others. The superfamily Cavioidae, family
Caviidae, contains those South American rodents that are
short-tailed or tailless, have only one pair of mammae,
and have four digits on the forefoot and three on the
hindfoot. The genus Cavia (Pallas, 1766) is in the subfamily Caviinae with the type species being Cavia porcellus (Walker, 1975b). The origin of the term "guinea pig"
is obscure and the subject of much speculation; however,
it is ingrained and undoubtedly will continue to be used
in preference to the more reasonable name, cavy.

General Characteristics

Guinea pigs are docile but vocal animals. They are easily handled and adapt well to the laboratory environment.
Guinea pigs have a normal body temperature of 39.0-39.5°C,
a respiratory rate of 110-150 per min, and a pulse rate
of 150-160 per min. For further information concerning
the general anatomy and physiology of the guinea pig,
Breazile and Brown (1976) and Sisk (1976) should be consulted. Clinical pathological indices have been reviewed
by Laird (1974).

Life Span

In 1958, Reid wrote that no data are available on the life
span of guinea pigs. The longest survival time that has
been reliably reported is 8 years; the average life span
is probably much less than this. Rogers has stated that

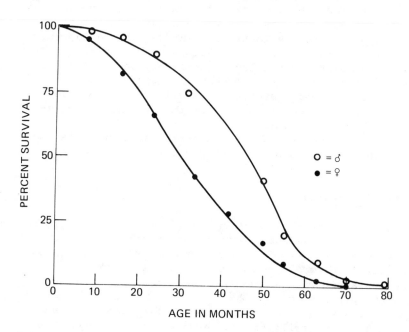

FIGURE 14 Survival curves for guinea pigs. Data from
Rust et al., 1966.

the median life span of guinea pigs is about 6 years
(Reid, 1958). In a study designed to evaluate the effects
of period gammaray exposure, 120 sham-exposed cavies were
allowed to live out their normal life span (Rust et al.,
1966). The oldest guinea pig lived until almost 7 years
of age. Approximately 50 percent of the males and females
died before 2.7 and 4.1 years, respectively (Figure 14).
Husbandry

The care and management of the guinea pig recently has
been reviewed and described by Ediger (1976). Management
procedures should comply with the recommendations of the
Guide for the Care and Use of Laboratory Animals (ILAR,
1978a) and Laboratory Animal Management: Rodents (ILAR,
1977).
     The guinea pig is a strictly herbivorous animal. This
species has an unusually high requirement for the amino
acids arginine, methionine, and tryptophan and is unique
among the laboratory rodents in that it requires an exogenous source of vitamin C (BARR, 1978c). Scurvy (hypo-
vitaminosis C) occurs in the guinea pig because of a
genetic deficiency of L-gulonolactone oxidase, which is
necessary for the synthesis of ascorbic acid from glucose
by the glucuronic pathway. While commercially available
guinea pig diets are fortified with ascorbic acid, this
vitamin is heat labile and loses potency over time, so
that even diets originally satisfactory when milled can
become deficient in this essential vitamin through im-
proper or prolonged storage. Details of the deficiency
state and known requirements for this vitamin have recently been reviewed by Navia and Hunt (1976), and the
relationship between dietary ascorbic acid and life span
has been discussed by Davies et al. (1977).

Ease of Breeding

Guinea pigs breed readily in the laboratory. A reproductive index of 0.7 and 1.0 young per female per month is
considered standard for inbred and outbred animals, respectively. Female guinea pigs are polyestrous, spontaneous ovulators with an estrous cycle of 15-17 days and a
gestation period of 59-72 days. The duration of gestation
is inversely related to the number of fetuses carried.
Young are born fully haired, have their eyes open, are
able to hear, and are unique among the rodents in their
ability to consume solid food almost at once. An average

litter size is 3 or 4. Weight at birth is in direct proportion to the size of the litter. In small litters,
the newborns may weigh 100 g, whereas in larger litters,
they may weigh 50 g or less. Young weighing less than
50 g frequently do not survive.

Males reach puberty and are fertile at 8-10 weeks of
age. Females reach sexual maturity at a very early age
and are known to mate prior to weaning at 33 days. One
way to maintain maximum productivity is to house the male
and female together so that the female is bred during
postpartum estrus. Approximately 80 percent of females
will conceive if bred at this time.

Genetic Stocks Available

Several outbred stocks of guinea pigs are available for
research; the most common is the short-haired, Dunkin-
Hartley stock. Many coat pattern variations of outbred
stocks are kept by fanciers, including the popular Abys-
sinian and Peruvian guinea pigs.

Only two inbred strains of guinea pigs, the Wright
Strains 2 and 13, are available commercially in the United
States. Other lesser known inbred guinea pigs listed in
the International Index of Laboratory Animals, fourth
edition, include the ALB, B, DHCBA, IMM/R 201, IMM/R 203,
IMM/S 209, IMM/S 740, JY-1, JY-2, OM3 and R9 (Festing,
1980). Two mutant stocks of guinea pigs also are available through the Veterinary Resources Branch, Division
of Research Resources, National Institutes of Health. The
Waltzer (Wz) shows a gradual atrophy and disappearance
of hair cells and the other cellular elements of the organ
of Corti along with cellular neuronal atrophy. The complement 4 deficient (c4d) guinea pig carries the recessive
gene that blocks the formation of the fourth component
of complement. The area of biochemical genetics, especially studies concerning various complement component
deficiencies, recently has been reviewed (Festing, 1976).

Factors Affecting Life Span

Infectious Diseases

Only the more common infectious diseases of the guinea pig
will be noted in this section. For a complete review of
these diseases consult Ganaway (1976).

A high incidence of respiratory disease is seen in guinea pigs and is generally precipitated by a combination of poor husbandry conditions and a vitamin C deficiency. Such agents as <u>Bordetella bronchiseptica</u> and <u>Klebsiella pneumoniae</u> usually are involved. The guinea pig is exquisitely susceptible to the tubercule bacillus and traditionally has been used in isolating and identifying strains of <u>Mycobacterium tuberculosis</u>. However, naturally occurring infection in well-managed colonies is unknown.

Salmonellosis, once a major disease problem in all laboratory rodents, still can cause disease and death in guinea pigs if they are fed natural supplements, such as kale, that are contaminated by wild rodent feces. Collibacillosis does not occur in well-managed colonies; however, where poor husbandry conditions exist, it can be a significant cause of disease and death.

<u>Streptococci</u>, particularly those in Lancefield's group C, can cause high morbidity and mortality. In addition to the respiratory infections, <u>Streptococci</u> are associated with cervical lymphadenitis, chronic nephritis, arthritis, and suppurative processes in a wide range of organs. Yersiniosis (<u>Yersinia pseudotuberculosis</u>) also can cause severe disease in guinea pig colonies. It is manifested as an acute septicemia with death occurring in 1-2 days, as chronic pseudotuberculosis with death occurring in 3-4 weeks, or as a nonfatal cervical lymphadenitis.

Van Hoosier and Robinette (1976) have described 17 naturally occurring virus infections in guinea pigs, but based upon a serological survey, indicate that only five are relatively common. The extent to which they affect life span in most cases is not known. Lymphocytic choriomeningitis (LCM) virus infection usually results in clinical disease and death. Consequently, guinea pigs have been recommended for use as biological sentinels in mouse colonies and other places where LCM virus contaminants may be a problem (J. Hotchin, New York State Department of Health, Albany, New York, Unpublished).

Dermatomycoses are among the most common infectious diseases in guinea pig colonies, but systemic fungal infections rarely occur (Sprouse, 1976).

Spontaneous Diseases

Female guinea pigs are subject to pregnancy toxemia. Aortic compression from the enlarged uterus reduces the blood pressure to 50 percent of normal posterior to the

stricture, resulting in a relative utero-placental ischemia (H. Hughes, Department of Comparative Medicine, Mil-
ton S. Hershey Medical Center, Hershey, Pennsylvania,
Unpublished).

The soft tissue calcification (STC) syndrome is characterized by poor growth, foreleg lameness, bony deformities, abnormal tooth formation, calcification of many
soft tissues, elevated serum phosphorus, and death. While
commercially available diets for guinea pigs purportedly
have the proper concentrations and ratios of calcium,
phosphorus, magnesium, and potassium, STC still occurs
(Galloway et al., 1964; Sparschu and Christie, 1968).

Naturally occurring neoplasms in guinea pigs are rare,
probably because guinea pigs are seldom kept into advanced
age when the incidence of neoplasms is highest in most species. One study, for example, has shown the overall incidence of tumors in guinea pigs to be only 1.4 percent. If
animals are allowed to survive to 3 years or more, however, the incidence rises to 14.4 percent (Rogers and
Blumenthal, 1960). Two recent reviews of guinea pig tumors can be consulted for more details (Manning, 1976;
Robinson, 1976b).

Rhabdomyomatosis is a frequently observed nonneoplastic lesion of the myocardium. While some regard this as
a congenital disease, since it is reported most often in
animals from 3 to 20 weeks of age, its etiology and pathogenesis remain obscure. Because of its relatively high
incidence in certain colonies, the guinea pig may serve
as a useful model for human rhabdomyomatosis (Manning,
1976).

Other Factors

Environmental factors can affect life span in a great variety of ways, but are poorly documented in the guinea
pig. Factors such as cage density, exercise, lighting,
temperature, humidity, and frequency of cage cleaning can
have profound effects on survival rates of animals in
the absence of intercurrent disease.

Research Use

The guinea pig is suitable for either single or multiple
use. Manipulations such as administration of materials
or blood withdrawal are easier than in rats, but more

difficult than in rabbits. For a review of methods of substance administration and collection of body fluids, see Hoar (1976).

In the past, long-term studies have been hampered by the relative unavailability of high-quality disease-free or specific pathogen-free (SPF) guinea pigs. Presently, however, investigators can procure such SPF cavies. The guinea pig, while susceptible to a wide host of infectious diseases, including those of possible zoonotic consequence, presents no particular problems for use in research if high-quality animals are purchased and are maintained in modern, well-managed facilities with good programs of animal health surveillance.

Use in Research on Aging

The guinea pig has received relatively little attention as a species for studies on aging. In the past, the guinea pig has been used extensively as a means of diagnosis of infectious diseases, especially tuberculosis, or in bioassays and basic research in bacteriology and pathology. The guinea pig, however, has an extensive history of use in auditory research (Finkiewicz-Murawiejska, 1972; Coleman, 1976; McCormack and Nutall, 1976) and studies of anaphylactic and other allergic phenomena and has been proposed as a model for experimental allergic neuritis and other neuropathies (Kraft, 1968). A model for ulcerative colitis has been reported in the guinea pig (Anver and Cohen, 1976). Some recent studies concerning age-associated changes are listed in Table 17.

HAMSTERS

The hamster is a relatively common laboratory animal species in biomedical research. The earliest use of the hamster dates back to 1930, when Professor Aharoni started the first laboratory colony of Syrian hamsters from one male and two females. They were introduced in the United States in 1938 (Hoffman et al., 1968). Today there are seven different species of laboratory hamsters and many different strains and stocks. The four major species of hamsters in common usage today are the Syrian or golden (Mesocricetus auratus), the European or common (Cricetus cricetus), the Chinese or striped-back (Cricetulus

TABLE 17   References for Age-Associated Changes in the Guinea Pig

Changes	References
Aging changes in collagens of skin	Kulonen and Pikkarainean, 1968
DNA-RNA changes in palate	Burzynski and Goljan, 1967
DNA synthesis in thymus	Blau, 1972
Cystic site ovaries in aged guinea pigs	Quattropani, 1978
Age changes in temporomandibular joint; shoulder joint	Karakasis and Tsaknakis, 1976; Silberberg et al., 1973
Nerve conduction velocity and aging	Kraft, 1972
Experimental allergic neuritis and other neuropathies	Kraft, 1972
Enterochromaffin cells in the gastrointestinal tract	Gandalovičova, 1974
Testosterone and androstenedione concentrations	Rigaudiere et al., 1976
Phospholipid content in submandibular salivary gland	Burzynski, 1971
Water loss-heat production	Calloway, 1971, 1974
Oral tissue changes	Burzynski, 1967a,b Burzynski and Rogers, 1965
Chromosome aberrations in liver cells	Curtis and Miller, 1971
Number of fibers in skeletal muscle	Maxwell et al., 1974
Glycosaminoglycans in heart valves	Hallgrimsson et al., 1970
Hair cell loss in the cochlea	Coleman, 1976
Hypothalamus	Hasan et al., 1974
Muscle action potential	Rumberger and Timmerman, 1976
Lipofuscin in cardiac muscle	Spoerri et al., 1974
Mast cell population	Buxton, 1966
Articular cartilage	Silberberg et al., 1970

griseus), and the Armenian (Cricetulus migratorius) (Hoffman et al., 1968; ILAR, 1979a).

General Characteristics

The use of the hamster in long-term research has been
primarily in the areas of cancer research, chemical
carcinogenesis, and experimental toxicology, especially
inhalation toxicology (Homburger, 1972; Mohr et al., 1972;
Brooks et al., 1974; Benjamin et al., 1976; Becci et al.,
1978a,b). Its use specifically for studies on aging has
been limited; however, despite this limited use, the hamster is certainly an appropriate animal species for such
studies. It can be developed as a potential model to
use for aging and long-term research to contrast experimental results with those results obtained in the more
commonly used rodents, such as the rat and the mouse.

Only a few strains and stocks of hamsters have been
studied in detail. Most physiological and clinical data
have been determined primarily from Syrian (Hoffman et
al., 1968; Laird, 1974; Frank, 1976; Dent, 1976; Benjamin
and McKelvie, 1978) and European (Emminger et al., 1975;
Reznik et al., 1975; Silverman and Chavannes, 1977) hamsters. Normal reproductive and developmental parameters
have been reviewed by Kent (1968), Mohr et al. (1973),
and Melby and Altman (1974a, b, 1976). Hamsters have
played an important role in hibernation research, and
physiological data from hibernating animals are available
(Kayser, 1961; Reznik et al., 1975). The average body
weight varies depending on the strain or stock of hamster.
For example, Haverland et al. (1972) has shown variations
in body weight in several different inbred lines of Syrian
hamsters. Some males have mean weights of less than 100
g, while others are greater than 130 g. These investigators have shown similar variability in body weights for
females.

The hamster has several unique anatomical characteristics, most of which have been reviewed by Homburger et
al. (1964) and Magalhaes (1968). A few of these characteristics are:

• cheek pouches (useful in tumor transplantation
research);
• an esophagus that enters closer to the glandular
stomach than in the rat;

- gastric compartments, each having a different ability to digest food and a different pH;
- an intestine adapted for water conservation;
- kidneys with long renal papillae extending into the ureter (useful in renal physiology studies); and
- fetal trophoblasts that migrate from the placenta into the mesovarium and mesometrial arteries in pregnant females (Burek et al., 1979).

Life Span

Longevity data have been reported from several colonies of hamsters. Most of these reports come from the Bio-Research Institute, Cambridge, Massachusetts (Bernfeld, 1979). Among 20 inbred strains, the mean survival varies from 12.4 months (BIO[®]1.26 strain[1]) to 25.9 months (male BIO[®]1.5 strain[1]). Males outlive females in 17 of the 20 strains. Mean survival ages of approximately 25.3 and 13.2 months in male and female Sch:(SYR) hamsters, respectively, have been reported (Redman et al., 1979). Figure 15 illustrates survival data from a recently completed chronic toxicity and oncogenicity study using Eng:ELA(SYR) hamsters (Rampy et al., 1979). The controls have mean survival times of 24 and 20 months for males and females, respectively. Figure 16 shows survival curves for Chinese hamsters raised at the Inhalation Toxicology Research Institute, Lovelace Biomedical and Environmental Research Institute, Albuquerque, New Mexico (Benjamin and Brooks, 1977). The mean survival time for male Chinese hamsters in this study is 38.8 months (maximum age 47.2 months) and for females is 35.3 months (maximum age 51.5 months).

Husbandry

Hamster husbandry has been reviewed adequately and should follow the guidelines in Guide for the Care and Use of Laboratory Animals (ILAR, 1978a) and Standards for the Breeding, Care, and Management of Syrian Hamsters (ILAR, 1960). For other reviews see Poiley (1950), Hoffman et al. (1968), and Melby and Altman (1974a,b, 1976). The nutrient requirements of hamsters have been discussed (BARR,

---

[1]BIO[®] is a registered trademark of the Bio-Research Institute, Cambridge, Massachusetts.

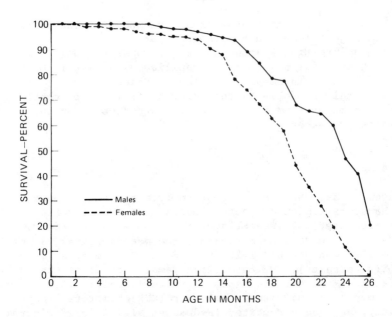

FIGURE 15 Survival Curves for Male and Female Eng:ELA (SYR) Hamsters. Figure Courtesy of J. D. Burek, Dow Chemical Company, Midland, Michigan. Data from Rampy et al., 1979.

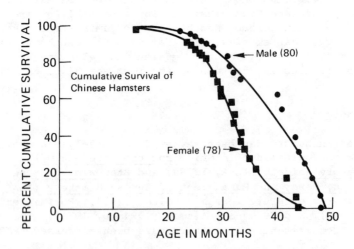

FIGURE 16 Survival Curves for Male and Female Chinese Hamsters. Adapted from Benjamin and Brooks, 1977.

1978c). Some hamsters are aggressive; however, with repeated handling most stocks adapt readily to experimental
manipulation.

Ease of Breeding

Hamsters have the shortest gestation period and most rapid development of the common laboratory rodents. The
gestation period is 16 days for Syrian hamsters, 19-21
days for Chinese hamsters. Hamsters are polyestrus, but
may undergo seasonal decreases in cycling; their normal
estrous cycle is 4 days (Orsini, 1961). Hamsters are
monogamous; however, fighting may ensue if a male and
female are housed together for extended periods. Breeding
can readily be accomplished by placing females with males
on the third day following estrus as determined by vaginal
smears. Hamster reproductive capacity decreases with age;
breeding life is approximately 1 year. Optimal breeding
performance can be obtained using light cycles of 14 hours
of light and 10 hours of darkness. Litter size is approximately 6-8 pups; weaning occurs at approximately 21 days.

Genetic Stocks Available

Currently, there are over 35 inbred strains and 30 known
mutations of Syrian hamsters (Yoon, 1979) and several
strains and mutations of the Chinese and other hamster
species. They have been developed for their usefulness
in many different facets of biomedical research, especially cytogenetics because the chromosome number for the
different species of hamster varies. For example, the
Syrian hamster has 44 chromosomes, while the other two
commonly used hamsters, the Chinese and the European,
both have 22 chromosomes (Benirschke, 1978).

Factors Affecting Life Span

Infectious Diseases

Hamsters have been used in various types of biomedical research on infectious diseases because of their susceptibility to many different types of these diseases. Despite
the number of diseases to which they are susceptible; however, only a few pose a real hazard to long-term studies.

Diseases that could potentially pose a serious threat are: profilerative ileitis (wet tail), salmonellosis, and Tyzzer's disease (Renshaw et al., 1975). Hamsters also are susceptible to Sendai and lymphocytic choriomeningitis viruses; however, infection with these viruses seldom results in extensive mortality. Antibodies to several other viruses also have been reported in hamsters (Schiff et al., 1973; Reed et al., 1974). Parasitic infections such as tapeworm (Hymenolepis nana) and pinworm (Syphacia obvelata) infections are also common. Parasitic mite (Demodex) infection can affect long-term studies involving the skin (Estes et al., 1971).

Spontaneously Occurring Diseases

The incidence of neoplastic and nonneoplastic diseases varies with the species and the genetic stock of hamster (Hoffman et al., 1968; Ward and Moore, 1969; Homburger, 1972; Melby and Altman, 1974a,b, 1976; Benjamin and Brooks, 1977; McMartin, 1977; Benirschke et al., 1978). Spontaneous neoplastic lesions have been reported by Handler (1965), Kirkman and Algard (1968), Pour et al. (1976a,b,c,d), Robinson (1976a), Benjamin and Brooks (1977), and Benirschke et al. (1978). Tumors of lymphatic tissues and endocrine neoplasms, especially adrenal cortical tumors, are the most common.

Amyloidosis or paramyloidosis is common in both males and females (Gleiser et al., 1971; McMartin, 1977). It is characterized by the deposition of hyalin-like material that often contains amyloid, in various parenchymal organs. The location of these deposits varies somewhat from stock to stock. The more commonly involved organs are the kidney, liver, adrenal glands, thyroid glands, and spleen. Biliary hyperplasia, biliary cysts (Handler, 1965), and hepatic hemosiderosis (J. D. Burek, Dow Chemical Company, Midland, Michigan, Unpublished) occur in the hamster in addition to amyloid deposits.

Dental caries in the hamster occur spontaneously and can be induced experimentally (Keyes, 1968). When caries are present, the teeth become dark and may erode to the gumline. Gingival inflammation and, occasionally, abscess formation may be associated with caries.

Many aged hamsters exhibit severe testicular atrophy (Handler, 1965) and depletion of abdominal and subcutaneous adipose tissue as a result of inanition (J. D. Burek, Dow Chemical Company, Midland, Michigan, Unpublished).

Miscellaneous pathological changes include subcutaneous edema, ascites, and hydrothorax associated with renal and hepatic amyloidosis. Dissecting aneurysms of the aorta, left atrial thrombosis, urolithiasis, pancreatic atrophy, hyperplasias of many endocrine organs, and radiculoneuropathy also are seen occasionally in aging hamsters (McMartin, 1977).

Nutrition

The relationship between nutrition and longevity in hamsters has been documented (Newberne, 1979). The incidence of many spontaneous, age-related diseases can be reduced by feeding semipurified diets. Reviews on hamster nutrition can be found in Granados (1968) and Melby and Altman (1976).

Other Factors Affecting Life Span

Additional factors affecting the life span of hamsters are poorly documented. Animals that are group housed tend to have shorter survival times than those that are individually housed. This probably is due in part to the fighting that occurs among group-housed animals and to cannibalism.

Research Use

Hamsters are appropriate animals for single or multiple uses and can be used for many of the same procedures as rats and mice. Frequent sampling of body fluids can be difficult, and measurements can be hampered by the relatively small volumes that are obtainable.

Use in Research on Aging

The hamster has several spontaneous age-associated diseases that are potential models of similar diseases in man. In addition, some chronic or age-associated diseases, such as chronic bronchitis and emphysema (Hayes et al., 1977), can be induced. Several of the major models are summarized in Table 18. Hamsters have a low background of spontaneous tumors, yet it is relatively easy to induce tumors in mammary, pancreatic, and respiratory tissues.

TABLE 18   Age-Associated Diseases Where Hamsters May
Serve as Animal Models

Disease	Reference
Amyloidosis	Gleiser et al., 1971
Angioimmunoblastic lymphadenopathy	Yerganian et al., 1978
Atrial thrombosis	Dodds et al., 1977; McMartin, 1977
Cardiomyopathy	Gertz, 1973
Chronic bronchitis and emphysema[a]	Hayes et al., 1977
Dental caries and periodontal disease[a]	Keyes, 1968
Diabetes mellitus[a]	Meier and Yerganian, 1959
Dissecting aortic aneurysms	Frenkel et al., 1959
Hydrocephalus	Yoon and Slaney, 1972
Prostatic hypertrophy[a]	Homburger and Nixon, 1970

[a]These diseases are described in detail in the section
entitled "Comparative Models of Problems of the Human
Elderly."

The major disadvantage of the hamster for research on
aging is the relatively poor survival of most colonies.
Few institutes have been able to maintain experimental
colonies consistently where males and females have 50
percent survivals of 24 months or more. A second major
disadvantage is the wide prevalance of amyloidosis or
paramyloidosis. The presence of this disease can
severely alter organ and tissue functions and interferes
with studies on aging.

MASTOMYS

The scientific name Praomys (Mastomys) natalensis is used
in accordance with the taxonomic designation of Davis
(1965). The brief term "mastomys" will be used in this

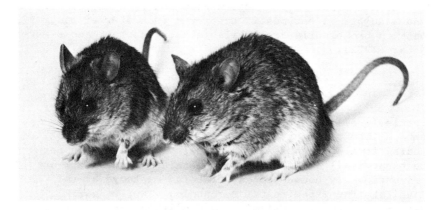

The mastomys, <u>Praomys</u> (<u>Mastomys</u>) <u>natalensis</u>. Photograph
courtesy of the Institute for Experimental Gerontology
TNO, Rijswijk, The Netherlands.

report because it has far greater common usage than the
larger scientific name. In the past, the terms "multimammate mouse" and <u>Rattus</u> (<u>Mastomys</u>) <u>natalensis</u> also have
been used (see Oettle, 1967; Isaacson, 1975; Soga, 1977a).
    Mastomys is one of the most common rodents in Africa,
being prevalent in bush, scrub, and cultivated lands of
the southern and northern savannah biotic zones. It forms
a link between human habitations and wild rodent populations
nearby, because it makes use of the burrows of other rodents
in preference to digging its own. For further information
on habits and ecology, see Oettle (1967) and Isaacson (1975).

General Characteristics

Mastomys is a rodent intermediate in size between mouse and
rat, with an average weight of 40 to 100 g, a body length
of 10 to 15 cm, and a tail length approximately the same as
body length. The species is characterized further by a
chromosome number of 36, the absence of a gall bladder,
well-developed prostate glands in both the male and female,
and a large number of mammae in the female (8 to 12 pairs,
distributed from the pectoral to the inguinal region).
    Baseline data are available on a number of immunological
parameters (van Pelt and Blankwater, 1972; Kozima, 1977),
hematological values (Martin and Rutty, 1969; Heitmann,

1971), and serum proteins (van Pelt and Blankwater, 1972)
and a number of enzymes in the serum (Schuster et al., 1972).
Data on proteinuria are available from van Pelt and Blankwater (1972).

Life Span

Oettle (1967) has observed that the life span in males may
extend into the fourth year, but is generally under 3
years; females do not attain 3 years. The mean (50 percent survival) and maximum ages obtained in a random-bred,
conventionally housed colony of aging mastomys at the
Institute for Experimental Gerontology TNO, Rijswijk, The
Netherlands (C. F. Hollander, Unpublished) are: males,
21 and 33 months, respectively (range 4-33 months); females, 23 and 38 months, respectively (range 12-38
months). The mean and maximum ages of the colony maintained at Argonne National Laboratory, Argonne, Illinois
(G. A. Sacher, Unpublished) are: males, 20 and 36 months,
respectively; females, 23 and 38 months, respectively.

Husbandry

Mastomys commonly are maintained under the same environmental conditions as mice and rats, and similar rodent
cages and bedding are adequate (Oettle, 1967; Soga, 1977b).
Cannibalism of young animals occurs in breeding colonies
and also is seen among adult animals housed more than
one per cage in long-term experiments. During long-term
research use, animals should be housed singly or should
be set up in groups of the same sex and age at the time
of weaning.

Initially, when starting a colony of mastomys, the animals may be so wild and aggressive they can be handled
only with forceps. Good laboratory animal practice can
tame them successfully; however, they still have a tendency to try to escape from the cage when it is opened
and great care is necessary to avert this.

Although little is known about specific nutritional requirements of mastomys, standard rodent pellets and tap
water ad libitum have proved adequate in most existing
colonies. Saito et al. (1977) have reported on the effects of diets of various composition on mastomys. Significant differences are observed in life spans of animals
on different diets, but the reasons are not clear. It

can be deduced, however, that nutritional requirements
of mastomys are similar to those of rats and mice.

Ease of Breeding

Depending on adaptation to the laboratory, as well as care
in handling, breeding can be conducted in a manner comparable to standard practices for mice and rats (for subtle
differences, see Oettle, 1967; Soga, 1977b). Experience in
different laboratories is that once a female mastomys has
demonstrated cannibalism, either by eating her own infants
or the male, she will not be successful in breeding and
should be discarded from the breeding program. Combined
data of reproduction performance from three sources are
given in Table 19.

Genetic Stocks Available

Random Bred

Most colonies maintained presently are random bred. Random bred colonies are located in Germany, Japan, The
Netherlands, South Africa, the United Kingdom, and the
United States. Most of these colonies either originated
directly from stock in Johannesburg, South Africa, or
from the colony established at the National Institutes

TABLE 19   Reproductive Performance of Mastomys

	Fujii et al. (1966), Random Bred	Soga et al. (1969), Random Bred	Hollander et al. (1978) Random	
			Bred	Inbred
Weaning rate (percent)	37.4	60.8	75.3	38.8
Average number of newborn per litter	6.3	5.4	5.6	5.7
Average number of young weaned per litter	2.3	3.2	4.2	2.2

of Health, U.S.A., which was also derived from Johannesburg stock (Soga, 1977a). These animals have the natural coat color (dark grey) and black eyes. However, agouticolored mastomys with red eyes exist. These are derived from one female caught around Pretoria, South Africa, with a natural coat color and red eyes (C. G. Coetzee, Director, State Museum, Windhoek, South West Africa, Unpublished). The agouti-colored colony in Durban, South Africa, has a direct linkage with this mutant and most probably also the agouti-colored colony in Giessen, West Germany. Presently, the genealogy of the different mastomys colonies is being studied.

Inbred

Inbred colonies are presently being maintained at:

- Institute of Medical Science, Tokyo University, Japan
- Institute for Experimental Gerontology TNO, Rijswijk, The Netherlands
- Institut für Parasitologie, Justus Liebig-Universität, Giessen, West Germany

Factors Affecting Life Span

Infectious Diseases

Ectoparasites such as those found in mice have not been observed in laboratory-reared mastomys. Pinworms have been found and outbreaks of Tyzzer's disease have occurred (C. F. Hollander, Institute for Experimental Gerontology TNO, Rijswijk, The Netherlands, Unpublished). Sendai virus and mycoplasma infections have not been described. Mastomys has been shown to be susceptible to plague, to a host of parasitic diseases, and a number of ectoparasites in the wild (Oettle, 1967; Isaacson, 1975; Soga, 1977a). The effects of these organisms on life span are, in most cases, not known.

Spontaneously Occurring Diseases

Mastomys is unique in that the occurrence of neoplastic and nonneoplastic diseases (Table 20) far exceeds, in

TABLE 20   Neoplastic and Nonneoplastic Lesions Found
in Aging Mastomys[a]

Neoplastic Lesions	Nonneoplastic Lesions
Thymoma	Glomerulopathy (various
Hepatocellular neoplasms	degrees of severity)
Adenoma	Osteoarthritis (moderate
Carcinoma	and severe)
Reticulum cell sarcoma	Intervertebral disc
Gastric carcinoid	herniation
Insulinoma	Liver degeneration
Adrenocortical adenoma	Prostatitis
Granulosa cell tumor	Vesiculitis seminalis
Parathyroid adenoma	Myocarditis
Sarcoma[b]	Myositis
Mesothelioma	Thyroiditis
Squamous cell carcinoma	Sialadenitis
Prostatic papilloma	Gastric/duodenal
Renal cortical adenoma	ulceration
Rete testis papilloma	Arteritis
	Osteodystrophy

[a]From Solleveld, 1978.
[b]Undifferentiated sarcoma, fibrosarcoma, rhabdomyosarcoma,
and osteosarcoma.

number per animal and variety, their prevalance in other
rodents, particularly mice and rats (for recent reviews,
see Snell and Stewart, 1975; Soga and Sato, 1977; Solleveld, 1978). The influence of these diseases on life span
is apparently small, because the survival curves observed
for random-bred males and females at the Institute for
Experimental Gerontology TNO, The Netherlands, show a more
or less rectangular form that fits an aging population undisturbed by any specific cause of mortality (Figure 17).

Research Use

Due to the small size and aggressiveness of mastomys, procedures involving frequent sampling of body fluids are
difficult to conduct. However, other procedures can be
done without much difficulty. Mastomys are useful for
experiments involving single or multiple treatments.

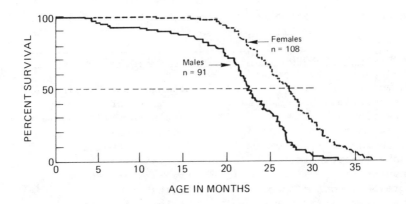

FIGURE 17 Survival curves of male and female mastomys.
Figure courtesy of the Institute for Experimental Gerontology TNO, Rijswijk, The Netherlands. The animals were
either found dead or were killed when they became moribund.

Positive titers for Lassa virus have been found in
wild-caught animals (Demartini et al., 1975), and mastomys
has been implicated in the epidemiology of naturally ocur-
ring Lassa fever in Africa. Because of this, restrictions
for its use in biomedical research have been initiated
in some countries. This hardly seems justified on the
basis of existing facts. Monath (1975) has stated that,
"since illness resembling Lassa fever has not been reported among scientists and auxiliary personnel working
with mastomys, it may be assumed with reasonable certain-
ty that the colonized animals do not harbor Lassa virus"
and, furthermore, "when the establishment of new colonies
of mastomys for biomedical research is contemplated,
breeder stock should be utilized from 'clean' colonies
already in existence." It seems, therefore, that established colonies of mastomys can be used safely for biomedical research. However, precautions should be taken
if, for any reason, capture of additional wild animals
for domestication is considered. It also is generally
recommended that precautions be taken to prevent animals
from escaping into geographical areas where they are not
naturally established.

Use in Research on Aging

Mastomys seems to be a promising animal for two areas of
research on aging. In this species, a broad variety of
auto-antibodies in combination with thymic abnormalities,
including hyperplasia and lymphoepithelial thymomas, have
been observed (H. H. Solleveld, Institute for Experimental
Gerontology, Rijswijk, The Netherlands, Unpublished).
Furthermore, no evidence for C-type virus production in
mastomys presently exists. Inbred strains are becoming
available; therefore, mastomys seems to be a more promising model for the study of autoimmunity than the NZB
mouse.

Sokoloff et al. (1967) have described, for the first
time in mastomys, degenerative joint disease and intervertebral disc herniation. These diseases also have been observed to occur spontaneously in the Rijswijk colony. It
seems warranted to exploit these lesions further, since
only limited information on these diseases exists in other
rodent species.

WHITE-FOOTED MICE

Peromyscus leucopus (the white-footed mouse), family
Cricetidae, is mouse-like in size and appearance. It is
ubiquitous throughout the United States, ranging from the
northeastern and north central United States through the
South and Southwest down to eastern Mexico and Yucatan.
The subspecies P. leucopus noveboracensis ranges through
the northeastern and north central United States about as
far west as the Missouri River. The high degree of speciation and subspeciation of the genus Peromyscus has made
it a favored taxon for students of population biology,
evolutionary genetics, and ecology. There is a large
literature on such topics as cytogenetics and enzyme
polymorphisms (Pathak et al., 1973; Zimmerman et al.,
1978).

General Characteristics

The external measurements of P. leucopus are: head plus
body length, 90-100 mm; tail length, 63-97 mm; hind foot
length, 19-24 mm; and ear length, 13-16 mm (Hall and Kelson, 1959). Young adult body weights are in the range of
20-30 g. In body dimensions and visceral organ weights,

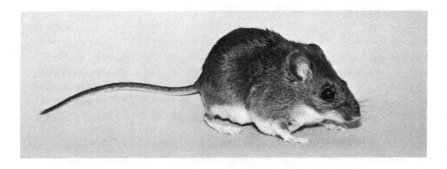

The white-footed mouse, <u>Peromyscus leucopus</u>. Photograph
courtesy of the Argonne National Laboratory, Argonne,
Illinois.

<u>P. leucopus</u> is not unlike a large laboratory mouse, but
there are major differences between the two species with
respect to brain weight and the size of the special sense
organs (Sacher and Hart, 1978). The brain of <u>P. leucopus</u>
weighs about 650 mg, approximately 50 percent more than a
typical mouse brain. The diameter of the eye is greater
in comparable degree, and the larger external ear suggests
that auditory acuity is also greater. This higher level
of neural and sensory endowment is characteristic for all
members of the genus <u>Peromyscus</u> and has made this genus
an important experimental resource for behavioral scientists (King, 1968).
  The external differences between <u>P. leucopus</u> and <u>P.
maniculatus</u> (the deermouse) are slight. <u>P. l. novebora-
censis</u> has a larger brain (650 mg) than <u>P. m. bairdii</u>
(600 mg) (King, 1965; G. A. Sacher, Division of Biological and Medical Research, Argonne National Laboratory,
Argonne, Illinois, Unpublished), and the eyeball is also
slightly larger. These differences may be related to the
more arboreal habitat of <u>P. leucopus</u>. Both species have
an unusual ability for adaptation and genetic differentiation, for <u>P. maniculatus</u>, which prefers grassland
habitats, ranges over most of North America below the
Arctic Circle and has a total of 45 subspecies, while <u>P.
leucopus</u>, which is confined to deciduous woodlands,
has 13 subspecies and covers most of the United States
east of the plains and the forested eastern side of Mexico (Hall and Kelson, 1959). The two species are about
equal in fecundity in captivity and superior to other
species of the genus in this respect. Both have maximum

life spans of about 96 months. They are widely used in laboratory and field research and are coming into prominence as indicator species for environmental pollution studies.

In biological terms there is little to choose between them, but P. leucopus has a large and growing documentation as a laboratory model for long-term toxicology studies and research on aging; it is already being used for the latter purpose in five laboratories: National Institute on Aging, Gerontology Research Center; Ohio State University; University of Washington Medical School; Michigan State University; and Argonne National Laboratory, which has separate colonies for research on aging and radiation toxicology. P. maniculatus, on the other hand, has been used extensively for behavioral research (King, 1968), but not for studies on aging.

Two closely related species of Peromyscus that deserve attention as possible laboratory species are P. polionotus (oldfield mouse) and P. gossypinus (cotton mouse). P. polionotus is native to the southeastern United States and is a member of the Maniculatus group, closely allied to P. maniculatus, while P. gossypinus, also native to the southeastern United States, is a member of the Leucopus group and is interfertile with P. leucopus. P. gossypinus is somewhat larger than P. leucopus (32 versus 22 g). Both P. polionotus and P. gossypinus are well adapted to laboratory breeding and maintenance. There are no lifetime survival data for P. polionotus, but P. gossypinus in the Argonne Laboratory colony is longer-lived than P. leucopus (average survival of 58.5 versus 46.4 months).

The differences in life expectation for captive populations of Peromyscus species seem to be due to differences in their vigor or disease resistance under the prevailing conditions of maintenance. It is entirely possible that the rank ordering of the longevities of these species will be considerably different in a different laboratory environment. The interfertile species pair P. leucopus and P. gossypinus are well suited for investigation of genotype-environment interactions governing survival in different artificial environments.

Life Span

Figure 18 gives survival curves for P. leucopus and three other Peromyscus species. The maximum attained longevity of P. leucopus in captivity is 100 months, and comparable

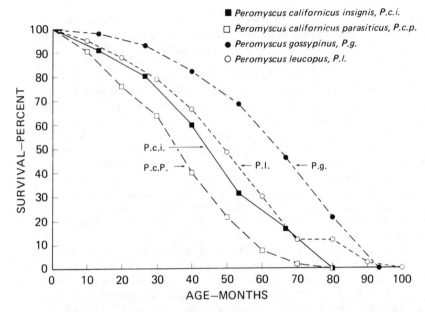

FIGURE 18   Survival curves for captive populations of
three species of Peromyscus.   Figure courtesy of G. A.
Sacher, Argonne National Laboratory, Argonne, Illinois.

maximum life spans have been recorded in other colonies.
The mean life expectation is 45.7 months for females and
47.7 months for males.   The longevity of P. leucopus is
consistent with data for six other Peromyscus species
maintained at Argonne National Laboratory.   Mean life
spans range from 34.6 months for P. californicus para-
siticus, which does not adapt well to the laboratory environment, to 64.6 months for P. eremicus (G. A. Sacher
and E. Staffeldt, Division of Biological and Medical Research, Argonne National Laboratory, Argonne, Illinois,
Unpublished).

Husbandry

The husbandry of the genus Peromyscus has been reviewed
by King (1968).   A satisfactory caging arrangement for
breeding and maintenance is the use of shoebox cages with
wood-chip bedding to a depth of 2.5 cm for breeding and
somewhat lesser depth for maintenance.   High cage

densities are not well tolerated. The standard at Argonne National Laboratory is to have no more than six white-footed mice in a shoebox cage that is 50 x 20 x 14 cm.

Health, fertility, and growth are adequately maintained with a good commercial laboratory rodent chow. Supplementation with natural foods has no perceptible beneficial effect. Breeding colonies at Argonne National Laboratory are maintained at 23°C on a light-dark schedule of 12 hours on and 12 hours off in spring and winter and with 15 hours on and 9 hours off in summer and fall. However, there is no evidence that these are the optimum conditions for breeding and maintaining this species.

In many ways, Peromyscus adapts to the laboratory environment within one generation better than some other species ever adapt. They are lively, but not overly excitable or aggressive, and they begin to breed readily. Wild-caught founder stocks are quickly freed of their ectoparasites, and subsequent generations remain free of ectoparasitic infestation. There are no indications of a stress syndrome in captivity. The absence of alopecia and dermatitis is a favorable feature.

Ease of Breeding

Sexual maturity is attained in about 6 weeks. Mating should be made at a later age than for laboratory mice, because matings made in early sexual maturity are more frequently infertile (Hill, 1974). Average litter size of P. l. noveboracensis is about five pups, and survival to weaning averages 80 percent in the Argonne colony. About 54 percent of the weanlings are males. P. leucopus and P. maniculatus are about equal in fertility and superior to all other Peromyscus species tested. A considerable proportion of matings are infertile, but interchanging partners will sometimes restore fertility. Breeding is best done by means of pair matings, with culling of infertile pairs after a few months. The interval between litters is about 28 days for a producing female.

Genetic Stocks Available

Breeding colonies of various Peromyscus species are maintained in several universities and research stations, but so far as is known, the colony of P. l. noveboracensis

maintained at Argonne National Laboratory is the only one
that has been defined in terms of actuarial and pathological characteristics of aging. No effort is presently
being made to produce an inbred strain of P. leucopus or
of any other member of the genus.

All species in the genus Peromyscus posseses a diploid
number of 48 chromosomes; however, the total number of
chromosome arms varies from 56 to 96 (Pathak et al., 1973).
Several coat color and other mutants have been described,
but few chromosome markers have yet been identified.

Factors Affecting Life Span

Infectious Diseases

Routine serological testing of P. leucopus for antibodies
to nine murine viruses has been carried out at Argonne National Laboratory for about 10 years, and until recently
P. leucopus has been found to be uniformly negative for
all nine. Recently, weak positive titers to Sendai virus
and pneumonia virus of mice (PVM) have been detected; however, no adverse health effects have been associated with
the appearance of these viruses (G. A. Sacher, Unpublished).

The only other potential pathogen routinely isolated
from P. leucopus at Argonne National Laboratory has been
Pasteurella pneumotropica. Again, no adverse health effects have been associated with it (G. A. Sacher, Unpublished).

Wild populations of P. leucopus are reservoirs for
babesiasis, a blood parasite (Healy et al., 1976), but
laboratory populations have not yet been implicated as
vectors for human or laboratory animal diseases.

Spontaneous Diseases

These disease categories in P. leucopus have been studied
in more than 200 histologically confirmed autopsies of
old animals. The following summarizes the tumor patterns
found in P. leucopus (Sacher and Hart, 1978).

The characteristic spontaneous tumors among Peromyscus leucopus maintained at Argonne National Laboratory include hepatocellular carcinoma, mammary ductal
carcinoma, and lymphoreticular and bone tumors. A

second type of liver cell tumor, hepatoblastoma, also occurs. The mammary carcinomas are commonly of the ductal type and are locally invasive, with metastasis most often to regional lymph nodes. This contrasts to mammary tumors in Mus, which metastasize primarily to lung. Other types of mammary tumors seen in Peromyscus include scirrhous carcinoma and undifferentiated carcinomas. Lymphoreticular tumors are predominantly of the solitary nonthymic type. The sole example of a generalized lymphoreticular tumor is the histiocytic lymphoma. Primary lung tumors are a rarity in Peromyscus. Only one minute subpleural alveologenic tumor nidus has been observed. Other types of tumors of interest for their potential use as models of human cancers include: papillary adenocarcinoma of the ovary with associated carcinomatosis and mineral concretions, endometrial adenocarcinoma, and choriocarcinoma. (p. 80)

There is no direct evidence that autoimmune disease in P. leucopus is a serious complicating factor in the aging processes of this species.

Research Use

All experimental procedures that can be carried out with laboratory mice can also be conducted with Peromyscus, for it is rather similar in body size. The somewhat larger brain and cranium of P. leucopus may make some neurosurgical procedures more convenient in this species.

A great advantage of the genus Peromyscus is that the wild-type genome always is available in the locality where the founder stock was collected. Also, the fact that one subspecies, such as P. l. noveboracensis or P. m. bairdii, is distributed over a dozen northeastern states means that populations can be collected in different parts of the range and yield a diverse pool of genes for eventual study. Thus, the real resource is not simply a closed laboratory population, but rather the entire gene pool available from the populations in their natural habitats.

Use in Research on Aging

P. leucopus seems to have a more deterministic growth in body length and weight than do the laboratory rat or mouse

(Duffy and Sacher, 1976). Head plus body length reaches a stable value at about 6 months of age and does not increase significantly thereafter. In comparison, head plus body length of laboratory rats and mice continues to grow for about two-thirds of their respective life spans. Concomitantly, body weight continues to increase until after cessation of linear growth, tending to decrease rather rapidly thereafter. This two-phase weight trend is not seen in P. leucopus, which maintains a constant or very slowly decreasing body weight throughout almost the entire adult life span. This skeletal growth pattern of P. leucopus resembles that of man and most large animal species, which suggests that P. leucopus or a comparable peromyscine may be a more appropriate model for lifetime metabolic and endocrinological studies than the laboratory rat or mouse.

P. leucopus, like the laboratory mouse, experiences a major loss of capacity for voluntary motor activity with age. Energy expenditure diminishes by more than 50 percent over the adult life span and, in this regard, P. leucopus may be quantitatively very similar to humans (Duffy and Sacher, 1976).

The basic reason for establishing P. leucopus as a laboratory model species is that P. leucopus is an intrinsically long-lived animal. The comparison of P. leucopus to short-lived, closely related rodent species may provide a basis for understanding the factors governing longevity (Sacher, 1966; Hart and Setlow, 1974; Sacher and Hart, 1978; Storer, 1978; Hart et al., 1979).

The following areas of research are appropriate for the comparison of Peromyscus and short-lived rodents:

● Analysis of the molecular basis for longevity, such as mechanisms for DNA repair, immune competence, and free radical scavenging systems.

● Analysis of the systemic mechanisms for physiological regulation and homeostasis to determine how long-lived and short-lived animals differ in the neuroendocrine regulation of growth, reproduction, and physiological adaptation.

● Analysis of the role of the central nervous system in behavioral homeostasis and in the maintenance of integrated rhythms and patterns of performance.

OTHER RODENTS

Two long-lived genera of the family Muridae, subfamily
Murinae, are Apodemus (from northern Eurasia) and Notomys
(Australian hopping mouse). In this same subfamily are
the short-lived genera, Mus and Praomys (Mastomys). Notomys has a longevity of 6 years or more and a 2.5-times
larger brain than Mus. The increase, beyond the values
for Mus, of brain size, and presumably of life span as
well, occurred during the Pleistocene period (a period of
2-3 million years). This makes the Notomys:Mus pair an
interesting model for the evolution of human longevity,
because almost the same factors of increase of hominid
life span and brain size occurred during the same geolog-
ical period.

Among North American rodents, the cotton rat, Sigmodon
hispidus, deserves attention as a model for aging. Its
short life span (Figure 19) is comparable to mastomys,
but it is more available than mastomys to American researchers. The size of the cotton rat (about 150 g)
makes it convenient for some biochemical procedures. A
closely related, long-lived rodent that is comparable in
body size is the wood or pack rat, genus Neotoma. These
animals live about as long as Peromyscus.

One feature of rodents that offers great potential for
research on aging is the presence of torpor and annual
hibernation. The hamster is widely used for studies concerning these phenomena, but rodents of the suborder Sci-
uromorpha (Figure 2), such as the chipmunks (Tamias) and
ground squirrels (Spermophilus), also have highly developed hibernation behavior. Pocket mice (Perognathus)
have the useful characteristic that the investigator can
modify the duration of daily torpor and the average daily
energy metabolism by controlling the food ration. However, rodents of this suborder are difficult to breed in
captivity. The small rodents also have strong daily cycles of activity and strong endogenous circadian rhythms.
This makes them good models for studies on the relation
of aging to physiological dyschronism of external and internal origin.

An advantage of using wild-type rodents is the great
degree of genetic polymorphism. This is useful, for example, in identifying new histocompatibility alleles or
in examining the genetic structure for specific kinds of
DNA repair. Lesser known rodents also offer good opportunities for the development of inexpensive models for

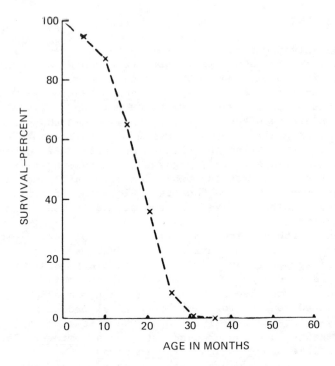

FIGURE 19 Survival curve for a captive
population of the cotton rat (Sigmodon
hispidus). Adapted from Sacher, 1977.

age-related diseases. For example, the sand rat, Psammomys, is an example of a rodent model for diabetes mellitus (Hachek et al., 1967; Strasser, 1968).

RABBITS

The laboratory rabbit (Oryctolagus cuniculus has not been
used widely in research on aging in the United States;
most publications concerning aging of rabbits are of European origin. Background information on the rabbit, including origin, domestication, taxonomy, genetics, breed
size, etc., has been reviewed by Fox (1974, 1975). The
text, The Biology of the Laboratory Rabbit (Weisbroth et
al., 1974), is a comprehensive review of what is known
about the rabbit and provides an extensive bibliography.

An update on the nutrition of the rabbit is given in
Nutrient Requirements of Rabbits (BARR, 1977).

General Characteristics

The rabbit is well adapted to the laboratory. It is large
enough to provide adequate quantities of tissue and can be
maintained economically. Baseline hematological, biochemical, and physiological data are available, and repeated
assays of these parameters are feasible throughout the
life span of the rabbit.

The published values for hematological, physiological,
and biochemical parameters vary with strain, age, sex,
and time of day (Fox, 1974, 1975; Kozma et al., 1974; van
Zutphen and Fox, 1977; Fox and Cherry, 1978; Fox et al.,
1978; and Skow et al., 1978). The rabbit neutrophil
(heterophil or pseudoeosinophil) has unique morphological
characteristics (Kozma et al., 1974). The eosin staining
granules of the neutrophil are much smaller than the granules in the rabbit's true eosinophils. The rabbit erythrocyte has a life span of about 50 days. Rabbit urine
contains much sediment, but many analytical tests can
still be performed (Kozma et al., 1974).

Some data on growth are available both for large and
small strains of rabbits. Crary and Sawin (1960) have
shown that three partially inbred strains of rabbits are
still growing at 210 days. This growth is based on
weight gain in grams and is probably due to an increase
in adipose tissue, and not necessarily to skeletal
growth. Mature weight may vary from 2 to 16 kg depending on factors such as breed and sex (Fox, 1974). In
general, growth rate is inversely proportional to the
adult size, but is also affected by season of birth.

Life Span

Good data on life span are very difficult to obtain since
most rabbit breeders cull animals as reproduction declines. It is difficult to find rabbits older than 5
years of age in most laboratories; however, some animals
still are fertile at this age. Good actuarial data are
nonexistent. Available data suggest a usual life span of
approximately 8 years (Weisbroth, 1974), although a report by Flower (1931) gives a possible life span of 13
years.

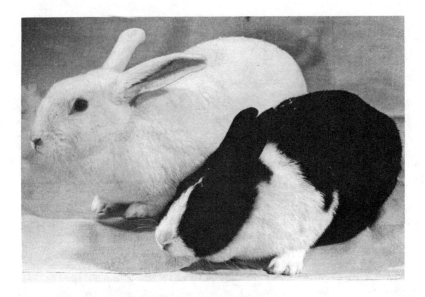

Two strains of rabbit (Oryctolagus cuniculus). Left,
fully inbred strain III/J; right, partially inbred OS/J.
Photograph courtesy of The Jackson Laboratory, Bar Harbor,
Maine.

Husbandry

Guidelines for husbandry and veterinary care for rabbits
are given in the Guide for the Care and Use of Laboratory
Animals (ILAR, 1978a). The rabbit, with its thick fur and
general lack of sweat glands, adapts much more readily to
a cool than to a warm environment; it will do well, even
while raising a litter, in an ambient temperature as low
as -18°C. An ambient temperature within animals quarters
of 16-19°C with low humidity is comfortable for rabbits.
Extreme heat can result in heat prostration and death.
If the temperature exceeds 32°C, temporary sterility may
result.
    There are several recent reviews of the nutritional
requirements of the rabbit (Hagen, 1974; Hunt and Harrington, 1974; BARR, 1977). There are marked strain differences in the rabbit's response to ad libitum feeding
(R. R. Fox, The Jackson Laboratory, Bar Harbor, Maine,
Unpublished); some strains add weight (as adipose tissue)

very quickly, others do not. Obesity can best be avoided by limiting the food intake. Guidelines on feeding are available from many food manufacturers. Water should always be available to rabbits ad libitum.

Ease of Breeding

The rabbit, unlike some other members of the order Lagomorpha, e.g., the hare (Lepus), breeds well in the laboratory. It is a reflex ovulator with ovulation occurring about 10 hours after copulation. The gestation period is approximately 31 days. The rabbit starts to eat solid food at about 14 days of age; weaning occurs between 4 and 8 weeks. Growth increases to a peak rate by about 40 days of age and then declines to maturity. General growth landmarks include the onset of fusion of the proximal tibia at approximately 60 days of age; beginning of follicular development at 90 days, with full follicular development and puberty at approximately 120 days; and complete fusion of the proximal tibia about 170 days of age (Crary and Sawin, 1960). Rabbits should be 5 to 8 months old before breeding. It is also recommended that a doe be rebred when the young are about 4 weeks of age. The female always should be brought to the male's cage for breeding and then returned to her own. Artificial insemination is accomplished easily with rabbits (Hafez, 1970; Hagen, 1974).

Genetic Stocks Available

Inbred, partially inbred, and hybrid rabbits currently are available from only a few research colonies (Institute of Laboratory Animal Resources [ILAR], National Research Council, National Academy of Sciences, Washington, D.C., Unpublished). Random-bred, line-bred, and a few partially inbred stocks of specific breeds of rabbit are available from reputable suppliers (ILAR, 1979a). Some rabbit vendors supply animals from several sources. This can influence the repeatability of experiments and can pose serious disease problems.

Factors Affecting Life Span

Infectious Diseases

The life span is increased in rats and mice that are freed
from the burden of infectious disease (Weisbroth, 1972).
It is likely, although not yet established, that this also
applies to rabbits. Among the common infectious agents
that affect studies on aging are Pasteurella multocida
(pasteurellosis), Bacillus piliformis (Tyzzer's disease),
and Eimeria stiedae (hepatic coccidiosis). These pathogens should be absent in any long-term study. Rabbits
that are free of specific diseases (specific pathogen
free or SPF) are available, but are more expensive than
conventionally reared rabbits. The term SPF is meaning-
less without knowing what organisms or diseases the animal is free of. Salmonellosis and Pseudomonas infections
are not major disease problems in rabbits. Ulcerative
pododermatitis (sore hocks), believed to be associated in
part with the type of flooring, should be treated as soon
as observed to preclude secondary infections (Flatt et
al., 1974).

Spontaneously Occurring Diseases

Neoplasms in the rabbit are related to age and sex (Weisbroth, 1974). Frequently observed tumors include malignant lymphomas and uterine adenocarcinomas. Atherosclerosis may develop as the animals age and may be modified
by both diet and genetic background (Clarkson et al.,
1974; van Zutphen and Fox, 1977). A genetic influence on
the prevalence of glomerulonephritis has been noted at
The Jackson Laboratory, Bar Harbor, Maine (R. R. Fox,
Unpublished).

Nutrition

Ad libitum feeding causes obesity, fatty liver, reduced
fertility, increased frequency of atherosclerotic plaques,
and premature death in rabbits of certain genetic backgrounds. Similarly, the feeding of a 0.5 percent cholesterol diet will result in a high serum cholesterol level
in some stocks, but not in others (van Zutphen and Fox,
1977). Trichobezoars (hairballs) in the stomach have been
associated with a lack of roughage in the diet. The

reason for the ingestion of hair is not clear (Flatt
et al., 1974), but it can occasionally result in death.

Other Factors

Inadequate ventilation may result in high ammonia levels,
drafts, and high humidity in room air and can predispose
to respiratory infections. Good data on the effects of
sound, extreme heat, and other stressors on the life span
of rabbits or other species are lacking. A low level of
background music may help minimize any adverse effects of
noise or other stressors. Calm and gentle handling of
rabbits also reduces stress. The handling should include
providing proper support to the rabbit's hind quarters to
prevent vertebral fracture.

Research Use

Techniques for Use

For surgical procedures, a variety of anesthetics are used
either singly or in combination. Anesthetic agents should
be given to effect, because individual responses are unpredictable (Bivin and Timmons, 1974). The most widely
used barbiturate, pentobarbital sodium (approximately 25
mg/kg), may be used safely for anesthesia provided it is
administered slowly. Another good regimen is ketamine
(44 mg/kg IM), followed 10 minutes later by xylazine (6-8
mg/kg IM). Administration of ketamine may be repeated if
required (A. L. Kraus, University of Rochester Medical
Center, Rochester, New York, Unpublished). Blood samples
can be obtained repeatedly from the marginal ear veins or
medial arteries, using a simple drip method, hematocrit
tube, vacuum ear bleeder (Hoppe et al., 1969), or a vacu-
tainer (Cohen, 1955). Intravenous injections are easily
accomplished using the marginal ear veins. Physiological
measurements such as blood pressure, heart rate, respiration rate, and electrocardiograms have been described
(Lepeschkin and Wilson, 1951; and Kozma et al., 1974).
Stereotaxic coordinates have been determined (Poisson et
al., 1974).

Use in Research on Aging

Some of the physiological and biochemical changes that
occur in the rabbit with increasing age are presented in
Table 21. Despite the fact that little information is
available on the life span of the rabbit, the physiological data presented here, based primarily on the first 5
years of life, indicate a use for the rabbit in research
on aging in areas where the rodents appear to be less
suitable.

TABLE 21 Changes in Physiological and Biochemical
Parameters in the Rabbit (Oryctolagus cuniculus) with
Increasing Age

System	Changes with Increasing Age	Reference
Blood		
Affinity of hemoglobin for oxygen	Decreases	Gladilov and Irzhak, 1975
Cholesterol level	Increases	Nasledova
β-lipoprotein content	Increases	and
Sugar level on fasting or 2 hours after glucose loading	Increases	Silnit-sky, 1972
Lymphocytes		Katosova, 1977
succinic dehydrogenase	Decreases	
acid phosphatase	Decreases	
β-glycerophosphate	Increases	
Vasopressin content	Increases	Frol'kis et al., 1976
Cardiovascular		
Arterial pressure	More sensi-tive to angiotensin administration	Pugach, 1975

TABLE 21 (continued)

System	Changes with Increasing Age	Reference
Atherosclerosis	Due to break-down in com-pensatory processes of repairing metabolic disorder	Gorev and Stupina, 1973; Kozhura, 1976a
Contractility of left ventricle myocardium	Decreases	Gorev and Cherka-ski^{V}i, 1976
Systolic blood pressure	Increases	
Hemodynamic parameters		Shevchuk,
cardiac output	Decreases	1973;
stroke volume	Decreases	Stroganova,
cardiac index	Decreases	1975;
contractility index	Decreases	Frol'kis
vascular resistance	Increases	et al., 1977
Enzymes of glucose oxidation	All increase after low	Mikhaylova and Na-
Breakdown from rabbit aortas	point at 1-2 years	dirova, 1977
hexokinase		
glucose-6-phosphate dehydrogenase		
6-phosphogluconate dehydrogenase		
cytochrome c oxidase		
Energy balance of the heart		Frol'kis
oxygen consumption	Decreases	and Bo-
muscle glycolysis	Increases	gatskaya,
adenosine triphosphate concentration	Decreases	1967
respiratory process with phosphorylation	Increases	
adaptive ability	Becomes restricted	

TABLE 21   (continued)

System	Changes with Increasing Age	Reference
Pulmonary arteries	Thicken from 3 months on. Also histological changes are evident	Grebenskaya, 1966
Vascular permeability	Decreases	Kozhura, 1967b

Endocrine

Adrenal gland	Degenerative changes	Lvovich et al., 1974
Fat mobilizing response to exogenous lipotropic hormone	Decreases	
Neuro-humoral sensitivity to catecholamines		Frol'kis et al., 1968
threshold responses	Triggered by smaller doses	
reactive ability	Decreased	
tolerance	Decreased	
Plasma testosterone	Decreases from peak at 90 days	Berger et al., 1976

Joints

Articular cartilage	Synthesis of chondroitin-4-sulfate decreases with respect to synthesis of chondroitin-6-sulfate	Mankin and Thrasher, 1977

TABLE 21 (continued)

System	Changes with Increasing Age	Reference
Nervous		
Catecholamine content of nervous fibers and ganglia of the sympathetic nervous system	Decreases	Klimenko, 1975
Hippocampus	Increased amplitude of epileptiform discharges in response to electrical stimulation	Gusel' and Grigor'eva, 1975
Hypothalamus and amygdala	Excitability changes	Frol'kis et al., 1974
Visual		
Choroid	Ultrastructural changes correlating with toxico-allergic uveitis	Kovalevsky and Stebaeva, 1973
Descemet's membrane	Progressively more laminated	Vo^{V}ino-Iasenetski^{V}i and Dumbrova, 1974
Uveal tract	Toxico-allergic uveitis with correlated changes in epinephrine and serotonin content	Proshina, 1973

Carnivores

INTRODUCTION

Only two species of the order Carnivora, which consists
of 7 families and 101 genera (Walker, 1975c), have great
popularity as pets and are widely used in research--the
domestic dog (Canis familiaris) and the domestic cat
(Felis catus). In the United States alone, there are an
estimated 41.3 million dogs and 23.1 million cats kept as
family pets (Pet Food Institute, 1978). The U.S. Department of Agriculture (USDA) records more than 197,000 dogs
and 65,000 cats used in research between October 1, 1977
and September 30, 1978 (USDA, 1979).

Dogs and cats are appropriate models for the study of
aging since many aspects of age-related changes in organ
structure and function mimic the aging process in man, and
many age-related diseases of these species are similar to
those of man. The pet population has an important place
in research on aging because these animals live under the
same environmental conditions as their owners throughout
their life spans. Retrospective data are available
through veterinary hospitals.

Dogs are used in many areas of biomedical research;
cats have been favored for certain types of research, particularly neurophysiological studies. Increasing attention has been given to the spontaneous and induced diseases of both dogs and cats that mimic human diseases.

BIOLOGY, HUSBANDRY, AND DISEASE

Because of their long history of domestication, much is
known about the biology, husbandry, and diseases of dogs
and cats (Andersen, 1970). The several breeds of dogs

and cats have a broad range of phenotypic characteristics, especially size, conformation, and hair coat. Some of these differences may be used to advantage in selecting animals of particular breeds for laboratory investigations.

The Code of Federal Regulations (CFR), Title 9, provides the minimum standards that must be met for the care and maintenance of dogs and cats. The Institute of Laboratory Animal Resources (ILAR), National Academy of Sciences, has prepared several publications that consider not only the general care and use of laboratory animals (ILAR, 1978a), but also specific information on dogs and cats (ILAR, 1973, 1978b). The Board on Agriculture and Renewable Resources (BARR), National Academy of Sciences, has published information on the nutritional requirements of dogs and cats (BARR, 1974, 1978a).

In the laboratory setting, most cats and dogs are fed commercial diets that conform to, or in some cases exceed, the minimum standards provided in the references noted above. If the dogs or cats are laboratory reared, it is quite likely that their nutritional history will be known, even if it is not controlled as an experimental variable. Companion animals presented at clinics or random-source dogs and cats may be fed commercially prepared diets, table scraps, or some combination thereof, and it is quite likely that the dietary history of a given animal will not be known.

Diseases of dogs and cats, oriented primarily toward the medical and surgical problems of pet animals, have been reviewed (Ettinger and Suter, 1970; Osborne et al., 1972; Archibald, 1974; Bojrab, 1975; Ettinger, 1975; Muller and Kirk, 1976; Kirk, 1977; Siegel, 1977). These texts have general applicability to dogs and cats maintained in the research environment, although, typically, the research environment provides a much greater degree of protection from accidental injury and exposure to infectious agents and environmental toxicants than is accorded companion animals.

SPECIAL STOCKS AVAILABLE

There are numerous breeds of dogs and cats; however, with the exception of Beagles and "Mill Hill" cats, or in situations where the genetics of a specific disease have been of interest, there has been little attention given to the genetic background of dogs or cats used for laboratory investigations. A major obstacle to developing

genetically defined stocks of either dogs or cats is their
relatively long gestation period (61-63 days) and age of
sexual maturity (6 months).

Perhaps the best genetically defined cats are the "Mill
Hill" cats, which were originated by the British Medical
Research Council in the 1960s. This colony of minimal
disease cats was established using cesarean-derivation/
barrier-maintenance methods to provide subjects with respiratory tracts free of indigenous disease for inhalation
toxicity studies. This project demonstrated the feasi-
bility of establishing and maintaining cats free from
significant infectious diseases for biomedical research
(Festing and Bleby, 1970). Since then, specific pathogen-
free and germfree cat colonies have been established at
several locations in the United States (Rohovsky et al.,
1966).

In the United States, the majority of dogs produced
specifically for laboratory use are Beagles. Major im-
petus for the use of the Beagle in laboratory investigations has come from their use in studies of radiation-
induced disease. Six major colonies have been initiated
for this purpose: in the early 1950s at the University
of Utah and Argonne National Laboratory, in the late 1950s
at the University of California-Davis and Battelle-Pacific
Northwest Laboratory, and in the early 1960s at Colorado
State University and Lovelace Inhalation Toxicology Research Institute. The early history of the University of
Utah colony has been described (Rehfeld et al., 1972).
In general, all of the colonies were started with breeders
selected primarily by phenotypic characteristics. Selection of successive generations of breeding stock has tak-
en into account not only the phenotype of the stock, but
also pedigree and reproductive performance of the parents.
Increasingly, as the colonies have become better established, more concern has been directed to the genetics
of the colony.

The Lovelace colony is an example of the use of a specialized breeding program to maintain a stable gene pool
as a basis for entry of dogs into a series of sequential
and interrelated experiments (Bielfeldt et al., 1969).
In 1967, a parental generation was selected to obtain a
broad genetic base relatively free of physical defects
and possible undesirable familial tendencies toward epi-
lepsy. Each breeding generation has included 20 males
and 40 females, with subsequent generations containing
one son and two daughters per sire and one daughter and
not more than one son per dam. With the exclusion of

brother-sister matings, initial breeding assignments are
randomized with lifetime pairing established between each
male and two females. The system has been used successfully for over 10 years.

Life Span

Dogs

Much anecdotal information on the life span of pet dogs
and cats is available. The maximum age reached by domestic cats and dogs is in excess of 20 years (Comfort,
1956). The longevity of pet dogs and cats is influenced
strongly by infectious diseases and trauma. It has been
shown that Beagles released to private owners (field dogs)
do not survive as long as female Beagles maintained in
the laboratory (Andersen, 1958). This early mortality is
related largely to accidental deaths such as from motor
vehicle accidents. When the accidental deaths are treated as if the dog is lost to follow-up, the life table
method of Cutler and Ederer (1958) shows the probability
of survival of the field and laboratory dogs through 10
years of age is nearly identical.
  The most useful life span data available have been obtained from observations of control populations of Beagles
in laboratories that have used dogs to study radiation effects. Birth data, clinical records, date of death, and
major findings at death have been available, because the
animals have been reared and maintained in the laboratories. Under these conditions, the 50 percent survival of
57 control female Beagles was 12 to 13 years (Andersen
and Rosenblatt, 1965). A later report (Andersen and
Rosenblatt, 1969) notes a median survival of 12.6 years
with some dogs living in excess of 15 years. Approximately half of the dogs have been bred and have whelped
litters between 1 and 4 years of age. The median survival
time of the bred and nonbred dogs is not different. The
major causes of death were acute diseases (14.6%), chronic
diseases (20.8%), reproductive disorders (2.1%), and neoplasms (62.5%).
  The survival of 409 male and 465 female control Beagles
from the University of Utah (Jee, 1978), Pacific Northwest
Laboratory (1979), University of California-Davis (Book et
al., 1979) and Lovelace Inhalation Toxicology Research Institute (Henderson et al., 1978) Beagle colonies has been
evaluated (Redman, 1980) using the method of Cutler and

Ederer (1958). Cumulative survival rates of Beagles are plotted in Figure 20.

Incidence rates for malignant and benign neoplasms in Beagles from colonies at the Lovelace Inhalation Toxicology Research Institute and University of California-Davis, and pet Beagles in the Animal Neoplasm Registry (1967-1974) of the University of California, Davis, are of interest in considering life span. The total gross tumor incidence rate for both sexes for the total population is 2,430 per 10^5 population, with 1,815 and 615 per 10^5 population for benign and malignant tumors, respectively. The total adjusted tumor incidence rate for the above population is 3,542 per 10^5 population with rates of 2,527

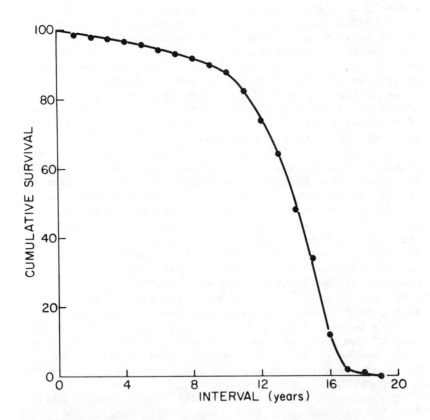

FIGURE 20 Combined male and female survival distribution for Beagles. Figure courtesy of H. Redman, Lovelace Inhalation Toxicology Research Institute, Albuquerque, New Mexico.

and 1,014 per 10^5 population for benign and malignant tumors, respectively. The total crude and adjusted population rate is lower for the privately owned dogs than for the laboratory colonies.

Equivalent age-grouped data on man and dog have been calculated (LeBeau, 1953). Human tumor incidence data from the Third National Cancer Survey (NCI, 1971) are compared in Table 22 with dog age-grouped data for all malignant neoplasms of the purebred Beagle study populations. Age-specific crude incidence rates for the Beagle and man increase with age for all systems. The adjusted rates for malignant tumors for all systems of the Beagle population and man are 1,011 and 364 per 10^5 population, respectively. For the crude incidence rate, there was an excess of malignant tumors in man in the respiratory, digestive, and urogenital systems, and for the adjusted rate, in the respiratory system.

As noted earlier, there are relatively limited survival data on dogs maintained under carefully controlled conditions and for a sufficiently long time period to allow detailed life table analyses. The most extensive data are for the Beagle, without comparable data for other breeds. Anecdotal data, however, do provide a basis for qualitative comparisons among breeds (Comfort, 1964). Larger breeds, such as Boxers and St. Bernards, have shorter life spans than the Beagle, whereas some of the very small breeds have longer life spans. The shorter life span of some of the larger dog breeds generally is related to a breed disposition to certain diseases, for example, osteosarcoma in the Boxer. Detailed life table analyses of survival and cause of death data on several breeds of

TABLE 22 Crude Incidence Rates of Malignant Tumors in Beagles and Man

Malignant Tumors	Crude Incidence Rate (per 10^5 population)	
	Beagle	Man
All systems	615	287
Mammary gland	261	39
All systems minus mammary gland	354	248

dogs might provide insight into the basis for the difference in life span.

Cats

Survival data on cats maintained under defined conditions
are even more meager than for dogs. The cause of death in
pet cats more than 10 years old and the pathological findings in aged pet cats from animal hospital populations
have been reported (Jones and Zook, 1965; Jones and Gilmore, 1968; Hamilton et al., 1969). Neoplasms (other than
leukemias) increase significantly with age. In cats between 4 and 9 years of age, trauma is a common cause of
death or disease. There is an age-related increase in
medial hypertrophy of the pulmonary arteries in cats.
Urolithiasis is a frequent cause of death in males. Castrated cats appear to live longer than intact males. The
oldest of the 30 surviving cats in the EPA colony at Research Triangle Park is approximately 15 years of age.
All members of this colony have been carefully necropsied,
and tissues are available for retrospective study (E.
Berman, Experimental Biology Division, Health Effects Research Laboratory, Research Triangle Park, North Carolina,
Unpublished), making this a potentially useful source of
material for histopathological study of organs from cats
of known age.

ADVANTAGES AND DISADVANTAGES OF USING DOGS AND CATS

Advantages in the use of dogs and cats for biomedical research, including research on aging, are: (1) an abundance
of information on normal biology, husbandry, and diseases;
(2) ease of evaluation as clinical subjects using many diagnostic procedures routinely used on man; and (3) ease of
handling because investigators and supporting staff are
familiar with these animals. In addition, the housing,
although space-consuming, need not be elaborate. Likewise, commercially prepared diets are readily available.
    Both animals have a relatively long life span. This
makes it hard to obtain data over the life span of a given
subject, but it permits subtle effects due to aging and
deleterious influences to accumulate and, ultimately, to
reach a level that may be detected. The long life span
and genetic heterogeneity of most dog and cat populations

allows most breeds to manifest a variety of natural
diseases not overshadowed by a single disease entity.
Ample amounts of fluid and tissue can readily be obtained
from a single subject. Sampling and observation can be
facilitated through the use of implanted catheters, physiological detectors, and various surgical procedures.
Serial sampling procedures usually are feasible.

The major limitations to use of the dog and, to a lesser extent, the cat for research are the cost and space
requirements for maintaining large numbers of individuals.
This sharply constrains the use of large groups of animals
and emphasizes the importance of using dogs and cats in
those situations where detailed observation of individuals is of greater importance than observations of a population.

Dogs of known parentage and that are well characterized
as to previous and current health are expensive to produce. Only a few research laboratories with special and
continuing needs have been able to develop breeding colonies. A number of commercial breeding establishments have
been started to meet the demand for high-quality dogs;
however, the supply and demand have fluctuated, so the
cost of individual dogs also has fluctuated substantially.

Recognizing that many procedures used to study aging in
cats and dogs do not require surgical intervention and do
not compromise the health of the subject, it is apparent
that many procedures could be performed on pets. Both
cross-sectional studies of animals of different ages and
longitudinal studies of the same individuals might be performed and yield useful information. Although the background (pedigree, diet, and health history) might not be
as well known as that of animals reared and maintained in
the laboratory, pets may offer an advantage in some situations due to their maintenance in an environment
essentially identical to that of the owner. Clinical observations made on pets at private and university veterinary clinics would result in the identification of large
numbers of animals with age-related diseases relevant to
studies on human aging. Such a screening approach has
been used successfully, as for example, in selecting animals with various genetically determined defects, which
have been used as breeding stock to produce affected offspring. Animals of differing age presented for necropsy
may provide a wealth of material for detailed pathological
evaluation. Studies of this type using pets not only can

yield information relevant to man, but also can result in
new knowledge about the diseases that affect pet animals.
This is important because of the role pets play as companions to aged people.

RESEARCH USE OF DOGS AND CATS

Studies of structure, function, and age-related changes
and diseases of dogs and cats are reviewed in the following pages. Special attention has been directed to comparisons to man and identification of potential models of
human aging. For convenience, the review is organized on
a system basis. Of necessity, it is selective, both as
to the items covered and the depth of coverage.

Central Nervous System

In spite of the medical and social importance of nervous
system disorders in old people, extraordinarily little has
been done to establish authentic analogs of these human
diseases in experimental animals. Indeed, little is known
about aging of the nervous system of animals (Wisniewski,
1979). A few morphological surveys of brains have been
conducted, but they have involved relatively few animals
at less than advanced age. This approach has produced no
extraordinary examples of animal models of CNS diseases
associated with aging. Dogs and cats are the species most
frequently studied as "old" animals. Dayan (1971) has
surveyed the brains from 47 vertebrate species. Only a
few animals of each species were studied; in many instances the exact ages were not known. In sixteen 10- to
14-year-old dogs and eleven 7- to 10-year-old cats, lipofuscin deposits and neuroaxonal dystrophy commonly were
found, but argyrophilic plaques or neurofibrillary tangles
characteristic of senile changes in man were not observed.
Vascular lesions in the brains of aged dogs have been described by Von Braunmuhl (Dayan, 1971), Dahme (1962), and
Osetowska (1966).
    Lipofuscin pigment often is found in human and animal
brains, and is thought to increase with age. The relationship between neuronal ceroid-lipofuscinosis (Kuf's
disease) and increased lipofuscin pigment deposits in the
brain associated with aging is unclear; however, the use

of well-defined models of ceroid lipofucinosis in dogs
(Koppang, 1973; Cummings and Delahunta, 1977) and cats
(Green and Little, 1974) may be useful to elucidate fun-
damental mechanisms and relationships, if any, to aging.

Argyrophilic plaques are considered to be concomitant
with advanced age in man. They usually are not found before age 65 to 75, but increase substantially thereafter
(Dayan, 1970a,b). Plaques are found less frequently in
older animals. Von Braunmuhl (Dayan, 1971) has found
plaque-like structures in 3 of 20 dogs, 14 to 20 years
of age. Dahme (1962) and Osetowska (1966) also describe
plaques in brains of dogs 15 to 18 years old. Wisniewski
et al. (1970b) have described senile plaques with cerebral
amyloidosis in aged dogs.

Neurofibrillary tangles have been found in brains of
several species, although they differ ultrastructurally
from those found in man (Terry, 1968). Spontaneous CNS
diseases have been described in dogs (DeLahunta, 1975)
and cats (Vandevelde et al., 1976) in which accumulation
of neurofilaments is prominent; however, in both instances
the disease has affected young animals. Spheroid swellings of terminal axons, known as neuroaxonal dystrophy,
are associated with aging in man as well as in dogs (Newberne et al., 1960) and cats (Friede and Knoller, 1964).

It is generally accepted that chronology of the aging
process of man and other animals is analogous regardless
of actual life span. It might be argued that the biology
and natural history of the neuron is sufficiently unique
that changes in man at 70 years may not occur in old animals of 3 to 20 years. This thesis cannot be evaluated
with current knowledge. However, morphological changes
that characterize senescence of the brain of man also are
found in aged animals. Furthermore, the concentration of
attention on the study of brain changes in animals by
morphological methods ignores the powerful, sophisticated
tools of inquiry that form the foundation of modern neuroscience. Therefore, it is not possible to provide an
accurate assessment of the value of animal models for
study of human age-related CNS disease. The eminent position of domestic cats as subjects for morphophysiologi-
cal studies of the CNS suggests that this species should
be considered for use in systematic evaluations of aging
on the nervous system. Moreover, spontaneous and induced
diseases in dogs and cats may prove to be valuable models
for elucidating neuronal dysfunction associated with advanced age in man.

Skeletal System

Comparison of Bone Structure of Carnivores and Man

The dog skeleton is an excellent model for studying age-related changes in bone. It differs from that of man only in having a more rapid rate of bone remodeling. The Beagle commonly is used for research in this area.

The skeletal weight of an adult Beagle is 850 g, of which 174.4 g is calcium. A 70-kg man has a skeletal weight of 10,000 g, of which 1,000-1,200 g is calcium. About 80 percent of the bone mass both in man and dog is made up of cortical bone (Snyder et al., 1975). The average surface-to-volume ratios for man and dog are similar, 50 and 66 cm^2/cm^3, respectively (Lloyd and Hodges, 1971; Beddoe, 1977, 1978; Jee et al., 1978); the surface-to-volume ratio for trabecular bone is 4 times greater than for cortical bone.

Microscopically, adult bone tissue in both species is identical. The skeletons consist of lamellar bone in which collagenous bundles are organized into bone lamellae. Briefly, lamellar bone can be described as layers of collagen fibers 3 to 7 μm thick. In any one unit, all collagen fibers run approximately in the same direction, but in adjacent units, the axis differs by about 90°. The layers may be arranged more or less concentrically around a small vascular canal to form a haversian system or osteon in cortical bone or around large vascular and soft tissue cavities (marrow) to form a trabeculus or spicule in cancellous bone (Hancox, 1972). Both cortical and trabecular lamellar bones possess the capacity to renew themselves (Frost, 1969; Parfitt, 1976).

Morphological evidences of bone renewal are observed as (1) interstitial lamellae that are remnants of haversian systems in cortical bone and (2) trabecular bone packets outlined by a scalloped cement line (reversal line) and the bone surface in cancellous bone.

The cellular distribution on bone surfaces of adult man and Beagle is also quite similar. Active osteoblasts occupy about 5 percent of the free bone surface, osteoid seams about 15 percent, active osteoclasts in Howship's lacunae about 0.5 percent, and Howship's lacunae, (resorbed bone surface), at which bone remodeling is either quiescent or arrested, about 5 percent. The remaining 80-95 percent of the free bone surface is covered by an envelope of thin flattened cells, called bone-lining cells, surface osteocytes, or resting osteoblasts. Bone tissue from dog differs slightly from that of man, having a higher population of osteoblasts and osteoclasts (Merz and Schenk, 1970; Parfitt, 1976; Kimmel and Jee, 1978a,b). This higher percentage of osteoblasts and osteoclasts indicates a higher remodeling activity.

Man, monkey, dog, rabbit, and probably other large animals, but not rodent, turn over their skeleton by bone remodeling. The cellular basis of cortical bone remodeling proceeds with the excavation by osteoclasts of a longitudinal tunnel that is refilled by osteoblasts forming a new haversian system or osteon. This discrete structure, called a cortical remodeling unit, consists of a cutting cone (resorption cavity) or osteoclasts in front and a closing or filling cone (forming a haversian system) of osteoblasts behind. Cortical bone remodeling involves the birth rate of new remodeling cycles called activation frequency, the duration of the resorption or excavation period, the quiescent interval between resorption and formation, and the formation period. By direct measurement within the dog, the rate of resorption is about 40 μm/day for longitudinal resorption, 7 μm/day for radial resorption, and the length of the cutting cone averages about 400 μm (Jaworski and Lok, 1972). Bone apposition rates are about 1 μm/day, and the thickness of an osteonal wall is about 50 to 72 μm. Estimates of these parameters in man are comparable (Frost, 1969). The time taken for a cortical remodeling cycle is estimated to be about 60-100 days in both species (Parfitt, 1976). A comparison of cortical bone in ribs from a 1.5-year-old Beagle and a 24-year-old man shows that there is a greater number of osteoid seams, resorption cavities, and remodeling sites per unit area of cortex, and a higher bone formation rate in dog (Frost, 1969; Anderson and Danylchuk, 1979a,b). These values all suggest a higher bone turnover rate for dog as compared to man.

Because cancellous bone occupies only 20 percent of the total skeleton by volume, but has a surface to volume ratio of at least 4 times that of compact bone (Lloyd and Hodges, 1971), it is of great importance to know the extent of trabecular bone remodeling. A reconstruction of trabecular remodeling surface in three dimensions indicates that the trabecular remodeling unit resembles a haversian system that has been cut open longitudinally and unfolded over the trabecular surface (Jaworski, 1971). Consideration of the extensive data on cortical bone and more limited data on trabecular bone suggests that the

cortical bone cellular activity model may be applied to
both types of bone.

A recent study of 36 normal subjects with a mean age of
50.9 years has shown a mean wall thickness of remodeling
packets of trabecular bone of 49.7 $\pm$ 8.7 μm. With a bone
appositional rate of 0.72 μm/day, the average formation
time of iliac trabecular bone packets is 69 days (Lips et
al., 1978). Average formation time for trabecular remodeling packets cannot be calculated for dog, because measurements for trabecular mean wall thickness do not exist.
A best estimate is that this value is quite similar to
that for man.

A variety of kinetic and morphologic data indicate that
the rate of bone turnover is about 4 percent per annum in
man. Marshall et al. (1973) estimate that the turnover
rate of compact bone is about 2.5 percent/year and of cancellous bone is about 10 percent/year. The average calcium
accretion rate using the method of Bauer et al. (1957) is
about 18 percent/year. This measurement takes into account
new bone formation, secondary mineralization, and the exchange processes and can overestimate bone formation by at
least a factor of two. Calcium accretion rate in an old
mongrel has been shown to average 30 percent/year (Shimmins
et al., 1971). Morphological measurements of the iliac
trabecular bone turnover rates in young adult men and 2-
year-old Beagles have been found to be 32 and 194 percent/
annum, respectively (Marshall et al., 1973; Marotti, 1976;
Kimmel and Jee, 1978a; Jee et al., 1978). It must be kept
in mind that the cancellous bone of the iliac crest pos-
sesses one of the highest rates of trabecular bone turnover
(Jee et al., 1978). A good working approximation of adult
cortical and trabecular bone turnover in Beagles is 10 and
50 percent/year, respectively. Although it is obvious that
more work needs to be done, the morphologic data all support the observation that the bone turnover in adult Beagles is much faster than in adult man.

It is not possible to compare the pattern and rates of
bone formation of specific bones and parts of bones in dog
and man, because data for man have not been collected.
Marotti (1973) has shown regional differences in 20 skeletal sites of adult Beagles. He assumes the rate of bone
formation in mid-diaphysis of the tibia to be one. The
ratios between the rate of a given bone and the rate in
the corresponding tibia mid-diaphysis are then: femur
0.8, metatarsal 1.2, humerus 0.7, ulna 1.2, radius 1.7,
metacarpal 0.9, rib 1.4, mandible 1.8, and thoracic vertebra 2.4. To derive the rates at the proximal epiphysis

and metaphysis region of a long bone, one must multiply their respective mid-diaphyseal values by 2.4 and 4.2, respectively. The distal end of long bones is often about half as active as the proximal end (Jee et al., 1978).

Comparison of Age-Related Bone Loss in Dog and Man

Loss of bone is recognized as a universal component of aging in man. Age-related bone loss has been described from prehistoric human specimens (Dewey et al., 1969; Van Gerven et al., 1969; Perzigian, 1973). Sir Astley Cooper, as early as 1824, stated "that regular decay of nature which is called old age, is attended with changes which are easily detected in the dead body, and one of the principal of these is found in the bone, for they become thin in their shell and spongy in their texture." More recently (see Meunier et al., 1973; Nordin, 1973; Morgan, 1973a,b; Parfitt and Duncan, 1975; Dequeker, 1975; Smith et al., 1975; Heaney, 1976; Garn, 1975; Avioli, 1977; Boyce et al., 1978), reviews of the subject matter suggest the following conclusions about the characteristics of age-related bone loss in man:

● With advancing age, bone is lost from all parts of the skeleton examined so far.
● Bone loss involves individuals in all geographic locations and of all races, but is slower in blacks than in whites.
● Bone loss begins about 10 years earlier and proceeds about twice as fast in women as in men. The rate of loss does not appear to increase with age in men. Although the onset of loss in females antedates the menopause, the rate of bone loss in females is accelerated after menopause.
● Both cortical and cancellous bone are thinned by endosteal (bone adjacent to marrow) bone loss.
● Cortical bone loss occurs predominately on the endosteal surface so that the cortex is removed from the inside as the marrow enlarges. This net endosteal loss is partly offset by net periosteal gain, which continues slowly throughout life in some bones. A small contribution to the total cortical bone loss is from the enlargement of haversian canals leading to increased porosity.

● Age-related cancellous bone loss is due to bone remodeling imbalance; the amount of bone replaced at endosteal remodeling sites decreases with advancing age.

● Recent reports consistently support the conclusion
that bone resorption remains unchanged while bone formation
is decreased with age.

The dog exhibits many of the same features of age-
related bone loss as man. Age-related bone loss has been
oberved in both sexes of Beagles and, as in man, the female loses bone about twice as fast as the male (Jee et
al., 1976). The rate of loss is about 4 times faster in
Beagles than in man; the rate of trabecular bone loss is
2 percent/annum in dogs as compared to 0.5 percent/annum
in man (Jee et al., 1976; Meunier et al., 1973).

Details of the mechanisms of bone loss with advancing
age in dogs are meager, especially for cortical bone.
Nevertheless, the available information suggests the dog
skeleton loses bone with advancing age in the same manner
as does man. More age-related bone apposition rate measurements are needed in both species (Frost, 1969; S. C.
Miller et al., 1978; Lips et al., 1978). It must also be
determined whether the dog exhibits a decrease of mean
wall thickness and an increased resorption of bone with
advancing age. If one can assume the mechanism of adult
bone loss is identical in dogs and in man, then it can
be said that the dog loses bone faster because it has
more endosteal surface area per net volume of bone that
is available for bone remodeling (Lloyd and Hodges, 1971;
Beddoe, 1978; Jee et al., 1978).

The loss of both trabecular and cortical bone in dogs
with advancing age can best be illustrated by comparing
microradiographs of cross-sections of rib from two young
adult (1.4 years old) and two aged (15 and 16.2 years old)
Beagles (Figure 21). The cross sections of the rib from
the aged Beagles exhibit thinned cortical and trabecular
bone mass, mainly due to endosteal bone loss with associated enlargement of the marrow cavity. There are slight
enlargements of haversian canal diameters and occasional
hypermineralized haversian canal plugs.

At autopsy, both aged dogs possessed enlarged parathyroid and adrenal glands. One of the aged dogs (whose rib
is shown in Figure 21D) had adrenal cortical hyperplasia
and an elevated plasma alkaline phosphatase level.

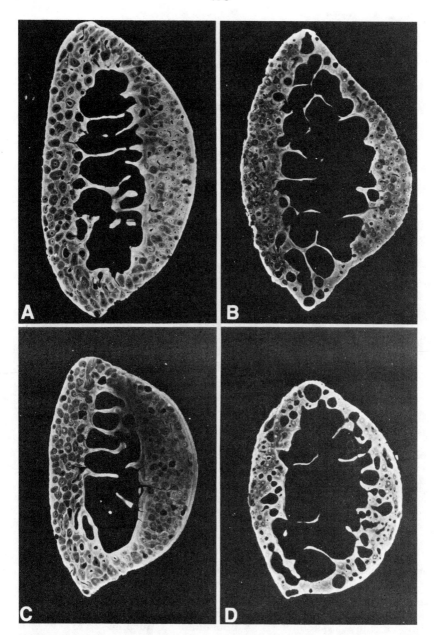

FIGURE 21 Microradiographs (magnified seven times) of rib cross sections from Beagles. (A) 1.4-, (B) 15-, (C) 1.4-, and (D) 16.2-year-old Beagles. Note the obvious reduction in bone mass in older dogs. Photomicrographs courtesy of W. S. S. Jee, Radiobiology Laboratory, University of Utah, Salt Lake City, Utah.

The Dog as a Model of Age-Related Bone Disease in Man

In man, when the loss of bone has progressed to the point where structural failure occurs, it is diagnosed as the disease osteoporosis. Age-related bone loss occurs in dogs, but fractures are not observed even though the dog loses bone much faster than does man. A possible reason for this is that the dog has a greater bone mass at maturity than does man. There are, however, experimentally induced canine adult bone loss models available. These are discussed in the section entitled "Comparative Models of Problems of the Human Elderly."

Appropriateness of the Dog Skeleton as a Model for Research on Skeletal Aging in Man

There are four principal reasons for using the dog as an experimental animal for studying age-related changes in bone:

1. The skeletons of adult man and dog are identical in composition, and both show bone remodeling and age-related bone loss. Females of both species have a more pronounced bone loss than males. The bone remodeling rate and rate of bone loss of the dog is about 5 times faster than the rates of man, which provides a means of completing experiments in a shortened time frame.

2. Much baseline data are available for the dog because it has been heavily employed in studies to predict the risk to humans from bone-seeking radionuclides. By comparing the metabolic parameters of these radionuclides in dog and man (uptake, distribution, retention) and knowing the toxicity in dogs, radiobiologists have sought to estimate the risk to man (Stover and Jee, 1972; Jee, 1976). Data concerning the metabolism of calcium compounds in dogs are available and compare favorably with similar data in man (Marshall et al., 1973). The dog also has been used to study the effects of nutrition, hormones, drugs, renal failure, and immobilization on the skeleton.

3. Repeated skeletal biopsy (rib or transilial) procedures can be performed, thus permitting longitudinal studies of the same dog, as is now done in humans. This eliminates interanimal variation, a significant problem when comparable longitudinal studies are conducted in smaller animals. In addition, the similarity of the procedures to those used in humans makes comparisons easier. Finally,

dogs as experimental animals for study of diseases of the skeletal remodeling system can be expected to display the same changes as humans, but at an accelerated rate.

4. Skeletal changes can be induced in dogs, thus permitting research on the prevention or arrest of bone loss and on the restoration of bone that has been lost.

Joints

Degenerative Joint Disease

Degenerative joint disease is a noninflammatory disorder of moveable joints characterized grossly by fragmentation and loss of articular cartilage and radiographically by the narrowing of the joint space, increased density of subchondral bone (sclerosis), and new bone formation at the joint margin (osteophytes). A detailed description of this disease is found in the section entitled "Comparative Models for Problems of the Human Elderly."

Inflammatory Joint Disease (Arthritis)

The inflammatory noninfectious arthritides of dogs may be divided into two general groups: the erosive and nonerosive (Pederson and Pool, 1978). Noninfectious, erosive, inflammatory arthritis of the dog is a condition similar to human rheumatoid arthritis. It is relatively rare, occurring mainly in small or toy breeds of dogs, with an average onset at around 4 years (range 8 months to 8 years) of age. This condition has been well characterized (Newton et al., 1975; Pedersen et al., 1976). The pathogenesis of this disease in the dog is not known. It is believed to be immunologic because it responds to therapy with potent immunosuppressive drugs (Pedersen and Pool, 1978). Whether the etiology of the canine disease is similar to human rheumatoid arthritis remains to be proven.

Noninfectious, nonerosive, inflammatory arthritis is seen frequently in dogs. Sixty-three dogs with this type of arthritis were examined at the University of California, at Davis, veterinary clinic over an 18-month period (Pedersen et al., 1976); 29 of these dogs had systemic lupus erythematosus, 15 had some chronic infectious disease process, and 19 cases were of idiopathic origin. This condition frequently is associated with diseases like ulcerative colitis and regional enteritis in man (enteropathic arthritis). The frequency of enteropathic arthritis in the dog is unknown (Pedersen and Pool, 1978).

Inflammatory joint disease tends to be cyclic. It affects the smaller, distal joints (i.e., carpus and tarsus). Radiographic changes tend to be minimal or nonexistent. Synovial membranes show a sparse mononuclear cell infiltration, with moderate-to-severe superficial inflammation, villous hyperplasia, and marginal erosions. Noninfectious, nonerosive inflammatory arthritis is believed to be caused by deposition of immune complexes in the synovial membrane resulting in an immune-mediated inflammation (Pedersen and Pool, 1978).

A recent review of canine joint disease by Pedersen and Pool (1978) touches upon the points covered in this brief survey and is recommended for comprehensive reading.

Hematopoietic System

Comparison of Structure and Function

The hematopoietic tissue of the dog and cat is in all general aspects identical to that of man with regard to embryonic development, maturation, and function. The blood forming tissue originates in the embryonic yolk sac; that function is then assumed by the spleen in the second trimester and by the liver in the third trimester. At the time of birth, the primary site of hematopoiesis is the bone marrow, with active hematopoiesis occurring in all marrow cavities (Schalm, 1964). The active marrow recedes as the animal matures and is replaced by fatty infiltration until, in the adult and aged animal, the active sites of hematopoiesis are limited to the ribs and pelvic bones (Spurling, 1977).

The cells of the hematopoietic tissue of the dog, cat, and man are alike both morphologically and functionally. Mature red cells are nonnuclear and biconcave; they carry the respiratory pigment, hemoglobin. The red blood cells of the dog and cat differ from those of man in two respects. They lack an active sodium pump, which is present in human red blood cells. Therefore, the intracellular sodium and potassium content is approximately equal to the levels of these ions in the plasma, while in human red blood cells sodium concentration is higher and potassium lower than in plasma (Romualdez et al., 1972). The other difference is that two types of hemoglobin (HbA and HbB) are present in cat red blood cells, while those

of the adult dog and man have only one type of hemoglobin.
HbA and HbB have identical alpha chains, but different
beta chains (Taketa et al., 1972). The myeloid cells,
i.e., neutrophils, eosinophils, and basophils, arise from
the hematopoietic tissue of the marrow and have identical
functions in all three species (Gilmore et al., 1964a;
Schalm, 1964, 1965; Coles, 1967; Bentinck-Smith, 1969).

Functionally, the lymphoid systems of the dog and cat
are similar to that of man (Hurvitz, 1975). In the dog,
there is a major histocompatibility-like complex that is
functionally similar to the major histocompatibility complex of man (Vriesendorp et al., 1973). Presumably there
is a similar system in the cat, although it has not been
characterized adequately.

Spontaneous Diseases

In the dog and cat, as in the human, primary hematological
diseases are uncommon; usually hematological manifestations are secondary to other diseases. A wide variety of
diseases may produce signs or symptoms of hematological
illness. The most prevalent hematological disorders of
the aged human are:

- lymphoproliferative disorders of all types, the most
common being chronic lymphocytic leukemia
- myeloproliferative disorders
- marrow suppression associated with
  a. rheumatoid arthritis
  b. chronic renal disease
- marrow hypofunctions secondary to
  a. iron deficiency
  b. nutritional deficiencies
- myelomas

Some diseases of dogs and cats are useful models of
these hematological diseases of the human elderly; however, in many instances disease identification is
difficult.

Lymphoproliferative Diseases

Canine Lymphosarcoma is characterized by neoplastic proliferation of lymphocytes (Chapman, 1975). It is, generally, a disease of mature dogs, usually between 5 and 10

years of age, with no specific sex preference (Dorn et al., 1968b). The etiology is unknown, but the evidence implicates a tumor virus (Chapman et al., 1967; Kakuk et al., 1968b). The clinical signs vary; generalized lymphadenopathy probably is the most characteristic and frequently seen lesion (Chapman, 1975; Dorn et al., 1968b). Other common clinical signs include anemia; hepatomegaly; splenomegaly; and digestive, renal, and ocular disturbances.

Feline Lymphosarcoma   Almost one-third of all feline neoplasms are lymphosarcoma (Nielsen, 1969). The disease has a much earlier onset in the cat than in the dog; approximately 50 percent of the cases appear by 3 years of age (Chapman, 1975). The etiology of feline lymphosarcoma is reported to be a C-type virus (Nielsen, 1969). Feline lymphosarcoma appears in three fairly distinct forms: multicentric, gastrointestinal, and thymic (Jarrett, 1970). The clinical signs vary according to the lymph nodes or organs involved. Hematological involvement occurs in about 15 percent of the cases (Holzworth, 1960).

Myeloproliferative Diseases

Myeloproliferative diseases are common in the cat but not in the dog. In man, it is usually possible to identify the morphological origin of the neoplastic myeloid cells, but in the cat and dog this is rare. Generally, in these carnivores, the disease is characterized by an abnormal proliferation of undifferentiated hematopoietic stem cells in the bone marrow and other organs of the reticulo-endothelial system (Gilmore et al., 1964b; Ward et al., 1969). A diagnosis of reticulo-endotheliosis frequently is made in these cases (Prasse, 1975). In the cat, as in man, the myeloproliferative diseases are progressive and fatal within a short period of time (Gilmore et al., 1964b). The clinical signs of myeloproliferative disease are relatively consistent (Prasse, 1975); the cat shows weight loss, listlessness, anorexia, pallor, and fever. Organ enlargement or lymphadenopathy is uncommon in feline myeloproliferative disease. Hematologically, anemia is the most constant finding, although the specific classification of the anemia varies (Prasse, 1975). Occasionally, as with man, the myeloproliferative diseases of dogs and cats involve only a specific cell type, such as neutrophils, eosinophils, or basophils. The more general

presentation in the dog and cat is of an undifferentiated
cell type (Schalm, 1971), and when this occurs, the diagnosis of reticulo-endotheliosis is frequently made (Prasse,
1975). This differs from man where it is usually possible
to identify the morphological origin of the neoplastic
myeloid cells.

Anemia

Anemia is a clinical sign of disease, not a disease per
se, and is due to blood loss or destruction. Some types
of anemia important in human medicine are:

• Nutritional anemia. This is frequently observed in
man, but is rare in the dog or cat with the exception of
iron-deficiency anemia (Schall and Perman, 1975). Folic
acid-deficiency anemia has been induced in the dog and cat
by various drugs that prevent folic acid absorption and
can be used as a model for the disease in man (Waxman,
1973).
• Pernicious anemia. This is not known to occur in
the dog and cat because neither animal appears to require
intrinsic factor for vitamin B_{12} absorption (Yamaguchi et
al., 1967).
• Iron-Deficiency anemia. In the dog and the cat,
iron-deficiency anemia is due primarily to chronic blood
loss caused by gastrointestinal parasites rather than to
nutritional deficiency as seen in man (Georgi et al.,
1969). It is more frequently a problem of the young animal than of the adult (Schall and Perman, 1975). Clinical
presentation of iron-deficiency anemia is variable depending upon the stage at which the anemia is recognized. In
the late stages of anemia, due to chronic blood loss, a
microcytic hypochromic anemia occurs (Harris and Kellermeyer, 1970).
• Parasitic anemias are all hemolytic in the dog and
cat, and are associated with intra-red cell parasites.
Canine babesiosis and hemobartonellosis; and, feline hemobartonellosis are examples of such diseases (Schall and
Perman, 1975).

Anemia also can be associated with feline leukemia virus (Hardy, 1974), resulting from a generalized bone marrow depression (Hoover et al., 1974). Feline leukemia has
been evaluated as a model for human leukemia (Hoover et
al., 1974).

Myeloma

The neoplastic proliferation of plasma cells occasionally
is observed in the dog and less frequently in the cat
(Hurvitz, 1975). Usually the animals are brought to the
clinic with an atraumatic fracture due to the osteolytic
effects of the proliferating plasma cells on bone (Osborne
et al., 1968b). Monoclonal production of one of the major
classes of immunoglobulin and Bence Jones proteinuria are
common clinical findings along with anemia and thrombocyto-
penia. The etiology of myeloma is not known. Myeloma in
dogs and cats has been evaluated as a model of human myeloma (Hurvitz, 1975).

Autoimmune Hemolytic Anemia

Autoantibody-induced destruction of red cells occurs in
the dog to the same extent as in man (Lewis et al., 1963).
It is most commonly a disease of the female, occurring in
midlife. Diagnosis is based on the demonstration of autologous gamma globulin coating on red blood cells by the
antiglobulin test (Bull et al., 1971). This protein coating appears to signal a red cell abnormality, resulting in
rapid destruction by the body's normal mechanisms (Lewis
et al., 1963). In the early stages, the anemia is a regen-
erative type, but can appear as a nonregenerative anemia
later in the disease when the hematopoietic reserves are
exhausted (Bull et al., 1971).

Hemorrhagic and Thrombotic Diseases

Carnivore models of the hemorrhagic and thrombic diseases
have been well described (ILAR, 1976a).

Alimentary System

Introduction

Diseases of the digestive system, such as gastric and colonic carcinoma, peptic ulceration, diverticulosis, consti-
pation, and intestinal obstruction, contribute significantly to health problems of old age (Andrew, 1961; McKeown,
1965). However, there have been surprisingly few studies
of age-related, morphological and physiological changes in

this system in man, and even fewer in carnivores. Nevertheless, features of several gastrointestinal disease syndromes in carnivores are comparable to the same diseases in man; therefore, this review will focus on these diseases.

Periodontal Disease

Periodontal disease, affecting the supporting tissues of the teeth, is common in man and is the most frequent cause of tooth loss. A discussion of this disease is found in the section entitled "Comparative Models of Problems of the Human Elderly."

Achalasia (Cardiospasm)

Cardiospasm or achalasia in man is a neuromotor disorder characterized by dysphagia associated with dilatation and tortuosity of the esophagus (Robbins, 1974b). The disease affects both sexes equally and usually occurs between the ages of 30 and 50 years. In cardiospasm, the lower esophageal region does not dilate in response to an oncoming wave of peristalsis and blocks passage of food into the stomach. This leads to vomiting and, in severe cases, to serious disability. Cardiospasm in man is believed to be the result of abnormal parasympathetic innervation of the myenteric plexus.

Esophageal dilatation occurs in low incidence (less than 1 percent of the population), but is associated with a high mortality rate in the dog (Guffy, 1975). The condition often has been diagnosed as achalasia and has been suggested as a model for the human condition (Sokolovsky, 1972). However, in-depth studies show that the canine disease is basically different from the human disease. So-called achalasia in the dog, rather than being caused by a blockage at the esophageal-cardiac junction, appears to be related to abnormal esophageal peristalsis (Sokolovsky, 1972; Diamant et al., 1973); lower esophageal sphincter function appears normal. Although the canine condition appears to be a neuromuscular disorder, ganglion cells of Auerbach's myenteric plexus are not abnormal (Clifford and Gyorkey, 1967) as they are in the great majority of human cases (Robbins, 1974b). Finally, the condition usually occurs in young dogs, is reversible, and is thought to relate to immaturity of innervation

and/or musculature, whereas in man, it occurs more commonly in midlife, is an acquired defect, and is irreversible.
All this suggests that the disease in dogs is not a good
model for the human syndrome. Acquired esophageal dilatation in dogs has been reported (Guffy, 1975) and may
represent a better model, although little information is
available presently on this syndrome.

Atrophic Gastritis with Achlorhydria

In man, atrophic gastritis is characterized by progressive,
irreversible atrophy of the gastric mucosa and is seen in
two populations of persons--those with pernicious anemia
and elderly persons without pernicious anemia (Robbins,
1974b). Achlorhydria and hypochlorhydria are conditions
in which there is lack of or decreased secretion of hydrochloric acid by the gastric mucosa. The functional capacity of the gastric mucosa declines with age, although
many persons with achlorhydria remain asymptomatic (Andrew,
1961). Chronic gastritis invariably results in some degree of achlorhydria (Robbins, 1974b). The etiology of
simple atrophic gastritis in elderly patients is not clear.
Ninety percent of patients with pernicious anemia have
circulating antibodies against gastric parietal cells,
but less than 60 percent of females and 20 percent of
males with atrophic gastritis--but without pernicious
anemia--have similar antibodies. There also is a strong
predisposition for persons with the atrophic gastritis
of pernicious anemia, but not for those with nonspecific
atrophic gastritis, to develop gastric carcinoma.
    Clinical cases of atrophic gastritis with achlorhydria
in dogs and cats have been reported, but are not well documented (Cornelius and Wingfield, 1975). Spontaneous cases
of atrophic gastritis are generally diagnosed at necropsy
and usually no information on the functional state of the
mucosa is available. On the other hand, atrophic gastritis
with achlorhydria had been induced in dogs immunized with
gastric juice or gastric mucosa (Smith et al., 1960; Krohn,
1968). Both specific antibodies to gastric mucosa and
cell-mediated responses to the antigen used could be found
(Krohn, 1968). Experimentally induced gastritis may be a
good model for the comparable lesions in pernicious anemia.
Since little is known about spontaneous atrophic gastritis
in the dog, it is harder to consider it as a model for the
human condition; however, it may well be worth further

evaluation to determine if any parallels exist with the nonspecific disease in elderly people.

Malabsorption Syndromes

Malassimilation is a broad term indicating failure of the gastrointestinal tract to supply nutrients to the body fluids (Kalser, 1976a). Malassimilation can be subdivided into two major categories: (1) maldigestion, referring to defective enzymic processes leading to impaired hydrolysis of fats, carbohydrates, and proteins and (2) malabsorption, referring to the failure of intestinal mucosal transport of nutrients from the intestinal lumen to the body fluids. Maldigestion will not be considered in this report; the emphasis will be on malabsorption in the dog and human as it relates to the aging process. Malabsorption generally is not considered a disease directly related to the aging process, but there are several conditions in man that have a high incidence in the later decades and that may have specific counterparts in the dog.

In the dog, about 75 percent of reported malabsorption cases are due to maldigestion secondary to pancreatic insufficiency; the remaining 25 percent are due to intestinal malabsorption (Schall, 1974). Celiac disease and lymphangiectasia due to Whipple's disease and intestinal lymphoma (discussed below) are the major causes of intestinal malabsorption in man for which there are possible experimental models in the dog. Malabsorption in the dog has not been intensively investigated and there may be potential for a much broader range of experimental models for malabsorptive disease in man.

In man, celiac disease (nontropical sprue, gluten enteropathy, ideopathic steatorrhea) is characterized clinically by steatorrhea, diarrhea, and weight loss. The etiology is thought to be either a toxic or hypersensitivity reaction to gluten or one of its fractions (Robbins, 1974b). The disease may manifest itself in childhood or middle age with the highest incidence in middle-aged adults. Kalser (1976b) states that celiac disease in man is a hereditary disease in which environmental factors play an equally important part in the pathogenesis. The primary lesion is marked jejunal villous atrophy, characterized histologically by blunted and distorted villi with an increased intervillous crypt depth and a marked chronic inflammatory reaction in the lamina propria with

infiltration of lymphocytes, plasma cells, and occasionally eosinophils (Robbins, 1974b). Clinical improvement
is seen within weeks after placing the patient on a
gluten-free diet; however, the villous atrophy responds
more slowly.

Malabsorption in dogs resembling celiac disease has
been reported (Vernon, 1962; Kaneko et al., 1965; Hill
and Kelly, 1974). The disease is characterized by marked
villous atrophy with a distinct deepening of the intestinal crypts and a chronic inflammatory response with lymphocytic and plasma cell infiltration of the lamina propria
in the jejunum and duodenum. This disease in the dog appears to be similar to human celiac disease and the dog
may serve as a good experimental model.

Whipple's disease is a chronic wasting disease of man
associated with intractable diarrhea, steatorrhea, weight
loss, polyarthritis, and generalized lymphadenopathy (Ruffin et al., 1976). The highest incidence of the disease
occurs in white males in the later decades of life. Clinically, the patient has a history of polyarthritis of
several years duration with diarrhea developing later in
the disease leading to steatorrhea, marked weight loss,
and a rapid deterioration (Ruffin et al., 1976). The disease is systemic with maximal inflammatory involvement in
the small bowel. Histologically, there are club-shaped
villi that are distended and blunted by masses of histiocytes in the lamina propria (Robbins, 1974b). These
macrophages are universally present in the proximal small
intestine and contain a periodic acid Schiff (PAS)-
positive material that often assumes a sickle form.
Ultrastructurally, they appear as masses of bacilli-like
bodies. The histiocytes are present in heart, lung,
spleen, pancreas, retroperitoneal tissues, and lymph nodes,
in addition to the gastrointestinal tract (Ruffin et al.,
1976). In most patients, there is a good response to antibiotic therapy suggesting an infectious agent; however, to
date, no organisms have been definitively isolated from
cases of Whipple's disease. The PAS-positive material
could represent a genetic abnormality in the function of
the reticuloendothelial system (Robbins, 1974b). There is
still a relative lack of knowledge concerning the etiology
and pathogenesis of Whipple's disease in man.

Granulomatous colitis (histocytic ulcerative colitis,
ulcerative colitis, colitis) of Boxers resembles human
Whipple's disease (Van Kruiningen et al.,1965; Koch and
Skelley, 1967; Sander and Langham, 1968; Russell et al.,
1971; Cockrell and Krehbiel, 1972; Ewing and Gomez, 1973).

Histologically, canine granulomatous colitis is characterized by diffuse distension of the lamina propria of the
colon with numerous large macrophages containing pink,
foamy cytoplasm. Small numbers of PAS-positive macrophages are present in some lymph nodes not associated
with the colon. An infectious etiology has been suggested
(Van Kruiningen et al., 1965); however, as in human Whipple's disease, no organisms have been isolated. The histologic resemblance between the two diseases has been
confirmed using ultrastructural techniques. Bacillary
bodies have not been seen in the dog; however, rod-shaped
granules have been reported (Cockrell and Krehbiel, 1972).
The presence of coccobacillary organisms within the macrophages has been confirmed, and Chlamydia has been suggested as the possible etiologic agent (Van Kruiningen, 1975).
In some respects, granulomatous colitis in Boxers is not
comparable with Whipple's disease (Russell et al., 1971).
In spite of the presence of the PAS-positive macrophages,
canine granulomatous colitis does not affect the small
bowel as in man. The PAS-positive macrophages are confined to the large bowel, not found systemically, and
are not identical ultrastructurally to those in the human
disease. In addition, ulceration is common in canine
granulomatous colitis, but not in Whipple's disease.

Because of the major differences between granulomatous
colitis of Boxers and Whipple's disease, the conclusion
that granulomatous colitis is a model for this human disease is tenuous. It is interesting to note, however, that
Whipple's disease is an infectious disease occurring in
older individuals, with the highest incidence in a rather
narrow population, and that granulomatous colitis appears
to be a similar process occurring in a single breed of
dog, the Boxer. This suggests that some common factors,
possibly immunologic in nature, may play a role in the
pathogenesis of the diseases. Enough similarities exist
to at least consider the canine disease for further studies of this intriguing condition.

Neoplasms

Oral and Pharyngeal Neoplasms Oral neoplasms commonly are
seen both in domestic carnivores and man. With the exception of the neoplasms of odontogenic origin, they are almost always malignant. Epidemiological studies indicate
that oral neoplasms account for about 6-7 percent of all
neoplasms in the cat and dog and have some similarities to

the human disease (Dorn et al., 1968a,b; Dorn and Priester, 1976).

The squamous cell carcinoma accounts for 90-95 percent of the oral neoplasms of man and 25-40 percent of the oral neoplasms of dogs (Brodey, 1960; Prier and Brodey, 1963; Bond and Dorfman, 1969). Oral neoplasms are seen more commonly in males both in man and the dog (Gorlin et al., 1959; Head, 1976). A higher incidence of squamous cell carcinoma of the tonsil has been reported in dogs from London, industrial cities in Scotland, and in Philadelphia (McClure et al., 1978). A possible relationship of carcinogenic air pollutants to carcinoma of the tonsils in city dogs is suggested, since a low incidence of tonsilar carcinoma has been reported in dogs from a rural population (Dorn and Priester, 1976). Whether such a relationship might apply to the human population is not known.

Other than the periodontal fibromatous epulis in the dog, odontogenic tumors are rare in domestic animals. The fibromatous epulis of periodontal origin is considered by most pathologists and veterinary clinicians to be the most common oral tumor of dogs. In a survey including benign lesions such as canine oral papillomatosis, transmissible venereal tumor, and salivary cysts, the fibromatous epulis has been found to represent 59 percent of the benign oral neoplasms (Gorlin and Peterson, 1967).

In summary, the canine appears to be afflicted by many of the same oral tumors as afflict man. In most cases, the biological behavior and histomorphological appearance of these tumors are similar in dog and man. Since these two species share a common environment, often consume similar diets, and appear to have the same relative age of oral tumor onset, the canine appears to be a good model for the study of oral neoplasia.

Salivary Gland Neoplasms   Salivary gland neoplasms in the dog may arise from either the major or minor salivary glands; involvement of the major glands, primarily the parotid, is twice as frequent (Koestner and Buerger, 1965; Brodey, 1970; Jubb and Kennedy, 1971a; Head, 1976). The histological structure of the salivary tumors in carnivores is as diverse as it is in man and the accepted human classifications apply (Willis, 1948; Jubb and Kennedy, 1970; Robbins, 1974b; and Thackray and Lucas, 1974). The variety seen most often in dogs is of acinar cell origin, although duct cell neoplasms also occur. The adenocarcinoma is the most common tumor reported in dogs and cats, accounting for 92 percent of the cases in one study

(Gorlin et al., 1959). Brodey (1970) suggests that salivary gland tumors are relatively more frequent in cats than in dogs.

In summary, although salivary gland tumors are rare, they do occur in dogs and cats and are similar to those seen in man. Therefore, carnivores may indeed be good models for study of these tumors.

Gastrointestinal Neoplasms Cancer of the stomach and of the colon and rectum rank fourth and sixth, respectively, in incidence of fatal lesions in elderly males (Timiras, 1972a). Malignant lesions of the small intestine are much less common, although they too increase with age. The dog and cat both develop gastrointestinal malignancies that bear some resemblance to the comparable lesions in man and, therefore, may be reasonable models for studying factors that could be important in the human diseases.

Gastric Carcinoma Gastric carcinoma is a disease that has been shown to increase in incidence continually from the third decade of life on in the human population (Timiras, 1972a; Robbins, 1974b). Geographic factors, probably environmental in nature, have a great influence on the prevalence of gastric carcinoma, having a higher incidence in some areas of the world (e.g., Japan and the Scandinavian countries) than in others (e.g., United States). Further, in the United States, there has been a dramatic decline in incidence over the past several decades, suggesting a changing environmental influence (Robbins, 1974b). Certain diseases, such as the atrophic gastritis of pernicious anemia and adenomatous polyps, seem to predispose to stomach cancer, and a familial tendency has been reported for this disease (McKeown, 1965; Robbins, 1974b). Gastric carcinoma is about twice as common in males as in females and is most frequently found in the pyloric region of the stomach.

Malignant tumors of the stomach are not among the more common lesions of the carnivore digestive system. There are a number of reports of such lesions, mainly adenocarcinomas, in the dog (Cotchin, 1954; Brodey and Cohen, 1964; Lingeman et al., 1971; Patnaik et al., 1977, 1978), but they appear to be rare in the cat (Brodey, 1966). While adenocarcinoma is the most common malignancy of the canine stomach, it represents only 1 to 2 percent of all malignant neoplasms in the dog, thus differing in prevalence from the human condition (Patnaik et al., 1978). Spontaneous canine gastric carcinoma has been reported

in areas of the world with both low and high human incidence, but no comparable geographic effect on incidence
of the canine disease has been reported.

Despite these differences, there are a number of similarities between the human and canine conditions. In both
man and dog, gastric carcinomas are more frequent in older
individuals (most affected dogs are between 5 and 10 years
of age) and males are most commonly affected. In both,
the majority of the lesions arise in the pyloric region
of the stomach, tend to infiltrate the stomach wall, and
metastasize widely. Finally, similar histologic types of
adenocarcinoma are found in man and dog, although the
relative incidence of the subtypes is not necessarily
comparable (Lingeman et al., 1971; Patnaik et al., 1978).

Malignant Lesions of Small Intestine In man, small intestinal malignancies, usually adenocarcinomas or lymphomas,
are relatively uncommon and tend to occur in older individuals. The greatest number of adenocarcinomas occur in
the jejunum, although the duodenum and ileum also can be
affected (McKeown, 1965; Robbins, 1974b). Primary intestinal lymphomas or lymphosarcomas approach adenocarcinoma
in frequency (McKeown, 1965; Robbins, 1974b), and occur
in both the stomach and the small intestine, especially
the lower small intestine.

In the dog, some investigators report a higher incidence of adenocarcinomas (Patnaik et al., 1977); to others
a higher incidence of lymphomas seems to be one of the
most predominant of all canine gastrointestinal neoplasms
(Cotchin, 1954; Brodey and Cohen, 1964). One problem in
evaluation of the true incidence of primary intestinal
lymphoma may lie with the criteria used for diagnosis of
this condition. In the strictest sense, only lymphoid
tumors in which there is little or no involvement of
organs or tissues outside the gastrointestinal tract are
considered to be primary at that site in man (McGovern,
1977). In the dog and cat these criteria are not necessarily followed, making direct comparison difficult. In
the cat, as in man, approximately equal numbers of small
intestinal adenocarcinomas and lymphomas are reported
(Brodey, 1966). Among dogs and cats with lymphoma, primary involvement of the intestine is about 3 times greater
in cats (Dorn et al., 1967). In cats, small intestinal
adenocarcinomas are most frequent in the ileum, whereas
in dogs, the duodenum is the main site (Patnaik et al.,
1976). Intestinal adenocarcinomas are more common in
the dog than the cat. Relatively little work has been

done comparing small intestinal adenocarcinomas in animals
and man; however, lymphomas both in dogs and cats have
been studied extensively and have been suggested as good
models for the human disease (Squire, 1966; Squire et
al., 1973).

Adenocarcinoma of the Large Intestine Carcinoma of the
colon is the second most common cause of cancer deaths in
the United States (Robbins, 1974c). This disease appears
to peak in the sixth to eighth decades of life, and there
are great variations in incidence associated with geographical location. This suggests an environmental etiology
factor, possibly dietary. Certain other conditions in
man seem to predispose to the development of colonic carcinoma, including ulcerative colitis, adenomatous polyps,
and a hereditary predisposition (McKeown, 1965; Robbins,
1974c).

In the dog, adenocarcinoma of the colon and rectum are
the most frequently occurring gastrointestinal neoplasms
(Brodey and Cohen, 1964; Patnaik et al., 1977). Colon and
rectal carcinomas tend to peak at slightly younger ages
(9-10 years) than do gastric carcinomas (11-12 years). In
dogs, cancer of the large intestine affects males more
than females, whereas in humans, the sexes are affected
equally. Since there is a hereditary predisposition to
cancer of the colon in man, it is interesting to note
that large intestinal adenocarcinomas, including those of
the rectum, appear to occur with a higher frequency in one
breed of dog, the German Shepherd Dog (Patnaik et al.,
1977). In the cat, colorectal cancers are not common and
most adenocarcinomas arise in the small intestine (Patnaik
et al., 1976). The high incidence of colorectal tumors
in man has been attributed to slow passage of intestinal
contents resulting in prolonged contact of the mucosal
surface with carcinogens in the diet. It has also been
suggested that colorectal cancer is caused by the action
of bacteria on bile acids, producing a carcinogenic agent
(Robbins, 1974c; Hill, 1977). The canine, especially the
German Shepherd Dog, might serve as a good model for explor-
ing the pathogenesis of this disease.

Respiratory System

Comparison of Lung Structure of Carnivores and Man

Lungs of all mammals share a common general structure consisting of a branching system of airways terminating in
thin-walled alveolar spaces where gas exchange occurs, but
there are variations among species. Species variations in
the subgross anatomic relationships of various pulmonary
anatomic components have been reported in detail (McLaughlin et al., 1961). Dogs and cats are included with monkeys as having a "type II" lung characterized by the absence of secondary lobules within lobes, ill-defined
intraparenchymal connective tissue support, and a thin
membraneous pleura. Distal airways consist of numerous,
well-developed respiratory bronchioles leading into large
alveolar ducts. The pulmonary artery supplies the distal
portion of the respiratory bronchiole, the alveolar duct,
alveoli, and pleura. The bronchial artery, except for a
few short branches near the hilum, contributes none of
the pleural supply, but does supply the hilar lymph nodes,
pulmonary artery and vein, bronchi and bronchioles, and
terminates in a common capillary bed with the pulmonary
artery at the respiratory bronchiole. In contrast, man
has "type III" lungs (as does the horse), which have partially developed secondary lobules with well-defined but
haphazardly arranged interlobular septae and a thick, vascular pleura. Distal airways are true terminal brochioles
and occasional, poorly developed respiratory bronchioles.
The pulmonary artery supplies the alveoli with only occasional anastamoses with the bronchial artery at the terminal bronchiolar level. The bronchial artery of man presents several contrasts to that of dogs and cats. As in
carnivores, it supplies the hilar lymph nodes, pulmonary
artery and vein, bronchi, and terminal airways, but it
also supplies the interlobular septae and pleura. The
bronchial artery of man also contributes blood directly
to the alveolar capillary network by three routes: the
terminal bronchiole, interlobular septae, and pleural network in areas lying close to the pleura.
    Other less comprehensive reports compare the lung struc-
ture of carnivores and man. The branching patterns of the
pulmonary arterial trees of dogs and cats are similar to
that of man, having a gradually tapered reduction in diameter rather than the abrupt changes in diameter found
in rabbits and rodents (Ferencz, 1969). The portion of
the bronchial wall of dogs occupied by mucous glands is

less than in man, but in both species the proportion is greater in distal than in central airways (Wheeldon and Pirie, 1974). Woolcock and Macklem (1971) have found similar rates of airflow through collateral channels in lungs from dogs and man. In spite of the differences in secondary lobulation, flow rates through collateral channels of both species are nearly as high as through the primary subtending airway. Martin and Sugihara (1973) have reported similar length-tension properties of cat and human lung parenchymal strips.

Structural Changes in Lungs of Carnivores with Age

The dog is the only carnivore, and in fact the only animal, for which significant information on age-related changes in lung structure has been reported. Robinson and Gillespie (1973a) have conducted histopathologic studies of lung tissue from Beagles that are 289 to 2,649 days of age, and Hyde et al. (1977) have studied the same lungs quantitatively using the point-count method. These reports indicate that the relative volume of alveolar ducts is larger, while the relative alveolar volume, tissue volume, and alveolar surface area are smaller in older dogs. The bronchial mucous glands also appear to be more active and bronchial cartilage calcified to a greater degree in lungs of older dogs (Robinson and Gillespie, 1973a). Wheeldon and Pirie (1974) have found no difference in the fraction of bronchial wall occupied by mucous glands in 10- to 14-year-old dogs as compared to 3- to 5-month-old dogs. Reif and Rhodes (1966) have reported an increased calcification of cartilage in lungs of dogs over 10 years of age. Fukuchi (1972a) has reported that the fractional area of bronchial wall cross sections occupied by muscle is less in dogs over 4 years of age than in younger dogs. In the same older dogs, there is also a greater vacuolization of the media, thickening of the intima, and narrowing of the lumena of bronchial arteries (Fukuchi, 1972b).

Additional radiological and morphological differences noted in lungs of older dogs include pleural thickening and an increase in nonvascular linear radiographic densities associated with fibrotic changes, nodular parenchymal densities from heterotropic bone growth, and a hyperlucency from focal emphysema (Reif and Rhodes, 1966). In a similar study (Reif and Cohen, 1979), chest radiographs of 1,994 dogs living in Ithaca, New York; Boston,

Massachusetts; and Philadelphia, Pennsylvania were evaluated for evidence of chronic lung disease. The incidence of chronic lung disease was positively correlated with age and with the degree of air pollution. Three groups of investigators have reported age-related increases in the deposition of pigmented granular material in dog lung tissue, and the nature of the sequestered material may be related to the locality in which the dogs have lived. Black pigment has been observed by Reif and Rhodes (1966) in lungs of dogs from the Philadelphia area, and "dark" particles have been observed in the lungs of dogs from the Los Angeles area by Catcott et al. (1958). Robinson and Gillespie (1973a) have reported detailed observations on the nature and location of pigmented material in lungs of Beagles from Davis, California. Macrophages in lungs of dogs of all ages contain both a golden-brown, nonrefractile, nonferrous material and black, angular, refractile particles. In dogs less than 1,500 days old, the pigment-containing macrophages lie beneath alveolar epithelium, primarily around alveolar openings. In older dogs, the macrophages are also found in interstitial tissue adjacent to blood vessels and airways and in walls of respiratory bronchioles, but form largest accumulations at the junctions of respiratory bronchioles and alveolar ducts. Focal inflammatory changes sometimes accompany the larger accumulations of pigmented macrophages in the older dogs.

Comparison of Structural Changes with Age in Dog and Man

The information available suggests many similarities and few differences in the effect of age on lung structure of dogs and man. Information on man is complicated by the difficulty of separating changes due to aging from those due to disease, since man is affected by factors such as smoking, air pollution, and recurring respiratory infections to a greater degree than dogs maintained in laboratory colonies. Some pulmonary structural changes that are similar in dog and man are age-related increases in relative volumes of alveolar ducts, alveolar sacs, and respiratory bronchioles (Heppleston and Leopold, 1961; Ryan et al., 1965), resulting in a decrease of alveolar surface area (Liebow, 1964; Hasleton, 1972; Thurlbeck and Angus, 1975); the thickness of the mucous gland layer of the bronchi (Hernandez et al., 1965); calcification of cartilage (Liebow, 1964); and accumulation of pigmented particles (Wright, 1961). It is presently uncertain whether there might be differences in the relationship between interalveolar fenestrae and age in dogs and man. Pump (1974) has reported an increase in the size and number of fenestrae with age in lungs of human subjects; however, it is not certain whether these changes are related to aging or to early emphysema. Martin (1963) has found no increase either in size or number of interalveolar fenestrae in dogs over 1 year old. At this time, there appears to be no reason to suspect major differences in the effect of age on lung structure of dogs and man.

Functional Changes in Lungs of Carnivores with Age

The number of reports of the effect of aging on lung function of animals is small, and the Beagle is the only carnivore for which such data have been published. Robinson and Gillespie (1973b) have measured the subdivisions of lung volume of 22 anesthetized Beagles ranging in age from 289 to 3,882 days. They found an increase in residual volume and no change in total lung capacity, resulting in a decreasing vital capacity with increasing age. No differences in functional residual capacity related to age were found. Mauderly (1974, 1979) has measured the lung function of 240 Beagles at 1 year, 10 at 3 years, 48 at 5 years, and 50 at 10 years of age, without anesthesia or sedation, and found that functional residual capacity increased progressively with the age of the groups. The distribution and mixing of inspired air was found to be less efficient, and the fraction of inspired air reaching the alveolar bed was found to be lower with increasing age in spontaneously breathing dogs (Mauderly, 1974, 1977, 1979). An age-related left shift of the quasi-static pressure-volume curve of anesthetized dogs (Robinson and Gillespie, 1973b) demonstrated a loss of elastic lung tissue recoil with a resulting increase in quasistatic lung compliance. Dynamic lung compliance was reduced with age in unsedated dogs (Mauderly, 1977, 1979). The efficiency of alveolar-capillary gas exchange reduced both in unsedated and anesthetized dogs. Robinson and Gillespie (1975) have found age-related reductions in diffusing capacity and capillary blood volume, but no change in the membrane component of gas diffusion in anesthetized Beagles. They reasoned that diffusing capacity was reduced because of the reduced blood volume and that the change was caused either by an actual difference in blood volume or flow or by an artifact introduced by uneven gas distribution. An age-related decrease in CO diffusing capacity also was demonstrated in unsedated dogs (Mauderly, 1974, 1979); however, the gas exchange impairment was not sufficient to increase the alveolar-capillary O_2 gradient or reduce arterial PO_2.

Little is known about the effects of age on respiratory reflexes and control mechanisms. Fukuchi (1972a) has found smaller contractile responses of bronchial muscle to directly injected acetylcholine and serotonin in dogs over 4 years than in those under 4 years of age.

Comparison of Functional Changes with Age in Dog and Man

The apparent qualitative changes in the lung function of dogs with age are remarkably similar to those reported for man. Several reviews of the alterations of human lung function with age and several recent reviews are available (Muieson et al., 1971; Klocke, 1977; Mauderly, In press). There is no significant age-related change in the total lung capacity of adult man, and the residual volume increases progressively, resulting in a decrease in vital capacity as seen in the dog. There are conflicting reports on the effect of age on the functional residual capacity of man, just as there are for the dog, but the majority favor a slight increase with age. Intrapulmonary gas mixing and distribution become less efficient with age. There is a decrease in elastic lung recoil with an associated increase of static lung compliance, but the dynamic lung compliance is reduced. The age-related, progressive loss of gas exchange efficiency in man has been repeatedly documented and results in a reduced CO diffusing capacity, as it does in the dog. Little more is known about the effect of aging on respiratory control of man than of carnivores. The reported reduction of ventilatory responses to hypoxia and hypercapnia in man (Patrick and Howard, 1972; Kronenberg and Drage, 1973) and the reduced contraction of bronchial muscle in dogs both constitute age-related reductions in a control response to stimuli, but the two effects are unlikely to be directly related.

The primary difference, if one indeed exists, in the effect of aging on the lung function of dogs and man, may be in the relative rate of functional decline with age. The present methods for determining relative ages of dogs and man are inadequate for an accurate comparison, but the best method presently available is that proposed by

LeBeau (1953). A graph presented in that report relates
the ages of dog and man in a nonlinear plot based on the
age of sexual maturity and average life span. According
to LeBeau's (1953) estimation, a 10-year-old dog has an
equivalent human age of approximately 56 years, an age
at which the pulmonary functional loss of man is much
greater than the slight alterations observed in dogs.
The extent to which environmental and disease factors may
be responsible for the apparent difference in the rate of
functional decline is uncertain. It is possible that
dogs simply do not live long enough for their lung tissues to undergo the magnitude of changes possible in man.

Spontaneous Lung Diseases of Carnivores Similar to Chronic
Lung Diseases of Man

A condition termed "feline bronchial asthma" is reported
to be a common clinical finding in cats (Head et al.,
1975). The etiology is unknown although allergies and
psychological stresses have been suspected. The condition
is characterized by a sudden onset of paroxysmal dry
coughing, which may be accompanied by dyspnea with wheezing and forced exhalation in severe cases. Radiographic
findings may include a "barrel-chested" appearance of the
thorax, increased radiolucency of the lung fields and
pronounced bronchial densities. High absolute and relative eosinophil counts are often found. Parasitic ova
are absent in bronchial washings and feces. Spontaneous
asthma-like conditions are uncommon among dogs.
  Chronic obstructive lung diseases, as they occur in
dogs and cats, have some similarities to chronic bronchitis in man. Emphysema, a common component of chronic obstructive lung disease in man, does not often occur spontaneously in carnivores; however, similar conditions have
been produced experimentally in dogs by several methods.
The appropriateness of the carnivores as models for studying these diseases is discussed in the section entitled
"Comparative Models of Problems of the Human Elderly."

Experimentally Induced Lung Diseases of Carnivores Similar
to Chronic Lung Diseases of Man

Bronchoconstrictive responses similar to those occurring
in human asthmatics have been produced in dogs via immunologic mechanisms. Transient episodes of bronchospasm with

dyspnea and altered respiratory mechanics have been induced in dogs having natural sensitivities to the parasite,
Ascaris suum, by inhalation of aerosols containing A.
suum extracts (Booth et al., 1970; Gold et al., 1972;
Cotton et al., 1977; Yamatake et al., 1977; Cohn et al.,
1978). Recent work at Northwestern University, Chicago,
Illinois (R. Patterson, Unpublished) has demonstrated similar responses in dogs experimentally sensitized by repeated inhalation of aerosols containing A. suum extract.
Dogs with natural sensitivities to grass pollen (Gold et
al., 1972) and passively transferred sensitivities to ragweed pollen (Patterson and Sparks, 1962) also develop
bronchospasm when challenged with aerosolized antigen.
Kepron et al. (1977) have sensitized newborn dogs to a
conjugate of 2,4-dinitrobenzene and ovalbumin with aluminum hydroxide as an adjuvant via intraperitoneal injection
and, subsequently, have elicited bronchoconstrictive responses by aerosol challenge. These induced models accurately reproduce the acute physiological responses during
an asthma attack in man and have been shown to be mediated
by reaginic antibodies similar to human immunoglobulin-E,
the type of mediator acting in certain forms of human
asthma (Patterson et al., 1969; Schwartzman et al., 1971).
However, the long-term pulmonary structural alterations
usually observed in chronic human asthmatics (Scadding,
1977) have not been produced in these dog models.

The chronic functional and structural effects of cigarette smoking have been studied by using dogs as models.
The relevance of the various smoking methods employed to
the smoking patterns of man is difficult to assess and has
made extrapolation of results difficult (Binns, 1975).
Park et al. (1977) have found that smoking for 6 months to
1 year induces a form of chronic bronchitis characterized
by basal cell hyperplasia in the tracheal epithelium, proliferation of goblet cells in the bronchi, and peribronchi-
olar inflammation. Depression of tracheal mucociliary
transport and the bacteriosupressive function of alveolar
macrophages also is observed. Longer exposures to cigarette smoke have resulted in the development of pulmonary
fibrosis and emphysema (Hammond et al., 1970; Binns,
1975).

Dogs have been used as models for studying the effects
of chronic exposure to air pollutants, both singly and in
combination. Exposure of dogs to 1-3 ppm of ozone daily
for 18 months results in fibrotic lesions at the terminal
bronchiole and alveolar duct level (Freeman et al., 1973).
Bullous emphysema has been observed in dogs after daily

exposure to 26 ppm of nitrogen dioxide for 191 days (Lewis et al., 1969), and subsequent exposure to sulfur dioxide and sulfuric acid for 225 days has resulted in several alterations of respiratory functions. Exposure of dogs daily for 61 months to various combinations of gasoline engine exhaust and other air pollutants has resulted in several chronic pulmonary functional and structural alterations (Lewis et al., 1974; Gillespie et al., 1976; Hyde et al., 1978). Because of the uncertainties regarding the etiologies of chronic lung diseases in man and their relation to air pollution, it is difficult to assess the accuracy with which these models represent the human situation. However, the functional and structural alterations induced in dogs are similar to those thought likely to be related to the long-term inhalation of air pollutants by man (American Thoracic Society, 1978).

Dogs also have been used in studies of the chronic effects of thoracic irradiation. Dose-response relationships and structural, functional, and biochemical alterations resulting from single or multiple irradiations of the lungs from external sources (Sweany et al., 1959; Schreiner et al., 1968; Hooykass et al., 1969), or from continuous irradiation from inhaled radionuclides (McClellan et al., 1970; Mauderly et al., 1973; Pickrell et al., 1976), have been studied. Dogs develop radiation pneumonitis and subsequent pulmonary fibrosis having the structural and functional characteristics of the disease in man (Rubin and Casarett, 1968), and the dog studies have been useful in defining the relationships between dose, time, and responses.

Appropriateness of the Dog Lung as a Model for Research on Lung Aging in Humans

There is almost a total lack of information on the effects of aging on the lungs of carnivores other than the dog, and information on the dog presently is derived only from cross-sectional studies. Current information, however, suggests that the lungs of dogs and man undergo structural and functional alterations that are qualitatively similar and possibly identical. Quantitative comparisons depend on the accuracy with which equivalent ages are determined, and only relatively crude comparisons have been possible to date. There are only a few spontaneously occurring lung diseases in dogs and cats that closely resemble chronic lung diseases common to man. One reason for this may be the differences in lung structure of carnivores

and man that may result in species differences in responses to pulmonary insults. Another factor may be differences in the insults encountered, such as cigarette
smoking and susceptibility to recurrent viral infections.
Differences in absolute life spans of carnivores and man
also may be important, since carnivores have a shorter
time to be affected by agents such as environmental pollutants. However, carnivores have proven useful as experimentally induced models for several chronic lung diseases found in man. Carnivores among the pet population
share a common environment with man, but there have been
few attempts to take advantage of this fact in epidemiological studies. Clearly, more information is needed regarding aging effects on lungs of carnivores, equivalent
ages between carnivores and man, and the age and environ-
ment-related incidence of spontaneous lung disease among
carnivores.

Cardiovascular System

Studies on aging in the cardiovascular system of carnivores are of two basic types; the first deals with age-
related changes in physiological parameters, the second
involves the characterization of specific, age-related
spontaneous diseases. This section will highlight and
briefly describe the important studies in each of the
two groups.

Physiological Studies

Cardiovascular changes associated with aging have been
evaluated in 37 Beagles studied nonlongitudinally at 1,
2, 5, and 12 years of age. Invasive and noninvasive ul-
trasound techniques have been used to evaluate the following parameters (Miller et al., 1976):

• Maximum blood velocity. Blood velocity declines
with age in the carotid artery, thoracic aorta, abdominal
aorta, and iliac artery. The largest, age-related decre-
ment occurs in the abdominal aorta.
• Blood flow. The average blood flow in the carotid
artery, thoracic aorta, abdominal aorta, and iliac artery
decreases to the greatest extent between 1 and 2 years of
age. At later ages, decreases are less obvious, although
the trend remains.

● Elastic modulus. The elastic modulus generally increases with age, although considerable variation exists
depending upon the vascular region and the age group.
Values for the elastic modulus are higher in the carotid
artery and abdominal aorta than the thoracic aorta.
● Pulse wave velocity. Pulse wave velocity increases
consistently with age in most arterial segments. Beagles
show an increased pulse wave velocity of 51 percent from
1 to 12 years of age. In comparison, pulse wave velocity
measurements in man show a 30 percent increase between 15
and 65 years of age.
● Blood pressure. Blood pressure remains fairly consistent as the dog ages. The values for systolic and
diastolic blood pressure average 101/75 mm Hg at the level of the aortic arch.

Esophageal and transcutaneous echocardiographic techniques have been used to study the atrioventricular valves
in five young and four old Beagles with atrioventricular
disease (Dennis et al., 1978). In two affected dogs a
reduction in EF slope has been found, and one affected dog
showed reduced valve motion.
Studies of contractile function in aged Beagles reveal
changes similar to those seen in man (Miller et al., 1976;
Shock, 1976; Templeton et al., 1978). Impaired function
is indicated by the development of lower pressure in the
left ventricle, a prolonged contraction duration, and an
increase in ventricular stiffness during diastole and
systole.

Spontaneous Disease

Hypertension and Atherosclerosis These diseases will
receive only brief attention here. Atherosclerosis is discussed in detail on pages 377-386. In general, the carnivores do not show spontaneous hypertension or atherosclerosis. The few reports of naturally occurring, essential
hypertension in the dog encountered in the veterinary
literature appear to be secondary to renal disease, a
common clinical problem, particularly in aged dogs (Valtonen and Oksanen, 1972).
Massive myocardial infarction due to occlusion of one
or more extramural coronary arteries by atherosclerotic
plaques comparable to that seen in man is rarely seen in
dogs. Atherosclerosis in the dog is limited to the intramural coronary arteries. The intramural coronary arterial

lesions are typically associated with chronic atrioventricular valvular fibrosis and insufficiency, as well as
myocardial necrosis and fibrosis. In a histopathological
study of 643 dogs, Jönsson (1972) has shown that 26.4
percent have coronary arterial lesions. The incidence is
age-related, and there is no sex or breed predilection.
The coronary arterial lesions include musculoelastic
thickening, intimal cushions, microthrombi, hyaline microthrombi, hyalinosis, and amyloidosis.

Chronic Valvular Fibrosis (Endocardiosis) A spontaneous
disease of dogs that may have the greatest potential as a
model for age-related changes in the human heart is chronic
valvular disease (CVD) (Ettinger and Suter, 1970). CVD is
a diffuse or nodular thickening of either or both of the
atrioventricular valves; the mitral valve leaflets are affected most often. CVD is the most common lesion found at
necropsy in dogs with congestive heart failure. Its etiology is unknown.

The prevalence and severity of CVD increases with age
(Detweiler, 1965; Detweiler et al., 1972; Whitney, 1974),
but data vary depending on whether the study is based on
clinical or necropsy examination (Hottendorf and Hirth,
1974). In a group of 9- to 12-year-old dogs, approximately
25 percent will have clinical and/or postmortem findings
compatible with CVD. In dogs 13 years of age and older,
the prevalence rises to about 35 percent. Male Cocker
Spaniels appear to be particularly susceptible to CVD.

Diagnosis depends on the specific valve involved and the
degree of congestive heart failure. In the typical case, a
systolic thrill and pansystolic murmur (band-shaped) are
detected in the mitral area. The murmur varies widely in
intensity (Grade I-V) depending on the severity of the insufficiency. Other physical findings may include a weak
and rapid femoral pulse, hepatomegaly, ascites, limb edema,
and weight loss. The EKG frequently is abnormal. Arrhythmias that are most commonly associated with CVD include
atrial and ventricular premature beats, atrial and ventricular tachycardia, and atrial fibrillation.

Lateral and dorsoventral radiographs of the thorax often
reveal pulmonary venous congestion and edema as well as
left ventricular enlargement. Tricuspid insufficiency results in right atrial and ventricular enlargement with the
subsequent development of the right heart failure. Cardiac
catheterization is not usually necessary to diagnose or
evaluate CVD.

CVD is classified according to gross pathological manifestations into four groups, as follows (Pomerance and Whitney, 1970):

Type 1: A few small discrete nodules are found on the leaflets in the area of contact and are associated with areas of diffuse opacity in the proximal portion of the valve.

Type 2: Larger nodules that tend to coalesce with their neighbors are evident in the area of contact. Areas of diffuse opacity may be present.

Type 3: Large nodules may be seen, but may have coalesced into irregular, plaque-like deformities. These lesions extend to involve the proximal portions of the chordae tendinae.

Type 4: There is gross distortion and ballooning of the valve cusp and the chordae tendinae are thickened proximally. Ruptured chordae tendinae are frequently identified.

Histologically, leaflets have increased amounts of acid mucopoly-saccharides in addition to dystrophic and proliferative changes. Less severe forms are characterized by fibroplasia and fragmentation of elastic fibers, especially in the spongiosa layer under the contact surfaces of the valves. In more severe forms, there is mucoid degeneration of the fibrosa layer, with disappearance of collagen and replacement of myomatoid connective tissue. The mucoid degeneration appears to be of utmost importance in both man and dog (Pomerance and Whitney, 1970). In some cases, amyloid is demonstrated.

Feline Cardiomyopathy Primary myocardial disease (cardiomyopathy) in the cat closely resembles the disease in man (Tilley et al., 1977). Typically, the problem occurs in a mature male cat with a history of dyspnea and aortic thromboembolism. Clinical examination usually reveals a systolic heart murmur, gallop rhythm, cardiomegaly, pulmonary edema, electrocardiographic abnormalities, elevated left ventricular and diastolic pressure, and angiocardiographic evidence of mitral regurgitation.

Pathological findings are primarily those of generalized cardiomegaly with either severe dilatation (congestive) or hypertrophy of the left ventricle. Histological study of the congestive type reveals muscle cells that appear thinner than normal and are separated by edematous extracellular ground substance or connective tissue. Areas of wavy muscle fibers are seen, and only a few fibers appear hypertrophied. The endocardium is thickened by the presence of dense collagen.

In the hypertrophic type of cardiomyopathy, the muscle cells are enlarged and have rectangular, hyperchromatic nuclei. Muscle bundles show bizarre disarrangement and are separated by increased interstitial connective tissue. Foci of endocardium are replaced by active fibroplasia and the atrioventricular Purkinje cells are frequently interrupted by or mixed with many dense collagen fibers.

Induced Disease

Myocardial Infarction   Although spontaneous myocardial infarction rarely occurs in dogs and cats, the disease can be induced readily in these animals. Many techniques are used to occlude the coronary arteries, thus producing symptoms comparable to those of human myocardial infarction. A survey of the literature shows more that 1.,800 articles have been published in the last 15 years concerning the use of dogs and cats as models for this disease. The use of these models has contributed to the progress made in the diagnosis and treatment of human myocardial infarction. Obviously, it will not be possible to present an extensive review here; only a few examples of the ways in which dogs and cats are used in the study of this disease will be discussed.

The techniques for producing myocardial infarction in dogs and cats include:

● acute coronary ligation in anesthetized, thoracotomized animals;
● two-stage coronary ligation in anesthetized, thoracotomized animals;
● gradual coronary occlusion using various types of materials implanted in anesthetized, thoracotomized animals; and
● the use of selective catheterization to deliver emboli to the coronary arteries in unanesthetized, closed-chest dogs.

The technique of acute coronary ligation has been in use for nearly 100 years (Cohnheim and von Schultess-Rechberg, 1881). A few recent studies using this model include those of Ceremużyński et al., 1969; Gillis, 1971; Lathers et al., 1977, 1978; Kennett and Weglicki, 1978; Fore et al., 1978;

Bissett et al., 1979. Many investigators employ the two-stage coronary occlusion method developed in the dog by Harris (1950) because this technique results in a larger number of animals surviving occlusion. The technique involves a partial coronary occlusion, followed by complete coronary occlusion in an anesthetized, thoracotomized dog. Experiments are carried out beginning 24 hours after the dog has recovered from anesthesia. Data obtained using this method have been reported by numerous investigators (Harris et al., 1971; Gillis et al., 1973; Heng et al., 1978; Reynolds et al., 1979; Ritchie et al., 1979; Hashimoto et al., 1979).

Employing techniques of gradual occlusion is thought to allow the development of collateral circulation, a situation similar to the prompt development of collaterals when human coronary blood flow is restricted in advanced coronary atherosclerosis (Baroldi et al., 1956). One technique employs Ameroid, a hydroscopic casein plastic, that is placed around a major coronary vessel. This material has a predictable rate of swelling when in contact with tissue fluids, and it gradually narrows the vessel diameter (Litvak et al., 1957). In another technique, wires of chromogenic alloy are placed around the coronary arteries to produce a gradual occlusion (Gage et al., 1956). Latex injection of hearts removed from cats following coronary occlusion aids in the evaluation of the possible protective contribution of coronary collaterals (Lathers et al., 1977, 1978).

One limitation of all these methods of coronary ligation is that thoracotomy is required for exposure and manipulation of the coronary artery. Neural and lymphatic pathways are altered during thoracotomy and opening of the pericardium and surgical follow-up procedures are more difficult. Variations in effects occur depending upon the size of the artery, the site and speed of the occlusion, the anatomy and preexisting state of the other major arteries and myocardium, the distribution and extent of the collateral circulation (Jobe, 1968), and whether the animal is conscious or anesthetized, since anesthesia appears to have a protective influence (Bland et al., 1976) and may decrease the probability of fatal ventricular fibrillation. To solve some of these problems, closed-chest techniques of coronary occlusion have evolved. Some of these methods involve selective catheterization to deliver multiple small emboli to the coronary arteries employing such agents as lycopodium spores (Guzman et al., 1962), glass or plastic beads (Agress et al., 1952), and clots. Use of these techniques produces countless obstructions of small vessels, but the changes are unpredictable and dissimilar to lesions generally seen in man. In addition, the interruption of flow is acute and collateral circulation does not have time to develop. Embolization also has been produced by injecting autologous clots into the left anterior descending coronary arteries of dogs until infarction or arrhythmia develop (Baumstark et al., 1978), using wire conductors to induce thrombus formation with electrical or thermal energy (Salazar, 1961) and infusing ADP into major coronary arteries to produce occlusive platelet aggregations and myocardial infarction (Rowsell et al., 1966). However, it is very difficult to regulate the size and location of the obstruction using these techniques.

A technique that has contributed greatly to our current knowledge of postinfarction arrythmias is the use of coronary microsphere embolization. The injection of latex microspheres (25-μm diameter) has been used to study the pharmacological alterations of different parts of the coronary circulation to further elucidate the hemodynamic relationships between the collateral and the nutritive microcirculation (Wichmann et al., 1978), the changes in collateral blood flow as a function of time and the relationship of these changes to myocardial necrosis (Reimer and Jennings, 1979), and the time course of ischemic cell death and the effectiveness of therapeutic interventions designed to contain the size of the infarct (Jugdutt et al., 1979). This area of research is extremely important because these arrhythmias account for most of the human deaths that occur in the hours immediately following myocardial infarction. Sixty to seventy percent of patients do not survive long enough to reach a hospital (Lown and Wolf, 1971).

It has been suggested that the autonomic nervous system is involved in the production of acute coronary occlusion-induced arrhythmias. Dogs and cats have been used to test this hypothesis (Costantin, 1963; Malliani et al., 1969; Gillis, 1971; Rotman et al., 1972; Webb et al., 1972; Levitt et al., 1976; Gillis et al., 1976) and to determine the mechanism by which antiarrythmic agents act upon this altered neural discharge (Kelliher and Roberts, 1974; Lathers, 1975; Levitt et al., 1976; Kupersmith, 1976). In particular, one factor thought to be involved in the production of ventricular arrhythmias after occlusion is altered sympathetic neural discharge to the heart and/or an imbalance between the sympathetic and parasympathetic nervous system (Webb et al., 1972; Levitt et al., 1976;

Schwartz et al., 1976; Lathers et al., 1977, 1978; Wehrmacher et al., 1979).

Other factors that are involved in cardiac susceptibility to ventricular arrythmias include the extent and intensity of ischemia, the severity of metaboic alterations
within the ischemic area, the perfusion gradient between
the nonischemic and ischemic cardiac muscle, and the extent
of coronary vascular collateralization (Corday et al.,
1977). It should be noted, however, that the first three
factors may be directly affected by the autonomic nervous
system. It has been suggested that pharmacological or
surgical interventions that correct regional ischemia,
and thus decrease the extent of ischemic injury, may also
decrease the incidence of ventricular fibrillation (Corday
et al., 1977). A review of the experimental and clinical
evidence supporting the roles of altered sympathetic discharge and acute myocardial ischemia in sudden cardiac
death following myocardial infarction has been published
recently (Lown et al., 1977).

Another area in which the dog and cat are employed as
models is in determining the effectiveness of drugs in limiting the area of necrosis following myocardial infarction
(Maroko et al., 1972; Reimer et al., 1973; Lucchesi et al.,
1976; Powell et al., 1976) and in developing techniques
to measure infarct size (Holman et al., 1976; Pitt and
Strauss, 1976). The therapeutic agents, their usefulness
often controversial, include practolol (Libby et al.,
1973a; Marshall and Parratt, 1974; Lathers et al., 1976),
methylprednisolone (Spath et al., 1974; Busuttil et al.,
1975; Brachfeld, 1976; Masters et al., 1976; Schneider
et al., 1976; Shatney et al., 1976a,b; Lathers, 1979),
hydrocortisone (Libby et al., 1973b; Braunwald and Maroko,
1976), acetylsalicylic acid (aspirin) (Jick and Miettinen,
1976; Ogletree and Lefer, 1976), and metoprolol (Sivam
and Seth, 1978; Lathers, 1980). The techniques developed
to measure infarct size include 99^mtechnetium pyrophosphate scans (Bonte et al., 1974; Bruno et al., 1976; Buja
et al., 1976, 1979; Willerson et al., 1979), thallium-201
myocardial perfusion imaging (Mueller et al., 1976; Wackers
et al., 1976; Bailey et al., 1977; Ritchie et al., 1977;
Botvinick et al., 1978; Umbach et al., 1978), indium-111
gamma-emitting radionuclide labeling (Thakur et al., 1979),
iodine-131 labeled antibody (Fab')$_2$ fragment imaging (Khaw
et al., 1978a,b), computerized axial tomography scans
(Siemers et al., 1978; Gray, 1979), intravenous administration of diatrizoate meglumine and sodium (Renografin-
76) (Higgins et al., 1979), reduced nicotinamide adenine

dinucleotide fluorescence photography (Barlow and Chance, 1976; Barlow et al., 1977; Harken et al., 1978; Simpson et al., 1979), serial creatine phosphokinase technique (Shell et al., 1971; Roberts et al., 1975), nitro-blue tetrazolium test (Nachlas and Schnitka, 1963), and two-dimensional echocardiography (Meltzer et al., 1979).

In summary, the dog and cat are useful models for studying myocardial infarction and its sequelae in humans. A few of the areas in which these models are useful include the study of the mechanisms of arrhythmia development, role of imbalance in the autonomic neural discharge, altered electrophysiology of the myocardium, size and location of the ischemic and/or infarcted areas, biochemical changes accompanying infarction, presence of coronary collaterals, pathophysiology of myocardial perfusion, and effects of pharmacological agents on the sequalae of coronary occlusion.

Urinary System

Structure and Function of Kidneys of Carnivores and Man

Physiologically and anatomically, the kidneys of carnivores are similar to those of man, made up of basic nephron units whose excretory and metabolic functions are necessary to maintain the body's homeostatic mechanisms. Grossly, the renal papillae in the dog are modified into renal crests that give the renal pelvis a different appearance from that of man. The kidney of felines also appears different from both the dog and man, being generally light tan to whitish in color due to a higher fat content (Bell and Scott, 1977). This higher fat content is also apparent at the histological level; the cortical tubular cells have a vacu-olated cytoplasm.

Changes in renal function with age in the carnivore have not been studied to any great extent; most reports have been concerned with specific disease entities without re-gard to age. Only fragmentary information is available on the changes in glomerular filtration rate (GFR) as a function of age. Miller et al. (1977) have reported no significant, age-related difference in the GFR (as meas-ured by the half-time clearance of sulfanilate and sodium iodohippurate) in annual tests of Beagles between 3 and 7 years of age. However, in single tests of Beagles from 2 to 13 years of age, renal clearance of sulfanilate has been shown to be significantly decreased in dogs between

5 and 8 years of age, with further significant decreases occurring in dogs between 11 and 13 years of age (Miller et al., 1977). This finding in older dogs is comparable to the continual decrease in GFR that occurs in man, beginning at 40 to 50 years of age (Wesson, 1969; Lindeman, 1975).

Pickrell et al. (1974) have provided some insight into the relationship of renal function to age by measuring the various constituents of serum from laboratory Beagles ranging in age from less than 1 year to 10 years. These investigators have observed no significant differences in serum urea nitrogen or serum ions (including potassium, chloride, and calcium) in dogs of different ages; serum phosphorus levels are actually lower in older animals than in dogs under 2 years of age. Lindeman (1975), in a review of age-related renal changes in dogs, states that changes do not occur in electrolyte concentrations when measured under basal conditions.

Spontaneous Diseases

Histologically, the kidneys of carnivores, particularly the dog, exhibit a number of changes that are generally age-associated. Pathologists routinely recognize these minor changes, although they have not been clearly quantitated or documented. Commonly, there is a thickening of Bowman's capsule, with or without concurrent lesions, which occurs focally or occasionally diffusely. Although not considered to be of clinical significance, the renal tubular epithelial cells frequently show accumulation of endogenous pigments. These pigments may occur in relatively young dogs, but are seen more frequently and in greater quantities in aged animals. Three pigments, lipofuscin, biliary pigments, and hemosiderin, are generally located intracytoplasmically in proximal convoluted tubules, but also occur in the straight tubular cells and cells of the distal convoluted tubules. One or all of these pigments may occur in the same dog, but generally only one predominates. Microscopically, focal mineralization in the renal medulla is relatively common in older dogs and cats. These minute accumulations of mineral salts may be seen within the tubular lumina, appearing as concretions, or occasionally involving epithelial cells.

In the clinically healthy dog, the most common renal change associated with aging is glomerulosclerosis, usually found during routine histologic examination of the kidney.

This lesion may appear as a focal change, affecting only some glomeruli, or may be diffuse appearing, at least segmentally, in essentially all glomeruli. It is characterized by an increase in the PAS-positive mesangial matrix and generally is accompanied by increased numbers of mesangial cells. Glomerular capillary loops show a variable increase in thickness of their walls.

The first systematic study of glomerulosclerosis in dogs was performed on laboratory Beagles up to 11 years of age by Guttman and Andersen (1968) utilizing histological, ultrastructural, and immunofluorescent techniques. Initial lesions were detectable at the ultrastructural level in dogs as young as 500 days of age, increasing in severity in older animals. There was an age-related increase in the amount of mesangial matrix and number of mesangial cells. In addition, collagen fibers were reported in some mesangial areas together with electron-dense deposits that were also present within the basement membranes and subendothelial areas of the glomerular capillaries. These investigators demonstrated that deposits of IgG were located within the affected glomeruli, primarily in mesangial areas, and they speculated that glomerulosclerosis is immunologic in nature, possibly a response to infectious agents or altered tissue components that occur during the life span of the dog. More recently, similar glomerular lesions were characterized by Stuart et al. (1975) in 4- to 6-year-old Beagles that had proteinuria but were clinically normal. In addition to the deposition of IgG within the glomerular lesions, the latter investigators also demonstrated that the lesions contained deposits of the third component of complement. Like earlier investigators, Stuart et al. (1975) felt that these glomerular changes had an immunologic pathogenesis of a nonprogressive nature.

Chronic renal disease occurs commonly in dogs. It may result from glomerular or interstitial lesions or from pyelonephritis or amyloidosis. The disease may occur in dogs of any age, but its frequency is higher in older animals (Osborne et al., 1972; Müller-Peddinghaus and Trautwein, 1977b).

Until relatively recently, canine glomerulonephritis has been considered rare, recognized only in those cases of a classical nature (Monlux, 1953). With the development of new techniques, however, it is now recognized as a relatively common disease (Kurtz et al., 1972; Murray and Wright, 1974; Müller-Peddinghaus and Trautwein, 1977b). Many of the cases called glomerulosclerosis in earlier

studies probably would be classified today as glomerulonephritis either of the mesangial sclerosing or mesangial
proliferative forms. All types of glomerulonephritis occur in the dog including the membranous and proliferative
forms, in addition to the mesangial types, and are considered to have an immunological pathogenesis (due to the
formation of antigen-antibody complexes). However, like
most cases of the disease in man, the antigens involved
in the immune-mediated lesions are unknown. Chronic viral
infection has been suggested as a possible etiologic factor. One piece of evidence supporting this is the unusually high frequency of membranous glomerulonephritis in
cats infected with feline leukemia virus.

Renal amyloidosis represents one of the most severe
clinical pathologic entities that occurs in the dog. The
incidence of renal amyloidosis is unknown; however, surveys made from necropsy cases indicate that from 0.5 to
1.0 percent of all dogs may be affected (Hjarre, 1933;
Runnells et al., 1965). The condition is considered primarily a disease of older dogs; mean ages of 9.4 and 9.2
years have been reported in studies of 28 cases (Osborne
et al., 1968a) and 44 cases (Slauson et al., 1970), respectively. Differences in the frequency of the disease
between sexes has not been established.

The etiology of amyloidosis is not clearly understood in
any species, including the dog, although it is frequently
considered associated with an altered immune response.
Traditionally, the disease is divided into primary and
secondary forms. Primary amyloidosis, also termed idiopathic amyloidosis, is not associated with any other specific clinicopathological condition and is considered the
most common form of the disease in dogs (Bloom, 1954b;
Jubb and Kennedy, 1971b). Secondary amyloidosis develops
in association with chronic infectious processes and is
also associated with neoplasms. A hereditary form of the
disease is recognized in several species, including man.
The hereditary form of amyloidosis has not been reported
in the dog or cats, but renal amyloidosis has been described in dogs with hereditary cyclic neutropenia (Cheville, 1968). It also has been described as occurring
with plasma cell myeloma in the dog (Jennings, 1949).

Clinically, amyloidosis in the dog (whether generalized
or renal) presents as glomerular disease with proteinuria
that may progress to the nephrotic syndrome (Osborne, et
al., 1968a). Proteinuria is the result of deposition of
amyloid in the subepithelial areas of the glomerular capillaries, which may progress to such an extent that the

capillary lumina are essentially obliterated. The three proteins recognized in amyloidosis of man--variable parts of monoclonal immunoglobulin light chains, fibril protein AA, and hormone-like polypeptides--have not been characterized in canine amyloidosis (Cornwell et al., 1977).

Chronic interstitial nephritis represents one of the most common and serious clinical entities of the dog (Bloom, 1954). The etiology of the disease is unknown; however, two infectious agents, Leptospira sp. and canine adenovirus type 1, have been suggested as possible causes since both agents are known to produce acute renal lesions (Wright, 1967; Platt, 1970). This lesion is unique to carnivores, principally dogs, and has no exact counterpart in man. It is characterized by extensive fibrosis centered at the cortical-medullary junction, frequently extending to the cortical surface and the pelvis, together with secondary tubular cysts and sclerotic glomeruli. There is also variable infiltration with immunocytes (Casey et al., 1978). As a result of the extensive tubular loss, reabsorptive functions are severely compromised, resulting in polyuria with a low specific gravity that may be accompanied by mild proteinuria. Müller-Peddinghaus and Trautwein (1977a) have shown that the frequency of the disease, although not the severity of the lesions, is age-related. In their study of 94 dogs, 90 percent of the dogs over 10 years of age had interstitial disease compared to 20 percent of the dogs under 5 years of age.

Both the dog and cat may develop pyelonephritis in mild to severe forms. Although the disease may occur in old animals, it is not considered age-related (Christie, 1971). Pyelonephritis in the dog, however, is recognized as occurring secondarily to conditions that are age-related, such as prostatic hyperplasia and degeneration of intervertebral disks resulting in secondary myelopathy (Casey et al., 1978).

Primary neoplasia of the canine kidney is not common; reports involving a significant number of renal tumors indicate that they represent from only 0.6 to 1.7 percent of all canine tumors (Flir, 1952; Baskin and DePaoli, 1977). Excluding embryonal nephromas, which generally occur in young dogs, renal neoplasia is considered a disease of middle- and old-aged dogs. Baskin and DePaoli (1977) have found that the mean age of 58 dogs reported to have primary renal neoplasia is 7.9 years when dogs with embryonal nephromas are excluded. Most reports suggest that the disease is more common in the male than the female (H. M. Hays, Jr., National Institutes of Health, Bethesda,

Maryland, Unpublished; Baskin and DePaoli, 1977). The majority of renal tumors are malignant; approximately half develop metastases (Baskin and DePaoli, 1977). Most primary renal neoplasms develop from the tubular epithelial cells and may show a variety of histologic patterns including tubular and papillary formations in either solid or cystic growths (Nielsen et al., 1976). Because of the mixed histologic patterns, the division of canine tumors by type often is arbitrary. The clear-cell carcinoma, frequently seen as a metastatic lesion in man (Oberling et al., 1960; Bennington and Beckwith, 1975), is apparently rare in the dog (Nielsen et al., 1976); however, areas of neoplastic clear cells frequently appear in many canine carcinomas (Baskin and DePaoli, 1977). Distinction between adenomas and carcinomas of renal tubular cell origin also is difficult on a histological basis and, as with the neoplasms in man, size is frequently used to divide these growths into malignant and benign types arbitrarily.

Transitional cell epithelial tumors arise in the canine renal pelvis and may either be benign papillomas or carcinomas. Histologically, these neoplasms are identical to those developing in the bladder and lower urinary tract. The kidney may also be the site of development of a variety of soft tissue sarcomas, including both benign and malignant types (Cadwallader et al., 1973; Nielsen et al., 1976; Baskin and DePaoli, 1977). Mesenchymal neoplasms of the kidney are similar to those developing elsewhere in the body and occur principally in older animals, but with less frequency than epithelial cell neoplasms.

Induced Models

A number of investigators have used the dog as a model to study glomerulonephritis. Bevans et al., (1955), Seegal et al. (1955), Steblay and Lepper (1961), and McPhaul et al. (1974) have used immunologic methods to produce Goodpasture's disease. Dogs readily develop antibasement membrane glomerulonephritis when they are administered nephrotoxic antiserum of heterogenous origin or autologous antibodies prepared from heterologous basement membranes and placental antigens. McPhaul et al. (1974), however, have been unable to produce these lesions by active immunization with autologous renal basement antigens. Guttman and Andersen (1968) have shown that the incidence of glomerulosclerosis approaches 100 percent and is increased in severity as a long-term effect of whole-body irradiation.

Summary

Chronic renal disease, with a variety of etiologies, is a common clinical entity in mid- and old-aged carnivores, particularly dogs. Glomerular lesions in the dog exhibit many of the morphological changes that occur in man. Glomerulonephritis in both man and dog is considered to have an immunologic pathogenesis, and definition of the antigens involved in the canine lesions should provide a better understanding of the possible etiology of these lesions in man. Likewise, renal amyloidosis is age-related in the dog as it is in man. This, coupled with the relatively high incidence of canine renal amyloidosis, makes the dog a unique animal model for the study of a disease associated with senility in man. Perhaps of greatest significance is the usefulness of dogs with chronic renal disease as models for the study of renal failure in man, particularly with regard to the effects of decreased renal function on other organs and functions of the body.

Genital System

Female Genital System

The carnivore female reproductive cycle differs considerably from that of the human female; the carnivore has an estrous cycle rather than a menstrual cycle. Dogs generally have an estrous cycle every 6-10 months, from puberty to approximately 8 years of age. Andersen and Simpson (1973) have reported that the mean interval between estrous cycles is approximately 241 days in Beagles up to 8 years of age. Similar timing has been reported by Taylor et al. (1976). A period of reproductive senescence (not comparable to menopause) is common in older dogs and is characterized by irregular estrous cycles with extended periods of anestrous. Andersen and Simpson (1973) have found that for dogs between 8 and 16 years of age, the mean interval between estrous cycles is 332 days, but can extend up to 20 months. A corresponding drop in fertility after 8 years of age has been noted (Andersen, 1957, 1965). At the peak of reproduction, approximately 3 years of age, Andersen and Simpson (1973) have reported a fertility rate of approximately 85 percent. In Beagles 4 to 8 years of age, the fertility rate is only approximately 47 percent, decreasing still further (to 30 percent) in bitches 8 to 12 years of age. This low rate of fertility has

also been observed in bitches over 8 years of age by
Strasser and Schumacher (1968). In addition to the low
fertility rate, pups borne of older bitches have been
shown to have a higher mortality rate than those borne
to younger bitches. The mortality rate for pups borne by
bitches 1 to 3 years old has been reported to be 22 percent versus 33 percent for pups borne to bitches from
4 to 8 years old and 66 percent for pups borne to bitches
from 8 to 12 years of age (Andersen and Simpson, 1973).

Morphological studies on aging of the carnivore female
genital tract have been principally limited to the canine,
specifically laboratory-reared Beagles. No gross changes
of the ovary have been observed in extensive studies of
aged Beagles conducted by Andersen and Simpson (1973); however, Stott et al. (1971) have reported an increase in
ovarian weights in Beagles up to 12 years of age that correlates with an increase in body weight. Similar observations also have been described by Das and Magilton (1971).
Despite the absence of gross morphological changes with age,
histologically, the canine ovary is remarkably different
in older bitches from that in young and middle-aged bitches
(Andersen and Simpson, 1973). In most areas, the simple
cuboidal epithelium becomes pseudo-stratified in a proliferative process that begins at approximately 5 years of
age. The epithelial proliferation also extends into the
parenchyma, forming clefts and tubular-like structures in
the surface of the ovary that may develop into cysts and
possibly neoplasms. Similarly, the rete ovarii undergoes
hyperplasia in approximately 50 percent of bitches over 8
years of age and may also become cystic. Cords of granulosa cells remaining from atretic follicles become very
prominent in the ovary of aged bitches. The most striking
histologic change with increasing age is the marked reduction in the number of follicles. Schotterer (1928) has
estimated that the number of follicles mixed-breed dogs
have at puberty is 355,000; 34,000 at 5 years of age;
and only 500 at 10 years of age. Andersen and Simpson
(1973) have made a somewhat lower estimate of follicles
in Beagles: 70,000 to 80,000 prior to puberty and 1,500
to 2,000 in animals 8-16 years of age.

In addition to ovarian changes, the uterus in bitches in
reproductive senescence frequently exhibits atrophic cystic
changes of endometrial glands. These changes are thought
to be the result of long periods of anestrus (Andersen and
Simpson, 1973).

Spontaneous Diseases   Pathological changes in the genital
system of aged bitches are primarily limited to cyst formation and neoplasia. Ovarian cysts of various pathogenesis
are common in the aged bitch (Andersen and Simpson, 1973)
and may arise from the tubular proliferations of the epithelium, the rete ovarii, or the atretic follicles. Andersen and Simpson (1973) consider most of these cysts nonfunctional in nature. Neoplastic diseases of the canine ovary
are of major importance; however, uterine neoplasia is relatively rare in the dog (McEntee and Nielsen, 1976; Andersen
and Simpson, 1973). Ovarian tumors most frequently arise
from the ovarian epithelium and may be either adenomas or
adenocarcinomas. Granulosa cell tumors are found less frequently. Andersen and Simpson (1973) have reported that
9 of 59 Beagles developed adenocarcinomas at a median age
of 13.5 years. Three of the fifty-nine dogs also developed
granulosa cell tumors. The subject of canine ovarian neoplasia has recently been reviewed by Moulton (1978).

Although not entirely limited to aged animals, the most
common pathological condition of the uterus in aged bitches
is pyometra or hydrometra (Whitney, 1967; Andersen and
Simpson, 1973). Andersen and Simpson (1973) have reported
that 4 percent of all Beagle bitches in their study exhibited either hydrometra or pyometra between 8 and 17 years
of age. Vaginal, fibromuscular polyps are also a highly
common pathologic entity in the aged bitch. Andersen and
Simpson (1973) have reported this disease in 25 percent of
Beagles over 10 years of age.

Summary   The canine offers an excellent model for the study
of the increased mortality and stillbirths that occur in
infants born to women in the latter part of their reproductive life. Defining the causes of the progressive mortality and stillbirths in pups born to 4- to 12-year-old
bitches could provide significant insights in addressing
the problem in human medicine.

Mammary Gland

The canine mammary gland differs in two major ways from
that of human females: It retains its secretory function
throughout life, not showing postreproductive atrophy,
and the lobular system undergoes atrophy during anestrus
and marked proliferation during estrus. Age-related
changes in the canine mammary gland are generally grouped
into dysplastic and neoplastic lesions.

Dysplastic lesions of the canine mammary gland are extremely common and are almost always multiple. They may involve both stromal and epithelial components of the gland, but the latter are more frequent. These lesions may be large and tumorous or small microscopic foci. Dysplasias are most common and larger in older bitches; however, they begin to develop relatively early in life. The large number and early nature of these lesions has become apparent only recently through study of subgross sections of mammary glands prepared by using whole mount techniques. In a study of 654 atypical mammary gland nodules in Beagles 7 to 8 years of age, 78 percent have been reported to be either focal or diffuse epithelial hyperplasia of the mammary lobule, 8 percent to be inflammatory in nature, and the remaining 14 percent to be early neoplastic lesions (Cameron and Faulkin, 1971).

The age at which these dysplastic lesions develop has been studied in 39 bitches 6 months to 4 years of age (Warner, 1976; R. Giles, Department of Veterinary Science, University of Kentucky, Lexington, Kentucky, Unpublished). Dysplastic lesions were not seen in bitches less than 2 years of age; however in bitches 2 to 3 years of age, the frequency of these lesions exceeded 50 percent. Of the 787 lesions examined in this study, 89 percent were classified as lobular dysplasias, the remainder as cysts, ductal ectasias, intraductal dysplasias, and inflammatory lobules. Neoplastic lesions were not described; however, five lobular dysplasias were described as atypical. Some investigators have suggested that mammary dysplasias represent preneoplastic lesions (Cameron and Faulkin, 1971; Warner, 1976; Giles et al., 1977; R. Giles, Department of Veterinary Science, University of Kentucky, Lexington, Kentucky, Unpublished). Definitive studies using transplantation techniques have not been undertaken because of the lack of inbred, histocompatible dogs.

Histologically, some dysplastic lesions bear a close resemblance to fibrocystic lesions of the human breast, having the hallmarks of fibrosis, cyst formation, and adenosis (Robbins, 1974d). However, most of the larger, tumor-like dysplasias contain significant areas of hyperplastic epithelium, consisting of both secretory and myoepithelial cells, with or without cyst formation and fibrosis (Bloom, 1954a; Hampe and Misdorp, 1974). The epithelial hyperplasia seen in the dog lesion may closely resemble adenosis of the human breast when composed of secretory epithelial cells; however, the canine mammary gland has a marked propensity for hyperplasia of myoepithelial cells, which is distinctly different from the human mammary gland. The distinction between dysplastic lesions, particularly those with a significant myoepithelial component, and complex adenomas and benign mixed tumors is frequently difficult to determine histologically, and some dysplasias probably represent a stage in the development of these benign tumors (Robbins, 1974d; Giles et al., 1977).

The most common age-related, clinical entity in bitches is mammary neoplasia, representing 10-15 percent of all neoplasms (Hamilton, 1974, Casey et al., 1979). Definitive incidence data for mammary neoplasms is limited due to the lack of defined populations at risk. A single study using a defined population shows the incidence of histologically malignant mammary gland tumors is approximately 200 per 100,000 dogs (Dorn et al., 1968b). The percentage of malignant versus benign mammary gland tumors in the dog varies from 40 to 60 percent (Hamilton, 1974; Casey et al., 1979). The peak age for the occurrence of mammary neoplasms is generally accepted to be around 10 to 11 years, with a sharp increase in their frequency at about 8 years of age. The median age reported in a variety of breeds of dogs from the general pet population is 10.5 years (Dorn et al., 1968b). Age-specific incidence rates continue to rise throughout life in laboratory-reared Beagles monitored for 15 years, (Taylor et al., 1976). Very few neoplasms are reported in bitches under 6 years of age.

Although the vast majority of canine mammary neoplasms develop at mid-to-old age, their occurrence apparently is dependent on normal ovarian function during the first two years of life. Numerous investigators have noted a lower frequency of mammary tumors in ovariectomized bitches, particularly if ovariectomy is performed at an early age (Bloom, 1954a; Mulligan, 1963; Brodey et al., 1966; Frye et al., 1967). In retrospective studies with matched controls, it has been shown that the risk of tumor development is 0.5 percent if ovariectomy is performed before the first estrus, 8 percent if performed after the first estrus, and 26 percent if performed after the second estrus. Ovariectomy after 2.5 years of age has no effect on the frequency of mammary tumor development. It may be significant that this age coincides with the age at which dysplasias become detectable in the mammary gland.

A wide variety of mammary neoplasms, from benign papillomas and adenomas to highly anaplastic carcinomas and sarcomas, occur in dogs. Approximately 50 percent of these neoplasms are designated as mixed or complex, which is not

true of the neoplasms of other species, including man
(Cotchin, 1958; Casey et al., 1979; Moulton et al., 1970;
Fowler et al., 1974). Mixed or complex tumors are composed
of two types of epithelial cells, secretory and myoepithelial. It is generally accepted that the myoepithelial cell
of the canine mammary tumor frequently undergoes metaplasia
into cartilage and/or bone (Cotchin, 1958; Moulton et al.,
1970; Pulley, 1973). Most studies indicate that over 90
percent of the mixed tumors are benign. The most common
malignant tumor of the canine mammary gland is the carcinoma (Mulligan, 1949; Cotchin, 1958; Moulton et al., 1970;
Misdorp et al., 1972; Fowler et al., 1974; Monlux et al.,
1977). These carcinomas readily metastasize to the regional lymph nodes and lungs and may disseminate throughout the
body. The dog also has a disproportionate number of sarcomas of the mammary gland compared to other species. Ten
percent of all malignant tumors are reported to be sarcomas
(Casey et al., 1979; Misdorp et al., 1971). Osteosarcomas
are the most common malignant mesenchymal neoplasm of the
canine mammary gland (Cotchin, 1958; Misdorp et al., 1971;
Giles et al., 1977), but fibrosarcomas and chondrosarcomas
are not uncommon. Many of these sarcomas are believed to
arise from the myoepithelial cells (Fowler et al., 1974).

In a number of ways, canine mammary neoplasms are suitable for the study of the human disease. The extremely high
incidence of mammary neoplasia in the dog provides a readily accessible source for neoplastic material. These neoplasms share many features with some types of human breast
neoplasias, the leading cause of cancer deaths in women.
The marked participation of the myoepithelial cells in
many of the mammary gland tumors of the bitch provides a
unique source of experimental materials for the study of
this type of cell and is directly applicable to the study
of metaplastic carcinomas in women. The abundance of the
myoepithelial cell in canine mammary tumors also offers a
highly desirable model for the study of the hormonal responsiveness of the different cell types within the mammary gland.

Testicles

Age-related, functional changes in the testicles of carnivores have not been investigated, and the limited number of
morphological studies that have been performed have dealt
principally with neoplasia. Most pathologists recognize
atrophy of the seminiferous tubules with aspermatogenesis

as a relatively common, age-associated change in the dog.
The atrophic tubules are considered the end result of degeneration of the germ cells primarily, with little effect
on the sertoli cells (Jubb and Kennedy, 1963). Tubular
atrophy may be focal or diffuse, and in severely affected
testicles the tubules may have a thickened basement membrane accompanied by interstitial fibrosis. Focal or diffuse hyperplasia of the testicular interstitial cells is
also a common finding in older dogs and may represent an
early stage of neoplasia.

Neoplasia of the testicles ranks second to tumors of
the skin in the frequency of their occurrence in male dogs
(Hayes and Pendergrass, 1976). Whereas the vast majority
of testicular tumors in man are seminomas, arising from
germ cells (Mostofi and Price, 1973a,b), the dog develops
approximately equal numbers of seminomas, interstitial
cell tumors, and sertoli cell tumors (Lipowitz et al.,
1973; Hayes and Pendergrass, 1976). The exact incidence
of testicular tumors has not been well defined, but is
considered extremely high. Studies have shown that the
frequency of tumors may vary with the breed (Hayes and
Pendergrass, 1976); the German Shepherd Dog is considered
to have a very high frequency of seminomas (Robinson and
Garner, 1973). In contrast, interstitial cell tumors
and sertoli cell tumors are rare in man (Mostofi and Price,
1973a). The seminoma of the canine also differs from that
of man in that it rarely metastasizes (Dixon and Moore,
1953). Another difference is that seminomas in man occur
principally in young men (Dixon and Moore, 1953; Mostofi
and Price, 1973b), while in the dog the risk of development of seminomas continues to rise throughout the life
span (Hayes and Pendergrass, 1976). Both human and canine
cryptorchid males are especially at risk (R) for the development of seminomas; R = 8 to 14 (man) and R = 13.6
(canine) (Hayes and Pendergrass, 1976; Morrison, 1976).

Summary Although studies on the age-related changes in
the testicles of carnivores are limited, the documented
high incidence of seminomas in older dogs suggests its
possibility as an animal model for the study of the second
leading cause of cancer deaths in men between the ages of
25 and 29 (Mason et al., 1975).

Prostate Gland

The canine model is of major interest in studying aging of
the prostate gland because only the dog routinely develops
spontaneous benign prostatic hyperplasia with an incidence
comparable to that occurring in older men. The prostate
is morphologically and functionally similar in both man and
dog. The gland surrounds the urethra at its emergence from
the bladder and when diseased frequently interferes with
micturation. In the dog, enlargement of the gland also may
cause difficulties in defecation.

The size of the normal canine prostate varies with the
weight of the dog, ranging from 1.9 to 2.8 cm in length
and 1.9 to 2.7 cm in height and having a ratio of 0.21 to
0.57 gm gland/kg body weight (Berg, 1958a). Slightly larger prostates (mean 0.66 gm gland/kg body weight) have been
reported by O'Shea (1962) for 57 dogs with histologically
normal prostate glands. This compares to the approximately
20-gram prostate and ratio of 0.27 gm gland/kg body weight
in normal adult men. In both man and dog, the gland is
surrounded by a fibromuscular tissue forming an irregular
capsular structure. Trabeculae from the fibromuscular capsule extend into the parenchyma, but distinct lobules are
not discernable. Some authors recognize five lobes (Moore,
1936; Mostofi and Price, 1973c) in the human prostate
gland, while others describe only three (McNeal, 1974).
Three ill-defined lobes (two lateral and one medial) have
been recognized in the dog (Schoetthauer, 1932; Berg,
1958a). In both the dog and man, the periurethral areas
of the gland contain abundant stromal elements. Histologically, the prostate is made up of tubuloalveolar glands
that have fewer branches in the periurethral area than in
the peripheral portion of the organ. These glands consist
of columnar epithelial cells generally in a single layer;
however, basal cells, giving a two-layer appearance, may
be present in some areas in both man and dog (Dermer,
1978; Timms, 1976). The columnar epithelium rests on a
basement membrane situated on a fine fibrovascular stroma.
Infolding may give a papillary appearance to the glands
of normal dogs.

Functionally, the prostates of the dog and man have been
shown to have similar rates of conversion and degradation
of dihydrotestosterone, the androgen thought to be related
to hyperplasia of the gland (Siiteri and Wilson, 1970;
Gloyna et al., 1970). Castration is known to produce prostatic atrophy in the dog (Huggins and Clark, 1940), and
exogenous estrogen administration decreases the size of the

gland and inhibits its secretions. Prolonged administration of estrogens produces squamous metaplasia of the glandular epithelium (Huggins and Clark, 1940; Huggins et al., 1940). Receptor sites for androgenic hormones have been documented in normal and diseased canine prostates (Shain and Boesel, 1978; Ofner et al., 1974). Prostatic disease in the dog is essentially limited to prostatitis, benign prostatic hyperplasia, and rarely, prostatic neoplasms. A discussion of the dog as a model for studying human benign prostatic hyperplasia is contained in the section entitled "Comparative Models for Problems of the Human Elderly."

Nonhuman Primates

INTRODUCTION

Nonhuman primates are of special importance as models in biomedical research because their phylogenetic proximity to man makes them more closely homologous to humans--in anatomical features, embryological and fetal development, physiological function, and biochemical mechanisms--than are other laboratory species. This relationship makes them particularly valuable for investigations of developmental processes and diseases relevant to human conditions.

The primates have been used infrequently in research on aging for several reasons. It has proved difficult to determine the age of wild-caught animals with acceptable precision, and aged captive animals have been scarce, widely dispersed, and of diverse species. Significant government support for facilities to maintain old animals has been available only since the early 1960s; thus, the numbers of older animals of known age available for study have been severely limited.

In 1974, the authors of a review article on animal models in research on aging (Getty and Ellenport, 1974) found too little information on nonhuman primates to merit discussion. A 1979 bibliography listing publications since 1940 in which primate aging is the focus of interest, or even in which the characteristics of individual aged animals are described, comprises only 193 references (Caminiti, 1979). Very few reports involve the study of more than one or two animals that could reasonably be regarded as in the last third of the life span of their species. The only species in which aging has been studied in any systematic way is the pig-tailed macaque (Macaca nemestrina) (Bowden, 1979).

Information on aging in nonhuman primates is limited but is consistent with the phylogenetic expectation that their aging is similar to aging in man. With increasing appreciation of this fact among biomedical researchers in the past two decades, and the accumulation of aged animals in primate research colonies, research on aging in these species has begun to increase. More than 95 percent of the published reports on aging in nonhuman primates have appeared since 1960, and more than 80 percent since 1970.

One of the major limitations to primate research is animal availability. Primates as an order have a relatively long gestation period, long generation time (time for the newborn to reach reproductive age), and, as a rule, single births. Even those animals that appear abundant in natural habitats, e.g., the rhesus macaque (Macaca mulatta), are easily depleted by habitat destruction, consistent trapping for commercial and biomedical use, and similar disturbances. In recent years, governments in the countries of origin have become alarmed at the depletion of endemic primate populations and have taken steps to slow exports or to stop them completely.

Such constraints make it essential that available animals be used wisely. In addition to the usual criteria used for judging the scientific merit of projects, the following considerations are important in judging proposals for research on aging with nonhuman primates:

● Nonhuman primates are appropriate subjects for studying aging phenomena and aspects of age-related diseases of humans for which no relevant model exists in phylogenetically more distant species.

● They are appropriate subjects for testing the generality of important findings in phylogenetically more distant species to the order Primates.

● They are appropriate subjects for the experimental testing of hypotheses that cannot be tested in man and for which there is sound scientific reason to doubt the relevance of other animal models.

When a project requires the use of nonhuman primates, the species used should be appropriate and available in sufficient numbers. Studies of nonhuman primates should use the smallest number of subjects necessary to produce acceptable scientific results, and each animal should be used in such a manner as to provide as much information as possible about aging processes and diseases of the human aged. For these reasons, we include here descriptions of the major genera and species that have been used in biomedical research, as well as information on the numbers of old animals that exist in U.S. institutions. Further information on the state of wild populations and degree of general use of the most widely used primate genera and species have been reviewed in Primate Utilization and Conservation (Bermant and Lindburg, 1975) and by the Institute of Laboratory Animal Resources (ILAR) Committee on Conservation of Nonhuman Primates (1976b); this report, Nonhuman Primates: Usage and Availability for Biomedical Programs, should be consulted for more information on the availability of a species of interest.

OVERVIEW OF TAXONOMY

The replicability of biomedical experimentation rests heavily on identifying subjects as precisely as possible using a standard scientific nomenclature. Recognizing that the taxonomy and nomenclature of the order Primates is not in final form, we recommend that Napier and Napier's (1967) Handbook of Living Primates be used as a provisional standard for identifying nonhuman primate subjects. It is generally available and already in wide use. The description of an experiment often reads most smoothly if the common name of the species, e.g., rhesus macaque, is used in the text; however, the common name should always be referenced at the outset using the Latin genus and species name, e.g., Macaca mulatta, followed by a subspecies name, if appropriate, and country of origin, if known.

Inasmuch as many species are composed of multiple subspecies, accurate identification of the animal used will be impossible unless the geographic origins are also indicated. Populations of a single species may differ from place to place in the very characteristics critical to the investigation concerned, and it is no more correct to assume that all individuals of a nonhuman species are interchangeable than to assume that all humans are identical in physiology, biochemistry, etc. (Wagner et al., 1978). Local populations of animals are generally more similar to each other than to individuals from other local populations, so that identificaton of geographic origin improves replicability of results of research on any animal species.

When attempting to identify a subject, the investigator cannot always rely on the identification or geographic

origin given by an animal dealer; it is not sufficient to
identify a subject as Macaca fascicularis simply because
the investigator ordered "cynomolgus monkeys" from the
dealer. When in doubt, the investigator should refer to
the Handbook of Living Primates or consult the Department
of Mammalogy of the National Museum of Natural History,
Smithsonian Institution, Washington, D.C. 20560, for assistance in proper identification. When there is a specific disagreement with nomenclature in the Handbook of
Living Primates, reference should be made to the source
of the genus and species names used to help others identify the subjects in a particular experiment.

The genetic history of the various nonhuman primate
species used in biomedical research is closer to the
"natural state" than that of any other commonly used animal model. Up to the present time, most primates in research laboratories have come directly from wild populations, whose gene pools have been subjected to minimal
manipulation by man. The impossibility of reconstructing
the genetic history of rodents, cats, and dogs that have
been bred for various characteristics by pet breeders and
scientists for tens or hundreds of generations often precludes answering questions about the genetic composition
of the "wild strains" from which they originated.

WHAT IS A PRIMATE?

The Handbook of Living Primates (Napier and Napier, 1967)
lists 52 genera and 182 species (excluding tree shrews)
in the order Primates. In general, the primates are recognized by common features of skeletal structure, reproduction, brain structure, and behavior (Napier and Napier,
1967; Schultz, 1969). The skeletal limb structure characteristic of primates includes the clavicle, which is absent in some mammalian groups. The hand and foot each
have five digits that tend to be more freely mobile than
in other animals, particularly the thumb and toe, which
are used for grasping. The digits terminate in flattened
nails rather than sharp, compressed claws, and the pads
of the digits have a considerably greater density of tactile receptors than in other mammals. Gestational processes contributing to the nourishment of the fetus are
elaborate, the duration of dependency of offspring on
their parents is long, and social relationships are
complex.

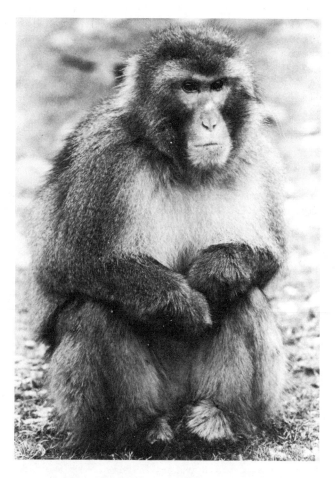

The Japanese macaque, <u>Macaca</u> <u>fuscata</u>. Photo-
graph courtesy of the Division of Research
Resources, National Institutes of Health,
Bethesda, Maryland.

A third group of features characteristic of primates concerns the phylogenetic development of the head and central nervous system. There is shortening of the snout with loss of certain elements of primitive mammalian dentition and relatively little development of the olfactory apparatus. The visual system is elaborate, with color vision and variable degrees of binocular vision. There is a bony ring around the orbits and the cranium is large in association with an elaboration of the brain, particularly of the cerebral cortex. The highly developed central nervous system no doubt contributes to the complexity of social behavior and accounts for the primates' ability to modify behavior as a function of experience.

Most of these characteristics of primates are general, i.e., neither universal nor exclusive. The only universal and exclusive characteristic of the living primates is the possession of a flattened nail on at least one digit. The bony ring around the orbits, retention of the clavicle, and retention of five digits are universal, but not exclusive, characteristics.

A representation of primate phylogeny focusing on the degree of separation between man and the major groups of nonhuman primates is presented in Figure 22. Man diverged from the chimpanzee and gorilla, his closest relatives on the phylogenetic tree, only a few million years ago. Given the rate of molecular evolution, some scholars postulate that only several hundred gene substitutions account for all of the differences between man and the great apes (Sacher, 1978). Depending on whether one dates by molecular indices or fossil records, the human and great ape lines diverged from the Old World monkeys 25 to 35 million years ago, from the New World monkeys 35 to 55 million years ago, and from the prosimians 60 to 65 million years ago (Cutler, 1976a). By way of comparison, our common ancestors with rodent and carnivore species widely used in biomedical research, lived 75 to 90 million years ago (Goodman, 1976).

The following is a simplified description of the major superfamilies and species within those families that have been used for biomedical research or that have obvious characteristics that could make them suitable subjects for studies of aging. Table 23 summarizes some of the characteristics of species commonly used in biomedical research that influence their suitability for particular studies.

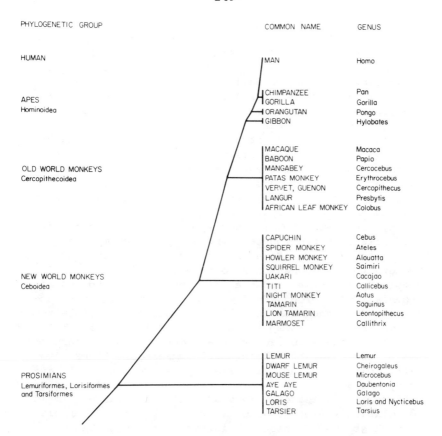

FIGURE 22 Phylogenetic distance between the human and various nonhuman primates. Nonhuman primates chosen for which maximal life span data are available (Bowden and Jones, 1979). Figure courtesy of D. M. Bowden, Washington Regional Primate Research Center, University of Washington, Seattle, Washington.

Apes (Hominoidea)

Humans share the superfamily Hominoidea with chimpanzees (<u>Pan</u> spp.), gorillas (<u>Gorilla gorilla</u>), orangutans (<u>Pongo pygmaeus</u>), and gibbons (<u>Hylobates</u> spp. and <u>Symphalangus syndactylus</u>). Characteristics of man and other hominoids that distinguish them from other primates include extreme mobility of the shoulder that allows relaxed overhead

suspension by the forelimb(s); long forelimbs relative
to trunk length; a broad, shallow thorax; shortened lumbar
region of the spine; and a common cusp pattern of the
molar teeth (Clark, 1959). There is considerable debate
over the exact dates of phylogenetic splits, but paleon-
tological data (Pilbeam, 1972; Simons, 1972) and comparative biochemical evidence (Goodman, 1976; Sarich and
Cronin, 1976) agree that chimpanzees, gorillas, and humans share the most recent common ancestor, that orangutans diverged somewhat earlier from the line, and that
gibbons separated still earlier. The most objective evidence on phylogenetic distance comes from biochemical
comparisons, and the phylogeny of primates in Figure 22
is based on such a comparison.

Pan, the genus of chimpanzees, includes the "common"
chimpanzee (Pan troglodytes) and the pygmy chimpanzee
(Pan paniscus). Found in Africa, their habitats vary
from dry forest and savanna to tropical rain forest. The
chimpanzee is the nonhuman animal most similar to humans
in overall morphology (Huxley, 1863) and molecular structure (Goodman and Tashian, 1976). Social lives of chimpanzees are highly complex (Lawick-Goodall, 1971). They
are rare in the wild, and natural populations are threatened by expansion of agricultural human populations into
their habitat. Chimpanzees are kept successfully in captivity and are the most common genus of great ape studied
in biomedical research. They are, however, large animals
and relatively expensive to maintain. The number of old
chimpanzees in U.S. research institutions is probably
less than 30 (Table 24), but they are concentrated in
a small number of facilities, enhancing their potential
availability for research on aging.

Pongo, the genus of orangutans, consists of a single
species, Pongo pygmaeus, occupying two distinct geographical areas, northern Sumatra and parts of Borneo. The
orangutan shares many morphological features with humans
and with the other great apes, but is phylogenetically
more distant from humans than the chimpanzee and gorilla.
It is an unusual primate in that it is often solitary
in the wild. Orangutans are almost exclusively arboreal.
Wild populations are sparse, threatened by destruction
of their tropical forest habitat by logging operations
and by increasing agricultural use of previously forested
land. Very few old orangutans exist in captivity (Table
24).

Old World Monkeys (Cercopithecoidea)

Morphological characteristics shared by Old World monkeys
that separate them from the apes and man are: generally
quadrupedal musculoskeletal anatomy, including a shoulder
that is relatively restricted in mobility; a deep, narrow
thorax and longer lumbar region of the spine; and "bilo-
phodont" cusp pattern of the molar teeth (Clark, 1959).
While there is no known fossil that is clearly a common
ancestor to the apes and Old World monkeys, comparative
morphology, fossil evidence (Simons, 1972), and a variety
of biochemical data (Goodman and Tashian, 1976) indicate
that they probably became distinct taxa between 25 and
35 million years ago. The 75 species (Napier and Napier,
1967) of Old World monkeys can be divided into two sub-
families: the Cercopithecinae and the Colobinae. Macaques (Macaca spp.), baboons (Papio spp.), and green
monkeys (Cercopithecus aethiops) are typical of the cer-
copithecines that are widely used in biomedical research;
the Colobinae are little used.

Baboons (Papio) may be divided into several species,
all of which are found in various parts of Africa. The
four species of savanna baboons are the guinea baboon
(Papio papio), olive baboon (Papio anubis), yellow baboon
(Papio cynocephalus), and chacma baboon (Papio ursinus).
The habitat of these species varies from arid savanna to
tropical forest. Hamadryas baboons (Papio hamadryas) are
found in Ethiopia and on portions of the Arabian penin-
sula. They are distinguished from the savanna baboons by
a lighter-skinned muzzle and a heavier mantle of hair on
the shoulders of males. They typically have a social organization comprised of one-male units that aggregate in
larger groups of variable size. The habitat of hamadryas
baboons is typically arid. Baboons are used moderately
in biomedical research where large hardy subjects are required and the topic of study does not require the use of
apes. More than 100 old baboons exist in U.S. research
institutions, and they are concentrated in a small number
of colonies (Table 24).

The genus Macaca consists of numerous species. They
share common body proportions with fore- and hindlimbs of
approximately equal length. They vary in size from 2 to
19 kg depending on sex and species (Table 23). This
highly adaptive genus is widely distributed from North
Africa to the Philippines and through habitats ranging
from the cold of northern Japan to the tropical rain
forests of Southeast Asia. Some macaques spend a

considerable portion of time on the ground, whereas others live predominantly in the trees. Because of their availability, moderate size, and ease of maintenance in captivity, the macaques are the most common nonhuman primates used in biomedical research. The rhesus macaque, Macaca mulatta, is the most common species of nonhuman primate in captivity. Other macaques commonly used in biomedical research include the pig-tailed macaque (Macaca nemestrina), bonnet macaque (Macaca radiata), and long-tailed macaque (Macaca fascicularis), otherwise known as the crab-eating macaque or cynomolgus monkey. The stump-tailed macaque (Macaca speciosa or arctoides) is found in some laboratories, although it is now an endangered species. The Celebes black ape (Macaca nigra; Fooden, 1969) is truly a macaque and is used occasionally in biomedical research. The macaques comprise the greatest numbers of old primates in U.S. research institutions (Table 24).

The green, vervet, or grivet monkeys (Cercopithecus aethiops) range over the savannas of subsaharan Africa; they are not found in tropical forests or arid regions. There is also a large population of green monkeys on St. Kitts Island in the Caribbean, where they were introduced several centuries ago. These animals are similar in body shape to a macaque, but are more gracile with more colorful pelage and a face that has a black muzzle surrounded by a ruff of white. They are moderately used in biomedical research, but few, if any, old ones exist in captivity (Table 24).

The patas monkey (Erythrocebus patas) is found in savannas of Africa. It is a colorful animal with a red coat on the back and outside of the legs, gray from the tips of the ears to the chin, and a distinctive white mustache. The patas' long legs give it a greyhound-like appearance, and it is in fact a fast-moving primate. It is used in some biomedical research, but is not a common primate in captivity, and few, if any, old ones exist in U.S. research institutions (Table 24).

New World Monkeys (Ceboidea)

All of the New World monkeys are native to Central and South America. They differ morphologically from the Old World monkeys, apes, and man in that they lack the downwardly directed nostrils, have a broader nasal septum, and have three premolars instead of two. Their phylogenetic line is believed to have diverged from that leading to the Old World monkeys, apes, and humans between 35 and 55 million years ago.

The New World monkeys are divided into two rather different families: the Cebidae and the Callitrichidae. Cebids resemble the Old World monkeys in general morphology and behavior. The callitrichids, in contrast, are smaller and differ in several aspects of morphology, most obvious of which are the claw-like nails of their fingers and toes. Examples of cebids used in biomedical research are squirrel monkeys (_Saimiri_ spp.), owl monkeys (_Aotus trivirgatus_, the only living nocturnal monkey), and cebus monkeys (_Cebus_ spp.). Of these, the squirrel monkey is by far the most common.

Squirrel monkeys were introduced into biomedical research in the United States during the 1950s and 1960s, because of their small size and ready availability. They consist of two species: _Saimiri sciureus_, the common squirrel monkey distributed widely through Central and South America, and _Saimiri oerstedii_, the red-backed squirrel monkey from Bolivia. Even squirrel monkeys of the same species can show behavioral and endocrinological differences that are significant. Like many smaller primates, they feed largely on insects. They are totally arboreal. Some squirrel monkeys are reported to live in large groups in which males are segregated from females except during the breeding season. They continue to be bred for research, and old animals of this genus are the second most common of all primate genera in U.S. research institutions. The fact that their maximal life span is 10 to 15 years shorter than that of the macaques (Table 23) may particularly suit them for certain studies of aging.

The callitrichids, including the marmosets (_Callithrix_ spp.) and tamarins (_Saguinus_ spp.), are smaller New World species. They are less studied than the squirrel monkey in U.S. laboratories, but several large breeding colonies have been established in Europe in recent years. Current evidence suggests (Table 23) that their maximal life spans may be half that of the squirrel monkey. If this proves true, the marmosets and tamarins will be the genera phylogenetically closest to the human that have life spans in the 10- to 15-year range. Tamarins are presently the fourth most common old primate in U.S. research institutions (Table 24).

Prosimians (Lemuriformes, Lorisiformes, and Tarsiiformes)

According to common practice in the United States, humans, apes, and Old World and New World monkeys are placed in the suborder, Anthropoidea, or "manlike" primates. The rest of the primates are assigned to the suborder Prosimii, or "premonkeys." They diverged phylogenetically from the Anthropoidea some 60 to 65 million years ago. Prosimians generally are nocturnal animals that are smaller and share more primitive mammalian characteristics than the anthropoids. Several prosimians of Madagascar, where there are no anthropoid primates, are diurnal and convergent with anthropoids in a variety of morphological and behavioral characteristics, i.e., they share features with man that have been selected for by similar environmental pressures, but the mechanisms of which may be more analogous than homologous to those found in the anthropoid species.

Prosimians that have been studied to a small extent in biomedical research include the lemurs (subfamily Lemurinae), lorises (subfamily Lorisinae), and galagos (subfamily Galaginae). Lemurs are found only on the island of Madagascar (Malagasy Republic), off the southeast coast of Africa. Lemurs are rare in captivity and seldom used in biomedical research. The lorises are found in Southeast Asia, Sri Lanka, southern India, and central and western Africa. They are slow moving, nocturnal animals with relatively short noses and small ears. The pottos (Perodicticus potto) of Africa and slow lorises (Nyctice- bus coucang) of Southeast Asia are commonly found in captivity, but rarely used in research. Galagos are found in subsaharan Africa. They are also nocturnal animals, but have elongated hindfeet, longer noses, and larger ears than lorises; they are capable of leaping and jumping, whereas lorises move about slowly on all fours. There are several species of galago, but only two are commonly found in captivity, Galago senegalensis and G. crassicaudatus. The latter is relatively large and is used in some biomedical research.

The tarsier (Tarsius, single genus of the family Tarsiidae) is found in the Philippines, Celebes, and some islands of the Malay archipelago. Although the tarsier has many features that are intermediate between prosimians and monkeys, it has certain specializations found in neither and, therefore, cannot be considered a direct link between prosimians and monkeys (J. H. Schwartz et al., 1978). Phylogenetic relations (and, therefore, the

taxonomic status) of tarsiers are currently under debate.
These animals are difficult to maintain in captivity.

The prosimians have seldom been used in biomedical research, although the short life span of some species,
particularly the dwarf lemur (Cheirogaleus) and the mouse
lemur (Microcebus) (Table 23), may make them useful for
studying certain problems of aging. Few, if any, old
animals of these genera exist in U.S. research colonies
(Table 24).

SUITABILITY AND AVAILABILITY

No one species can be expected to qualify as a perfect
model of human aging in all its aspects. At the same
time, only a small number of nonhuman primate species
have been studied sufficiently to generate a body of
knowledge allowing selective decisions regarding suitability for many problems of biomedical research. Information concerning species that have been studied with
regard to certain diseases of the human elderly is discussed later in the section, "Comparative Models for
Problems of the Human Elderly." Current bibliographies
of research on particular topics, with categorization by
species, can be obtained from the Primate Information Center at the University of Washington, Seattle, Washington
98195.

A 1973 survey by the Institute for Laboratory Animal
Resources (ILAR) reveals that less than a dozen species
account for 98 percent of primates used in biomedical
research (ILAR, 1976b). Those and several other species
that have been little used, but which are small and
short-lived and, thus, which may be particularly suited
for research on aging, are presented in Table 23. The
genera are listed in order of increasing phylogenetic
distance from man and described in terms of a number
of general factors that influence suitability and availability. In addition to phylogenetic proximity to man,
some of the major characteristics that influence the
suitability of species for particular studies are longevity, body size, diet, and reproductive mechanisms.

Life span (Table 23, col. 1) is a characteristic that
can greatly influence the choice of primate species for
research on aging. Many questions about aging can only
be answered by studying the same animal over a significant
portion of its life span. Different systems may age at
different rates, but if 10 percent of the maximum life

span of the species is taken to represent a significant
fraction, human subjects must be studied for a decade or
more to observe many changes. By the same token, a chimpanzee must be studied for more than six years, or a
macaque for more than three. It has been argued that the
study of aging would be considerably advanced by identifying those species of primate that offer the best balance of short length of life and phylogenetic proximity
to man. Longevity statistics currently available for
nonhuman primates (Bowden and Jones, 1979) would suggest
that such species might be found among the prosimians,
e.g., the mouse lemur, dwarf lemur, and galago, few of
which have been maintained in captivity beyond 15 years,
or, even closer to man, among the marmosets and tamarins,
New World genera that appear to have similarly short life
spans.

Body size is a second characteristic that can influence choice of species. Weights range from less than 1
kg for some of the New World and prosimian species to
45 kg or more for some of the apes (Table 23, col. 2).
In general, the closer the species is to man phylogenetically, the larger and more difficult it is to work with.
The smallest primate species are the dwarf lemurs and
mouse lemurs, which are about the size of rats and mice,
respectively. These animals have not been used as models
in biomedical research. In many primates, there is sexual dimorphism in weight; the mean adult weight of the
male exceeds that of the female in many species by a
ratio greater than 2 to 1.

A third general characteristic that may influence
suitability is diet (Gaulin and Konner, 1977). The more
than 50 genera of primates have adapted to a variety of
diets (Table 23, col. 3), and such adaptations have resulted in a variety of masticatory, digestive, and metabolic differences among species. The type of diet can
influence how easily the animal is maintained in captivity and its suitability for certain kinds of study. Five
feeding patterns are recognized among primates: frugivory, folivory, gramnivory, omnivory, and insectivory.
The predominant feeding patterns of different species are
presented in column 3 of Table 23. Significant adherance
to a second pattern is indicated in parentheses. It
should be noted that, regardless of dietary classification, all primates include some quantity of animal protein in their diet, usually in the form of insects.

The most common pattern is frugivory, defined as a
diet composed of more than 65 percent fruit. Leaf eating

TABLE 23 Characteristics of Primates that Influence Suitability and Availability for Research on Aging

	Life Span (yr)[a]	Adult Wt. (kg)[b]		Diet[c]	Menstrual Cycle[d]	Captive Survival[e]	Captive Breeding[e]	Geographical Distribution	Status[f]
APES									
Pan troglodytes (Chimpanzee)	49	M	49-57	Om(Fr)	+	G	G	Forests of East, Central, and West Africa	V
		F	41-44						
OLD WORLD MONKEYS									
Macaca speciosa (stump-tailed macaque)	33	M	11-13	Fr	+	G	G	Assam to Szechwan Province, China, south to peninsular Thailand	U
		F	7-10						
Macaca fascicularis (long-tailed macaque, crab-eating macaque, cynomolgus monkey)	33	M	4-10	Fr(Om)	+	G	G	Lower Burma to Cochine, China; south through Maylay Peninsula; most islands of Maylay Archipelago; Luzan, Mindanao; Angaur Islands	U
		F	2-6						
Macaca fuscata (Japanese macaque)	33	M	11-18	Om	+	G	G	Japanese Islands (Honshu, Shikoku, Kinshu, Yakushima)	U
		F	6-16						

TABLE 23 (continued)

	Life Span (yr)[a]	Adult Wt. (kg)[b]	Diet[c]	Menstrual Cycle[d]	Captive Survival[e]	Captive Breeding[e]	Geographical Distribution	Status[f]
Macaca mulatta (rhesus macaque)	33	M 6-11 F 4-11	Fr(Om)	+	G	G	Eastern Afghanistan to China south of Yangtze River; Ottar Pradesh India to Hainan Islands, China	U
Macaca nemestrina (pig-tailed macaque)	33	M 9-19 F 5-10	Fr(Om)	+	G	G	Upper Burma, South to Maylaya, Sumatra, Borneo, and other islands	U
Papio spp. (baboon)	31	M 18-30 F 5-10	Om	+	G	G	Subsaharan Africa	U
Cercopithecus aethiops (green, vervet, or grivet monkey)	28	M 3.2-6.4 F 1.8-3.9	Om	+	G	G	Subsaharan Africa	U
NEW WORLD MONKEYS								
Cebus spp. (capuchin)	43	M 1.2-3.3 F 0.9-2.5	Fr-Om[g]	+	G	G	Central and South America to 30°S	U
Saimiri spp. (squirrel monkey)	18	M 0.6-1.1 F 0.4-0.8	Om(Fr)	-	G	G	Central and South America	U
Aotus trivirgatus (night or owl key)	17	M 0.8-1.0 F 0.8-1.2	Fr(Om)	-	P	P	Central and South America	U

Saguinus spp. (tamarin)	12			In	-	F	P	South America and southern Panama	E
Callithrix spp. (marmoset)	9	M	0.2-0.4	Om		F	P	South America	R
		F	0.2-0.3						
PROSIMIANS									
Cheirogaleus spp. (dwarf lemur)	7	M	0.30	Fr	-	F	?	Malagasy Republic	V
		F							
Microcebus spp. (mouse lemur)	8	M	0.06	Fr	-	F	?	Malagasy Republic	V
		F	0.06						
Galago spp. (galago)	14	M	0.3-1.2	Fr-In	-	G	G	Subsaharan Africa	U
		F	0.2-1.0						

a Mean of 5 oldest animals reported (Bowden and Jones, 1979)
b M = male; F = female
c Fr = frugivorous; In = insectivorous; Om = omnivorous
d + = present; - = absent
e G = good; F = fair; P = poor
f E = endangered; V = vulnerable; R = rare; U = unlisted (Thornback, 1978)
g Species dependent

(folivory) is usually associated with anatomic, physiological, and behavioral adaptations. Due to their specialized diet, leaf eaters are difficult to keep in
captivity and are seldom used in biomedical research.
Gramnivory (grass seed eating) is a diet typical of only
a few primates, such as the gelada (Theropithicus gelada).
This diet is of interest because it is presumed to be the
dietary adaptation of early hominids. An eclectic diet
(omnivory) is typical of many of the most common primates
used in biomedical research. The rhesus macaque (Macaca
mulatta), for example, is predominantly frugivorous in
forest areas, its "natural" habitat; it survives quite
well, however, as an omnivore in areas of dense human
habitation. Feeding on insects (insectivory) is common
to small primates, many of which are nocturnal. Some
species feed on substances that do not fit easily into
the five major dietary categories. For instance, the
gum of cashew trees is an important element in the diet
of marmosets (Callithrix).

A fourth major characteristic that may influence selection of primate species, particularly for studies relating to reproductive senescence and menopause, is the
nature of the female reproductive cycle (Table 23, col.
4). Only the apes, Old World monkeys, and some New World
monkeys exhibit the kind of menstrual cycle characteristic of the human female. The implications of this and
related characteristics for research on reproductive senescence are explored in the section entitled "Reproductive Decline and Menopause."

Two factors that determine the availability of the
most studied species, whether the species can be maintained and bred in captivity and the location and conservation status of wild populations, also are presented in
Table 23. Such factors change rapidly and are generally
outside the control of individual investigators. Populations of wild animals of some species have declined markedly in recent decades, due largely to the influx of the
human population into their habitats. At the same time,
the ability of research institutions to maintain and
breed certain species in captivity has increased. Two
sources of information on the availability of different
species for biomedical research are the ILAR (1979a) publication, Animals for Research--A Directory of Sources,
10th edition, and the Primate Supply Information Clearinghouse operated by the Primate Information Center at
the University of Washington, Seattle, Washington.

While questions of demography, husbandry, and politics impinge strongly on the supply of primates, the most important constraints on primate research on aging for the coming decade are likely to be imposed by the numbers and distribution of old primates already in captivity. There is presently no way to determine accurately the age of a monkey that enters captivity as an adult. Thus, in order to know that an animal is in the second half of its life span, it must have been in captivity for many years. For species whose longevity is more than 30 years, which includes most of the Old World monkeys and the apes, the minimum number of years an animal must have lived in captivity to meet that criterion is 15. Few of the research breeding colonies in the United States have existed for more than 15 years, and even fewer have been able to afford to maintain older, often nonreproductive animals for that length of time. Nevertheless, the number of such animals is not minuscule. Table 24 presents the results of a 1979 census of aged nonhuman primates in U.S. research institutions. Several features of the population of aged nonhuman primates are clear from this survey. The total number of primates in the second half of the life span is well over 700; about 60 percent are females, 40 percent males. Although 13 genera are represented, 4 account for 90 percent of the total: macaques (49 percent), baboons (17 percent), squirrel monkeys (17 percent), and tamarins (7 percent). Of the six macaque species represented, 86 percent belong to one of two species: Macaca mulatta (65 percent) and Macaca nemestrina (21 percent). There are 18 collections of 10 or more animals of a given species, located at 15 different institutions.

AGED NONHUMAN PRIMATES

Very little is known about aged primates in the wild. Lack of means for determining the age of adult animals has prevented accurate studies of longevity in the wild or of the time course of biological changes with age. Investigators who have studied old animals in the wild have relied on characteristics such as hair loss, wrinkled facial skin, absence of teeth, and loss of reproductive function as signs of old age. Many observers of primates in the wild have noted a paucity of animals that look old. Some of the reasons are not difficult to identify. Two independent demographic studies have reported high rates of mortality in the first years of

TABLE 24 Census of Nonhuman Primates in the Second Half of Life Span[a]

	Number of Insti-	Number of Animals		
Common Name (Genus)	tutions	Female	Male	TOTAL
Aye aye (Daubentonia)	--	--	--	--
Baboon (Papio)	2	103	24	127
Capuchin (Cebus)	--	--	--	--
Chimpanzee (Pan)	2	16	3	19
Colobe (Colobus)	--	--	--	--
Galago (Galago)	3	9	6	15
Gibbon (Hylobates)	--	--	--	--
Gorilla (Gorilla)	1	1	--	1
Green monkey (Cercopithecus)	--	--	--	--
Howler monkey (Alouatta)	--	--	--	--
Langur, leaf monkey (Presbytis)	--	--	--	--
Lemur (Lemur)	2	7	6	13
Lemur, dwarf (Cheirogaleus)	--	--	--	--
Lemur, mouse (Microcebus)	--	--	--	--
Loris (Loris or Nycticebus)	1	5	3	8
Macaque (Macaca)	14	207	160	367
Mangabey (Cercocebus)	1	6	1	7
Marmoset (Callithrix)	1	2	3	5
Night or owl monkey (Aotus)	1	3	--	3
Orangutan (Pongo)	1	2	1	3
Patas monkey (Erythrocebus)	--	--	--	--
Spider monkey (Ateles)	--	--	--	--
Squirrel monkey (Saimiri)	8	56	70	126
Tamarin (Leontopithecus)	--	--	--	--
Tamarin (Saguinus)	4	26	26	52
Tarsier (Tarsius)	--	--	--	--
Titi (Callicebus)	--	--	--	--
Uakari (Cacajao)	--	--	--	--
TOTAL		443	303	746

[a]Included are genera for which maximal life span data are available (Bowden and Jones, 1979). Current age of wild-born animals conservatively estimated as time in captivity plus 1 year. Report based on numbers supplied by more than 130 of 250 U.S. institutions contacted (Primate Supply Information Clearinghouse, University of Washington, Seattle, Unpublished).

life. Among Toque macaques (M. sinica), 90 percent of all males and 85 percent of all females die before adulthood (Dittus, 1975). Among yellow baboons (Papio cynocephalus) of the Amboseli Game Preserve, 67 percent of infants die before the age of 20 months (Altmann, et al., 1977). With such losses, only a very small proportion remain to fill the ranks of the aged. Infrequent observations of old animals may also result, in part, from misperception of age. Wild primates are constantly active throughout life and, with the exception of some temple-dwelling macaques of India, probably live on a relatively healthy diet with little or no surplus. In addition, it seems likely that when they become at all weak, the aged animals are immediately susceptible to disease or predation. Aged animals, therefore, probably are culled quickly.

Several authors have focused attention on nonreproductive females as a subgroup of older animals that is relatively easily identified in the wild. Reproductive output of females in provisioned colonies of macaques decreases with age (Koyama et al., 1975; Sade et al., 1977). Waser's (1978) review indicates that postreproductive survival is rare. However, some nonreproductive females are found in groups of Hanuman langurs (Presbytis entellus), which tend to live in large female groups attended by a single male (Hrdy, 1974). Dittus (1975, 1977) has reported the presence of three nonreproductive females in a population of 446 wild Toque macaques (Macaca sinica) in Sri Lanka. He also has reported that females do not often live more than three years after last reproduction. Goodall (Waser, 1978) has reported that the oldest chimpanzee female that she observed in Tanzania died within two years after cessation of cyclic perineal swelling.

Maxim (1979) has reviewed possible social roles and fates of aged members in primate species that exhibit different kinds of social organization. He notes that aged monkeys have been identified in greatest numbers in species whose social organization goes beyond immediate family ties and includes both male and female affinity ties, linear dominance hierarchies, and kinship ties. This may be because such species have been studied most closely; however, it is also postulated that such complexity of social organization may allow for adult roles that go beyond the reproductive function of younger adults. Several investigators suggest that older animals may function as reservoirs of information about how to cope with rare problems, such as the location of a water supply outside the group's normal territory (Kummer, 1971; Waser, 1978). Nevertheless, the nonhuman primates appear to lack the well-developed set of cooperative patterns characteristic of all human societies. Even when some benefit derives from the presence of an aged individual (Waser, 1978), there are relatively few social mechanisms to improve chances of survival of that individual if it becomes weak or socially withdrawn.

Although the literature is small, more is known about aging in captive primates. Caminiti's (1979) bibliography, The Aged Nonhuman Primate, indicates that more than half of the literature relates to aging of the nervous system, reproductive senescence, and neoplasia. Major, long-term studies of the nervous system and behavior have focused on lipofuscin accumulation and neuron and glial cell packing densities in the cortex (Brizzee et al., 1976), neurochemical changes (Ordy et al., 1975), the histochemistry of primate neuromelanin (Barden, 1975), and changes in cognitive functions with age (Davis, 1978; Bartus et al., 1978). Most of these studies have been carried out in the rhesus macaque. Extensive studies of reproductive senescence have focused primarily on the chimpanzee (Graham, 1979) and the rhesus macaque (Hodgen et al., 1977). The literature on neoplasias in nonhuman primates has been extensively reviewed in recent years (Chapman, 1968; Lapin, 1973; Seibold and Wolf, 1973; Mc-Clure, 1975; Effron et al., 1977). The most comprehensive study of aging in one species of primate is reported in Aging in Nonhuman Primates (Bowden, 1979). In that large collaborative study, more than 250 behavioral, morphological, physiological, and biochemical indices were evaluated in pig-tailed macaques (Macaca nemestrina) 4, 10, and 20+ years of age. The volume also contains an extensive report on aging in macaques and baboons from the Soviet primate center at Sukhumi (Lapin et al., 1979).

The answers to many questions of comparative aging across species require knowledge of the maximal life span of those species. For example, we now know that females of certain macaque species undergo menopause late in the third decade of life. The maximal recorded life span of those species is about 30 years. If 30 years is a true estimate, then reproductive senescence occurs proportionally much later in the life span of the macaque female than in the human female. Our knowledge of maxmal life spans in primates other than man remains woefully inadequate. Virtually all of the information we have comes from zoo records. This source of information may disappear, for in 1978, the American Association of Zoological Parks and Aquariums adopted a resolution to discourage the tendency toward unnatural prolongation of life of some animals in search of "longevity records."

Comprehensive baseline studies of biological and behavioral changes during aging in nonhuman primates are necessary to identify aging processes that are unique to primates and that predispose the aging primate to particular losses of adaptive functions and diseases. As yet, relatively little is known about aging in nonhuman primates compared with other phylogenetic orders. The greatest methodological deficit in the present literature on aging in nonhuman primates is the general lack of studies capable of distinguishing characteristics that result from age-related changes in individual subjects from characteristics of animals that happen to have survived to old age, i.e., a lack of longitudinal or cross-sequential studies.

Because old primates are rare and scattered, most studies are simply case reports of old individuals, with no systematic comparison to younger animals. A few are cross-sectional studies with small numbers of animals of different ages. Even fewer are longitudinal or cross sequential. The major reason for such lack of information is that potential investigators are hindered by lack of access to groups of animals in different age groups of a given species for adequate periods of time to carry out the cross-sequential studies essential for identifying age-related biological and behavioral changes. Most colonies with old animals of known age suitable for entering studies of aging have had no funding mechanism for support of such animals once their productivity as breeders begins to decline.

Nonhuman primates are particularly useful as models for research on age-related human diseases in which the clinical expression requires considerable similarity to the human in terms of structure and function of the organ systems concerned, e.g., disorders of the aging brain, such as Parkinson's disease, depression, and neuronal degeneration of the Alzheimer's type, and disorders of the menstrual cycle. The endocrinological similarities of menopause offer the opportunity to study its relationship to a number of pathological processes believed to be influenced by reproductive senescence in the human, e.g., osteoporosis and loss of protection against coronary heart disease.

Nonhuman primates offer particularly good models for disorders in which the problem of interest results from disease processes in other organ systems. For example, a major complication of diabetes mellitus is the accelerated development of atherosclerosis, particularly in the coronary and cerebral arteries. Another example is the effect of hypertension on cardiovascular disease. The study of diabetes and hypertension using rodent and canine models that do not share with humans a reasonable susceptibility to arteriosclerosis is not useful in defining the interrelations of these two diseases.

Investigators in many fields of biomedical and behavioral research have grappled with the problem of effective identification and use of animal models for solving specific problems of human disease. There is a widespread impression that, because some of the most spectacular successes have emerged from unexpected sources, a systematic approach to species selection is as likely to miss the answer by excluding serendipity as it is to find the answer by adhering to an ostensibly rational approach. While serendipitous observations have contributed immensely to medical science, the growth in knowledge of basic biological principles and the accumulation of information about biological mechanisms in specific strains, species, and phylogenetic orders allows a more rational, comprehensive, and effective strategy for identifying and exploiting animal models than was the case earlier in this century. Good examples are the systematic screening and model development strategies that have resulted in improved understanding of coagulation disorders and atherosclerosis. Information on diseases of nonhuman primates that are relevant to some problems of the human aged are discussed in the section entitled "Comparative Models for Problems of the Human Elderly."

Effective animal model development requires screening of potential models by investigators who are thoroughly familiar with the human disorder to identify species in which the disorder occurs, the accumulation of sufficient animals with the disorder to allow scientific studies to be carried out, and the assurance of access to the animals by qualified, motivated scientists. The National Institutes of Health currently support a large number of nonhuman primate breeding colonies. These colonies vary in their emphasis. The seven primate centers supported by the Division of Research Resources, Animal Resources Branch, produce animals for a wide array of on-site research projects; other colonies supported by the same

agency are primarily production colonies, which provide
research animals to other institutions. In addition,
there are a number of mission-oriented colonies, such as
those supported by the National Heart, Lung, and Blood
Institute, for the long-term maintenance of animals with
arteriosclerosis and hypertension and those supported by
the National Institute of Child Health and Human Development with a major emphasis on providing fetal specimens
and infants of known gestational age for perinatal and
developmental research. While most of these colonies include some aged animals, few have as a current objective
to maintain animals beyond their reproductively active
years so that they might be available for research on
aging and age-related diseases.

METHODS OF DETERMINING AGE

The only way to be fully confident of a monkey's age is
to know when it was born. This information is usually
available only for colony-born animals. Only one-third
of the animals listed in Table 24 were colony born. The
most conservative estimate of age for an imported adult
animal is the number of years in captivity plus one year
for its age at entry. Using this criterion, a wild-born
animal must have been in captivity for at least 10 to 20
years (for most Old World and New World monkeys) for one
to judge whether it is in the last third of the presently
estimated maximal life span of its species. Because most
primate research colonies were small or nonexistent 10 to
20 years ago, the number of imported animals identifiable
by the time-in-captivity criterion is limited. Undoubtedly, when better means are developed for identifying old
animals accurately, many more old animals will be found
in present breeding colonies than are represented in
Table 24.
    Fortunately, for many studies in which aging is an im-
portant independent variable, it is not necessary to have
an exact knowledge of chronological age. Accurate assign-
ment of subjects to experimental groups, in which the
mean ages differ by a significant fraction of the life
span, may be adequate for purposes of experimental design.
If by evaluation of various developmental characteristics
it becomes possible to determine with a high degree of
statistical confidence that individual animals belong to
a certain age group, e.g., over 20 years of age, it will

not be necessary to know their exact chronological ages to perform valid experiments of many kinds.

For animals captured as juveniles, weight, dentition (Bowen and Koch, 1970; Gavan, 1967; Hurme, 1961; Nissen and Riesen, 1964; Long and Cooper, 1968; Siegel and Sciulli, 1973; Tappen and Severson, 1971), calcification and closure of epiphyses of the bones (Bramblett, 1969; Thurm et al., 1975; Michejda, 1978), and sexual development may be used to assign ages accurate to within a year, provided sex-referenced normative data are available for the species (Wintheiser et al., 1977; Reed, 1973; Levy et al., 1972; Gavan and Hutchinson, 1973). Unfortunately, few of the records on animals that entered breeding colonies over a decade ago are sufficiently detailed to judge the age of juveniles entering the colony; most of the animals of interest entered as breeding adults.

We currently have no adequately tested method for determining the age of nonhuman primates that were captured as adults. The ideal measure would be one that changes at a known rate with time and that is totally insensitive to environmental or experiential influences, similar to the carbon isotope measure used by archeologists to determine the age of objects composed of once living material. The racemization of aspartate in teeth is currently being investigated as a possible measure of this kind (Helfman and Bada, 1976). The proteins in living animals are made up almost exclusively of L-amino acids. These spontaneously convert to their D-enantiomers at a relatively constant rate. Analysis of protein extracted from teeth of humans of various ages has revealed that D-aspartic acid racemization increases approximately 0.1 percent per year. Using human tooth dentine, age can be estimated with a maximum error of plus or minus 10 percent. Data on nonhuman primates are not presently available.

Another approach to assessing the age of adult animals is to measure characteristics that are more susceptible to influence by time-independent factors, but that, nevertheless, correlate strongly with chronological age. Some of the criteria for measures of this sort have been set forth by investigators who use time-free indices of age to measure rates of biological aging in different human populations (Comfort, 1969). Because of individual variation in rate of change of particular indices and the fact that any particular index in a given individual may be distorted by accident or disease, a battery of measures is likely to be much more useful than any one measure.

Among the criteria that should be considered in developing a battery of tests for determining biological aging for primates are the following. The indices must correlate closely with chronological age, change sufficiently rapidly to assure significant differences over a 3- to 5-year period of time, be differentially responsive to experiences specific to the individual, be measurable without endangering the life of the animal, and be minimally influenced by experimental factors such as stress and diet. In addition, if they are to be used for screening large numbers of animals, the tests must be inexpensive.

A recent collaborative study of aging in the pig-tailed macaque (Macaca nemestrina) has identified about 14 measures that correlate sufficiently with chronological age to merit consideration for use in a biological aging test battery (Bowden, 1979). Five of the fourteen represented enough independent anatomical and functional characteristics to constitute a relatively nonredundant set. They are bone thinning (percent cortical area of the second metacarpal; Garn, 1970), tactile corpuscle density in the thumb (Bolton et al., 1966), serum level of brain reactive antibodies to cortex or cerebellum (Nandy, 1972), white cell count, and the ratio of HDL- to LDL-cholesterol. Another measure that has been proposed as an index of aging in the living animal is the degree of cross linkage in connective tissue obtained by biopsy (Hamlin and Kohn, 1972; Cannon and Davison, 1977). Such indices no doubt vary considerably in the extent to which they may be influenced by environmental factors and diet, but for a stable colony of animals in similar surroundings and on a common diet, they were found to correlate well with age. The findings must be validated on a second sample of animals of known age before this set of measures can be confidently incorporated into a test battery that will provide a single index of biological age in the pig-tailed macaque. The same set of measures may not be suitable for measuring biological age of different species, or even of the same species under different living conditions. It illustrates, however, a legitimate approach to solving a very practical research problem, viz., to identify nonhuman primates of appropriate age for prospective studies of aging processes.

The test-battery approach can also be applied in determining the age of animals that come to necropsy. The much larger variety of specimens that can be taken from the dead animal should allow a statistically more reliable estimate of age. Among the indices that have been

suggested in this context or for which some data are
available in various species of nonhuman primates are
the accumulation of lipofuscin (Brizzee et al., 1974);
changes in neuronal and glial packing density in certain
areas of the brain (Ordy, 1975); changes in numbers of
osteons, osteon fragments, and other histological characteristics of bone (Kerley, 1965); structural change of
the pubic symphysis (Rawlins, 1975); lens weight (Malinow
and Corcoran, 1966); wearing of the teeth (Miles, 1963);
and a variety of measures taken on the pig-tailed macaque
(Bowden, 1979). For investigators seeking a broad perspective on measures that have been shown to correlate
with age in mammalian species ranging from mouse to man,
the Handbook of the Biology of Aging (Finch and Hayflick,
1977) contains an excellent review of changes at the
molecular, cellular, tissue, organ, and systems levels.

HUSBANDRY

Although few investigators have had much experience with
aged animals, many have well-established, successful protocols for laboratory maintenance of various nonhuman primate species. Many aspects of animal husbandry represent
a combination of good common sense and the results of
experience that have generated a laboratory "folklore" as
to how to keep primates. As with most folklore, the recommended procedures are more often right than wrong, but
the arbitrary elements are not readily distinguishable
from the necessary ones. A good source of information
of this kind is, Laboratory Animal Management: Nonhuman
Primates (ILAR, 1980).

Diet

Three sometimes conflicting considerations enter into the
selection of diet for captive primates, viz., nutritional
adequacy, practicality, and appropriateness for establishing models of diseases in which diet is believed to play
a role. Most information on nutrition in laboratory primates is based upon a compromise between the first two
factors.

This information has accrued from experiences with lab-
oratory-formulated and commercial diets that have been
shown to be economical, yet adequate for growth, maintenance, and reproduction. Limited controlled studies have

also been done on the requirements for certain nutrients
by a few species, most notably the rhesus macaque, Macaca
mulatta (Harris, 1970; Kerr, 1972; BARR, 1978b). Most
controlled studies have been of short duration and have
been concerned with growth, biochemical change, or pathological change associated with specific nutrient deficiency or excess. Nonhuman primates have been maintained
for relatively long periods of time on laboratory-formu-
lated and commercial feeds, but there are no reported
data that would indicate that any specific diet or nutritional regimen is superior with regard to promoting longevity. It is presumed that the nutrient requirements
of old, nonhuman primates are the same as those for
younger, adult animals, although again, there is no definitive information in this regard.

Recent years have brought an increasing awareness of
the extent to which health problems of the human elderly
may derive not from aging per se, but from long exposure
to particular diets or an interaction between vulnerability factors associated with aging and exposure to such
diets. Atherosclerosis, diabetes, and certain forms of
cancer all increase in incidence and severity with old
age, but they may not be found in old animals unless the
animals are subjected to diets similar to those of the
modern human populations in which they represent such
serious problems. Thus, in seeking nonhuman primate models of human disease, the investigator should consider
not only the natural diet of the species and the most
economical diet that will maintain the species in good
health, but nutritional factors that might be manipulated
to induce or exacerbate the pathological phenomenon of
interest. This approach has been applied most compre-
hensively in the attempt to identify nonhuman primate
models of atherosclerosis (see section entitled
"Atherosclerosis").

Housing

Nonhuman primates are social creatures. They are similar
to man in that the expression of many of their normal behavioral and physiological functions depends upon contact
with other individuals. For instance, testosterone and
corticosteroid levels in male macaques are greatly influenced by changes in social environment (Bernstein et
al., 1974). Changing an animal from one living group to
another is stressful and increases the likelihood of

trauma and disease. Thus, for many studies, particularly
for longitudinal studies of changes in social, emotional,
and cognitive behavior that may occur with age, it may be
important to maintain animals in stable social groups as
much of the time as possible.

Aged monkeys left in a social context often physically
cannot compete with younger, more robust individuals, but
in long-established groups they are seldom challenged by
younger individuals and are usually allowed to continue
to function in a diminished capacity in the group. Older
individuals are sometimes found associated with immature
animals, and old females often interact primarily with
their own mature young. Anecdotal observations indicate
that irritable behavior on the part of some elderly individuals is tolerated by other group members beyond usual
expectations. On the other hand, aged monkeys, like aged
humans, may be ostracized by their living groups. Some
colony managers report that aged primates do best when
housed with other aged individuals or with very young
animals.

Aged primates are certainly more vulnerable than young
adults to disease and, perhaps, to social stress. They
are at a time in life when age-specific mortality rates
are high and when the repeated stresses of injury and disease may have produced permanent weakening and increased
susceptibilities. Aged individuals may no longer have
the resources to recover from comparatively minor stresses
or they may take longer and require more nursing care to
recover. These factors or experimental requirements may
demand that they be housed in individual cages. More detailed information on housing appropriate to different
species of nonhuman primates is provided by the Guide for
the Care and Use of Laboratory Animals (ILAR, 1978a).

Four basic kinds of housing are ordinarily used for
primates in biomedical research: single indoor caging,
small group outdoor caging, small group indoor/outdoor
caging, and field cages. The following is a description
of the four kinds of housing features that are important
for different aspects of biomedical research and features that may make them more or less appropriate for old
animals.

Individual indoor caging provides an environment where
food intake and other factors can be controlled, where
the animal can be carefully monitored for medical or behavioral problems, and where it is easily accessible for
research activities, e.g., obtaining blood or urine samples or administering test drugs. Obesity occurs in some

old animals caged singly and on an ad libitum diet. For
weak, old animals who are unable to survive the competition of group living, single caging can add several years
to the life span, but it must be recognized that such
housing may produce depression in a social primate that
has lived all of its life in a social context. Depression, the most common psychiatric complaint in the human
elderly, has not been studied in aged nonhuman primates
(see section entitled "Depression"). An environmentally
controlled room may be advantageous for the older animal,
whose ability to thermoregulate may deteriorate with age.
Maintenance of animals in indoor individual caging is expensive and limits opportunity for exercise, but is often
justified on the basis of research requirements.

Small group outdoor caging, e.g., in corn cribs, provides a less costly environment that still allows for
monitoring of medical or behavioral problems and adequate
access to animals for many research needs. Acquisition
of blood or urine samples or administration of test agents
are facilitated by training the animals to enter a small
squeeze cage or by training the animals to permit sampling. Temperature control may have to be implemented
to some degree, depending on local climate.

A combination of indoor/outdoor caging for small groups
may be the most economical and manageable housing for older animals. A large indoor cage that is climatically
controlled and has modifications to facilitate obtaining
blood specimens for research constitutes the primary living quarters, and an outdoor run is available when weather
conditions are favorable for greater freedom of movement.

Field cages (0.5 to 2.0 acres in area) provide greater
opportunity for the patterns of social interaction that
are seen in the wild. Research in such enclosures is often limited to behavioral observations. At this time we
have limited knowledge of the ability of the aged primate
to adapt to group field caging, especially if the animal
previously spent much of its life in an indoor individual
cage.

Because of the scarcity of aged nonhuman primates and
the long lead time required to increase their supply, they
are extremely valuable animals for biomedical research.
Their best use will involve multiple studies over long
periods of time. At the same time, their age makes them
more vulnerable to the stress of experimentation and to
diseases than younger animals. Little is known about the
caging and housing arrangements that are most conducive to
good health in very old monkeys.

Animal Records

The quality of research on aging, perhaps more than any
other aspect of primate research, depends upon accurate
record keeping over long periods of time. Because accurate information on the old animal's age depends on its
having been in captivity for many years, and because most
animals in captivity have been subjected to experimental,
therapeutic, and husbandry oriented procedures that can
influence their behavior and physiological functions in
old age, it is essential that records of such experiences
be maintained. Furthermore, the records should be maintained in a manner that permits ready access by investigators who may need the information. Because the establishment of an experimental group of old monkeys may
involve the collection of animals from several institutions, it is desirable that important information be
recorded in a manner that is sufficiently consistent from
institution to institution to allow comparison and combination of data. The ILAR Committee on Laboratory Animal Records has recently published recommendations and
examples of standardized records for primate breeding
colonies (ILAR, 1979c).

AREAS OF RESEARCH

Research on aging in nonhuman primates should be concentrated in areas where they are likely to be uniquely
useful as animal models. Some of these areas are high-
lighted below.

Aging in Natural or Seminatural Environments

The biological and behavioral significance of much information obtained from aging animals in captivity can only
be fully understood if one knows how it compares with
aging in the wild. Some aspects of function may only
make sense when viewed in the natural environment. There
are presently no survivorship curves for wild populations
of any nonhuman primate species beyond the first few years
of life. Although menopause has now been demonstrated in
some captive species, there is no information on whether
females survive to menopause in the wild. A number of
hypotheses have been proposed regarding possible social

roles of aged, nonhuman primates with very few observations by which to test them. To the extent that life is more satisfying when lived consistently with inherited roles, such roles should be studied in the relatively culture-free models provided by nonhuman primates in the wild. There is no information on possible natural shifts in diet or use of habitat with respect to age, and very little demographic information on wild populations of the primate species most used in biomedical and behavioral research (birthrates, death rates, rates of in and/or out migration, sex, and age composition of natural groups). The wild populations of most species are rapidly decreasing, largely because of habitat destruction. Some governments in the countries of origin are beginning to express interest in establishing nature reserves that would serve both primate conservation and research needs without distorting the natural demographic characteristics of wild populations. Isolated groups in seminatural surroundings provide opportunities to study certain aspects of aging in the wild.

Genetics

Because of their long intergeneration times and expensive maintenance, nonhuman primates are not presently suitable for genetic studies that require inbred strains. Several kinds of genetic study, however, are feasible and should be encouraged. Among those are the identification and breeding of animals with biochemical mutations that may occur only in primates and predispose to diseases of the elderly, studies of genetic markers that may correlate with maximal longevity or the process of aging, and studies of environmental-genetic interactions that may influence maximal longevity and vulnerability to disease in primates. Genetic considerations should be given due weight in the design of all studies on the biology and pathology of aging.

Immunosenescence

Immunogerontology is a relatively new science, but already some investigators theorize that aging is largely the result of progressive loss of immune competence. This hypothesis is reasonable since so many manifestations of senescence involve immune phenomena, notably autoimmune diseases, diminished efficiency of protection against infectious diseases, drastic reduction in capacity to mount an effective primary humoral antibody response, atrophy of the thymus, and several age-related malignancies that may be associated with loss of immune surveillance. Very little is known about the immune system in nonhuman primates. The immune systems of the primate species that are likely to be objects of intensive research on aging should be characterized, and observations on immunosenescence that have been obtained from species phylogenetically more distant from man should be tested for their generality to the primate order.

Nutrition

With the drastic reduction of primary bacterial disease as a cause of death in affluent societies, diet has emerged as one of the most important environmental determinants of life span. Diet is believed, almost exclusively on the basis of epidemiological correlational studies, to play a crucial role in many of the most common diseases of the elderly, and may influence the rate of biological aging as well. The manner in which primates metabolize various dietary elements differs considerably from that of other phylogenetic orders. Thus, studies in species phylogenetically more distant from man than the nonhuman primates have failed to yield adequate models for the correlations between dietary factors and specific pathological processes that are hypothesized on the basis of human epidemiological studies. Furthermore, the major hypotheses generated from rodent nutritional studies, such as the efficacy of caloric restriction in extending life span, are impractical, if not unethical, to perform on human subjects.

Hundreds of epidemiological studies have led to consensus among nutritionists regarding several worthy and eminently testable hypotheses. Most generally stated, they are that human morbidity and mortality are accelerated by diets high in calories, high in lipids, high in salt, low in fiber, and low in ratio of vegetable-to-animal protein. Again, the necessary experimental studies cannot ethically be performed in man. While such studies may be time-consuming, they are not incompatible with a broad range of other essential studies of biological and behavioral aging in nonhuman primates, and many could be carried out in the same groups of animals under study

from other points of view. This is particularly pertinent
to longitudinal studies of biological and behavioral aging
where the dietary variable would not compromise the interpretation of results regarding other variables under
test and to comprehensive studies of disease models where
there is reason to believe that the dietary variable might
be critical for manifestation of the disease.

Reproductive Senescence

Inasmuch as the only animals that show true menstruation
are a few of the primates phylogenetically closest to man,
the nonhuman primates will be the models of choice for
many studies of female reproductive senescence. While
less is known about the male climacteric, there is reason to expect, on phylogenetic grounds, that the changes
in hormonal patterns and their sequelae in nonhuman primates may also be more homologous to those of man than
changes that occur in other orders. The similarity of
reproductive senescence in nonhuman primates to that of
the human elderly should be exploited to further our understanding of the metabolic and behavioral consequences
of reproductive senescence and its contribution to health
problems of the human elderly.

Diseases of the Human Elderly

While the nonhuman primates have received relatively little attention as objects for the study of aging per se,
there is considerable literature on primate models of specific diseases of the human elderly. The advantages and
limitations of existing models for a number of those diseases are discussed in the section "Comparative Models
for Problems of the Human Elderly." Useful models that
already exist should be exploited, and screening programs
and research projects to identify and analyze the mechanisms of those and other diseases of the human aged
should be pursued.

Brain and Behavior

While the basic processes that mediate aging of the human
brain may be shared by a wide range of mammalian and
even nonmammalian species, their expression in terms of

cognitive and affective changes can only be assessed in
species similar enough to the human to allow comparison.
Only certain nonhuman primate species are sufficiently
similar to the human in brain structure, cognitive capacities, and complexity of socio-emotional behavior to meet
that need. Determining the relative contributions of biological aging and disease to such problems of the human
elderly as dementia and depression will require the study
of normal changes with aging of cognitive and affective
behavior in relevant animal models. Nonhuman primate
models provide the opportunity to analyze the neural
mechanisms of such changes, to evaluate the possible
roles of social stress, as well as other factors, in
bringing them about, and to test the efficacy and safety of pharmacological and behavioral interventions that
have potential for ameliorating them.

Pharmacokinetics

Age-related changes in pharmacokinetics can greatly influence required dosage, duration of action, therapeutic
ratio, and side effects of drugs. Large species variation
in rates and modes of drug metabolism have made it necessary to test drug effects in nonhuman primates before
their potential therapeutic effects can be evaluated in
clinical studies. The response of elderly patients to
pharmacological therapy can be quite different from that
of younger patients. It is reasonable to expect that nonhuman primate models will be necessary to study how aging
influences the absorption, distribution, metabolism, and
elimination of particular classes of drugs in primates,
including man.

Culture Systems

Culture Systems

INTRODUCTION

It is generally accepted that some age-related changes of
the organism as a whole have a cellular basis and can be
expressed by certain cell types in culture. Perhaps the
evidence cited most often in support of this view is the
inverse relationship between replicative life span in culture and donor age for cells derived from several human
tissues (Martin et al., 1970; Cristofalo, 1972; Le Guilly
et al., 1973; Schneider and Mitsui, 1976; Hayflick, 1977;
Bierman, 1978). Aging in cell culture is useful for the
study of senescence, not because aging in culture is identical to aging of cells in vivo, but because sequential
changes in the functional, particularly the replicative,
capacity of cells can be analyzed with a degree of experimental control that is impossible to achieve in the living
organism. The use of cell culture systems will achieve
even greater importance in research on aging if specific,
differentiated cells with well-defined properties, which
can be correlated in culture and in situ, can be
developed.

Until recently, the major thrust of research on aging
in cell cultures has involved the use of proliferating
cultures of fibroblast-like cells derived from vertebrates, mainly human and chick. However, the utility of
culture methods for studying problems of aging is broader,
ranging from the short term explant of organoid cultures
to cultures that can be serially propagated for long periods of time and display specific differentiated
properties.

TYPES OF CULTURES

Tissue Explants

The prolonged maintenance in culture of organ or tissue
explants in which tissue organization and, especially,
epithelial-mesenchymal interactions are retained is a
practical and potentially useful preparation for studying
aging. For example, explants of human peripheral lung,
bronchus, bladder, and kidney have been maintained without
great difficulty in a standard medium for periods up to
one year (Autrup et al., 1977; Stoner et al., 1978a).
Long-term culture of amphibian tissue has also been described (Balls et al., 1976). Precocious aging as a result of rapid growth is less likely in organ and tissue
explants than in proliferating cell cultures. This type
of culture provides a reasonable basis for studies that
cannot be approached in the more widely used proliferating
cultures, such as forming epithelial-mesenchymal tissue
chimeras using old and young cells; of culturing tissue
explants in fluids (possibly by reimplantation) of young
and old donors and comparing functional changes; or of
testing explant responses to a variety of stimuli as a
function of donor age.

Cell Cultures

The most widely used cells in studies on aging have been
proliferating cells, such as skin fibroblasts. Small
pieces of tissue are explanted into a culture environment
that will support cell proliferation. Initially, cells
migrate from the explant, attach to the substrate, grow,
and divide. Cells can be subcultivated serially for a
varying number of times depending on the species, donor
age (Martin et al., 1970; Schneider and Mitsui, 1976;
Hayflick, 1977), and culture conditions (Cooper and Goldstein, 1977). For human skin, the first cells that migrate from the explant are epidermal cells; these are
followed by polar fibroblast-like cells that divide rapidly and outgrow other cell types within several passages.
The polar fibroblast-like cells apparently are derived
from the connective tissue, but definitive markers are
lacking. Eventually, the culture enters a phase of
declining proliferative capacity that is accompanied
by a number of physiological changes, including the accumulation of lysosomes and an increase in cell size

(Cristofalo, 1972). It is pertinent to note, however, that cell cultures are very heterogeneous and the proliferative capacity of individual fibroblasts in a population varies widely (Smith and Hayflick, 1974; Martin et al., 1974).

The loss of proliferative potential with time in culure is suggested to be a manifestation of aging at the cellular level (Hayflick and Moorhead, 1961). It is a characteristic of fibroblast-like cells from many vertebrates. Cultures from large, long-lived animals, such as man, tend to be longer-lived than those from smaller, shorter-lived animals, such as rodents, i.e., populations of human fibroblast cultures will double in number 60-70 times compared to 8 times for those of rodents (Hayflick, 1977). Although the doubling potential of any given cell population is reproducible under specific conditions (Cristofalo, 1972), the relevance to aging of any but large interspecies differences is still uncertain.

Although fibroblast-like cells from all vertebrates can be cultured, technical restrictions currently limit both the type and replicative capacity of cells displaying differentiated markers. When such cell lines do grow, the specific cell type often is identified only roughly. Also, comparative studies of the sort carried out with fibroblasts have not been done because it often has not been possible to grow the same cell type from many different species. It is interesting, although perhaps fortuitous, that three of the bovine cell types cultured, arterial endothelial cells (Schwartz, 1978; Mueller et al., 1980), epithelial cells from the prostatic duct (Stoner et al., 1978b), and fetal lung fibroblasts (Lithner and Ponten, 1966), all have comparable life spans in culture (roughly 50 population doublings). Bovine adrenal cells (Hornsby and Gill, 1978) and nasal epithelium (Carbrey et al., 1971) apparently show a shorter replicative life span in culture.

Aside from fibroblasts, normal human cells that have been cultured include skin epithelial cells, which have a shorter lifetime in culture than expected on the basis of their in vivo properties (Rheinwald and Green, 1975; Peehl and Ham 1978); fetal striated muscle cells, which have been grown for about 30 doublings (Hauschka, 1977); fetal kidney epithelial cells, which have been grown for about 10 doublings (W. Nichols, Department of Cytogenetics, Institute for Medical Research, Camden, New Jersey, Unpublished); prostatic epithelium, which has a culture life span of 35 doublings (Lechner et al., 1978); and trophoblast cells, with a culture life span of about 12 doublings (Stromberg et al., 1978).

Monolayer cultures of differentiated cells that normally proliferate infrequently, such as liver hepatocytes (Williams et al., 1979; Michalopoulos and Pitot, 1975) or lung type II cells (Mason et al., 1977), can be prepared, and changes in functional capacity with time in culture could be followed as possible models for research on aging; however, there are difficulties in defining whether changes observed reflect aging in the usual sense or are related to physiological deficiencies in the environment.

Criticism has been leveled at these systems because of the artificial nature of the culture environment. The arguments, pro and con, have been discussed elsewhere (Cristofalo, 1972); however, the potential for a cell to carry out a number of rounds of a complex, highly integrated, physiological process, such as mitosis, is evidence that this functional capacity is not grossly distorted by the growth conditions used. Understanding the basis for the ultimate instability of the proliferative capacity in culture, and determining to what extent the loss of expression of this capacity reflects life span-related genetic function, may help us understand how senescent changes arise in the cells of an organism.

Most fibroblast lines studied show clear evidence of irreversible loss of proliferative potential with serial passage, unless the cells undergo transformation; however, some normal cell lines apparently are immortal in culture. One example is a cell line established from larval Rana pipiens (ICR-2A) that has undergone well over 100 doublings in culture without showing obvious chromosomal change (Metzger-Freed, 1977). There are similar reports for several lines of rat cells (Hay, 1970) and Drosophila imaginal disc cells (Hadorn, 1965).

CHOICE OF ANIMALS AS SOURCES OF CELLS

Longevity is, at present, the primary correlate in selecting animals as sources of cells in studies of vertebrate aging. However, aging is not correlated in a simple way with longevity (Cutler, 1976b; Sacher, 1976), and more refined parameters must ultimately be defined. One approach is to select material for comparative purposes. By pairing closely related animal species that differ markedly in life span, one can try to characterize other significant correlates.

This approach has been pioneered by Sacher and Hart (1978) using two different species of outbred mice: Mus musculus and Peromyscus leucopus. These animals are similar in cellular DNA content, body and organ size, metabolic rate, and body temperature, yet they differ in average life span by a factor of 2.4. Fibroblast cell cultures from the longer-lived Peromyscus have been shown to have 2.5 times the proliferative capacity of those from from Mus. In addition, the level of DNA synthesis following ultraviolet (UV) irradiation is greater in the long-lived Peromyscus. These results are in agreement with the earlier work of Hart and Setlow (1974) indicating that the the level of repair synthesis observed in fibroblast cultures from a variety of animals, including elephant and man, correlates well with the logarithm of maximum life span.

The advantages of cell culture are particularly apparent in instances where the methods of molecular biology can be applied readily to defining the nature of lesions, the biochemical events involved in repair, and those factors regulating the level of repair capability. The relationship of the properties observed in culture to those of the organism is still tenuous, but these results are at least consistent with the general thesis that aging results, in part, from cumulative damage to DNA (Strehler, 1977).

A similar approach in selecting material for comparative purposes is to use different strains of the same species that differ markedly in life span. The life span order of three inbred mouse strains with average life spans of approximately 1, 2, and 3 years has been found to correspond to the culture replicative life span order of fetal fibroblasts and also to the level of UV-initiated DNA repair (Paffenholz, 1978). Criticism of this type of study centers on the question of whether the time of death for cells from closely related animals is unique to the strain rather than to the species and is determined by discrete factors acting in a much narrower range than in outbred populations (Russell, 1979). This can be a criticism in using any related animal species, but the problems in using unrelated animals are even greater.

SOME DEFINED CULTURE SYSTEMS DERIVED FROM NONHUMAN
VERTEBRATES

A recent comprehensive study of aging, cell transformation, and tumorigenicity in mouse and rat fibroblast cultures as a function of time in culture shows a time-
related decrease in growth of cells from both species
(Meek, 1978). This decrease is interpreted to be in vitro
senescence, analogous to that of human and chick cell systems. For mice, the decrease starts shortly after explan-
tation. It is followed by a period of slow growth for
about 1 month and then evidence of culture transformation
after about eight population doublings (rapid growth,
presence of mouse leukemia virus antigen, karyotypic
changes, and, later, tumorigenicity). This is comparable
to the behavior of cultures from Mus musculus (Sacher and
Hart, 1978) and agrees with earlier observations by Rothfels et al. (1963) and Todaro and Green (1963). Similarly, cultures of fibroblast-like cells from F344 rat
embryos show a change in growth rate at about 18 population doublings followed by recovery not associated with
an overtly changed karyotype.

Another rodent fibroblast system that may be useful
for research on aging is the Syrian hamster fibroblast
culture (Williams et al., 1979). Loss of growth potential
in this culture is greatly affected by subcultivation
frequency (cell density) and other growth conditions.
This behavior clearly is not seen with human lung fibroblasts (Smith and Braunschweiger, 1979).

The chick embryo fibroblast culture is another well-
studied system that shows a clear loss of growth potential
and increase in cell size after about 20 doublings. The
number of population doublings in culture is sensitive
both to cell density and to serum concentration (Hay,
1970; Ryan, 1979). Recovery due to transformation does
not occur.

The in vitro replicative life span of nonfibroblastic
bovine endothelial cells has been studied in several laboratories (Schwartz, 1978; Mueller et al., 1980). These
lines grow well in standard media and undergo a well-
defined decrease in proliferative potential at a population doubling level of 50 (calf: PDL 45, Schwartz, 1978;
fetal calf: PDL 80, Mueller et al., 1980) without evidence of frequent transformation. In addition, characteristic cell functions, such as factor VIII production,
provide additional parameters to follow on serial

cultivation. Thus, loss of proliferative capacity can be correlated with specific loss of differentiated function.

The loss of proliferative capacity in cultures of human and chick fibroblast-like cells usually terminates the culture, although the cells may live for some time in the postmitotic state. However, the cultures of fibroblasts from most other species can undergo transformation (Cristofalo, 1972; Hayflick, 1977), giving rise to one or a few cells with essentially unlimited proliferative potential whose progeny take over the cultures. Transformation is particularly common in rodent, especially mouse, cultures and may have a viral etiology (Rothfels et al., 1963; Todaro, 1973; Meek, 1978). It is often correlated with obvious chromosomal changes (Rothfels et al., 1963). Transformation is, by far, the most restrictive aspect of using rodent cell cultures for studies that require the cells to senesce.

CULTURE AND MEDIA

Cell functions are integrated in the organism to a large extent by humoral factors such as hormones, nutrients, and probably other, as yet undefined, factors. This circulating milieu, although highly regulated during short-term homeostasis, apparently varies with age. The fluids from animals of different ages might, therefore, affect cells differently both in terms of immediate physiology (Adelman, 1976) and gradual changes in cellular functional capacity in situ, as has been described for the loss of proliferative potential in human fibroblast-like cultures.

In recent years, the emphasis in research with cell cultures has been on developing simple media that support prolonged survival or maximal growth and that are chemically defined (Ham and McKeehan, 1978). The use of complex, chemically undefined fluids, such as whole plasma and lymph from young and old animals, has been virtually ignored as an approach in studies on cellular aging. However, on the basis of earlier work (Carrel and Ebeling, 1923), this approach appears worthy of further experimental study.

Of perhaps more significance in exposing cells to a young versus an old milieu are attempts to develop sites for cultured cell implantation into syngeneic animals. The cleared fat pad (DeOme et al., 1959), irradiated marrow and spleen sites (Till and McCulloch, 1961), skin grafts (Billingham and Hildeman, 1958), and peritoneal chambers are potential sites. An ideal situation would permit long-term implantation (possibly with superimposed growth), cell recovery, and redevelopment of the cell culture to permit testing of functional capacity under defined conditions. The experimental advantages of genetically defined material of the sort most readily available in mice and rats are apparent in this area. An invertebrate prototype, growth of imaginal disc cells in Drosophila larva for prolonged periods by serial passage, followed by a rigorous functional test of developmental potential when the larva metamorphoses, has been described (Hadorn, 1965).

SUMMARY

Cell culture techniques provide powerful tools for research on aging in terms of developing model systems for the study of physiological regulation and for direct studies on mechanisms of aging. Two types of studies are particularly relevant for animal aging: serial observations, in which changes in culture based either on donor or culture age or on subcultivations are related to aging changes that occur in vivo and comparative studies, in which cell cultures from closely related species or strains with differing life spans are compared. In the former instance, it is difficult to relate the data to specific in vivo effects that are intrinsic to the cell. Therefore, other than freedom from transformation and the presence of suitable markers, there is little basic reason to select one organism over another except for differences in replicative life span. For example, biochemical studies on cloned lines at varying times in culture may require cells with a long culture life (50 or 60 population doublings), so that ample material is available. Studies on the effects of life span moderators are perhaps done most readily with cells having a short culture life. For comparative studies, the animals used as sources for cells may be closely related phylogenetically and differ in longevity or may have similar life spans but be more distantly related. The technology is now available to use culture systems to provide new insights into animal aging.

Comparative Models of Selected Problems of the Human Elderly

Comparative Models of Selected Problems of the Human Elderly

INTRODUCTION

Health problems faced by the elderly are numerous and diverse. Leading causes of disability are presented in Figure 23. The purpose of this section is to consider how animal models have been used to further our understanding of some of these and other age-related problems in the interest of curing or preventing them. Several considerations have entered into the selection of the conditions to be discussed. All are significant causes of morbidity or mortality in people over 60. Some are important because they kill; others because they cause chronic discomfort or disability. Some are primary diseases; others occur as secondary manifestations of several disorders, but are sufficiently burdensome to merit attention in their own right. An attempt has been made to include disorders representing a broad range of physiological systems and a number of different experimental models. Finally, the selection is designed to illustrate relationships between aging and disease. Some diseases that occur primarily in the elderly, such as cancer, are omitted because relevant animal models and the relation to the aging processes have been well reviewed in recent years (Pontén, 1977). For information on disorders not included here, the reader is referred to the Comparative Pathology Bulletin, which is published quarterly by the Registry of Comparative Pathology, Armed Forces Institute of Pathology, Washington, D.C. and a recent, two-volume book, Spontaneous Animal Models of Human Disease (Andrews et al., 1979). These and other sources are valuable, though they may not specifically emphasize the relation between the disease and aging processes. For more information on aging of particular organ systems, the reader is referred to the Handbook of the Biology of Aging (Finch and Hayflick, 1977).

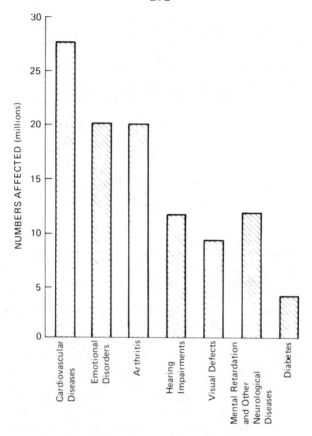

FIGURE 23   Leading causes of disability
in the United States (1974).   Data are
from the National Health Education Committee (ILAR, 1979b).

Most reviews of animal models of disease present a plaus-
ible picture of a particular human disease by piecing together observations derived from a variety of species; discussion of species differences is limited to a pro forma
acknowledgement that differences exist and are important.
Reports on individual models discuss the issue more extensively but tend to extoll the virtues and neglect the limitations of the model in hand.   Both kinds of report are
important, but they often do not meet the needs of the investigator in the position of choosing the animal to which
he is preparing to dedicate several years of his research
career.

Taxonomic Considerations

In seeking an animal model of a human process or characteristic, it is important to recognize that evolution creates
two different kinds of structural and functional similarity among species--analogy and homology. The wing of a
bird is analogous to the wing of a butterfly. Both are
structures that evolved in adaptation to particular features of the atmospheric environment and they perform similar functions. The bird wing, however, is more homologous to the paw of the cat, in that both evolved from the
five-digit appendage of a common ancestor. One of the
major challenges to the development of a phylogenetic
taxonomy of animal species is to differentiate between
analogous and homologous similarities. The same challenge,
to some extent, faces the investigator seeking relevant
animal models of various pathological human conditions.
    Degree of genetic similarity to man is one of the con-
siderations to be taken into account in seeking animal
models of a human disease. All other things being equal,
one is more likely to find a spontaneous condition homologous to the human phenomenon in a nonhuman primate than
in a more distant species, simply because nonhuman primates
share a greater proportion of the human genome than members
of other phylogenetic orders. Figure 24 illustrates the
relative distances of different phylogenetic groups from
man as indicated by molecular and immunologic indices of
homologic distance. It indicates that, while the apes,
Old World monkeys, and New World monkeys are considerably
closer to man than other orders, there is little basis
for choice among other mammalian species on this criterion.
The rodents may be somewhat more distant than the prosimians and the carnivores more distant than the rodents, but
by the criteria of molecular genetics, the differences in
relative distance of those phylogenetic groups from man
is not great. The most important aspect of the nonhuman
primates as models of human disorders is the opportunity
they offer for studying as closely homologous conditions
as exist in nature.
    Because of the limited numbers, expensive maintenance,
and large size of most nonhuman primates, the investigator
seeking a model of a particular condition is always faced
with a strategic trade-off between the likelihood of finding the phenomenon he seeks, which is maximized by studying
man's closest relatives, and the availability of subjects
for study (see pages 243-278). In general, he will choose
the cheapest, most readily available, smallest, most

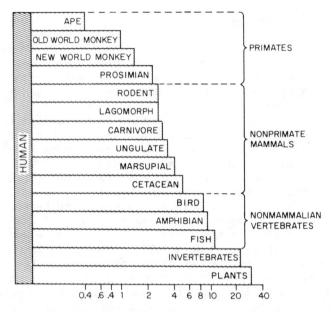

Mean Homologic Distance from Human (OWM)

FIGURE 24 Homologic distance between man and
various phylogenetic groups. Estimates of homologic distance are based on the time estimated
to have elapsed since the different phylogenetic
groups diverged from the human line. Because
the absolute time estimates for a given evolutionary branch point vary with the method on
which the estimate is based, all estimates are
referenced to the estimated time of divergence
of the Old World monkey group from man. This
branch point has been chosen as reference because the Old World monkey group is close to
man phylogenetically, and it is the only group
other than man represented in all of the nine
studies from which data were drawn.

The mean of the estimates of homologic distance for each phylogenetic group across the
nine studies is presented. The measures of
dissimilarity are based on studies of amino
acid structure of cytochrome-c, α-hemoglobin,
β-hemoglobin, carbonic anhydrase, and other
proteins or on immunologic characterization
of albumin, transferrin, or total serum proteins. The estimates for invertebrates and

widely studied species that exhibits the phenomenon of interest. For studies of aging, one should add shortest-
lived to this list of criteria, because meaningful longitudinal studies of animals with a 30-year life span may
require 3 times the investment of time and resources that
are required for studying the same fraction of the life
span in an animal whose maximum longevity is 10 years.

Of course, an animal model need not simulate a spontaneous disease in man to be relevant in the search for a cure
(Beveridge, 1972). A solution to the problem of osteoporosis in the aged may ultimately lie in a better understanding of the normal coupling of bone formation and bone re-
sorption--a basic phenomenon of vertebrate biology that
may be more successfully studied in tissue from chick embryos than from senescent mammals. Identification of more
effective pharmacological agents for treating depression
in the elderly may better be achieved by screening procedures based on their effects on rodent behavior than on
work with animals more clearly susceptible to human-like
depression. Even the understanding of specific lesions
can be greatly aided by studying related phenomena in quite
different animals. For instance, it has been observed that
aging rodent brains show reactive glia and degenerating
synaptic elements in the absence of the amyloid characteristic of the human lesion. This has been interpreted by
some to suggest that the degenerating neurite component of
the senile plaque is the primary lesion of aging in the
mammalian brain and that the amyloid is a peculiarity of
aging in primates and certain other phylogenetic groups
that complicates analysis of the basic phenomenon. Therefore, the rodent may provide a simpler model than the primate for clarifying the etiology of synaptic lesions.

---

plants are based entirely on analysis of
cytochrome-c. For example, analysis of dissimilarity in the amino acid sequence of the
hemoglobins between man, Old World Monkey,
and carnivore indicates that the branch point
of human from the monkey group occurred 40
million years ago, and from the carnivore
group 75-90 million years ago; thus, the
carnivore is assigned a homologic distance
from man of 2-3 Old World Monkey (OWM) units
on the basis of the hemoglobin measure. From
Goodman and Tashian, 1976.

Models more similar to the human lesion would no doubt
be necessary to determine the pathogenesis of the amyloid
component.

The purpose of this section is to cite and discuss the
animal models available for studying several major problems
of the human aged. The primary focus is on their scientific relevance to understanding the human problem. The
coverage is not intended to be exhaustive, but to define
and illustrate key kinds of information to be considered
in selecting a model for studying different aspects of a
disease. One of the goals is to cite authoritative sources
regarding aging in the system affected. A second major
goal is to discuss important aspects of available models
about which there is sufficient information to compare
among species.

SENILE DEMENTIA OF THE ALZHEIMER TYPE

Definition

Senile dementia of the Alzheimer type (SDAT) is a disease
of mid- or late life characterized by a decline in cognitive ability and adaptive skills due to primary neuronal
degeneration of the Alzheimer type. At present, the diagnosis can only be made after a postmortem, neuropathological examination demonstrating large numbers of neuritic
plaques and neurofibrillary tangles in the frontotemporal
cortex and hippocampus. A description of the behavioral
syndrome that accurately predicts the neuropathological
diagnosis, particularly in the early stages of the disease,
does not currently exist.

Clinical and Pathological Manifestations

SDAT is the most common form of dementing illness in the
aged (Terry and Wisniewski, 1972, 1977; Tomlinson et al.,
1970), accounting for 50 percent or more of the dementias
that come to autopsy (Jellinger, 1976; Terry, 1978). The
clinical diagnosis is presumptive, i.e., made by elimination of all other causes of intellectual impairment that
are known or for which there are tests. For a clinical
diagnosis of SDAT, patients should be over 50 years of age
with a deterioration of general cognitive functions that
compromises self care and adaptation to the environment
(Eisdorfer and Cohen, 1978). They should meet the following diagnostic criteria (Eisdorfer and Cohen, In press):

● impairment of at least two of the cognitive abili-
ties: attention, learning, memory, or orientation (as
judged, for instance, by performance on the Mini-Mental
Status Exam, the Wechsler Adult Intelligence Scale
(WAIS));
● impairment of at least one of the following symbolic skills: calculation, abstraction, or comprehension
(as judged by performance on the WAIS); and
● problems in at least one of the following life
areas: ability to work, to relate to family, to relate to
peers, to function socially (as judged by psychosocial
examination).

The onset of the disorder should be gradual and progressive with at least a 6-month history of symptoms. Because
the diagnosis is based upon elimination of other causes
of intellectual impairment, it is important to rule out
the following conditions before a diagnosis of SDAT can
be made: multiinfarct dementia, Jacob-Creutzfeldt's disease, focal neurologic disorders, Parkinson's disease,
Huntington's chorea, Pick's disease, primary affective
disorder, cerebrovascular accident, or pseudodementia
secondary to any of a number of physical disorders, metabolic disorders, or drug toxicity.
The primary microscopic lesions of SDAT are cell loss,
particularly in the hippocampus (Ball, 1977), neuritic
plaques, and neurofibrillary tangles. Other lesions that
appear to be more common in patients with senile dementia
than in normal aged individuals include reduced dendritic
arborization, neuronal granulovacuolar degeneration, and
perhaps changes in neurochemical characteristics of certain areas of the brain.
Neuritic (senile) plaques are the most conspicuous
pathological change found in people with SDAT. Morphological studies have revealed that the plaque consists
primarily of three elements: amyloid, degenerative neuronal processes, and reactive glial processes (Wisniewski
and Terry, 1973, 1976). The plaques appear to develop in
three stages:

● Primitive plaques. In between wisps of amyloid,
degenerating neuronal processes are seen, many of which
are packed with electron-dense mitochondria.
● Typical or classic plaques. These plaques have a
central core of amyloid surrounded by degenerating neurites and reactive cells.

● Compact or burned-out plaques. These are made up predominantly of the amyloid central core alone.

At least two types of amyloid are found in neuritic plaques: amyloid A, a nonimmunoglobulin protein, perhaps local in origin (Powers and Spicer, 1977), and amyloid B, believed to be a complex of light-chain immunoglobulins (Glenner et al., 1972, 1973; Glenner and Page, 1976). Almost all of the abnormal neuronal processes in plaques are axonal terminals or preterminals. In spite of the enlargement of the terminals due to the accumulation of normal and pathological cytoplasmic organelles, the plasma membrane is well preserved. Even in terminals that are depleted of synaptic vesicles, the specialized membranes and cleft are still identifiable (Wisniewski et al., 1974). Thus, it appears that the majority are alive and have not lost contact with their perikaryon. Such data may offer some hope of functional recovery of the terminals if it were possible to reverse the primary pathological process.

The neurofibrillary tangles found in brain cells of humans with senile dementia are readily demonstrable by light microscopy. The features specific to the neurofibrillary tangles of SDAT, however, can only be seen by electron microscopy. They consist of paired, helically wound filaments with an intertwist interval of 80 nm. They are found, for the most part, in the neuronal cytoplasm, but they can also appear in the cellular processes (Wisniewski and Soiser, 1979). Application of the Golgi technique to brain tissue from patients with SDAT has revealed marked loss of the dendritic apparatus (Scheibel et al., 1975; Machado-Salas et al., 1977; Buell and Coleman, 1979). Granulovacuolar degeneration in pyramidal cells in the hippocampus has been demonstrated using a variety of methods (Hooper and Vogel, 1976; Tomlinson and Henderson, 1976; Ball and Lo, 1977).

Studies of SDAT have focused for the most part on the morphology of the lesions, and to a lesser extent on their distribution. As interest in the pattern(s) of cognitive deficit grows, however, correlative studies become increasingly important. The great involvement of the frontotemporal cortex and hippocampal areas in SDAT has long been known, but the extent of involvement of other areas is not known, and there is some evidence that the different lesions of SDAT are distributed differentially. Neuritic plaques are found most frequently in the neocortex and amygdala and are also present in the hippocampus;

however, they do not show exactly the same regional preferences as do the other neuropathological lesions (Dayan, 1970b; Corsellis, 1962; Tomlinson and Henderson, 1976). Granulovacuolar degeneration is greatest in the hippocampus (Ball and Lo, 1977), particularly area H1 (Tomlinson and Henderson, 1976). Neurofibrillary tangles occur more often in the hippocampus and brain stem than in the neocortex (Hirano and Zimmerman, 1962; Hooper and Vogel, 1976; Dayan, 1970a,b; Ball, 1978).

There is a large body of data that implicates the cholinergic system in memory functions; therefore, the search for possible neurochemical correlates of SDAT has focused primarily on that system. Postmortem samples from cortical regions show decreases of greater than 50 percent in the activity of cholineacetyl transferase (CAT)--the enzyme that catalyzes the final step in the synthesis of acetylcholine (Davies and Maloney, 1976; Perry et al., 1977a,b; White et al., 1977; Davies, 1978; Reisine et al., 1978; Bowen et al., 1979). Loss of CAT activity in the caudate nucleus and putamen also has been reported (Davies and Maloney, 1976; Perry et al., 1977a; Reisine et al., 1978), but these data are controversial (Perry et al., 1977b; Bowen et al., 1979). There is a linear decline in human hippocampal CAT activity between 46 and 93 years (Davies, 1978), and neurologically normal individuals as they near 90 years of age may have CAT activity comparable to that seen in SDAT patients. Acetylcholine esterase (AChE), the primary degradative enzyme for acetylcholine in the mammalian brain is decreased by 90 percent in the hippocampus of patients with SDAT (Davies and Maloney, 1976). Data on muscarinic cholinergic receptor binding in the hippocampus of patients with SDAT are contradictory, perhaps because of differences in the age ranges sampled (Davies and Veith, 1978; Reisine et al., 1978). Muscarinic cholinergic receptor binding in the cortex remains constant (Perry et al., 1977a; White et al., 1977; Davies and Veith, 1978; Reisine et al., 1978; Bowen et al., 1979).

In addition to the other areas of the brain affected in SDAT, there are indications that the basal ganglia may also be involved. Levels of homovanillic acid, a major dopamine metabolite, are lower in the cerebrospinal fluid, caudate nucleus, and putamen of SDAT patients, but not in cases of dementia of vascular etiology (Gottfries et al., 1969, 1970).

Etiology and Pathogenesis

While SDAT is clearly a disease of old people, the relationship between genetic and epigenetic factors in its
etiology is unclear. Since all of the brain lesions of
SDAT are seen to some degree in all aged humans, some
investigators regard it as an inevitable end point of
normal biological aging in man. The incidence of SDAT increases rapidly above age 65 (Larsson et al., 1963; Kay,
1972) and may rise as high as 15 to 20 percent in some
age categories if mild and severe dementias are combined
(Kay, 1972). However, the often rapid course of the disease and the fact that the incidence of new cases declines,
rather than increases, in humans beyond age 80 (National
Center for Health Statistics, 1979) has led others to
question whether the condition is a normal phenomenon of
aging or is instead an age-associated disease. The human
population may be genetically heterogeneous in its vulnerability to the disease (Constantinidis, 1978).

Current evidence suggests that multiple factors may be
involved in the development of SDAT (Wisniewski and Terry,
1976). Cytotoxic immune factors (Nandy, 1977; Cohen and
Eisdorfer, 1980; Eisdorfer et al., 1978; Chaffee et al.,
1978; Rapport and Karpiak, 1978), deterioration of cholinergic mechanisms (Ball, 1978; Davis and Yamamura,
1978; McGeer and McGeer, 1978), transmissible viruses
(Gajdusek, 1977; Gibbs et al., 1978), aluminum deposition
(Crapper et al., 1978; Trapp et al., 1978), hereditary
factors (Larsson et al., 1963; Heston, 1977; Heston and
Mastri, 1977), and trisomy 21 and myeloproliferative disorders (Heston, 1977) may play a role in the etiology of
the disease. Further, Alzheimer's patients exhibit elevated cortisol levels (Müller and Grad, 1974), which have
been hypothesized to play a role in the development of
brain glial changes during aging (Landfield, 1978). If,
from a pathogenetic point of view, the important amyloid
in neuritic plaques is of immunologic origin, the factors
that trigger its formation also may be responsible for
neurite degeneration (cf, Wisniewski, 1978).

Much of the speculation regarding pathogenesis of the
disease has focused on the combinations and distributions
of the different lesions. For example, a possible explanation for the marked regional distribution of neurofibrillary tangles, granulovacuolar changes, and Hirano
bodies in the hippocampus may relate to deterioration of
the microvasculature there (Ball, 1978). In contrast to
the binary dividing pattern of terminal arterioles in the

rest of the brain, the hippocampus has a rake-like config-
uration that may be more susceptible to hypotensive episodes. Some speculate that lesions in the subcortical
nuclei that project to the cortex may have a role in
the initiation of the more classical cortical lesions.
Most patients with primary neuronal degeneration occurring
before age 60 have tangles in the locus ceruleus compared
to only one-third with disease of later onset (Forno,
1978).

Animal Models

In spite of the medical and social importance of several
diseases involving primary neuronal degeneration in old
people, extraordinarily little has been done to establish
authentic analogs of these human diseases in experimental
animals. In many respects then, the sequence of aging
changes in other animals is similar to that of man regardless of great differences in life span and the fact that
neurons do not replicate during the life of the organism.
Broad reviews of the fragmentary knowledge currently
available on aging of the nervous systems in animals are
presented by Brizzee et al., (1978) and Wisniewski (1979).
The present review focuses on those changes that are most
similar to those seen in SDAT.

No known animal model mimics all or even most of the
behavioral and neuropathological defects of SDAT. Investigators have studied the behavior and neuropathology of
old animals of a variety of species to identify characteristics that in one way or another are similar to the
changes characteristically seen in people dying of SDAT,
viz., nerve cell loss, neuritic plaques, and neurofibrillary tangles, particularly in the frontotemporal cortex,
the hippocampal gyrus, and certain brainstem nuclei.
Each of these characteristics has been identified in aged
animals of some species, but none have been identical in
all respects to the lesions of SDAT.

Nerve Cell Loss

There are only a few quantitative studies of age-
associated neuronal cell loss in animals (Brizzee, 1975);
several focus on the cortical and hippocampal areas. The
hippocampus of aged F344 rats is reported to show a reduced density of pyramidal neurons (Ordy and Brizzee,

1977; Landfield et al., 1977), and the neocortex may lose granule cells (Landfield et al., 1977). However, no neuronal loss has been seen in the dentate gyrus of the hippocampus in these rats (Geinisman et al., 1977).

Genetic control of the number of neurons in the dentate gyrus of the hippocampus has been demonstrated in a variety of inbred mouse strains (Wimer et al., 1976). If central cholinergic mechanisms also are influenced genetically, this mouse model may offer the possibility of testing hypotheses about the interaction of age and genetic factors in the etiology of senile dementia.

Neuritic Plaques

Neuritic plaques have been noted in a number of mammalian species. Some have developed spontaneously with increased age, others have been induced by viruses. Some are quite similar to those seen in aged humans, i.e., contain amyloid, degenerating axons, and reactive glial cells; others are made up predominantly of amyloid.

Neuritic plaques are known to occur in aged nonhuman primates, dogs, and horses. Among nonhuman primates, they have been observed in rhesus macaques (Macaca mulatta) over 20 years of age (Alekandrovskaia and Shirkova, 1960; Wisniewski and Terry, 1973) and bushbabies (Galago spp.) over 11 years of age (H. M. Wisniewski, New York State Institute for Basic Research in Mental Retardation, Staten Island, New York, Unpublished). Von Braunmuhl (Dayan, 1971) has found plaque-like structures in 3 of 20 dogs, 14 to 20 years of age. Dahme (1962) and Osetowska (1966) also describe plaques in the brains of dogs 15 to 18 years old. Wisniewski et al. (1970b) have described senile plaques with cerebral amyloidosis in aged dogs.

Light and electron microscopic studies of the neuritic plaques in the macaque reveal that they are similar to those in humans. They are composed of three major elements: amyloid, degenerating neuronal processes, and reactive (glial) cells. The primary mechanism leading to amyloid formation and terminal degeneration is unknown. It also is unclear whether there is an invariable association between plaques and blood vessels. In studies on the pathogenesis of the plaque formation in Alzheimer's disease, the impression is that there is no necessary topographical relationship between blood vessels and plaques; however, in the aged nonhuman primates, many plaques have been found in proximity to small blood vessels and perivascular amyloid (Wisniewski and Terry, 1973; 1976). One might infer from this that congophilic angiopathy is responsible for degeneration of the neurites and subsequent plaque formation. However, it is unlikely that amyloid deposits are the precipitating factor in the formation of neuritic plaques (Divry, 1934; Schwartz, 1976), because, as noted above, perivascular deposits of amyloid have been seen without associated degeneration of the neurites in aged nonhuman primates. Furthermore, cerebral deposits in familial amyloidosis are not associated with the formation of neuritic plaques.

Neuritic plaques apparently do not occur in the rat. However, age-associated changes in the rat brain are similar in some respects to those of aged humans in that they apparently consist of degenerating neuronal processes, reactive astrocytic and microglial processes, and probably lost neurons. The hippocampus of aging rats, as of aging humans, is particularly affected. In the hippocampus of aging F344 rats, a major hypertrophy of astroglia is seen (Geinisman et al., 1978b; Landfield, 1978; Landfield et al., 1977, 1978a); in some cases, the astroglia cluster in dense synaptic terminal fields (Landfield et al., 1978b; Lindsey et al., 1979). Degenerating neuronal elements, apparently enveloped by reactive microglia, have been found in the neocortex of aging SD rats (Vaughan and Peters, 1974b), and degenerating neuronal elements, apparently enveloped by astroglial processes, have been reported in the hippocampus of aging F344 rats (Landfield, 1978). At present, however, large clusters of degenerating neurites, as occur in senile plaques, have not been reported in rats. Amyloid plaque deposition also has not been observed in the brains of aged rats. The changes in rodents, then, may provide a less complicated model than the nonhuman primate or dog models for investigating the etiology of the synaptic-glial alterations that appear to be the fundamental lesions in plaque formation.

Neuritic plaques are not spontaneously present in the brains of C57BL/Icrf and C57BL/6J mice as old as 35 months (Dayan, 1971; Machado-Salas and Scheibel, 1979). There are, however, changes in the hippocampus of aged C57BL/6J mice consisting of swollen neurons with a loss of apical branching of the cells and appearance of reactive astrocytic processes (Machado-Salas and Scheibel, 1979).

Although over 250 inbred strains of mice are recognized at present (Staats, 1976), few other than the C57 line have been examined as models for aging. The different

strains of the C57 line have been used primarily because
of their low incidence of overt pathology as they age.
It is unfortunate that investigators have ignored other
mouse strains that may be more susceptible to neuropathological changes. Specific scrapie agents in certain
strains of mice can induce amyloid and neuritic (senile)
plaque formation (Wisniewski et al., 1975). Scrapie is
a naturally occurring disease of sheep and goats, caused
by a replicating agent that can be transmitted to a variety of species by using infected tissues. Morphologica-
ly, scrapie is often accompanied by vacuolar degeneration,
which may include a severe spongy change. There are different strains of scrapie agent, distinguishable on the
basis of incubating periods and topography of the brain
lesions in inbred mice (Fraser and Dickinson, 1973). Neuritic plaques observed in female VN mouse brain following
long-term (20 to 22 month) infection with scrapie agent
provides an interesting model for senile plaques (Wisniewski et al., 1975). Control brains of mice up to 33 months
of age show no plaques, but large numbers of plaques are
seen in mice injected with the scrapie agent. These
plaques are similar to, if not indistinguishable from,
naturally occurring plaques in human SDAT.

Neurofibrillary Tangles

Neurofibrillary tangles have been found in brains of several species; however, they are relatively uncommon compared to neuritic plaques and vary in ultrastructure from
neurofibrillary tangles in man (Wisniewski and Terry,
1973). Spontaneous diseases of the central nervous system in dogs (DeLahunta and Shively, 1975) and cats (Vandevelde et al., 1976) have been described in which accumulation of neurofilaments was prominent; however, the
animals affected were young.
    Several compounds cause the accumulation of fibrillary
tangles in nerve cells. The best known are the spindle
inhibitors and aluminum salts (Wisniewski et al., 1970a).
Electron miscroscopic studies of neurons from animals
treated with these compounds reveal, however, that the
experimentally induced neurofibrillary tangles are made
of 10-nm filaments and not of the paired helical filaments
found in humans (Wisniewski et al., 1976). To date, small
aggregates of paired, helically wound 10-nm filaments with
a twist about every 50 nm have been found in only one
rhesus macaque (Macaca mulatta) (Wisniewski et al., 1973).

This intertwist distance differs from the 80-nm distance
characteristic of human neurofibrillary tangles. The fact
that one aged monkey has been found to show spontaneous
neurofibrillary pathology so similar to the human lesion,
however, indicates that nonhuman primates may eventually
prove to be useful models for research on age-associated
spontaneous or experimentally induced neurofibrillary
tangles.

Other Aspects of SDAT

In addition to the animal models of the lesions that classically define SDAT, a number of models have been investigated representing aspects of the disease that have only
come to light or begun to be defined in recent years,
e.g., the loss of dendritic spines from cortical neurons,
neurochemical changes, and behavioral deficits that may
be specific to the disease.

The complexity of dendritic arborization in cerebral
neurons correlates inversely with the degree of a variety
of dementias, including senile dementia. The loss of dendritic arborization correlates more strongly with decline
in psychomotor performance than with chronological age
(Scheibel, 1978). Using Golgi techniques, Mervis (1978)
has reported loss of dendritic spines and shrinkage of
dendritic shafts in the frontal cortex of dogs 12 to 18
years of age. These changes appear to be highly similar
to those seen in Golgi preparations of cortical tissue
from patients with senile dementia (Scheibel, 1978). Aging F344 male rats show a decreased density of both axo-
dendritic (Geinisman et al., 1977) and axosomatic (Geinisman, 1979) synaptic contacts in the dentate gyrus of
the hippocampus; similar changes in the hippocampus have
been observed in aged C57BL/6J mice (Machado-Salas and
Scheibel, 1979). Aging SD rats show a loss of dendritic
spines and atrophy of the dendritic shafts of neocortical
neurons (Feldman, 1976; Vaughan, 1977).

The relation of changing neurochemical indices is less
clear than the relation of morphological changes to dementia in the human. Nevertheless, the apparent role of
cholinergic processes in memory and the role of memory
deficits in dementia have led to a number of animal studies on changes in cholinergic systems with age. These
have focused on the activity levels of two major enzymes
involved in cholinergic metabolism: cholineacetyltransfer-
ase (CAT), which catalyzes the last step in acetylcholine

synthesis, and acetylcholinesterase (AChE), which catalyzes the breakdown of acetylcholine. In C57BL/6JN mice,
hippocampal CAT activity is constant from 3 to 8 months
and then declines by 50 percent by 24 months of age
(Vijayan, 1977); cerebellar CAT activity is constant between 3 and 24 months of age in these mice. Hippocampal
and cerebellar AChE activities also are constant between
3 and 24 months of age in this strain (Vijayan, 1977).
CAT and AChE both decline with age in the forebrain of
some rat stocks (Hollander and Barrows, 1968; McGeer et
al., 1971; Moudgil and Kanugo, 1973). In the rhesus
macaque, AChE levels in the caudate nucleus increase progressively up to about 15 years of age (40 to 50 percent
of maximal life span) and decline markedly in animals
over 20 years of age. No age group differences have been
seen in various cortical areas of the rhesus macaque
(Ordy, 1975) or in the cerebellum of the pig-tailed macaque (Macaca nemestrina) (Nandy and Vijayan, 1979).

Because of the involvement of the locus ceruleus and
other catecholaminergic nuclei of the brainstem in the
histopathology of senile dementia, some investigators
have postulated a role for the catecholaminergic systems
in SDAT. The literature relating changes in the catecholamine systems to Parkinson's disease is discussed on
pages 308-315.

While the relation of primary neuronal degeneration to
dementia is clear, there is presently no specific pattern
of behavioral deficit that is known to characterize the
disease (Cohen and Dunner, In press). The most important
aspects of cognition that are included in the research
diagnostic criteria and that are amenable to study in
animals, i.e., that are not dependent on symbolic processes, are attention, learning, and memory functions.

There have been numerous studies of behavioral change
in aging rats (see reviews in Elias and Elias, 1976; Gold
and McGaugh, 1975). These studies have consistently shown
age-related impairment in avoidance retention, in the
learning of complex, as opposed to simple tasks, in reversal or extinction of responses once learned, and in
the retention of avoidance responses. In view of the known
morphological, age-related hippocampal changes in some
rat strains, it is interesting to note that experimental
hippocampal lesions in young rats produce a syndrome that
includes impaired learning of avoidance (but not escape)
tasks, complex mazes, and reversal and extinction tasks
(Isaacson, 1974). Thus, there appears to be a similarity
between age-associated behavioral impairment and the

behavioral deficits produced by hippocampal lesions in rats (Landfield, In press). In this regard, it may be of interest that a specific neurophysiological monosynaptic hippocampal deficit has been found to be highly correlated with an active avoidance deficit in aging F344 rats (Landfield, 1979, In press).

The common factors, if any, between hippocampal function in rats and humans are ill-defined. In some respects there are clear differences (Isaacson, 1974). For example, the global anterograde amnesias found with hippocampal lesions in humans (Milner, 1970) apparently do not occur in the rat. Nevertheless, since hippocampal lesion-like behavioral changes (e.g., memory deficits) are prominently seen in humans with SDAT, aging rats might provide useful models for the study of hippocampal-dependent, age-related behavioral changes, regardless of species-specific behavioral patterns (Landfield, In press).

There are no reports of the extreme cognitive disintegration of senile dementia in nonhuman primates. This may be simply because so few nonhuman primates have been maintained to a sufficiently old age to develop the brain lesions characteristic of the human disease. Changes in learning and memory functions with age have, however, been described in nonhuman primates. Behavioral studies of a 27-year-old rhesus macaque, in which neuritic plaques have since been demonstrated, indicate a decline in the proficiency of discrimination learning and stimulus reversal tasks and failure to withold responses during operant extinction (Aleksandrovskaia and Shirkova, 1960). Some of these findings have been substantiated in a group of pig-tailed macaques more than 20 years of age (Cohen et al., 1979). A unique 24-year longitudinal study of a small group of rhesus macaques has demonstrated distinct deficits in "recent" memory function during the third decade of life (Medin and Davis, 1974). More recent studies on rhesus macaques (Bartus et al., 1978) indicate that the deficits in short-term memory of older animals are more likely attributable to impairment of information storage or retrieval mechanisms than to motivational or sensory-perceptual impairment. The deficit seen in the older macaques is more nearly simulated in young animals by the administration of scopolamine, an anticholinergic drug, than of haloperidol, an antidopaminergic agent (Bartus, 1978).

PARKINSON'S DISEASE

Definition

Parkinson's disease (PD) is a disorder of later life characterized by degeneration and loss of neurons from the
substantia nigra with resulting bradykinesia, postural
tremor, and muscular rigidity. It is a common neurologic
disease in the elderly, affecting 1 percent of people over
50 years, to some degree.

Clinical and Pathological Manifestations

The bradykinesia of parkinsonism consists of difficulty
in initiating movement or in altering an existing movement
pattern. Muscular rigidity is reflected in resistance
to passive movement and a mask-like facial expression.
The postural tremor ("tremor at rest," "alternating trem-
or," "reciprocal tremor") occurs at a rate of 3 to 8
cycles/s and is present at rest; it is interrupted by
voluntary movement and by sleep. It is more pronounced
in the distal than the proximal portions of the limbs,
and the arms are more involved than the legs. Disturbances of speech, swallowing, and muscular strength are
also present. The abnormalities may lead to marked inability to move and helplessness. Depression is common;
intellectual deterioration occurs rarely. Relief of symptoms can be produced by anticholinergic drugs, L-dopa, or
ablation of certain thalamic nuclei.

It is generally agreed that, regardless of the etiology, most of the signs of PD result from the loss of
neuromelanin-containing dopaminergic nerve cell bodies in
the zona compacta of the substantia nigra (Hornykiewicz,
1972; Alvord et al., 1974). Depending upon the etiology,
the predominant histological lesion is loss of neurons,
depigmentation of some of the remaining neurons, inclusion bodies (Lewy bodies or Alzheimer's neurofibrillary
tangles) in some of the remaining nerve cells, and gli-
osis where nerve cells have disappeared. The biochemical
profile is one of drastically reduced dopamine (DA) levels
in the caudate nucleus and putamen (Bernheimer et al.,
1973). The loss is particularly great in the latter,
where DA levels may be less than 10 percent of normal
(K. G. Lloyd et al., 1975; Lee et al., 1978; Price et al.,
1978). This is consistent with a greater cell loss in

the rostral zona compacta; these cells project primarily
to the putamen. The activity of enzymes involved in DA
syntheses also is reduced by more than 90 percent (Hornykiewicz, 1972). Homovanillic acid (HVA), the main catab-
olite of DA in human brain, also is reduced in the caudate nucleus and putamen (Bernheimer et al., 1973; K. G.
Lloyd et al., 1975; Lee et al., 1978; Price et al., 1978).
However, the extent of HVA depletion (60 to 90 percent)
is not as great as that of DA, and it has been suggested
that the remaining nigral neurons increase their rate of
turnover of DA to HVA to compensate for the loss of nerve
cell bodies (Bernheimer et al., 1973).

DA receptors (as measured by 3H-haloperidol binding)
have been reported to increase 50 percent in the putamen
of patients with parkinsonism (Lee et al., 1978). This
has been interpreted as a compensatory mechanism to
counter the effects of reduced anatomic dopaminergic pro-
jections to that structure. Dopamine-sensitive adenyl
cyclase activity is another index of DA receptor activity
(Kebabian et al., 1972). Data, based on only a few cases,
indicate an increase in DA-sensitive adenyl cyclase in
the caudate nucleus of PD patients (Nagatsu et al., 1978).

The interpretation of results of DA receptor binding
studies is a complex undertaking. The rodent striatum
contains DA receptors in at least three locations: post-
synaptically, on intrinsic striatal neurons, and presynap-
tically, on both cortical and nigral afferents to the
striatum (Kebabian and Calne, 1979). While it is attractive to suggest that the increased DA receptor binding
seen in PD is postsynaptic, more data will be needed to
assess this hypothesis. More information on the specific
locus of receptor losses with age will be useful, albeit
difficult to obtain, in assessing the interaction between
normal aging changes and other etioligical factors in
Parkinson's disease.

Treatment with L-dopa appears to suppress the increased
receptor binding observed in the putamen of patients with
PD (Reisine et al., 1977; Lee et al., 1978).

Etiology and Pathogenesis

Idiopathic PD has its onset between the ages of 40 and 50.
Its etiology is unknown; however, even in neurologically
normal individuals, there appears to be an age-associated
loss of neurons in substantia nigra (McGeer et al., 1977)
and a loss of DA in the putamen (Carlsson and Winblad,

1976; Riederer and Wuketich, 1976). Several authors (e.g., Finch, 1978a) have suggested that the symptoms of PD become manifest only after individuals who, for some reason, have a low number of nigral neurons lose more neurons through the aging process. In idiopathic PD, the distribution of cell loss is focal within the zona compacta (Bernheimer et al., 1973; Price et al., 1978), and Lewy inclusion bodies in the remaining cells of substantia nigra, as well as other catecholaminergic nuclei of the brainstem, are common (Alvord et al., 1974). Postencephalic PD develops following infections, possibly even subclinical infections, of viral encephalitis lethargica (von Economo's encephalitis), major epidemics of which occurred between 1918 and 1925. Widespread cell loss and neurofibrillary tangles in the zona compacta of the substantia nigra are characteristic of patients with the postencephalitic syndrome (Alvord et al., 1974). In addition, there is an arteriosclerotic or presenile PD that is postulated to result from focal vascular damage in the substantia nigra (Bernheimer et al., 1973). There is an almost random distribution of asymmetric lesions and milder damage than is observed in the first two forms of the disease. Drugs, such as the antipsychotics (dopaminergic antagonists), and toxins, such as carbon monoxide, also can produce transient or chronic parkinsonism.

Animal Models

There is presently no spontaneous animal model of Parkinson's disease. Extensive studies in rodents, particularly mice, and a few in nonhuman primates suggest that the normal decline in functional status of the nigrostriatal-dopaminergic system, which is postulated to interact with other mechanisms to produce parkinsonism, is a phenomenon common across disparate mammalian species. None have been studied to determine whether the cell loss or characteristic pathology is present in the substantia nigra of aging animals. Nonhuman primates have been used extensively to study the neuroanatomic basis for the postural tremor of parkinsonism using the lesion method. Rodents have been widely used to study neurochemical aspects of aging in the dopaminergic systems and to explore the neuropharmacological basis for the parkinsonian syndrome induced by neuroleptics.

Nonhuman Primates

All relevant research in nonhuman primates has been done
in Old World monkeys, largely in rhesus macaques (Macaca
mulatta), with a few studies in long-tailed macaques (Macaca fascicularis) and African green monkeys (Cercopithecus aethiops). The majority of research in nonhuman
primates relating to parkinsonism has been based on the
brain lesion-induced model of postural tremor first reported by Ward et al. (1948); there has been little if
any investigation of relevant spontaneous changes in aging monkeys. Neurophysiological recording techniques
have been used to explore the role of the motor cortex,
globus pallidus, ventrolateral nucleus of the thalamus,
and cerebellum in the generation of the tremor induced
by ventromedial tegmental lesions in monkeys (Cordeau et
al., 1960; Lamarre, 1975; Ohye and Albe Fessard, 1978).
　　Postural tremor, one of the salient signs of parkinsonism in man, has been more convincingly demonstrated
in nonhuman primates than in any other species. It is
similar to the human tremor in that it consists of a 3
to 7 cycle/s, reciprocally organized pattern of agonist-
antagonist contractions that can be interrupted by voluntary movement, anesthesia, and natural sleep (Cordeau et
al., 1960). Unlike the human tremor, it tends to involve
the proximal more than the distal limb musculature (Cordeau et al., 1960). Since the early 1950s, a number of
investigators have used this model to analyze the neural
mechanism underlying the tremor, to identify brain structures in which lesioning eliminates the tremor, and to
test the efficacy of pharmacological agents in suppressing
tremor.
　　Because Parkinson's disease is associated with degenerative changes in brainstem catecholaminergic nuclei (Alvord et al., 1974) and with neuroleptic drugs that act as
dopaminergic antagonists (Dreyfuss et al., 1972; Bedard
et al., 1977; Hornykiewics, 1975), it is suggested that
the cause of the disease is anatomic or functional disruption of dopaminergic pathways. Numerous studies involving lesions of the substantia nigra in monkeys have generally supported this hypothesis in a modified form, viz.,
that physical or pharmacological disruption of the nigrostriatal pathway is a necessary but not sufficient condition for producing postural tremor in monkeys (Duvoisin,
1976). Postural tremor is most consistently produced by
a lesion of the ventromedial tegmentum of the rostral
pons and midbrain along the dorsomedial part of the

substantia nigra (Poirier, 1960). Disruption of nigro-striatal function, however, is consistently effective in producing the tremor only if accompanied by disruption of a more caudal neural system variously described as a rubro-olivo-cerebellorubral loop (Poirier et al., 1975a,b), lateral cerebellar system (Lamarre, 1975), or ventrome-dial tegmental and brachium conjunctival system (Lamarre, 1975). A study in which 6-hydroxydopamine injections into the substantia nigra have been used to achieve selec-tive destruction of its dopaminergic cells, indicates that while greater than 70 percent depletion of dopamine yields postural tremor for a few days, greater than 85 percent depletion is required to produce tremor lasting 6 months or more (Kraemer et al., 1976).

Parkinsonian tremor is generally regarded as resulting from a loss of neural suppression that, in the intact or-ganism, is imposed by the combined function of nigrostri-atal and more caudal mechanisms. Studies of the neural mechanisms that generate the tremor have focused on the motor cortex, globus pallidus, and ventrolateral nucleus of the thalamus. Lesions in these areas reduce or elimi-nate tremor produced by lesions in the ventromedial teg-mentum (Battista et al., 1969; Poirier et al., 1975a,b). Prior to the introduction of pharmacological therapy, destruction of the ventrolateral thalamus was widely and successfully used in humans to alleviate parkinsonian tremor. L-dopa, the drug most commonly used in treating parkinsonism in the elderly, reduces the tremor in mon-keys subjected to a lesion in the ventromedial tegmentum. Further, drugs that influence dopamine metabolism by in-creasing its extraneuronal concentration, potentiate the tremor-suppressant effect of L-dopa (Goldstein et al., 1976).

Studies on spontaneous age changes in the substantia nigra during aging in monkeys have been limited by the lack of availability of aged nonhuman primates. There is a single study that suggests nigral changes may accompany the normal aging process in a nonhuman primate. Dopamine content of individual cells in the substantia nigra of healthy pig-tailed macaques (Macaca nemestrina) over 20 years of age is reported to be about 40 percent lower than in 4-year-old animals of the same species (Sladek et al., 1979).

Rodents

Aging rodents have been widely used as models for studying changes in the nigrostriatal-dopaminergic pathway that occur in PD. However, neurochemical alterations observed in aged rodents, in general, have not approached the large changes observed in humans with PD. This points out the large safety factor in the human nigrostriatal system; 75 percent of the system must be damaged before behavioral effects are observed. This also may suggest that the rodent is not the best model for PD, because of the relatively small changes that occur in its nigrostriatal function during aging. Most research relevant to parkinsonism using rodents has been carried out in mice. It has concentrated largely in two areas: characterization of neurochemical changes that occur with aging in the nigrostriatal-dopaminergic pathway of normal animals and investigation of the neuropharmacological mechanisms of action of neuroleptic drugs that produce parkinsonian side effects in the human.

Rodent striatal DA has not been shown to consistently decline with age. In the mouse and rat, some investigators have found a 30 to 50 percent age-related decline (Finch, 1973a; Joseph et al., 1978), but others have shown that striatal DA remains constant during aging (Ponzio et al., 1978). High-affinity DA uptake in the striatum of C57BL/6J mice declines with age, which suggests that dopaminergic nerve terminals are being lost (Jonec and Finch, 1975). Although no losses of the key synthetic enzymes have been demonstrated in the striatum of aged mice for DA, tyrosine hydroxylase (TH) (Reis et al., 1977) and aromatic L-amino acid decarboxylase (DDC) (Finch, 1973a; Reis et al., 1977), the conversion of L-dopa or L-tyrosine to DA in the striatum of aged C57BL/6J mice is reduced by 25 to 30 percent (Finch, 1973a), and the conversion of radiolabelled precursor into DA is reduced in the striatum of aged Wistar rats (Ponzio et al., 1978). Furthermore, striatal DA turnover, as determined by the loss with time of precursor-labelled DA, is slowed by 25 to 30 percent between 10 and 28 months of age (Finch, 1973a), and DA uptake by striatal synaptosomes is reduced in aged C57BL/6J mice (Jonec and Finch, 1975).

While changes in DA concentration in the striatum of normal aging animals resemble those in patients with PD, the data with respect to DA receptors, differ markedly from those in human patients. Spiroperidol binding increases in patients with PD, but declines by 60 to 70

percent between 3 and 28 months of age in the C57BL/6J
mouse (Severson and Finch, 1978). Several studies in
aged rats indicate that DA-stimulated cyclic-AMP synthesis in the striatum is reduced (Walker and Boas-Walker,
1973; Puri and Volicer, 1977; and Schmitt and Thornberry,
1978).

Interpretation of the discrepant DA-receptor binding
data in normal aging rodents and humans with PD is hampered by lack of information on the course of change in
DA-receptor binding in normal human aging. It may well
be that a compensatory increase in postsynaptic receptor
binding only occurs when nigrostriatal input is reduced
by more than 80 percent, as in the case where cell loss
due to a second process is superimposed on that due to
a normal aging process. It is possible that the gradual
loss of dopaminergic afferents to the striatum is the
neural substrate of a normal, developmental change in the
behavior of the mature animal against which counteraction
by a compensatory mechanism, as by increasing numbers of
DA receptors, would be nonadaptive.

Attempts to induce a syndrome in rodents similar to PD
in the human have involved disrupting the function of the
nigrostriatal pathway in various ways and looking for behavioral changes characteristic of PD and for changes in
DA receptors in the striatum. Disruption of nigrostriatal
function has been induced by physical ablation, electric
current, 6-hydroxydopamine, or by functional blockade,
using neuroleptic drugs.

The use of neuroleptics, i.e., antipsychotic drugs, can
produce a parkinsonian syndrome in the human. The acute
effect of neuroleptics on rodents is a cataleptic akinesia
similar in some respects to the akinesia of PD. When
placed in unusual postures, rodents remain immobile in
those positions for a length of time that is directly correlated with the dose and antipsychotic potency of the
drug. Chronic neuroleptic treatment in rodents results
in tolerance to the acute cataleptogenic dose. This is
thought to be due to an increase in the number of receptors because neuroleptic binding has been observed to increase both in vivo and in vitro in the striatum of mice
chronically treated with haloperidol (J. G. Schwartz et
al., 1978), and L-dopa treatment suppresses such an effect in rats (Friedhoff et al., 1977). These data suggest
that the chronic neuroleptic-induced supersensitivity in
rodents may be a good model for DA receptor supersensitivity seen in PD. It should be noted, however, that the
behavioral tolerance produced by chronic treatment with

neuroleptics occurs only in young animals. Aged mice do
not show such tolerance (Randall et al., 1978), suggesting that the old mouse may not be able to produce the
increase in receptors necessary for tolerance to develop.

Chronic neuroleptic treatment of several strains of
mice (Von Voigtlander et al., 1973, 1975; Hyttel, 1978)
and the Wistar rat (Friedhoff et al., 1977) has not resulted in any alteration in DA receptors as measured by
DA-sensitive adenyl cyclase activity. Von Voigtlander
et al. (1973) have not found increases in DA-sensitive
adenyl cyclase in mice following unilateral lesions of
the nigrostriatal tract. On the other hand, Tang and
Cotzias (1977) have reported large increases (50 to 75
percent) in striatal DA-sensitive adenyl cyclase activity
in mice following chronic administration of the DA
precursor L-dopa; a similar study in rats showed no effect (Friedhoff et al., 1977).

L-dopa treatment has been suggested to increase the
life expectancy of PD patients (Sweet and McDowell, 1975;
Markham et al., 1974). L-dopa fed to female Swiss mice
results in a 41 percent (7-month) extension of life expectancy (Cotzias et al., 1977). The dose required to
extend life, however, is about 30-fold higher than that
used to treat PD patients; a dose comparable to that used
to treat PD has no effect on life expectancy. It should
be noted that a significant portion (13 percent) of the
mice treated with life-extending doses of L-dopa die
within the first 2 to 3 months of treatment are not included. This removes a possibly less vigorous subset of
the mouse population that could bias the results. In
spite of these complications, these studies represent an
interesting facet of research on aging that merits further consideration.

DEPRESSION

Definition and Clinical Manifestations

Like many diseases of unknown cause, depression has been
variously defined by a number of theorists based upon
their concepts of its etiology. For research purposes,
depressions are classified as primary or secondary, depending on whether the signs and symptoms occur alone or
in combination with other, preexisting psychiatric or severe medical conditions.

A major depressive disorder (Spitzer et al., 1978) lasts at least one week and consists of a dysphoric mood, expressed by introspective accounts of feeling depressed, without hope, irritable, worried, or discouraged and at least five of the following:

- a change in appetite or weight;
- sleep difficulty (insomnia or hypersomnia);
- loss of energy (fatigability, tiredness);
- motor changes (agitation or retardation);
- loss of interest or pleasure in usual activities, including sex;
- feelings of self-reproach or guilt;
- inability to concentrate or think clearly;
- recurrent thoughts of death or suicide.

Primary depression is subclassified as bipolar if it occurs in a person with a history of manic illness and as unipolar if it does not. Secondary depression is diagnosed if the syndrome develops against a background of other psychiatric conditions, such as schizophrenia, anxiety neurosis, phobic neurosis, hysteria, alcoholism, drug dependency, antisocial personality, homosexuality and other sexual deviations, mental retardation, organic brain syndrome, or any medical conditions of a life-threatening or incapacitating nature. A minor depressive disorder is defined similarly, but is without the full depressive syndrome. A full description of psychiatric subclassifications of depressive disorders can be found in the research diagnostic criteria developed by Spitzer et al. (1978).

At one time, depression in the elderly was regarded as a specific, "involutional depression." However, there is little evidence that the clinical manifestations of depression in the elderly are qualitatively different from those in younger patients (Post, 1968; Epstein, 1976; Gurland 1976). While geriatric psychiatrists generally agree that depression is the single most common psychiatric problem in the elderly (Epstein, 1976), estimates of its incidence and prevalence vary from 10 to 65 percent (Pfeiffer and Busse, 1973). Much of this variability may be traced to differences in operational definitions of depression, depending upon whether the questions under study relate primarily to public health, clinical treatment, or etiology (Gurland, 1976). Epidemiological studies have shown that while clinical diagnosis of depression is most frequent in middle-aged adults, symptoms

of depression are most common in those aged 65 and over
(Gurland, 1976). In addition, elderly patients with a
broad spectrum of depressive complaints respond favorably
to antidepressant medication, suggesting that depression
is seriously underdiagnosed in the over-65 age group
(Epstein, 1976).

Etiology and Pathogenesis

There are at least 10 major theories concerning the etiology of depression, classified according to the disciplinary perspectives from which they derive as biological,
behavioral, sociological, psychoanalytical, and existen-
tial (Akiskal and McKinney, 1975). Among the theories
most amenable to testing in animal models are the theories
that regard depression as resulting from generalized mammalian behavioral factors (e.g., disruption of social attachments, loss of status, learned helplessness) or from
biological factors (e.g., functional derangement of neural mechanisms that mediate behavioral reinforcement,
functional dominance of cholinergic mechanisms in the
central nervous system, impaired monoaminergic neurotrans-
mission, or hyperarousal secondary to intraneuronal sodium
concentration). Age-related changes in these factors may
account for the increased prevalence of depression with
age (Salzman and Shader, 1978a,b). Behavioral stresses
of bereavement, social isolation, or changes in social
role increase in frequency in old age. Also, age-related
changes have been found to occur in the metabolism of neurotransmitter (e.g., catecholamine) substances in the human central nervous system, and these may predispose to
depression in the aged (Lipton, 1976; Carlsson, 1978). In
addition, there is a preferential loss of catecholamine-
containing neurons in the human brain stem during aging
(Brody, 1976; McGeer et al., 1977). However, unlike the
lesions of the substantia nigra that underlie parkinsonism, the specific location of possible lesions directly
involved in depression are at present completely unknown.

Animal Models

The evidence for depression in animals has been reviewed,
the need for appropriate experimental models noted, and
the following minimal requirements for a useful animal
model of depression suggested (McKinney and Bunney, 1969):

- The symptoms of depression should be reasonably analogous to those seen in human depression.
- Behavioral changes should be defined so as to allow objective measurement.
- Independent observers should agree on objective criteria for evaluating the subjective state.
- Treatments effective in reversing depression in humans should reverse behavioral changes in animals.
- The system should be reproducible.

Although these criteria have been reconsidered and qualified (Suomi and Harlow, 1978), they have been little modified since 1969.

Nonhuman Primates

Primate models of depression have been recently and thoroughly reviewed (McKinney, 1977; Suomi and Harlow, 1978). Most research has focused on the anaclitic depression model in infant monkeys; their behavioral response to separation from mother, mother surrogate, or peers; and the influence of environmental factors and drug manipulation of central neurotransmitter systems on that response. Some of these studies are summarized here, because they may provide good models for similar studies in adult and aged nonhuman primates.

When separated from their mothers, a certain proportion of rhesus macaques (Macaca mulatta) less than 1 year old goes through a two-stage reaction: a "protest" stage lasting about 1 day, consisting of motor excitement and vocalization, followed by a "despair" stage lasting from 5 days to several weeks, consisting of reduced activity, self-mouthing, self-clasping, reduced food intake, huddling, and reduced response to social and inanimate stimuli. Preseparation levels of activity return after reunion with the mother, a mother-surrogate, or peers. The biphasic protest-despair pattern resembles and is considered to be an appropriate model of anaclitic depression in human infants (Spitz, 1946; Bowlby, 1960: Suomi and Harlow, 1978).

In designing experiments using the separation model it is important to note that, as in humans, there is considerable individual variation in response to separation under uniform experimental conditions. This may require the use of individuals known to be predisposed to depressive disorders. There is also an interspecific variation in response to separation. Although some other macaques, such as the pig-tailed (M. nemestrina) and the long-tailed (M. fascicularis) macaques, exhibit a similar biphasic response to separation, bonnet macaques (M. radiata) do not. This may be because there is a closer relationship between infants and adult females other than the mother in this species, and such females have the ability to act as substitute mothers. Neither patas monkeys (Erythrocebus patas) nor squirrel monkeys (Saimiri sciureus) show the full biphasic response to separation from the mother.

Studies of depressive reactions in juvenile and young adult monkeys are rare. Separation after the first year of life normally does not induce the biphasic protest-despair reaction. Rhesus macaques of 2 to 4 years of age respond to peer separation with protest, but without subsequent despair. It has been suggested that disappearance of the despair reaction may be due to maturation of frontal lobe function (Bowden and McKinney, 1974). Since the frontal lobe shows relatively high rates of age-related neuronal loss in humans, it is possible that there is an age-related shift back to an infantile separation response.

Social separation and confinement of rhesus macaques in a vertical chamber designed to produce learned helplessness (W. R. Miller et al., 1978a,b) can induce a despair response in older animals. This response can be partially suppressed by electroconvulsive therapy. When rhesus macaques are reared to 5 years of age in nuclear families (i.e., with constant access to mother and father), separation with isolation, but not separation with either strange or familiar companions, induces protest-despair. Even after reunion with the family, residual effects on social behavior persist.

Several pharmacological studies suggest that the brain mechanisms underlying depression in monkeys may be similar to those in humans (McKinney, 1977; Suomi and Harlow, 1978). Treatment with compounds that reduce the production of biogenic amines (α-methyl-p-tyrosine, reserpine, 6-hydroxydopamine, and p-chlorophenylalanine) can induce depressive behavior similar to that exhibited by rhesus macaques in response to separation. Indeed, treatment with α-methyl-p-tyrosine, at doses that do not affect the behavior of infants in a normal social setting, greatly sensitizes them to separation depression (Kraemer and McKinney, 1979). Imipramine, a drug commonly used to treat clinical depression in humans, can reduce symptoms of depression in infant rhesus macaques subjected to peer separation (Suomi and Harlow, 1978).

Results of most pharmacological studies of depression
in nonhuman primates are consistent with the view that
impairment of central monoaminergic mechanisms predisposes
to depression. A recent study in pig-tailed macaques indicates that intraneuronal monoamine levels are considerably
lower in aged animals (more than 20 years old) compared to
animals 4 to 10 years old (Sladek et al., 1979). If impairment of monoaminergic mechanisms causes increased susceptibility to depression, one would predict that old monkeys, like old people, would show increased vulnerability
to the syndrome.

Rodents

Common laboratory rodents do not exhibit the kinds of af-
filiative and emotional behavior necessary for establishing
behavioral models of depression clearly relevant to the
human syndrome. Nevertheless, it is fair to say that most
of our knowledge regarding the neural mechanisms of depression is based on studies in rodents. The research strategy
has been to study in rodents the mechanism of action of
drugs known to alleviate or exacerbate depression in man.
As neurochemical and neuropharmacological studies in rodents clarify the mechanisms of action of these drugs in
neural tissue, the behavioral implications are tested in
human subjects or in animal models with affective behavior
similar enough to that of man to allow relevant studies
to be made.

Because monoaminergic systems appear to be particularly
involved in depression, many of the same studies discussed
in the section on rodent models of parkinsonism also are
relevant here. For example, there is evidence for decreased concentrations and reduced breakdown of norepinephrine and dopamine in the hypothalamus of aging rats
(Simpkins et al., 1977; Riegle and Miller, 1978), and for
decreased numbers of dopaminergic receptors or decreased
receptor sensitivity in the corpus striatum of aging rats
(Walker and Boas-Walker, 1973; Puri and Volicer, 1977;
Schmitt and Thornberry, 1978), rabbits (Makman et al.,
1978), and mice (Finch, 1978). In addition, there is evidence of reduced synthesis of catecholamines in the hypothalamus and striatum of aging rats (Ponzio et al., 1978).

The use of aged rodents to study the interaction of age-
related changes in central monoaminergic mechanisms and
drugs used to treat clinical depression may throw some
light on the mechanisms of human depression. For example,

there is a small, age-related reduction of L-dopa and 5-hydroxytryptophan (5-HTP) in rat brain (McNamara et al., 1977). Electroshock treatment elevates levels of L-dopa, but not 5-HTP, significantly less in old than in young rats. It is not clear presently whether depressed elderly patients are less responsive to electroshock therapy than younger patients; however, this rodent study does suggest an important method of interspecies comparison using a treatment that is highly effective in treating depression.

Better characterization of the behavioral changes associated with deterioration of monoaminergic systems in rodents may provide a behavioral handle for studies relevant to human depression. Reduced motor activity is characteristic of depression in both aging rats and humans; in fact, reserpine-induced depression in rodents was used as a model system in the initial development of early antidepressant agents. Perseverative and stereotyped behaviors also have been observed in both aging rats (Elias and Elias, 1976) and depressed humans. However, it must be cautioned that many different brain lesions can affect activity level and perseveration and, in all likelihood, do so by a variety of underlying mechanisms. To date, reduced motivational or "hedonistic" drives have not been clearly demonstrated in aging rats (Jakubczak, 1977), although studies on self-stimulation might be of interest in this regard.

A useful approach to establishing a behavioral model in rodents relevant to depression may be to identify rodent genera other than rats and mice that form long-lasting personal bonds and study the behavioral and neurochemical responses to separation (McKinney and Bunney, 1969). If such a model could be established, much of the exploratory research that is so time-consuming and expensive to carry out in nonhuman primates could be well performed on cheaper, shorter-lived animals.

SENILE CATARACTS

Definition

Cataracts are opacifications of the crystalline lens sufficient to cause visual impairment. They are the leading cause of human blindness throughout the world; approximately 15 percent of legally blind persons in the United States have cataracts. Ninety percent of all cataracts are age-associated, and 98 percent of persons over 65 years

of age are affected to some degree. The disease is managed
surgically and/or optically; prophylaxis and medical treatment do not exist.

Clinical and Pathological Manifestations

The clinical manifestations of cataracts depend on age of
onset, location, and extent of the lesion. They may be
genetically determined (primary cataracts) or result from
concurrent or antecedent ocular or systemic disorders (secondary cataracts). Senile cataracts are usually primary,
and the only relevant history may be that of a familial
occurrence. However, underlying factors such as diabetes
mellitus may accelerate their development.

Cataracts may be classified pathologically by the degree
of opacification. Such classification is important for describing the cataract's effect on vision and, particularly,
for describing the development of the common senile cataract. The terms used to describe the progressive stages
of opacification are early immature, immature, or advanced
immature; mature; morgagnian; and hypermature.

Cataracts are classified as immature if the opacification of the lens is not complete and vision is only mildly
to moderately impaired. Immature cataracts also may be
classified according to their location, e.g., cortical or
nuclear, and according to the type of opacity, such as
zonular or punctate. The mildest senile cataract is one
in which there is nuclear sclerosis (a disproportionate
hardening and a yellow or brown discoloration of the lens
nucleus) with a reduction in visual acuity. Sclerotic nuclear changes are caused by compression of the lens. Opacification of the cortex may accompany or occur independently of nuclear changes. Cortical opacification progresses
relatively rapidly and is caused by increased lens hydration. The posterior subcapsular cataract is the cortical
cataract that causes the most troublesome reduction in
vision due to distortion of light. It begins in the visual
axis and progresses peripherally until the entire lens becomes involved. It is frequently related to chronic intra-
ocular inflammation or prolonged use of drugs, such as
topical steroids.

When the lens is entirely opaque, the cataract is considered mature. Mature senile cataracts are usually white,
often with a yellow nucleus, or they may become brown or
black in color. Imbibition of fluid and liquefaction of
cortical material may occur in the mature cataract.

A morgagnian cataract represents one of two possible progressions from the mature stage. It results from dissolution of the lens material. The impermeability of the lens capsule prevents leakage, a tense bag of milky fluid is created, and the freely movable, hard nucleus sinks to the bottom of the capsule.

The hypermature cataract is the second possible progression from the mature stage or may be a progression from the morgagnian stage. The lens capsule becomes permeable to liquefied lens substance, fluid leaks out of the capsule, and the cataract loses volume. The capsule becomes wrinkled and the cataract appears as a sac filled with a yellow brown nucleus and grayish white, insoluble, cortical debris. As a result of lens shrinkage, the depth of the anterior chamber increases.

Etiology and Pathogenesis

As the lens ages, changes occur that precede clinical evidence of cataracts. There is a decrease in water concentration, resulting in insolubility of some of the lens protein, and a progressive hardening (sclerosis) that is related to the continued growth of the lens tissue throughout life without a signficant increase in lens size. Etiopathogenesis involves alteration of normal lenticular metabolism; however, with the exception of a few types of cataract, the specific changes in metabolism are unknown.

Animal Models

Nonhuman Primates

There are few reports of naturally occurring cataracts in nonhuman primates. Congenital cataracts have been reported in one rhesus macaque (Macaca mulatta) and one chimpanzee (Pan troglodytes) (Schmidt, 1971), and cataracts of traumatic, nutritional, or toxic origin have been described in several species (Schmidt, 1971; Peiffer and Gelatt, 1976; Peiffer, 1978). Natural selection against affected animals may account for the low frequency of spontaneous cataracts. More likely, the short life span of nonhuman primates in the wild relative to their maximal life span allows insufficient time for cataracts to appear, especially those of a suspected senile origin. To increase the likelihood of finding animals with spontaneous senile cataracts, routine screening should be carried out in nonhuman primate colonies using pharmacological dilation and slitlamp biomicroscopy.

Several lens proteins of normal nonhuman primates and humans have been compared including, prealpha (Manski, et al., 1964; Maisel, 1965; Maisel and Goodman, 1965), alpha (Maisel and Goodman, 1964, 1965; Mehta and Maisel, 1967), beta (Maisel and Goodman, 1964, 1965), and gamma (Maisel and Goodman, 1964, 1965) crystallin. The nonhuman primate shows lens protein patterns that are characteristically mammalian, with significant similarities to human lens protein patterns, as well as subtle differences. Subtle differences also exist in the lens protein patterns among different species of nonhuman primates.

Cataracts can be induced in the nonhuman primate by a variety of chemical or physical insults; however, the biochemical and ultrastructural similarities to human senile cataracts have not been studied. Cataract is a general term that represents the end stage of a multitude of possible etiopathological factors. Thus, it is reasonable to say that no good nonhuman primate model fo· senile cataracts presently exists.

Carnivores

The dog may be a good model for senile cataracts for a number of reasons: the canine lens/globe ratio is nearly comparable to that of man; diagnostic procedures used to visualize, photograph, and document cataracts in man can be readily adapted to the dog; and cataracts occur commonly in the dog and are inherited in a large number of specific breeds. Table 25 summarizes the genetic and clinical manifestations of spontaneous cataracts in the dog. Histological studies of these cataracts have not been reported.

Lagomorphs

Cataracts in the rabbit arise as a result of two inherited conditions. The first is due to an autosomal, recessive mutant gene, symbolized cat-1 (Nachtsheim and Gürich, 1939; Ehling, 1957). It is manifest at birth as an isolated opacity of the horizontal posterior lens suture that is not visible macroscopically. Opacification of the posterior cortex begins at about 3 days and involves the entire

structure by 2 weeks. During this stage, the opaque subcapsular zone extends to involve the equator, while the
nucleus remains clear. The lens nucleus becomes opaque
as the cataract matures between the fifth and ninth weeks.
Lens fibers that form after maturation of the cataract are
normal, so that a transparent zone arises around the opaque
nucleus. If the cataract has not fully matured by 12
weeks of age, the development of the cataract stops.

The second inherited cataract is due to an autosomal,
incompletely dominant mutant gene, symbolized Cat-2 (Ehling, 1957). Three forms of this cataract are reported.
Type c is a nuclear cataract that progresses with a variable degree of cortical opacification to maturity and
hypermaturity. It is comparable to a posterior pole cataract. Type b is a cataract limited to the central embryonic nucleus. The lens may be completely opaque or have
multiple, focal opacities. Type a is a cataract consisting
of punctiform axial opacification with or without cortical
involvement. In a few cases, the punctiform opacities may
coalesce. Usually Cat-2 cataracts occur bilaterally.

Rodents

Rats Several outbred stocks of rats have been shown to be
useful models for the study of precataractous changes
that occur in the aging lens (Sherman rats, Balazs et
al., 1970; SD rats, Balazs and Rubin, 1971). Cytological
bindings in the lens of the aging rat that are similar to
bindings in the aging human lens include:

● increased irregularity of the cortical cell surface
in WI rats (Gorthy and Abdelbaki, 1974);
● segmental swelling of the superficial lens fibers
(Gorthy and Abdelbaki, 1974);
● structures thought to be the submicroscopic equivalent of lamellar separations (Nordmann, 1972; Philipson,
1973);
● cortical globular bodies (Gorthy and Abdelbaki,
1974);
● cortical multilamellar bodies (Philipson, 1973);
● increased prevalence of cells with a dense cytoplasm
and complex endoplasmic reticulum within the lens epithelium (Gorthy and Abdelbaki, 1974); and
● swelling of epithelial mitochondria (Gorthy and Abdelbaki, 1974).

TABLE 25 Summary of Inherited Cataracts in the Dog

Breed	Age of Onset	Cataract Characteristics	Mode of Inheritance	Reference
Miniature Schnauzer	Congenital	Nuclear; cortical; usually progressive	Autosomal recessive	Rubin et al., 1969
Old English Sheepdog	Congenital	Nuclear; cortical; usually progressive	Familial; probably autosomal recessive	Koch, 1972
Beagle	Congenital	Nuclear; cortical	Dominant with incomplete penetrance	Anderson and Schultz, 1958; Heywood, 1971; Hirth et al., 1974
American Cocker Spaniel	1-6 yr	Posterior cortical; variable progression	Autosomal recessive or polygenic	Yakely et al., 1971; Olesen et al., 1974; Yakely, 1978
Boston Terrier	2-12 mo	Posterior cortical; progressive	Autosomal recessive	Barnett, 1978
Staffordshire Terrier	2-12 mo	Nuclear and cortical	Autosomal recessive	Barnett, 1978
Golden Retriever	6 mo-3 yr	Triangular; posterior cortical; usually non-progressive	Dominant with incomplete penetrance proposed	Gelatt, 1972

Breed	Age	Description	Inheritance	Reference
Labrador Retriever	6 mo–3 yr	Entire posterior cortex; variable progression	Dominant with incomplete penetrance proposed	Gelatt, 1972
	1–3 yr	Posterior cortical; variable progression	Dominant with incomplete penetrance proposed	Barnett, 1978
Afghan Hound	6 mo–3 yr	Equatorial cortical progression	Autosomal recessive proposed	Roberts and Helper, 1972
Standard Poodle	6 mo–3 yr	Equatorial cortical progression	Autosomal recessive	Rubin and Flowers, 1972
Chesapeake Bay Retriever	6 mo–6 yr	Cortical-posterior axial and equatorial variable progression	Autosomal dominant with incomplete penetrance proposed	Gelatt et al., 1979
Siberian Husky	9 mo–3 yr	Posterior subcapsular axial opacity and equatorial vacuolation with slow progression	Probably autosomal recessive	R. L. Peiffer, University of North Carolina, Chapel Hill, unpublished
German Shepherd Dog			Dominant	von Hippel, 1930
Pointer			Dominant	Host and Sveinson, 1936
Welsh Corgi	9 mo–6 yr	Equatorial feathering and vacuolation; posterior subcapsular axial opacity and equatorial vacuolation with slow progression	Probably autosomal recessive	R. L. Peiffer, University of North Carolina, Chapel Hill, unpublished

Two types of cataract are found in aged WI rats: supranuclear and posterior subcapsular (Gorthy, 1977, 1978). Cortical alterations occurring early in cataractogenesis include segmental, cellular swelling and formation of globular and multilamellar inclusions. Histochemical analyses support the concept that the swelling and degeneration of cortical fibers may be caused by intercellular hydrolases.

Spontaneous congenital cataracts occur in some SD rats. The condition is inherited as an autosomal recessive trait and has been proposed as a potential model for the study of inheritance of congenital cataracts that resemble some human forms, e.g., those that occur in Down's syndrome. There is an overproduction of lens capsule and a proliferation of lens epithelium suggesting that the primary lesion is in the lens epithelium (Smith et al., 1969). Lens abnormalities are present at 20 days of age, but cataracts are not evident until 70 days of age or later, when, in one-third of cases, the polar posterior lens capsule ruptures and the lens extrudes into the vitreous chamber (Gorthy and Abdelbaki, 1974). Vascular attachments to the lens suggest that abnormalities may be initiated by inflammatory adhesions between the lens and pupillary margin (Gorthy and Abdelbaki, 1974).

Cataracts can be induced in rats using a number of experimental procedures, including x-irradiation (Poppe, 1942; Worgul and Rothstein 1975); bleomycin, a cancer chemotherapeutic agent that concentrates in epidermal tissues (Edwards et al., 1975); triethylene-thiophosphoramide (Thiotepa) (Robertson and Creasman, 1972); and bromodeoxyuridine (BUdR) (Gasset et al., 1975). Thiotepa and BUdR in particular produce cataracts with few side effects. Bilateral, congenital, nuclear cataracts develop between the sixteenth and twentieth day of gestation in fetuses of Wistar rats injected with BUdR. This appears to be a useful model for congenital nuclear cataracts.

Cataracts can be produced in rats maintained on a diet high in certain sugars, particularly galactose (Mitchell and Dodge, 1935). Feeding a diet high in lactose for 1 month can induce minor changes (Korc et al., 1970); feeding a diet high in sucrose produces no changes. Major alterations in the crystallin fraction of the lens, with an increase in proteins of high molecular weight and decrease in proteins of low molecular weight, are produced by diets containing 40 percent galactose. The biochemical events associated with the development of galactose cataracts involve saturation of hexokinase in the anaerobic glycolytic pathway, resulting in the formation of polyalcohols. The bioflavonoids, inhibitors of aldose reductase, are effective in preventing the development of this cataract. As in cataracts associated with diabetes mellitus, galactose-induced cataracts show increased incorporation of ^{32}P into phosphatidic acid and phosphatidylglycerol without alteration of the phospholipid component of the lens (Broekhuyse, 1971). It has been suggested that cataracts cannot be altered by systemic treatment without altering galactose levels in the diet (Van Heyningen, 1971); however, the development of galactose-induced cataracts has been reversed by providing the "sugar diet" rats with a well-balanced diet, enriched with nutrients (Heffley and Williams, 1974).

Mice Cataracts in mice are predominately congenital; however, mice are useful models for studying biochemical mechanisms of cataractogenesis that may relate to senile cataracts. Cataract formation with rupture of the posterior lens capsule in Swiss mice is inherited as a recessive trait (Fraser and Herer, 1950). First detectable at 2 to 3 weeks of age, when the hyaloid artery is normally present, the early cataract is manifested histologically as a subcapsular aggregation of homogeneous eosinophilic droplets at the posterior pole of the lens. As the number of droplets increases, the posterior sutures widen distorting and tearing the posterior lens capsule. The lens substance then extrudes into the vitreous chamber. The subsequent course is variable; the process may halt or the nucleus may become completely extruded into the vitreous chamber to be wedged between the remaining lens and retina. Occasionally it enters the anterior chamber. Similar syndromes have been described by Smelser and Von Sallman (1949), Verrusio and Fraser (1966), and Beasley (1963).

A uni- or bilateral cataract that is inherited as an autosomal dominant factor also occurs in Swiss mice (Davidorf and Egilitis, 1966; Tissot and Cohen, 1972). Beginning at 14 days of embryonic life, there is a progressive total degeneration of the primary lens fibers and laying down of abnormal secondary fibers. The cataract usually progresses to maturity, the nuclear region consisting of a clumpy eosinophilic mass with scattered, calcified areas and a vascularized epithelium. Progression to hypermaturity may occur in the adult mouse.

Congenital cataracts are inherited in A/J mice as an autosomal dominant with high penetrance (Paget and Baumgarter-Gamauf, 1953; Fraser and Schabtach, 1962; Verrusio and Fraser, 1966; Zwaan and Williams, 1968a,b, 1969; Hamai and Kuwabara, 1975). The cataracts begin as the nuclear type, later involving the entire lens, and finally becoming shrivelled. The first abnormality is detectable postnatally on the fourteenth day. The cell nuclei of some of the primary lens fibers become pyknotic and the cytoplasm degenerates. In general, cells of the posterior layer of the developing lens elongate normally but contain great numbers of dilated, rough endoplasmic reticulum, vacuoles, and mitochondria and smaller than normal amounts of crystalline substance and polysomes. With further differentiation, apical portions of these cells begin to swell and the lens becomes opaque. The swollen lens cells then degenerate.

A small nuclear cataract is inherited as an autosomal recessive trait (Nakano et al., 1960; Brown et al., 1970; Iwata and Kinoshita, 1971). This cataract appears to result from a deficiency of Na-K ATPase. At 13 days of age the lens is clear and the electrolyte levels are normal. However, by the twentieth day, the sodium content of the lens increases, inducing a hydrophilic osmotic change that results in swollen, granular, or liquified cortical lens fibers. Subcapsular cataracts in conjunction with microphthalmia in young mice of unspecified stock have been described by Tust (1958).

A developmental cataract is inherited in deermice (Peromyscus maniculatus) as an autosomal recessive trait progressing to a complete bulbus (Burns and Feeney, 1975). The earliest microscopic change is vacuolation in and near the nucleus just inside the lens bow at the equator. Posterior, subcapsular opacities originate with the posterior migration of equatorial cells. Large round epithelioid cells (bladder or "Wedl" cells) occur in the posterior, subcapsular region. With involvement of the anterior or posterior cortex, the lens nucleus disappears, producing a total, mature cataract. Progression to hypermaturity follows with iritis and phthisis bulbi.

Discussion

Senile cataractogenesis in animals is difficult to compare with that in the human, because the human processes are almost impossible to study progressively and to control

adequately. Throughout the spectrum of mammalian species
discussed, lens structure and metabolism are remarkably
similar. This fact points out the potential for valid interspecies extrapolations in the study of cataractogenesis.
Data from animal models may provide guidelines for genetic,
structural, chemical, and functional studies in human
lenses, as they become available.

The lens is a unique tissue with respect to its anatomy
and physiology; while the genetics and morphology of cataracts merit investigation, investigational research should
also emphasize the biochemical alterations that occur in
the lens and surrounding tissues before and during cataract
formation. Major biochemical processes include energy metabolism, primarily anaerobic glycolysis; transport mechanisms that are essential for the transparency and normal
function of this avascular tissue; amino acid, peptide,
and protein metabolism; and phospholipid metabolism.

SENILE MACULAR DEGENERATION

Definition

Senile macular degeneration is a progressive, bilateral
degeneration of the macular region of the retina, resulting in a loss of central vision. It is the most common
of the macular diseases affecting people 60 years of age
and older (Vision Research, 1978-1982).

Clinical and Pathological Manifestations

Senile macular degeneration may be divided into two phases.
The first, the predisciform phase, is characterized ophthalmoscopically by the presence of drusen (i.e., hyaline
excrescences of Bruch's membrane and pigment epithelium)
in the macular area, pigment mottling in the macular
epithelium, and/or serous detachment of the retinal pigment epithelium. During this phase, Bruch's membrane is
intact although it may show microscopic morphological alterations. The second or disciform phase is characterized
by degeneration of the macular photoreceptor elements and
development of scar tissue in the macular area. It may
arise by one of two different mechanisms: dry atrophic
or wet exudative Kuhnt-Junius macular degeneration.
Atrophic macular degeneration is a slow insidious process

in which the choriocapillaris degenerates, causing a secondary degeneration of the overlying retinal pigment epithelium and photoreceptors in the macula. Wet exudative macular degeneration develops more rapidly, and its effects are more acutely noticed by patients. Breaks in Bruch's membrane are characteristic of this form, and blood vessels from the choroid grow through the breaks into the subpigment epithelial and subretinal spaces. Fluorescein angiography is used to detect clinical vascular abnormalities. Hemorrhage occurs from the new vessels, and an organized plaque of scar tissue forms (Gass, 1967; Sarks, 1976), leading to end-stage or disciform macular degeneration. There are no truly effective therapy or preventive measures for this disease.

Etiology and Pathogenesis

Senile macular degeneration appears to be a choroidal disease involving degenerative changes in the choriocapillaris and Bruch's membrane, with secondary alterations in the pigment epithelium and retina. Changes in the permeability of the choriocapillaris and Bruch's membrane may result in exudative and hemorrhagic disciform detachment of the overlying neuroepithelium. The etiology of the abnormal permeability in Bruch's membrane is unknown.

Animal Models

Nonhuman Primates

Most higher order primates, along with certain avian species, possess a foveate retina and, thus, are more likely than other mammalian species to offer models most similar to the disease seen in the human. There are three reports in the literature concerning drusen or drusen-like abnormalities with pigment mottling in the macula in rhesus macaques (Macaca mulatta) (Stafford, 1974; El-Mofty et al., 1978; Fine and Kwapien, 1978). A survey of animals in a closed breeding colony at the Caribbean Primate Center has shown a high incidence of suspected macular degeneration in older monkeys (16-21 years old). In many cases there is a decreased cone-flicker response as revealed by electroretinography, suggesting abnormalities in macular photoreceptors. Macular degeneration comparable to the human

syndrome must still be demonstrated histologically; if
this can be done, the potential for studying the developmental phases of the disease is promising.

Fine and Kwapien (1978) have ophthalmoscopic evidence
of drusen or drusen-like bodies in the macular area of
rhesus macaques in a long-term study of contraceptive drug
safety. The condition has been seen in both treated and
control animals and, thus, is not attributable to a drug
effect. Histological and electron microscopic studies
show many retinal pigment epithelial cells in the macular
area filled with lipidlike material that the authors designate a lipoidal degeneration associated with aging. Typical drusen also have been observed on occasion, but no
breaks in Bruch's membrane nor abnormalities of the photoreceptors have been evident.

A similar clustering of small, sharply delineated, hypopigmented spots has been observed in another colony of
rhesus macaques (Bellhorn, et al., 1980), but the incidence
is much lower than that reported by El-Mofty et al. (1978).
Further, electroretinography and visual evoked potentials
of monkeys with these hypopigmented spots are within normal limits. This indicates that pigment epithelial degeneration may be spontaneous in aging rhesus macaques, but
that more time is necessary for abnormalities of Bruch's
membrane to occur in order to produce a macular degenerative phase.

A maculopathy of suspected hereditary origin has been
described in baboons (Papio papio) in a closed colony at
the Chicagoland Zoological Park, Chicago, Illinois (Vainisi, et al., 1976). Pigmentary abnormalities of the macula
have been observed ophthalmoscopically in several older
members of the colony. This disease has been characterized
as a cone-rod degeneration because the electroretinographic
abnormalities are present in both cone and rod responses
to light stimuli and there is a diffuse retinal abnormality, a feature that is more akin to hereditary cone-rod
dystrophies than to senile macular degeneration in man.
However, since maculopathy is a part of the syndrome, studies of these baboons will provide insight into photoreceptor disease. Also, senile macular degeneration may occur
in these animals as they grow older. Since the disease
in baboons is apparently of hereditary origin, this model
provides the potential opportunity to investigate the developmental phases of the disease.

Carnivores

Like primates, the domestic cat (Felis catus) and dog
(Canis familiaris) have duplex retinae, i.e., they have
both cones and rods. The area centralis has a high density
of cones (Koch and Rubin, 1972; Steinberg et al., 1973);
however, there is no macula with a pure population of
cones such as exists in man and other higher order primates. The feline retina has a delineated area in which
the proportion of cones to rods is higher than in the
canine retina and the retinal vascular pattern, as in
man, is decidedly thinner. A central retinal degeneration, characterized histologically as a loss of photoreceptors, has been reported in the feline area centralis
(Bellhorn and Fisher, 1970). This spontaneous lesion involves a diffuse retinal cone abnormality as revealed
both electroretinographically and ultrastructurally (Bellhorn et al., 1974). In addition, cats affected with this
condition show reduced visual acuity proportional to the
size of the lesion (Blake and Bellhorn, 1978). A similar
disease process has been shown to result from taurine deficiency (Schmidt et al., 1976). This induced retinopathy
progresses from a central to a diffuse retinal disease,
but does not appear to be associated with abnormalities
of the retinal pigment epithelium, Bruch's membrane or
choriocapillaris. Thus, there is no evidence of the precursor events that accompany senile macular degeneration
in the human. Because it is reproducible, however, this
lesion provides a means of studying photoreceptor degenerative processes, and, most importantly, the photoreceptor
degeneration in taurine deficiency can be halted, and
even reversed, by adding taurine to the diet (Hayes et
al., 1975; Berson et al., 1976).
    Hereditary retinal degenerations occur in certain
breeds of dogs. Those most thoroughly investigated are
found in the Irish Setter, Miniature Poodle, and Norwegian
Elkhound (Aguirre, 1976). The pathogenesis of the lesions
varies in the different breeds; the Irish Setter shows a
rod-cone dysplasia, the Miniature Poodle a rod-cone atrophy, and the Norwegian Elkhound a rod dysplasia. Recently, the Collie also has been shown to have a rod-cone
dysplasia with retinal pigment epithelial abnormalities
(Wolf, et al., 1978). Abnormalities of the retinal pigment epithelium are also seen in the Irish Setter and
the Norwegian Elkhound, but not until the later stages
of the disease, and no abnormalities of the choroid or
choriocapillaris have been reported. Finally, the Alaskan

Malamute suffers from a day-blindness syndrome (Rubin,
1976) that is characterized by a developmental abnormality
of the cones. These diseases appear to have relevance to
such conditions as retinitis pigmentosa and monochromatism
in man and provide the opportunity to study photoreceptor
cell degeneration in reproducible models. Unless late-
stage pathology is shown to include degenerative changes
in the choriocapillaris/Bruch's membrane/retinal pigment
epithelium complex, however, these diseases are not likely to be relevant to the study of senile macular
degeneration.

The canine retinopathy that may prove most relevant for
the study of human senile macular degeneration is a progressive dystrophy in the central, retinal pigment epithelium that occurs in several breeds of dogs (Aguirre
and Laties, 1976). Retinal degeneration in the Labrador
Retriever begins in the area centralis and develops secondarily into a pigment epithelial dystrophy characterized
by accumulation of autofluorescent, lipid-ceroid material
in the pigment epithelial cells. Thus, the disease has
at least one parameter in common with senile macular degeneration, viz., a pigment epithelial defect. It may be
relevant to senile macular degeneration in man, especially
if late-stage pathology proves to include disease of
Bruch's membrane and neovascularization of the subretinal
space. This progressive dystrophy occurs sporadically,
and no established breeding program for its perpetuation
exists.

Rats

There is no specialization of the central retina of the
laboratory rat (Rattus norvegicus) resembling a fovea
centralis or macula lutea; therefore, retinal degeneration
in the rat cannot replicate human senile macular degeneration. However, the retina is composed of rod and cone
photoreceptors and the rat has demonstrable color and
black-white vision.

Spontaneous retinal changes that occur in the aging,
specific pathogen free Chbb:THOM rats have been well described (Weisse et al., 1974). Abnormal retinal findings
in 2.5- to 3-year-old animals include rarefication of nuclei in the outer (36 percent) and inner (27 percent)
nuclear layers. Retinal capillaries have increased diameters, thicker vessel walls, and show the presence of
acid mucopolysaccharides when stained with periodic acid

Schiff (PAS) stain. Age-dependent changes in the choroid
are relatively few (4 percent) and consist mainly of vascular occlusions.

Valuable basic structural and functional information
can be gained by inducing destruction of photoreceptors,
either independently of or together with destruction of
the pigment epithelium; modification of choriocapillarial
fenestration; and neovascularization of the retina by
varying the light intensity (O'Steen et al., 1972), duration of exposure to light (Anderson and O'Steen, 1972,
1974), the animal's body or environmental temperatures,
and other factors (Noell et al., 1966; O'Steen, 1970,
1979). In retinopathies induced in rats by urethan administration (Bellhorn et al., 1973; Rabkin et al., 1977)
and exposure to light (Rabkin et al., 1977), the photoreceptor cells degenerate and deep retinal capillary vessels
proliferate, extending into the retinal pigment epithelium. Ultrastructurally, these vessels are fenestrated due
to neovascularization or modification of existing vessels
(Bellhorn et al., In press). Such changes may serve as
models of the vascular component of senile macular
degeneration.

Considerable basic research information has been derived from studying two hereditary models of rat retinal
dystrophy: the Royal College of Surgeons (RCS) strain
(Bourne et al., 1938; Dowling and Sidman, 1962) and the
WAG/Rij strain (Lai et al., 1975). The RCS strain shows
a rapid destruction of photoreceptors by 60 days of age
with accompanying loss of electroretinographic responses;
the production of outer segment lamellae and function of
pigment epithelial cells have been described in detail.
The retinal dystrophy of the WAG/Rij strain has an early
onset and follows a slow progressive course as the animal
ages. This disorder involves mainly the photoreceptor
cells, although there is some reduction in the number of
bipolar and ganglion cell neurons as well. Retinal vessels invade the pigment epithelium and vitreous humor,
and migration of pigment epithelial cells in the retina
is prominent. The disease mechanism in RCS rats apparently involves an abnormal phagocytic function of the pigment epithelium, but a different, unknown mechanism is
involved in the retinal dystrophy of the WAG/Rij strain.

Summary

Nonhuman primates offer the greatest potential for providing a model of human senile macular degeneration because the higher order primates have a macula and foveate retina and a retinal vasculature similar to those of man. These lesions may be identified by screening captive primate populations. Certain avian species also have a foveate retina, but spontaneous retinopathies have not been reported. The feline has a more highly developed area centralis than the canine and may, therefore, be the better model for studies concerning focal central retinopathies. It must be recognized, however, that none of the presently available animal models of retinal disease (with or without foveal or macular manifestations) meet the important criterion of exudative senile macular degeneration in man, viz., vascular invasion of the subretinal space through defects in Bruch's membrane and pigment epithelium. These vessels are involved in the precipitous hemorrhages and scar formation that occur in the human disease. Thus, models that focus on the process of neovascularization induced by whatever means, such as the induced rat models, may be of value in understanding the human condition, by providing the opportunity to investigate the anatomic and physiological parameters of vessels proliferating in the retina.

A recent report discusses the implications to senile macular degeneration of the histological and ultrastructural characteristics of the aging Bruch's membrane/retinal pigment epithelium complex in man (Grindle and Marshall, 1978). This report verifies and expands the light microscopic studies of Sarks (1976) and further notes that the fenestrated choroidal vessel loses its fenestrations on entering the neural retinal tissue. This suggests that the morphology of the neovascularization associated with senile macular degeneration is dependent upon which tissue the vessel is subserving. If neovascularization induced by various methods in different species shows a similar vascular metamorphosis, the resultant models could provide a means of investigating this most interesting phenomenon. Basic information regarding the normal physiology and pathophysiology of the choriocapillaris and Bruch's membrane with regard to the blood-retinal barrier is likely to be necessary before the aberrations that develop in senile macular degeneration will be fully understood.

PRESBYCUSIS

Definition

Presbycusis is the progressive loss of hearing that occurs with old age. It is not a direct threat to life,
but does lead to a sense of isolation and frustration for
the patient and reduces his or her ability to cope in
ways that become major problems for clinicians, family,
and friends.

Clinical Manifestations and Pathology

Although there is some disagreement about applicability
to the clinical situation (Bredberg, 1967, 1968; Johnsson
and Hawkins, 1972, 1979), it has been suggested that there
are four main types of presbycusis (Schuknecht, 1964,
1974):

• sensory presbycusis, characterized by a loss of hair
cells from the basal cochlear turn and abrupt high-tone
hearing loss;
• neural presbycusis, characterized by severe degeneration of the neurons of the central auditory pathway and
cochlea and a decreased ability to discriminate speaking
sounds;
• strial presbycusis, characterized by strial atrophy
of the cochlear turns and a flat audiometric curve; and
• cochlear conductive presbycusis, characterized by a
descending audiometric pattern that begins in middle age,
attributed to a disorder in motion mechanics of the
cochlear duct.

Although not dealt with specifically here, dysequilib-
rium due to vestibular receptor and nerve degeneration in
the inner ear is also a complication of aging (Ross, 1979).
It is unclear whether such degeneration is a concomitant
of presbycusis. Comparative models for human vestibular
degeneration have been little sought and represent a fertile field for future investigation.

Etiology and Pathogenesis

The causes of presbycusis are unknown; however, degeneration of the auditory system appears to be a continual

process beginning early in life. There is evidence of outer hair cell degeneration in infants and newborns (Johnsson and Hawkins, 1972), and changes typical of the aged inner ear can be demonstrated by the second decade of life (Bredberg, 1968).

Genetic determinants for presbycusis are being sought. Certain tribes in Africa and India, living in a quiet environment, hear better in old age than do persons of the western world (Rosen et al., 1962, 1964; Kapur and Patt, 1967). Whether this is a result of lack of exposure to noise, or to the degree of pigmentation (Bunch and Raiford, 1931; Post, 1964; Lyttkens et al., 1979), or other genetic differences is not clear. The specific role of the pigment-containing melanocytes in the inner ear is unknown; however, many defects in pigmentation are part of a constellation of signs, including various degrees of deafness and vestibular disturbances (see, for example, Marcus, 1968).

The causes of hearing loss among elderly Americans almost certainly involve both genetic and epigenetic factors. The relative contribution of genetically determined changes in the auditory system that unfold as a natural accompaniment of increasing years, as opposed to changes induced by ototoxic drugs or chronic exposure to noise, particular diets, or other external factors, is unknown. Animal models offer the opportunity to sort out these factors and to clarify the mechanisms by which they individually contribute to the problem of deafness in the aged.

Animal Models

Nonhuman Primates

With the exception of one pilot study using the squirrel monkey (Saimiri sciureus) (McCormick et al., In press), the nonhuman primate has not been explored as a model for presbycusis. For several reasons, however, nonhuman primates should make good models for studies of this disease. First, the nonhuman primate has an auditory anatomy and physiology similar to that of the human. The comparative vascular anatomy of human and nonhuman primates has been worked out (Nabeya, 1923; Axelsson, 1968), and cochlear potentials of the nonhuman primate (Wever et al., 1958) are remarkably like those of the human (Ruben et al., 1959). Considerable baseline behavioral and electrophysiological auditory data and sophisticated methods for auditory research also are available (Gourevitch, 1970; Moody et al., 1970; Stebbins, 1973; Beecher, 1974; Pugh et al., 1974; Dewson and Burlingame, 1975; Pfingst et al., 1975, 1978). The advent of computer-averaged brain stem auditory recording techniques has made noninvasive electrophysiological studies possible. Light microscopic observations of the inner ear of humans and nonhuman primates have been compared (Hawkins and Johnsson, 1968), and the reaction of the nonhuman primate inner ear to noise and drug damage has been shown to be very much like that for the human (Stebbins, 1970).

Human studies have shown that, in addition to auditory damage caused by noise, hearing loss may result from direct or indirect damage due to high levels of blood lipids, elevation of systemic blood pressure, and vascular disease (Rosen and Olin, 1965; Spencer, 1973). A controlled experiment using nonhuman primate and avian models of human atherosclerosis (McCormick et al., In press) has demonstrated a direct relationship between the loss of inner ear function and vascular disease, high blood pressure, elevated serum cholesterol, and blood coagulation defects. Animal species without vascular disease do not show the great magnitude of age-related hearing loss seen in humans (Crowley, 1975; Lawrence, 1979), indicating that the inner ear does not necessarily deteriorate as a function of age itself, but rather concomitantly with a disease process (Lawrence, 1979).

The long-tailed macaque (Macaca fascicularis) may also be an excellent model for research on presbycusis, because this nonhuman primate develops vertebral vascular disease (Alexander and Clarkson, 1978), and the ear receives its blood supply from the vertebral system. This macaque also is more prone to intracranial atherosclerosis than other nonhuman primates (Clarkson et al., 1976a).

Carnivores

Deafness is a common occurrence in old dogs, and although studies have been limited to a few animals, sensorineural degeneration, strial atrophy, and vascular changes similar to those in humans have been demonstrated (Johnsson and Hawkins, 1979).

Rodents

The chinchilla (life span about 20 years) has been studied
as a possible model for human presbycusis. Chinchillas
13 and 14 years of age have essentially normal thresholds
for hearing and normal cochlear microphonic activity, although there is an approximate 30 percent ganglion cell
loss in the 14-year-old animal (Miller, 1970). Loss of
hair cells in the cochlea is insignificant (B. A. Bohne,
Department of Otolaryngology, Washington University, St.
Louis, Missouri, Unpublished). There is no documentation
on the condition of the stria vascularis or the nerve
fibers throughout the cochlea. These studies suggest
that the chinchilla may not be a good model for human
presbycusis.

Studies have shown that 2-year-old SD rats experience
a high frequency-specific loss in nerve action potential
(AP) that is analogous to the descending audiogram of human presbycusis (Crowley et al., 1972a,b, 1973). Cochlear
microphonic losses are also registered. More outer than
inner hair cells are lost; however, compared to losses
encountered in aged humans, both the electrical and the
hair cell changes are very small. It will be necessary
to study the rat further to determine whether it is a
good or poor model for human presbycusis. It has been
suggested that the rats used by Crowley et al. may not
have been truly old (Hoffman, 1979). Another study has
demonstrated a 25 percent reduction (most pronounced
basally and apically) in spiral ganglion cells of 34-
month-old SD rats and ultrastructural changes in the
eighth cranial nerve and nerve fibers central to the
spiral ganglion (Feldman and Vaughan, 1979). In addition, there are a number of signs of degeneration in the
central auditory pathway and nuclei, even at the cortical
level. Thus, losses in hearing ability cannot be attributed solely to structural changes in the cochlear tissues
in these animals. Related behavioral studies have failed
to demonstrate differences in behaviorally determined
auditory thresholds between young and old rats, although
minor differences do occur (Crowley, 1975).

It is unclear at the present time whether the laboratory mouse, Mus musculus, will provide a good model for
presbycusis. In behavioral testing, outbred NMRI mice
show an age-related rise in auditory threshold (Ehret,
1974). The magnitude of the hearing loss is approximately the same as that occurring in man; however, unlike
man, low rather than high frequencies are most affected.

NMRI mice have an average life span of 18 months, and no pathological abnormalities in the middle ear or in behavior have been observed. There have been no studies of morphological changes in the inner ear.

Several inbred strains of mice show hereditary, progressive loss of hearing soon after birth with a corresponding loss of hair cells from the organ of Corti beginning in the basal coil. Mikaelian et al. (1974) have reported such a defect in C57BL/6 mice. These and other mice with inner ear defects of the Scheibe type should be extremely useful in better understanding the basic mechanisms pertaining to age-related degeneration of the human inner ear. The fact that the degeneration noted is genetically determined should be a stimulus to further investigations using these animals.

Cochleas of 4-year-old Peromyscus maniculatus bairdii (deermice) have been studied by scanning electron microscopy. Aged animals show a striking loss of outer hair cells that is most severe basally, with a few outer hair cells persisting near the apex. Many inner hair cells of the basal cochlear region are absent, and the stereocilia may be clumped or abnormally elongated and reduced in number. These changes appear comparable to those described for human presbycusis.

A mutation called "epileptic waltzer" is found in Peromyscus maniculatus bairdii. These mice develop hearing after birth, but within a few months their hearing acuity, particularly for high-frequency sounds, begins to decline and deafness ensues. These animals show a severe degeneration of the organ of Corti beginning at the base of the cochlea and spreading apically with increasing age (Ross, 1965). Indeed, the organ of Corti sometimes disappears near the base of the cochlea. Ganglion cells of corresponding cochlear regions degenerate, and there may be a second focus of degeneration far apically. Strial atrophy and some degeneration of the saccular neuroepithelium are also noted. This complex of degenerative signs corresponds to those observed in human presbycusis. This mutant may prove invaluable as a model for this disease, because the process of "aging" of the cochlea appears to be accelerated. Severe degeneration occurs so rapidly that deermice as young as 1 year of age may show a relatively complete pattern of presbycusis.

Nearly all signs of presbycusis can be reproduced by the administration of ototoxic drugs (Johnsson and Hawkins, 1979). The end result of treatment with these drugs is referred to as "galloping presbycusis," an apt description that could be applied as well to the genetic defects of the inner ear. A better understanding of the primary site of action of ototoxic drugs, as well as of the basic mechanisms involved, may undoubtedly help us to understand the processes underlying age-related inner ear degeneration.

The investigator should be aware that human presbycusis represents a constellation of anatomical, physiological, and related electrical signs and is of unknown etiology. The use of aged animals as models for presbycusis in man is one approach toward understanding the basic mechanisms underlying the disease. Equally valid avenues toward the same end appear to be the use of carefully selected animals showing genetically determined inner ear degeneration and the use of normal animals in which presbycusis is induced by exposure to factors (such as ototoxic drugs, noise, or other environmental factors) that are experienced by aging humans.

GINGIVITIS AND PERIODONTITIS

Definition

Gingivitis is a relatively innocuous inflammation of the gums, with associated bleeding and exudation. It may progress, however, to periodontitis, a destructive, aggressive disease, characterized by resorption of alveolar bone, destruction of collagen with fibrosis, formation of acute abscesses and deep pockets around the necks of the teeth, and tooth loss. These diseases are the principal causes of tooth loss in adults (Page et al., 1978).

Clinical Manifestations and Pathology

In most individuals, gingivitis appears within 3 to 4 days after all means of oral hygiene are withdrawn (Page and Schroeder, 1976). The clinical manifestations of gingivitis include redness, swelling, and slight bleeding from the gingival sulcus upon gentle probing. Although gingivitis is usually painless, patients may express concern that their gums bleed during tooth brushing. A diagnosis of periodontitis is made when, in addition to the signs of gingivitis noted above, there is also evidence of involvement of the alveolar bone and deepening of the gingival sulcus with formation of a periodontal pocket.

Histologically, as periodontitis develops, an infiltrate, made up predominantly of plasma cells and lymphocytes, forms and the cells of the junctional epithelium proliferate and extend into the adjacent connective tissues and apically along the root surface. The attachment of the gingival tissue to the root surface is lost and a pocket filled with microorganisms, white blood cells, and sloughed epithelial cells forms. Finger pressure on the marginal gingival tissues may cause pus to exude from around the neck of the tooth. If the opening of the pocket lumen to the oral cavity becomes blocked, pus accumulates, and a periodontal abscess may develop. Associated with these clinical changes in the gingival tissues are resorption of the alveolar bone, destruction of the periodontal ligaments leading to loosening of the teeth, loss of function, and ultimately to loss of teeth.

Etiology and Pathogenesis

Gingivitis and periodontitis are caused by bacterial colonization of the region of the gingival sulcus (Page and Schroeder, 1976). The amount of microbial and calculus correlates with the severity of gingivitis (Löe et al., 1965) and bone loss (Schei et al., 1959). The microorganisms are generally considered to be gram negative, motile, assychrolytic rods including Bacteroides, Fusiformis, and "Capnocytophaga." Various spirochaetes and organisms of the genera Actinobacillus and Actinomyces may also be involved. Gingivitis and periodontitis are not infections in the usual sense of the word. Except in specialized cases, such as acute periodontal abscess, the microorganisms do not invade the tissues (Page, 1977). The exact mechanism by which they induce periodontal destruction is unknown; however, possible mechanisms include activation of immunopathological and inflammatory responses that lead to the destruction of the intracellular matrix of connective tissue or epithelial cells, death of cells, and bone resorption.

Although microorganisms are essential for inducing the disease in humans, there are also predisposing and precipitating factors that are not well understood, such as defects in various host defense mechanisms; psychological stress; bruxism; use of certain drugs (e.g., the anticonvulsant, diphenylhydantoin); and periods of hormone imbalance occurring at puberty, during pregnancy, and in some women taking oral contraceptives. It should be

emphasized that such predisposing factors by themselves
do not cause gingivitis or periodontitis; microorganisms
must be present.

Animal Models

Periodontal disease has been found in virtually every
species of dentate animal studied. Several excellent reviews and a recent book are available on this subject
(Cohen and Goldman, 1960; Dreizen and Levy, 1977; Navia,
1977).

Nonhuman Primates

Nonhuman primates have been used as models to study several aspects of normal structure (Skougaard and Beagrie,
1962; Skougaard and Levy, 1971; Ammons et al., 1972;
Caffesse and Nasjleti, 1976). Periodontal disease with
clinical and radiographic features comparable to that
seen in humans occurs spontaneously and can be induced
in nonhuman primates. The flora of the periodontal
region of nonhuman primates, although not well studied,
seems comparable to that found in humans (Cock and Bowen,
1967; Krygier et al., 1973). Spontaneous periodontitis
has been studied in numerous nonhuman primate species but
the prevalence and the histopathological characteristics
of the disease have not been well defined. In addition,
nonhuman primates have been used to investigate the role
of occlusion trauma in periodontitis (Polson, 1977).
Pathological alveolar bone loss has been found in one
of 17 skulls from long-tailed macaques (Macaca fascicularis) (Cohen and Goldman, 1960). Periodontal pockets,
but no evidence of generalized periodontitis as seen in
humans, have been found in 16 of 106 formalin fixed and
65 defleshed skulls of wild howler monkeys (Aloutta spp.)
(Hall et al., 1967). On the other hand, bone lesions
have been observed in 76 percent of 292 gorilla (Gorilla
gorilla) skulls studied (Kakehashi et al., 1963), although this high percentage may be misleading since
fenestrations and dehiscences counted as lesions in this
study are now considered to represent normal anatomical
variation. In a study of 40 healthy baboons (Papio
anubis), ranging in age from 7 to 10 years, gingivitis
has been found in 33 and periodontitis in only 3 (Hodosh
et al., 1971).

Periodontitis also has been studied in four chimpanzees (Pan troglodytes) 6 to 12 years of age and two chimpanzees 39 and 44 years of age (Arnold and Baram, 1973). The young animals exhibited gingivitis, but not periodontitis. Bone loss and pockets characteristic of periodontitis were found in the old animals. In a group of eight chimpanzees varying in age from 27 to 47 years, masses of calculus and plaque were found, and there were clinical and radiographic manifestations of periodontitis around most teeth (Page et al., 1975). Most lesions were not severe, however, indicating that chimpanzees are remarkably resistant to destructive spontaneous periodontitis.

Colony-maintained marmosets (Callithrix spp.) have a high prevalence of severe periodontal disease comparable to the human disease, with pocket formation and enlarged gingiva (Shaw and Auskaps, 1954; Page et al., 1972). Preliminary investigations indicated that wild-caught animals also have the disease (Levy, 1963); however, subsequent studies have shown that the prevalence is very low (Ammons et al., 1972).

The same features of chronic peridontitis are seen in both nonhuman primates and humans, i.e., formation of an inflammatory cell infiltrate, conversion of junctional epithelium to pocket epithelium, alterations in the connective tissue substance, and resorption of the alveolar bone. Changes in epithelium, connective tissue, and bone are fairly consistent from one species to another, but the nature of the inflammatory cell infiltrate varies significantly among primate species. This fact is likely to be significant. In humans, plasma cells and, to a lesser extent, lymphocytes (especially B cells) predominate in the lesions (Page and Schroeder, 1976). This is also true for chimpanzees (Pan troglodytes) (Arnold and Baram, 1973; Page et al., 1975), baboons (Papio spp.) (Avery and Simpson, 1973; Simpson and Avery, 1974), and probably for galagos (Galago senegalensis) (Grant et al., 1973), but not for some other species. In both wild and colony-maintained marmosets, periodontitis is manifested clinically as a hyperplastic, acutely inflammed granulation in which neutrophils and mononuclear cells predominate and vascular proliferation is apparent (Page et al., 1972; Schectman et al., 1972). Plasma cells are not found, even in the terminal stage of the disease (Page et al., 1971). Still another pattern, the predominance of macrophages in diseased tissues, is seen in the squirrel monkey (Saimiri sciureus) and the long-tailed macaque (Macaca fascicularis) (Hopps and Johnson, 1974; Johnson and Hopps,

1974; Heijl et al., 1976; Adams et al., 1979). These observations have major implications for investigators selecting primate models for study of pathogenic mechanisms.

Periodontitis may be induced in nonhuman primates in
several ways, including:

• placement of a ligature around the cervix of the
tooth inside the gingival sulcus, causing the accumulation
of bacteria; formation of an inflammatory infiltrate; and
tissue damage, including alveolar bone resorption characteristic of chronic periodontitis (Kennedy and Polson,
1973; Heijl et al., 1976; Adams et al., 1979);
• surgical creation of periodontal pockets around the
molars by opening a flap, removing a portion of the alveolar bone from between the roots, and placing a foreign
object into the wound, followed by feeding on a soft,
plaque-enhancing diet for 6 weeks (Ellegaard et al.,
1973); and
• manipulation of the immunological responses in various ways (Ranney and Zander, 1970; Levy et al., 1976;
Wilde et al., 1977; Asaro et al., 1978).

Each of these methods provides a reasonable model for
studying some aspect of human periodontitis.

Carnivores

The dog is a widely used model for periodontal disease
(Navia, 1977). The etiology and histopathology of the
diseased periodontium to some extent resembles that of
man, and the dog is of sufficient size to allow manipulation of the oral tissues. The incidence of the spontaneous disease in dogs is unknown, but is believed to
be high. The disease is responsible for more tooth loss
in dogs than any other factor and increases in incidence
and severity with age (Hamp and Lindberg, 1977).

Progressive periodontal disease in the dog is characterized by dense subepithelial inflammatory infiltrates
consisting predominately of plasma cells intermingled
with lymphocytes, epithelial proliferation and migration, and loss of alveolar bone (Hamp and Lindberg,
1977). The extent of periodontal disease varies considerably in dogs of the same breed and age (Hull et
al., 1974; Hamp and Lindberg, 1977). The histological
features of normal and diseased periodontium are to some
extent similar to those in humans (Melcher and Bowen,

1969; Löe and Listgarten, 1973; Stahl, 1973; Page and
Schroeder, 1976); however, it has been shown radiographically that periodontal disease in dogs usually originates
at the furcation (Hull et al., 1974; Page and Schroeder,
In press), whereas in man the interproximal regions usually show the first signs of alveolar bone loss (Lovdal
et al., 1959).

There is an association between the number of microbial deposits and the degree of gingivitis and periodontal
disease (Rosenberg et al., 1966; Saxe et al., 1967; Gad,
1968; Hamp and Lindberg, 1977). Removal of these deposits
retards the disease process (Saxe et al., 1967). Dogs
given a soft diet accumulate and develop more bacterial
plaque and gingivitis than dogs given a hard diet (Egelberg, 1965a,b; Saxe et al., 1967). The flora of the
Beagle has been assessed, but the data are incomplete,
Krasse and Brill, 1960; Saxe et al., 1967; Courant et al.,
1968). At least 15 different genera of microorganism
have been isolated from the plaque of Beagles (Wunder
et al., 1976); gram-positive organisms predominate in
incipient lesions and gram-negative anaerobic rods predominate by at least 2:1 in advanced periodontal disease
(Newman et al., 1977). There is a quantitative similarity
in flora between the dog and man (Crawford et al., 1975;
Newman et al., 1976).

Dogs are used extensively as models for gingivitis and
periodontal disease. A few of the many aspects of these
diseases that have been studied are:

● clinical and morphological features (Attström,
1970; Schroeder et al., 1973; Attström et al., 1975;
Lindhe and Rylander, 1975; Schroeder et al., 1975);

● vascular changes (Egelberg, 1967; Meyer, 1969;
Ranney and Montgomery, 1973; Söderholm and Egelberg,
1973; Kaplan et al., 1975, 1978a,b,c; Söderholm and
Attstrom, 1977);

● inflammatory response (Egelberg, 1964);

● fine structural changes (Garant and Mulvihill,
1972);

● enzyme histochemistry (Hamp et al., 1972);

● effect of decomplementation (Attström and Larsson,
1974; Attström et al., 1975; Kahnberg et al., 1977);

● conversion of stable gingivitis into destructive
periodontitis (Schroeder and Lindhe, 1975);

● fate of collagen fibrils (Soames and Davies, 1977);

● effects of chlorhexidine (Briner and Wunder, 1977);

- prevention of bone loss by indomethacin (Nyman, et al., 1979);
- neutrophil destruction of collagen (Attström and Schroeder, 1979);
- serum antibodies in plaque (Ahlstedt and Rylander, 1975);
- sensitivity of plaque microoganisms to chlorhexidine (Hamp and Emilson, 1974; Briner and Wunder, 1977);
- relationship of plaque formation to the development of gingivitis (Egelberg, 1965a,b);
- identification of cultivable bacteria in plaque (Wunder et al., 1976);
- attraction of crevicular leukocytes by human dental plaque factors (Helldén and Lindhe, 1973);
- clinical radiography and scintigraphy (Saxe et al., 1967; Lindhe et al., 1973; Kaplan et al., 1975, 1978a,b,c);
- bacterial flora (Newman et al., 1977);
- plaque-induced periodontal disease (Lindhe et al., 1975);
- conversion of stable, established gingivitis into destructive periodontitis (Schroeder and Lindhe, 1975, 1980);
- surgical induction of periodontal disease (Lindhe and Svanberg, 1974); and
- alveolar bone resorption secondary to nutritional manipulation (Henrikson, 1968).

Rodents

Although periodontitis in rodents is not analogous to that in humans, these animals can be used successfully as models to study some aspects of the disease, e.g., acute inflammation, the role of neutrophils, and genetic factors.

Rats The rice rat (Oryzomys palustris) is the only rat that spontaneously develops a form of periodontitis in high incidence (Gupta and Shaw, 1956). The disease occurs in varying degrees of severity in all rice rats more than 15 days old. The periodontal lesion is characterized by gingival recession, periodontal pockets filled with hair and food debris, severe alveolar resorption, and mobility of the teeth. The severity of the disease is enhanced by feeding a high carbohydrate, hard consistency diet (Auskaps et al., 1957). The disease

progresses more rapidly in the rice rat than in humans
(Mulvihill et al., 1967).

The gnotobiotic Norway rat (Rattus norvegicus) has
been used as a model for investigation of the microbial
aspects of periodontitis. Gnotobiotic rats innoculated
orally with some kinds of bacteria from periodontal
pockets develop a form of periodontitis (Jordan et al.,
1965). Bone destruction is observed by day 42 and severe
periodontal destruction by day 92 after induction of
periodontal disease with actinomycete strains from human
periodontal pockets (Socransky et al., 1970; Jordan et
al., 1972; Irving et al., 1974). The induced disease
differs from the spontaneous human form in that bone
destruction is inordinately rapid. There is little
inflammation, and plasma cells usually are not present.
Both gram-positive and gram-negative organisms have been
assessed in the rat system (Sharawy and Socransky, 1967;
Irving et al., 1974, 1975). One shortcoming of this technique is that human oral bacterial flora is usually complex, and it is not known to what extent other oral bacteria can modify the periodontal changes observed in
monoinfected animals.

Periodontal disease also has been induced in rats by
manipulation of systemic factors, such as cold stress and
cortisone administration. Changes in the periodontium
due to cortisone administration (Stahl and Gerstner,
1960; Labelle and Schaffer, 1966) are not as typical of
human periodontal disease as are those due to cold stress
(Shklar, 1966).

Mice A number of strains of mice (Mus musculus) spontaneously develop periodontal disease (Baer and Lieberman, 1959, 1960). This indicates that there is a genetic
predisposition to periodontal disease in some mice and
that, in using mice as models, strain and substrain
variations must be taken into account.

Lesions of the periodontium are first manifested in
STR/N mice at 30-50 days of age (Baer and White, 1960).
Both severity and incidence increase with advancing age,
and by the age of 170 days all animals have some degree
of alveolar bone loss. Whether an inflammatory response
is associated with this loss is unclear, as is the relationship of sex to periodontal bone loss (Baer and
Lieberman, 1960; Baer and White, 1960; Glickman and
Quintarelli, 1960).

The physical consistency and fat content of the diet
influence the incidence of periodontal lesions in STR/N

mice. Mice fed Purina Chow in pellet form develop more
severe periodontal disease than if fed the same diet in
powdered form or a synthetic diet with similar composition, but of much finer consistency. This indicates that
the hardness of the diet influences development of the
disease (Baer and White, 1960). In this regard, the
mouse appears to differ from humans and other species
such as the dog and nonhuman primate, where the reverse
is true. Mice maintained on a diet high in fat have less
periodontal disease than mice fed a stock diet (Baer et
al., 1961).

Periodontal disease can be induced in Mus musculus by
repeated administration of cortisone. This treatment enhances destruction of interdental gingiva and causes
osteoporosis of alveolar bone in albino mice of unspecified stock (Glickman et al., 1953), while in phenotypically normal mice with the heterozygous gene mutation,
gray-lethal (gl), it induces apical proliferation of attachment epithelium, periodontal pocket formation, and
alveolar bone loss (Cohen et al., 1969). In both these
stocks, the loss of alveolar bone is associated with a
decrease in osteoblastic activity rather than the increase in osteoclastic activity that is usually characteristic of human periodontitis.

Summary

Currently there is no animal model of gingivitis or periodontitis that precisely duplicates the human disease.
For example, unlike the human disease, the degree of inflammation in rats and mice is relatively minor and poly-
morphonuclear leukocytes (PMN), rather than lymphocytes,
and plasma cells predominate. In dogs, the disease occurs first in the furcations of the premolar region,
whereas in man it occurs first interproximally in the
molar region. Fibrosis is not a dominant feature of periodontitis in dogs. Periodontitis occurs rarely in nonhuman primates, and when present, a diversity of forms is
seen. For example, in marmosets, there is predominance
of mononuclear cells and PMNs, while in chimpanzees and
baboons, plasma cells predominate.

None of the models presently used to study gingivitis
and periodontitis have been sufficiently characterized.
Nonetheless there are good models for various aspects of
these diseases. Rodents are excellent models for survey-
ing potential pathogens and genetic factors. The

potential of the rodent model for the study of human periodontal disease is discussed by Jordan (1971). The dog, especially the Beagle, is useful in the study of etiology and pathogenesis, and some nonhuman primates provide an excellent opportunity for similar investigation as well as research into treatment methodology.

DEGENERATIVE JOINT DISEASE

Definition

Degenerative joint disease (osteoarthritis, osteoarthrosis) is characterized by deterioration of the joint cartilage and sclerosis of the subchondral bone. There is radiologic evidence of degenerative joint disease in 85 percent of people over 70 years of age. Many are asymptomatic; others have stiffness, pain, and decreased motion of the affected joints.

Clinical and Pathological Manifestations

Degenerative joint disease is usually a benign condition with only mild symptoms. Knee, hip, and distal phalangeal joints and the vertebral column are affected most often. Laboratory findings are usually normal, and the radiographic appearance of degenerative joint disease can be indistinguishable from that of the arthritides. Flaking of the cartilage surface is one early sign. Damage then progresses to fissuring, abrasion, thinning, and loss of cartilage. At the edges of the joints, cartilage and bone proliferate to form spurs, and cystic areas appear in the bone adjacent to the joint. Responses to the damage include increased production of chondrocytes and osteophytes and an increase in thickness of the joint capsule. Joint erosion is associated with enzymatic breakdown of proteoglycans and collagen. In some patients, this joint degeneration leads to severe disability. Treatment is nonspecific; acetylsalicylic acid (aspirin) and local heat are used for pain, and corrective surgery increases mobility of the joints.

Degenerative changes in the spinal column affect two discrete intervertebral articular systems: the posterior diarthroideal (apophyseal) joints and the intervertebral disks. It may be useful to distinguish apophyseal disease from osteophysis of the vertebral bodies, reserving

the term spinal degenerative joint disease for the former
and spondylosis for the latter (Sokoloff, 1969).

Etiology and Pathogenesis

The causes of degenerative joint disease are unknown.
The abnormalities are associated with a combination of
prolonged wear and tear and loss of compressibility of
the joint cartilage. They also may develop secondarily
to such stresses as fractures, infections, or developmental abnormalities.

Animal Models

Several excellent review articles are available on comparative models of joint diseases (Sokoloff, 1959, 1960,
1969; Alspauth and Van Hoosier, 1973; Loewi and Stasny,
1974; Pedersen and Pool, 1978; Young et al., 1979).

Nonhuman Primates

Spontaneous degenerative joint disease has not been reported in nonhuman primates; however, the knee joint of
the nonhuman primate is similar to that of man with respect to both function and anatomy and, thus, can serve
as an experimental model. The disease has been induced
in four nonhuman primates (species not given) by placing
pins transversely through the bones above and below one
knee joint, then immobilizing and compressing the joint
by squeezing the pins together with a clamp (Salter and
Field, 1960). Changes in the joint were compared with
the opposite, untreated joint and with joints immobilized
without compression. Degenerative changes occurred only
in the presence of compression. This is comparable to
the degeneration in human joints associated with immobilization in a "forced" position. It provides indirect
evidence that continuous compression of opposing joint
surfaces causes pressure necrosis of articular cartilage.

Carnivores

Degenerative joint disease is common in the knee (stifle)
of dogs (Zahm, 1965). Twenty percent of randomly selected

dogs in one study have been shown to have degenerative
stifle joint disease at autopsy with no recognizable cause
in 61 percent of the cases (Tirgari and Vaughan, 1975).
In the Beagle colony at the University of Utah, a 35
percent incidence is observed at autopsy in dogs over 12
years of age (W. Jee, Radiobiology Laboratory, University
of Utah, Salt Lake City, Unpublished).

Dogs with primary degenerative joint disease usually
do not manifest signs until late in life. The earliest
clinical sign is a reluctance to perform certain maneu-
vers; late in the course of the disease, stiffness and
lameness are consistent features. The synovial fluid is
usually normal, but in severe cases, the total cell count
is slightly elevated due to an increase of mononuclear
cells. Characteristic radiographic changes are present
(Pedersen and Pool, 1978).

The earliest lesion observed in an affected joint is
an area of dullness in the articular cartilage accompanied by a color change or a velvety disruption. As the
cartilage deteriorates, the underlying subchondral bone
reacts by becoming thicker and and denser (sclerosis).
The resulting osteochondral defect heals with granulation
tissue, fibrocartilage, and loss of normal contour of the
articular surfaces. This leads to bone proliferation
(osteophytes) on the periarticular bone surface adjacent
to or within the joint capsule. Changes in the joint
capsule are unremarkable; villous hypertrophy and inflammation in the synovium are uncommon (Pedersen and Pool,
1978).

Spinal osteophytosis first appears in dogs when they
are 3 years old, and almost all are affected by the age
of 10 (Morgan, 1967; Knecht, 1970; Gage, 1975; Brown et
al., 1977). Eighty percent of the Beagles at the University of Utah colony have been observed at autopsy to
have osteophytes in the thoracolumbar region by 12 years
of age (W. Jee, Radiobiology Laboratory, University of
Utah, Salt Lake City, Unpublished). Males are more often
affected than females (Hansen, 1952; Hoerlein, 1956;
Knecht, 1970). Similarly, the majority of old cats have
osteophytes in the thoracic region (Beadman et al., 1964).
Spinal lesions can be induced experimentally; making a
small surgical incision into the annulus results in marginal osteophyte formation of the vertebral body (Morgan,
1967). Structurally, this experimental lesion resembles
degenerative changes in the human vertebral column; however, more thorough studies are required to determine

whether it is analogous to the human condition biochemically.

Rodents

Rats A detailed histological study of knee and ankle
joints of eight inbred strains and one outbred stock of
rats has shown lesions in only 3 out of 157 knees (Sokoloff, 1956). These findings suggest, and it is now generally accepted, that rats are resistant to development of
degenerative joint disease. However, this disease can be
induced in a number of ways. One procedure is to immobi-
lize the knee joint in an extended position for a long
period of time. Histological examination of the knee
after 23 and 116 days reveals death of cartilage cells
followed by loss of staining characteristics, distortion
of cartilage matrix, fissure formation, and thickening of
the subchrondral plate in the pressure-bearing zone. In
the peripheral, non-weight-bearing areas, there is an increase in the size and number of cells and an overgrowth
of the synovium. While effective in producing degenerative joint disease, this technique probably does not produce a suitable model for the human disease because the
changes in the knee joints are preceded by cell death,
in contrast to the human disease where the initial changes
appear to occur in the matrix (Hall, 1964).
     The relationship of weight-bearing, non-weight-bearing,
and rigidity of fixation to degeneration of immobilized
joints has also been studied in rats (Thaxter et al.,
1965). One knee was immobilized by denervation or by
pin fixation, in a manner such that the knee was either
weight-bearing or non-weight-bearing. Histological and
autoradiographic examination of animals after 15, 45, or
90 days showed no significant change in cartilage attributable to denervation alone. In contrast, in immobilized, weight-bearing knees, there was flattening of
the tibiofemoral surfaces, an increase in the synovial
and connective tissues, progressive chondrocyte death,
and decreased chonodrocyte activity with persistent intact matrix devoid of fibrillation. Similar changes were
seen in immobilized, non-weight-bearing knees and in immobilized, denervated, non-weight-bearing knees, although
the degenerative changes in the latter group were less
extensive. The degenerative joint disease seen in these
animals also differed from those seen in humans. The
findings indicate that the rat is probably not a suitable

animal model for human degenerative joint disease; indeed, there are few studies in this area that use rats.

Mice Certain strains of mice have been shown to have a genetic predisposition to spontaneous degenerative joint disease. A study of 18 strains of 12- to 22-month-old mice has shown the incidence of this disease to range from as high as 93 percent in STR/1N mice to as low as 2 percent in AL/N mice (Sokoloff and Jay, 1956). More recently, a high incidence of this lesion has been found in the STR/Ort substrain, derived from the STR/N substrain (Figure 25) (Walton, 1977 a,b,c). The incidence of degenerative joint disease in male C57BL mice increases with advancing age; 39 to 61 percent of the males are affected after 17 months of age, compared to only 19 percent at 15.5 months of age (Wilhelmi and Faust, 1976). The mutant designated "blotchy" (bl) carries a gene causing inadequate cross-linking of collagen and develops degenerative joint disease at a much earlier age than do other mice. Significant degeneration of the knee has been observed at 3.5 months of age, and at the time of death at 5-6.5 months of age, 88 percent of the animals are reported to have degenerative joint disease (Silberberg, 1977).

Male mice appear to be more susceptible to spontaneous degenerative joint disease than female mice (Silberberg and Silberberg, 1945; Sokoloff and Jay, 1956). The incidence of histologically identifiable degenerative changes of the knee is 14 percent in 16-month-old female mice compared to 56 percent in 17-month-old males (Wilhelmi and Faust, 1976). This difference in susceptibility is apparently related to the action of the sex hormones, because the incidence of the disease is greatly increased in female mice when they are treated with the male hormone testosterone propionate (Silberberg and Silberberg, 1963b) and is significantly inhibited in males if they are treated during early adulthood with the female hormone estradiol benzoate (Silberberg and Silberberg, 1963a). Breeding accelerates the development of degenerative joint disease (Silberberg and Silberberg, 1945). A single pregnancy, occurring in early life appears to have more adverse effect than several pregnancies occurring later in life.

Increasing the fat content of the diet increases the incidence of degenerative joint disease in mice. An increase of fat from 5 to 29 percent causes a twofold increase in incidence and significantly accelerates onset

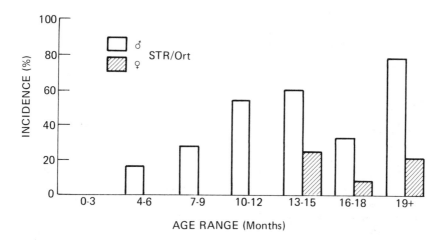

FIGURE 25 Incidence of degenerative joint disease in different age groups of STR/Ort mice. The presence of the disease was assessed radiologically. A positive diagnosis was made when there was a full depth sclerosis of the medial tibial epiphysis. From Walton, 1977a.

of the disease in C57BL mice (M. Silberberg and R. Silberberg, 1950). The exacerbating effect of fatty diet appears to be dependent on the type of fat and the strain of mouse. A diet containing 25 percent cotton seed oil fed to C57BL mice causes a 47 percent incidence of degenerative joint disease, while if 25 percent lard is used, there is an incidence of 73 percent (Silberberg and Silberberg, 1960). In DBA mice, a high-fat diet does not change the incidence of the disease (R. Silberberg and M. Silberberg, 1950).

Mastomys Degenerative joint disease has been described in a number of different joints in mastomys (Sokoloff et al., 1967). The incidence observed in the colony of aging mastomys at the Institute for Experimental Gerontology TNO, Rijswijk, The Netherlands, is given in Table 26. Degenerative joint disease has been observed in the vertebral column, knee, and sternum, and herniation of the nucleus pulposus has been seen relatively frequently.

TABLE 26   Incidence and Mean Age of Occurrence of Degenerative Joint Disease and Herniation of the Nucleus
Pulposus in Mastomys[a]

Disease	Number Affected	Percent Affected	Mean Age (Range) in Months
Degenerative Joint Disease			
Males (n = 91)	28	31	23 (6-31)
Females (n = 108)	27	25	27 (19-34)
Herniation of nucleus pulposus			
Males (n = 91)	32	39	24 (5-33)
Females (n = 108)	4	4	31 (30-31)

[a]C. F. Hollander, Institute for Experimental Gerontology
TNO, Rijswijk, The Netherlands, Unpublished.

Summary

Degenerative joint disease appears to be a common finding
in mice, mastomys, dogs, and cats. In mice the incidence
depends upon the strain, degree of inbreeding, sex, and
genetic factors. Although these lesions are morphologically similar to those in man, more research is required
to determine additional similarities and dissimilarities
between degenerative joint disease in these animals and
that in man.

OSTEOPOROSIS

Definition

Osteoporosis is most commonly a disease of the elderly,
characterized by an abnormal loss of bone mass (osteopenia) accompanied by pain, spinal deformity, loss of
height, and fracture. Its onset is earlier, and it progresses faster in women than in men and in Caucasians
than in Negroes. About 25 percent of all white women
over the age of 60 suffer spinal fractures, and the risk
of hip fracture in both sexes is 20 percent at age 90

(Urist, 1960; Alffram, 1964). Approximately one-sixth of all patients with hip fracture die within 3 months of injury (Alffram, 1964).

Clinical and Pathological Manifestations

Bone is lost progressively with increasing age beyond 45 years. Whether this loss results in osteoporosis is dependent on the amount of bone reduction and on the quality of the bone remaining. Most osteoporotic patients are asymptomatic, even in the presence of vertebral fractures. When back pain is present, it is usually localized. The patient may lose height over a period of months or years due to lumbar and thoracic vertebral compression. Radiographic changes include cortical thinning and a decrease in cancellous bone. The pattern of trabecular bone loss in lumbar vertebrae, pelvis, and femoral necks is according to the structural line of stress. There is an extensive body of literature on this disease (Rowland et al., 1959; Jowsey, 1960; Merz and Schenk, 1970; Urist et al., 1970; Eddy, 1972; Morgan, 1973a,b; Nordin, 1973; Aaron et al., 1974; Dequeker, 1975; Parfitt and Duncan, 1975; Smith et al., 1975; Heaney, 1976; Lips et al., 1978; Melsen and Mosekilde, 1978), from which the following characteristics can be summarized:

● Bone is lost from all parts of the skeleton with increasing age.
● The rate of loss does not increase with age, except in the case of postmenopausal women.
● The amount of bone remaining in an elderly individual appears to depend on the amount of bone present at maturity.
● After about 45 years of age, there is an imbalance in bone remodeling; the rate of bone loss remains constant, but less bone is formed. This imbalance occurs mainly at the endosteal surface of the bone.
● The endosteal loss in cortical bone is offset by a net periosteal gain. No such compensating event occurs in trabecular bone.
● The reduction in the amount of bone is the main contributory cause of fractures.
● The frequency of fracture of the vertebra is much greater than the frequency of fracture of the femur.

Etiology and Pathogenesis

The etiology of osteoporosis is unknown, although certain
contributing factors have been identified. One major
factor is the deficiency of estrogen that accompanies
menopause. During the first 10 years after menopause,
the rate of bone loss in women is accelerated to about
twice that of men. There is an increase in urinary calcium and hydroxyproline excretion (Heaney, 1976), a
slight rise in plasma calcium and inorganic phosphate
(Heaney, 1976), a modest drop in N-terminal immunoreactive parathyroid hormone (Riggs et al., 1973) and in
plasma 1,25 dihydroxy-vitamin D (Riggs and Gallagher,
1977), and an increase in bone turnover (Heaney and
Recker, 1975). The slight rise in plasma calcium and
phosphate has been interpreted to mean that the calcium
homeostatic system in bone is more sensitive than normal
to parathyroid hormone (PTH) or needs less PTH to maintain normocalcemia (Heaney, 1974). The sensitization of
the bone-remodeling system to PTH by estrogen deficiency,
coupled with the age-related decrease in bone formation,
may account for the accelerated bone loss seen in women
(Melsen and Mosekilde, 1978). The reduction of PTH may
also have an adverse effect on bone formation (Heaney,
1974).

Animal Models

Nonhuman Primates

Age-related osteopenia has been demonstrated in at least
one species of nonhuman primate. A cross-sectional study
(Bowden et al., 1979b) of 20 pig-tailed macaques (Macaca
nemestrina), ranging in age from 4 to more than 20 years,
showed a decline in thickness of cortical bone of the
second metacarpal, similar to that seen in the human
aged. The rate of thinning was about 1 percent per year
between the ages of 10 and 20 years, corresponding to an
approximate 30-year age span in man. Bone thinning occurred in both males and females. Mineralization indices
measured from tibial samples showed age-related differences similar to those seen in man. Within a given age
group, cortical bone thickness was greater in females of
high parity than of low parity. Despite the fact that
most of the females were premenopausal, the rate of thinning was comparable to that seen postmenopausally in the

human female. Current information on maximal life span
in macaques suggests that menopause may occur later in
the life span than it does in the human. If so, this
macaque model may provide an opportunity to study the
mechanism of age-related osteoporosis dissociated from
menopause.

Carnivores

The comparative aspects of skeletal aging in man and dog
are discussed on pages 190-197. Fractures have not been
observed in dogs, even though the dog loses bone mass
faster than does man. This may be because the dog has a
greater bone mass at maturity than does man (roughly 30
percent versus 20 percent vertebral trabecular bone mass).
A dog losing bone at a rate of 2 percent per year (Jee
et al., 1976) has a trabecular bone mass of 20 percent at
the end of 15 years. A man losing bone at a rate of 0.5
percent per year (Bromley et al., 1966; Merz and Schenk,
1970; Meunier et al., 1973) has a trabecular bone mass of
only 16 percent at the end of 40 years, an equivalent
period with regard to life span, and is approaching the
fracture threshold bone mass level of 12 percent.
    There are three methods for experimentally inducing
adult bone-loss models in dogs: feeding a calcium-
deficient diet, administering corticosteroids, and
immobilizing limbs. All of these factors may contribute
to osteoporosis in man. Feeding a diet that is low in
calcium, has a low calcium-to-phosphate ratio, or is high
in phosphate induces a reversible bone loss by causing
secondary hyperparathyroidism (Jowsey and Gershon-Cohen,
1964; Jowsey and Raisz, 1968; Krook et al., 1971; Laflamme
and Jowsey, 1972; Jowsey et al., 1974). This method has
been used to study the influence of estrogen (Ferguson
and Hartles, 1970) and the administration of calcium
(Jowsey and Gershon-Cohen, 1964; Krook et al., 1971),
fluoride (Adams and Jowsey, 1965), or calcitonin
(Jowsey, 1969) in preventing, arresting, or restoring bone
loss. It has potential as a model for studying the efficiency with which the aged skeleton can reverse this type
of osteopenia.
    Corticosteroid-induced osteopenia in dogs has been
shown to be similar to osteopenia in man arising from
Cushingoid states or from treatment with corticosteroids
for more than 6 months (Collins et al., 1962; Jett et

al., 1970; Bressot et al., 1976). There is a marked reduction in bone formation, resulting in a bone-remodeling
imbalance. It is not clear whether bone resorption is
also altered.

Experimentally induced immobilization osteopenia using
a variety of methods has been studied in cats as well as
in dogs (Burdeaux and Hutchinson, 1953; DeNayer 1969;
Burkhart and Jowsey, 1967; Uhthoff and Jaworski, 1978).
This is a very effective bone-loss model; however, more
detailed work is needed in both man and animal to determine the course and site of bone loss in trabecular and
cortical bone (Minaire et al., 1974; Uhthoff and Jaworski,
1978). The influences of parathroidectomy, thyroidectomy,
and thyroparathyroidectomy (Burkhart and Jowsey, 1967);
fluorides (Milicic and Jowsey, 1968); and diphosphonate
(Ellsasser et al., 1973) on immobilization osteopenia
also have been studied.

Rodents

The occurrence of osteopenia in aging rodents has only
recently been documented, and the histology of the associated changes remains largely unknown. In particular,
there is no information regarding the incidence of fractures, if any, that may ensue, and there is no documentation of adult bone remodeling. Nevertheless, it is
apparent that cortical thinning and bone fragility are
characteristic of both aged mice and rats.

Interest in the occurrence of age-related bone loss
has been stimulated by the need for suitable animal models
to test the hypothesis that nutrition is a factor in the
etiology of human osteoporosis. This hypothesis has been
put forward to explain the reduced skeletal mass recorded
in some populations of elderly people who habitually
consume a diet low in calcium (Matkovic et al., 1979) or
high in phosphorus (Mazess and Mather, 1974). A possible
relationship between the use of phosphate food additives
and bone loss in humans consuming a mixed "western diet"
is a subject of current interest in clinical nutrition.
Rodents appear to be useful models for testing these
hypotheses.

Rats Age-associated changes in rat bone have been
poorly characterized. The available evidence indicates
that although rat bones are subject to cortical thinning,
they do not undergo a significant decrease in bone mass.

Calcified bone appears to accumulate in the epiphysis of
the rat tibia until about 1 year of age and to be undi-
minished until at least 2 years of age (Hansard and
Crowder, 1957). Nevertheless, the rat has been useful in
evaluating the influence of various nutritional factors
(e.g., calcium, phosphorus, excess protein, dietary acidity, fluoride) on bone mass at senescence. In general,
the long-term effects of these factors observed in rats
have been compatible with the short-term effects seen in
humans.

Ovariectomy of young, adult female rats leads to increased bone resorption and a net reduction in bone mass
of aged animals that can be suppressed by estrogen administration (Shin et al., 1976). Ovariectomy also increases
the influence of dietary calcium and phosphorus on bone
resorption. In female rats over 16 months of age,
neither ovariectomy nor estrogen administration has a
significant effect on bone resorption and the influence
of dietary calcium and phosphorus is greatly diminished.
These observations are in general agreement with the results of calcium and estrogen administration to oophorec-
tomized and postmenopausal women.

The theory that the "titratable acidity" of human
diets is a factor in osteoporosis has been a subject of
controversy for a number of years. Administration of a
1.5 percent solution of ammonium chloride (NH_4Cl) to
adult rats in place of drinking water causes calciuria
and a reduction in bone mass that has been attributed to
the utilization of the alkaline salts of bone as buffers
(Barzel and Jowsey, 1969). However, this effect may be
due to the concomitant decrease in food consumption and
body weight caused by acid loading. In subsequent studies, neither feeding 2 percent NH_4Cl in the diet for 9
months nor hydrochloric or lactic acid loading for 1 year
has been found to have any effect on bone mass (Ellis
et al., 1974; Newell and Beauchene, 1975), raising doubt
about the relationship between dietary acidity and bone
loss. Further, osteoporosis among vegetarians, whose diet
is neutral or alkaline, is as frequent as among omnivores,
whose diet is typically acid (Ellis et al., 1974).

The calciuric effect of high-protein diets is apparently due to endogenous sulfate production arising from
the catabolism of excess sulfur-containing amino acids
(Whiting and Draper, 1980). In the rat, this calciuria
is offset by a decrease in endogenous fecal calcium and
is not accompanied by increased bone resorption (Bell et

al., 1975). In adult human subjects fed a high-protein
diet, however, a negative calcium balance may ensue and
persist for several weeks (Hegsted and Linkswiler, 1980).

Mice Thinning of the vertebral and femoral cortices
in B6D2F1 female mice fed an apparently adequate stock
diet is extensive between 6 and 18 months of age (Krishnarao and Draper, 1969). Decreases of 59 percent and 48
percent are observed in the cortical thickness of the
lumbar vertebrae and femoral midshaft, respectively.
The tibias are less affected. Further thinning is seen
at 30 months of age; no additional change occurs in mice
surviving to 40 months.

Despite the decrease in the cortical thickness of the
femoral midshaft, there is a progressive increase in
width (Krishnarao and Draper, 1969) and a net increase in
total mineral content (Shah et al., 1967). These observations indicate that, during aging, the mouse femoral
shaft undergoes active endosteal bone resorption accompanied by a moderate incidence of intracortical porosity.
These changes in cortical bone are generally similar to
those seen in man. Like the human, the female mouse is
subject to greater cortical bone loss than the male
(Silberberg and Silberberg, 1962).

Cortical porosity does not seem to be related to diet
(Shah et al., 1967), and cortical thinning is not significantly affected by calcium intake unless the diet is
grossly deficient in this element (0.1 percent of the
diet). Excess dietary phosphorus or an adverse calcium:
phosphorus ratio (i.e., 1:2 as opposed to 2:1) accelerates
cortical bone loss. The effect of excess phosphorus has
been shown to be due to parathyroid stimulation (secondary
hyperparathyroidism), and similar parathyroid responses to
dietary phosphate have been observed in the rat (Sie et
al., 1974), dog (Laflamme and Jowsey, 1972), and human
(Bell et al., 1977).

Hamsters Syrian hamsters have been found to have a
greater bone loss and negative calcium balance in old age
than do rats (Lovelace et al., 1958). Various diets modify, but do not prevent, this loss. This model may be
useful in determining the dietary, hormonal, and other
effects on age-related osteopenia.

Summary

There is no animal other than man that develops osteoporosis, although the skeletons of all species appear to lose bone with age. For example, rodents lack lamellar bone and the capacity to remodel bone. The dog and cat have a skeleton similar to that of man, but do not lose sufficient bone mass during their life spans to develop fractures. There is insufficient information about the skeletons of nonhuman primates to evaluate the relevance and appropriateness of these animals as models of osteoporosis. Nonetheless, there are good experimental models for studying various aspects of this disease. The roles of various factors in arresting and preventing bone loss can be studied in rats and mice. The dog and cat are useful in studying the mechanisms of age-related bone loss and bone remodeling, and the efficacy of drugs and other factors in the prevention of age-related bone loss and restoration of previously lost bone.

CHRONIC BRONCHITIS

Definition

Chronic bronchitis is a condition associated with prolonged exposure to nonspecific bronchial irritants, accompanied by mucous hypersecretion and structural changes in the bronchi (American College of Chest Physicians-- American Thoracic Society, Joint Committee on Pulmonary Nomenclature, 1975). Sputum production and a cough persisting for at least 3 months of the year are often accepted as critera for diagnosis (American Thoracic Society, 1962; Medical Research Council, 1965). Chronic bronchitis affects 10-25 percent of the adult population, primarily middle-aged and elderly individuals, significantly limiting activity in 5 percent of affected individuals (Wilson, 1973). When the disease is accompanied by a reduction in air flow rate during forced expiration, it is called chronic obstructive bronchitis.

Clinical and Pathological Manifestations

The predominant symptom of chronic bronchitis is a cough of long standing that produces sputum; wheezing, shortness of breath, and cyanosis appear as the condition worsens.

Pulmonary function studies may demonstrate a reduction of
vital capacity and forced expiratory flow rates that may
be moderately improved by bronchodilators. The residual
volume may be increased in the presence of a normal total
lung capacity. As the disease progresses, hypoxemia may
occur, followed by carbon dioxide retention and acidosis.
Chest roentgenograms are of little use in identifying
chronic bronchitis, but help in ruling out other disorders. Congestive right heart failure, abnormal electrocardiograms, and secondary polycythemia may be found in
advanced cases.

Enlargement of the tracheobronchial mucous glands
(Reid, 1978), and increased numbers of goblet cells in
peripheral airways (Thurlbeck et al., 1975) are characteristic findings. The ratio of bronchial gland thickness
to total thickness of the main and lobar bronchial wall
(Reid index) increases, and small airways become narrowed
and plugged with mucus. Other morphological changes include fragmentation and destruction of cilia, inflammatory
cell infiltration of epithelial layers, basal cell hyperplasia, and squamous metaplasia of columnar epithelium.
The structural changes are poorly correlated with symptoms (Thurlbeck, 1976).

Etiology and Pathogenesis

Chronic bronchitis is related to several intrinsic and ex-
trinsic factors (Bates et al., 1971a; Barnett, 1972;
Mitchell, 1974; and Welch, 1977). It is more common among
males than females, among urban populations than rural,
among smokers than nonsmokers, and among the socioeconom-
ically disadvantaged than the more affluent. There is a
strong epidemiological relationship between bronchitis and
cigarette smoking and similar, but less definitive, relationships to urban air pollution and occupational exposure
to inhaled toxic particles and gases. Bacterial or viral
lung infections, allergies, and natural or induced ineffi-
ciencies in mucociliary clearance are thought to be associated with its development. Certain individuals are
thought to be predisposed to the condition because of acquired or genetically determined biochemical defects.
Although the disease appears primarily in middle-aged and
older subjects, it is uncertain whether aging itself predisposes the lung to the disease or whether the increased
incidence with age results simply from the cumulative effects of other causative factors.

Animal Models

There is little clinical evidence of spontaneous chronic bronchitis in nonhuman primates, rodents, or lagomorphs. Rats and mice are frequently afflicted with chronic respiratory diseases of infectious origin that affect the airways and cause morphological alterations of secretory elements (Elmes and Bell, 1963; Richter, 1970; Iravani and van As, 1972); however, they feature too much inflammation and involvement of the parenchyma to qualify as models for chronic bronchitis.

The term "chronic bronchitis" defined as a chronic, productive cough, has been applied to the dog and cat (Suter and Ettinger, 1975; Wheeldon and Breeze, 1979). The term, chronic obstructive bronchitis, has not been applied to animals because appropriate techniques for assessing airflow obstruction during forced expiration have only recently been developed. Therefore, information on animal models for chronic bronchitis is limited primarily to conditions involving morphological alterations of airway epithelium, such as enlargement or proliferation of mucus-secreting elements. The definition is further complicated by species differences in secretory elements of the airway epithelium. There is some quantitative information, for instance, regarding species differences in the occurrence, size, and location of mucous glands, goblets cells, and Clara cells (Breeze and Wheeldon, 1977; Goco et al., 1963). Available data suggest that man has the greatest number of tracheobronchial mucous glands; pigs slightly fewer; sheep, monkeys, dogs, and guinea pigs significantly fewer; and horses and rats none. The portion of the bronchial walls occupied by mucous glands in the dog appears to be less than in man, although the distribution of glands is similar (Wheeldon and Pirie, 1974). In general, dogs and cats have airway secretory elements similar to those of man, although the mucous glands are fewer and smaller than in man. Rodents and lagomorphs have mucous glands in the trachea, but few if any in intrapulmonary airways. The type, size, and distribution of mucus-secreting elements of nonhuman primates have not been documented. Clara cells have been observed in the airways of the stump-tailed (Macaca arctoides) and bonnet macaques (Macaca radiata), but not in the rhesus macaque (Macaca mulatta) (Castleman et al., 1975). There are no reports of noninfectious conditions resembling chronic bronchitis of man that have been experimentally induced in nonhuman primates, rabbits, or mice.

Carnivores

Spontaneous, chronic, obstructive lung diseases that are
similar in some respects to chronic bronchitis in man
have been reported in a few dogs and cats. As in man,
the etiologies are uncertain, but are thought to include
viral and bacterial infections, parasitic infestations,
allergies, foreign body aspiration, and air pollutants
(Suter and Ettinger, 1975). In dogs, such cases have been
observed most frequently in middle-aged and older animals
of the smaller breeds, with no difference in incidence
between urban and rural settings (Wheeldon et al., 1974).
The major sign of chronic bronchitis in dogs and cats is
a continuing or recurrent intractable moist cough, often
followed by retching and swallowing. The cough may produce expectoration of greenish or blood-tinged mucus, and
nasal or ocular discharge may be present. A variety of
bacteria have been isolated from bronchial washings. Radiographs often reveal a thickening of bronchial walls
and a flattening of the diaphragm. A thickening of bronchial mucosa with excess mucus in the lumen and chronic
inflammation of bronchi and bronchioles are observed histologically. Bronchial mucous glands are increased in
size and number, and there is a proliferation of goblet
cells in the bronchial epithelium (Wheeldon and Pirie,
1974; Wheeldon et al., 1974). Histochemical studies have
demonstrated that shifts in the composition of mucosubstances in lungs of dogs with naturally occurring chronic
bronchitis are similar to changes in mucus composition
observed in the human disease (Wheeldon et al., 1976).
A form of chronic bronchitis resembling mucoid bronchial
impaction in man also has been observed in the dog (Castleberry et al., 1965). In this condition, impaction of
bronchi and bronchioles with mucus and debris is accompanied by mucosal inflammation, hyperplasia and metaplasia
of bronchial glands, and proliferation of goblet cells in
bronchioles.

A disease having characteristics very similar to those
of human chronic bronchitis can be induced in the dog by
inhalation of sulfur dioxide (Chakrin and Saunders, 1974).
Beagles exposed to 500-600 ppm of sulfur dioxide for 2
hours, twice weekly, for 4-5 months develop abnormal lung
sounds on ausculation and periodic episodes of productive
coughing that last for several weeks after exposure. Histological changes include an increased number of goblet
cells in the bronchioles and considerable hyperplasia of
the bronchial glands. Metaplastic changes are found in

the mucosa of larger bronchi and inflammatory changes in the bronchioles. Inflammatory lesions also have been found in bronchioles of dogs after chronic inhalation of cigarette smoke, but no changes in bronchial glands or goblet cells have been reported (Hernandez et al., 1966). The inhalation of 11 ppm of nitrogen dioxide for 1 year induces bronchiolar changes in cats, including an increase in number of goblet cells and in amount of intraluminal mucus (Kleinerman et al., 1976). These cats also have an increased bronchial gland mass in the small bronchi.

Rodents

Rats Hypertrophic and hyperplastic changes in secretory elements and mucus hypersecretion have been induced in the rat by using inhaled irritants. Young rats exposed chronically to 300-400 ppm sulfur dioxide develop hypertrophy and hyperplasia of mucus-secreting cells (Reid, 1963; Lamb and Reid, 1968). Rats inhaling cigarette smoke for 6 weeks develop dose-related increases in goblet cell numbers, hypertrophy of tracheal mucous glands, and alterations of goblet cell glycoproteins (Lamb and Reid, 1969; R. Jones et al., 1973). The drugs pilocarpine and isoproterenol cause increases in the number of goblet cells and size of mucous glands in rats, in addition to other systemic effects (Sturges and Reid, 1973).

Hamsters Intratracheal instillation of elastase has been reported to cause an increase in the size and number of goblet cells in airways of Syrian hamsters (Christensen et al., 1977; Hayes et al., 1977; Hayes and Christensen, 1978), presumably accompanied by mucous hypersecretion. Although the model is complicated by emphysematous changes in the parenchyma, it may be a useful model of chronic obstructive lung disease of man because the goblet cell alterations persist for up to a year after instillation (Christensen et al., 1977).

PULMONARY EMPHYSEMA

Definition

Pulmonary emphysema is an anatomic alteration of the lung, characterized by abnormal enlargement of air spaces distal to terminal, nonrespiratory bronchioles, accompanied by destructive changes of alveolar walls (American Thoracic Society, 1962). The term "emphysema" is often used to describe the clinical syndrome that may accompany the disease, including breathlessness, coughing, and sputum production. However, because many people with appreciable emphysema are asymptomatic, and because this syndrome may occur in the absence of emphysema, it now generally is agreed that use of the word be limited to the pathological definition.

Clinical and Pathological Manifestations

The anatomical diagnosis of human emphysema is usually made from whole-lung slices or "Gough sections" (Gough, 1952) of lungs fixed while inflated. There are four major types of emphysema, named for the primary anatomic location of lesions (Thurlbeck, 1976): centrilobular, panlobular, paraseptal, and paracicatrical. Emphysematous lungs frequently display a mixture of types and are classified by the type that predominates.

In centrilobular (centriacinar) emphysema, respiratory bronchioles become dilated and confluent, forming enlarged airspaces at the center of lobules. Classically, the alveolar ducts, alveolar sacs, and alveoli at the periphery of the lobule are unchanged, giving the appearance of punched-out holes surrounded by normal tissue. Frequently, however, the peripheral structures are also somewhat abnormal. The upper zones of the lung are usually more severely affected than the lower zones, there is often evidence of chronic inflammation, and the lumina of bronchioles subtending the emphysematous lobules often are narrow.

In panlobular (panacinar, diffuse, or diffuse-generalized) emphysema, the entire acinus distal to the terminal bronchiole (i.e., the alveolar ducts and alveoli) is involved. In the early stages there is a coarsening of the normal honeycomb structure of the cut lung surface. As the disease progresses, the parenchyma may assume a "cotton candy" appearance due to the loss of tissue around remaining bronchioles and blood vessels. The lesions are usually randomly distributed, but there is a tendency toward greater involvement of the lower zones of the lung. The incidence of both centrilobular and panlobular emphysema is higher in men than in women. Individuals with alpha$_1$ antitrypsin deficiencies who develop the disease all have panlobular emphysema. In paraseptal emphysema

there is destruction of respiratory epithelium along lobular septae, and in paracicatrical emphysema the lobule
is irregularly involved, and destruction is found adjacent
to scars in the lung.

The diagnosis of emphysema is based on anatomic alterations rather than symptoms, clinical signs, or functional
abnormalities. Many older people with appreciable amounts
of emphysema are asymptomatic. As much as 30 percent of
the lung may be involved without overt symptoms (Pratt
and Klugh, 1967). As the lung is damaged further, or as
complications and other pathological changes appear, a
progressive dyspnea or shortness of breath occurs, sometimes accompanied by coughing. Patients with advanced
emphysema may have breath sounds that are difficult to
hear or absent, an abnormal breathing pattern including
active expiration, and a "barrel-chested" appearance.
Thoracic radiographs may show hyperlucency, attenuation
of vascular markings, and a flattening of the diaphragm.
Pulmonary function measurements are variable, but a rather
typical pattern emerges as emphysema progresses. Total
lung capacity may increase; however, there is also an increase in residual volume resulting in a decreased vital
capacity. Flow rate during forced exhalation is reduced,
and there is little or no improvement after treatment with
bronchodilators. Progressive loss of elastic recoil leads
to an increase in lung compliance, best reflected in static or quasi-static compliance. Local differences in expansion and surface area of the alveolar bed result in
an imbalanced ventilation-perfusion relationship that may
result in hypoxemia, carbon dioxide retention, and respiratory acidosis. Right heart enlargement and congestive
heart failure are observed in some advanced cases.

Etiology and Pathogenesis

The specific cause of pulmonary emphysema in man is unknown. There are several theories concerning factors
influencing the incidence and severity of the disease,
and since there are several forms, it is likely that diverse causative factors are involved (Bates et al., 1971b;
Barnett, 1972; Mitchell, 1974; Welch, 1977). Emphysema
is more common with advancing age, and the panlobular
type is often difficult to distinguish from the ductec-
tasia that normally accompanies aging. At present, there
seems to be little basis for ascribing the disease to a
genetically determined process of structural change with

age. The increased incidence with aging may result from
the cumulative effects of repeated insults to the lung
over a long period of time. Injurious factors may include cigarette smoking, air pollution, occupational exposure to inhaled toxic materials, allergies, and abnormalities of mucociliary clearance. For example, the incidence of emphysema is reported to be as much as 10 times
greater in heavy smokers than in nonsmokers (Thurlbeck,
1976). A contributing factor currently receiving much
attention is an unfavorable balance between naturally occurring proteolytic enzymes and serum antiproteases such
as alpha$_1$ antitrypsin (Laurell and Erickson, 1963). These
antiprotease deficiencies are thought to be, at least in
part, hereditary. It is unclear whether the higher incidence of emphysema in males is due to a difference in
susceptibility or to a greater exposure to exogenous
etiological factors.

Animal Models

The following discussion summarizes the available information on animal models of emphysema, focussing on the relevance of these models in studying the relationship between
emphysema and aging. For recent reviews of spontaneous
and induced emphysema in animals, consult Chrzanowski and
Turino (1977), Karlinsky and Snider (1978), and Breeze and
Wheeldon (1979).

Defining and Characterizing Emphysema in Animals

The characterization of emphysematous changes in lungs of
laboratory animals using terminology applied to human
lungs is complicated by several interspecies differences
in subgross anatomy (McLaughlin et al., 1961). In human
lungs, the gas-exchanging units distal to the terminal
bronchiole comprise a primary lobule. Secondary lobules
are formed by the grouping together of several primary
lobules within connective tissue septae. Rodents, lagomorphs, carnivores, and nonhuman primates have a paucity
of interlobular connective tissue preventing the definition of lobules. In addition, human lungs have several
orders of branching respiratory bronchioles, as do the
lungs of dogs, cats, and nonhuman primates. In contrast,
respiratory bronchioles are rarely found in lungs of rats,
hamsters, and mice where the terminal bronchioles lead

directly into alveolar ducts. Species differences in the terminal bronchioles of nonhuman primates have been reported (Castleman et al., 1975). Bonnet macaques (Macaca radiata) have long terminal bronchioles similar to those of man, while rhesus (Macaca mulatta) and stump-tailed macaques (Macaca arctoides) have shorter terminal bronchioles. The terminal bronchioles of rhesus macaques also have been noted to have "transitional" areas in which there are mixed epithelial cell types characteristic of both terminal and respiratory bronchioles and occasional alveoli.

It is questionable whether the term "centrilobular," as it applies to the enlargement and coalescing of respiratory bronchioles in man, can correctly be applied in species (rodents and lagomorphs) without well-developed respiratory bronchioles. However, these species can develop emphysematous lesions most prominent in the structures immediately distal to the terminal bronchioles with preservation of alveoli at the periphery of the ventilating unit. There is a similar problem with the term "paraseptal"; only those animals with well-defined lobular septae can serve as models. Panlobular and paracicatrical emphysema can be observed in all of the animals mentioned.

It is uncertain whether the pathogenesis of pulmonary emphysema is affected by species-related anatomic differences. Contributing factors, such as local mechanical stresses, may have different effects on lungs with and without extensive connective tissue lobulation. Factors related to blood supply may have diverse effects because of variation in the branching patterns and level of termination of the bronchial arterial system (McLaughlin et al., 1961). On the other hand, these structural differences are likely to be less important in studies of the effects of antiprotease deficiencies or injurious agents on lung tissue.

The methods used to identify emphysema in lungs of animals present another interpretive difficulty. Functional assessments may detect changes that are consistent with the presence of emphysema, but do not provide a diagnosis. Measurements of excised lung volume at standardized inflating pressures, evaluation of terminal airspace size by calculating mean linear intercepts, and estimations of terminal airspace surface area are useful in determining abnormal expansion of airspaces. However, these indices do not directly detect alveolar destruction and, therefore, do not differentiate between emphysema and other causes of hyperinflation or increased lung compliance.

Thus, many reports of spontaneous or experimentally induced emphysema in animals do not demonstrate the anatomic
features of emphysema. Whole lung sections, similar to
those obtained from human lungs, should be made from the
larger experimental animals and evaluated in the same
manner as in man. Sections of inflated lungs from smaller
animals should be observed microscopically for evidence
of alveolar wall disruption. The number and size of interalveolar communications also may be described, although
the extent to which methods of inflation, fixation, and
tissue preparation may influence the appearance of these
channels is largely unknown.

Spontaneous Emphysema

At present, it is not certain whether uncomplicated emphysema exists in animals as a single, age-related disease
entity, although emphysematous changes have been observed
in lungs of most species in association with other disease
processes. Thirty-eight-week-old rats have been reported
to have a larger terminal airspace size than do 10-week-
old rats; however, alveolar wall disruption has not been
documented (Bell et al., 1974). Twelve cases of naturally occurring emphysema among 776 nonhuman primates necropsied have been reported at the Oregon Primate Center
(McNulty, 1973). Similarly, emphysematous changes have
been reported in two of three necropsied female pig-tailed
macaques (Macaca nemestrina) over 18 years of age, but
not in animals under 10 years of age (Boatman et al.,
1979). Both reports show concomitant infestation of the
emphysematous lungs with the lung mite, Pneumonyssus sim-
icola. Ischemia resulting from pulmonary capillary lesions has been suggested as a cause of emphysematous
changes in rabbits (Boatman and Martin, 1965).
    Inflammation is a common cause of emphysematous le-
sions. Destruction of the alveolar walls and large bullae
at the edges of the lobes has been seen in dogs after
inflammation of the bronchioles and alveolar ducts. Emphysema also has been observed in rats in the presence
of inflammation of airways and parenchyma (Casarett, 1953;
Palecek and Holusa, 1971). "Spontaneous" emphysema has
been reported in 52 percent of rabbits over 2.5 years of
age (Strawbridge, 1960), but associated inflammatory
changes and lack of control of the degree of lung expansion throughout the fixation period make the interpretation questionable.

The blotchy mouse (mutant symbol, Mo^{blo}) has a genetically determined defect that prevents the generation of
the lysine-derived aldehyde necessary for cross-linking
of collagen and elastin (Rowe et al., 1974; Hunt, 1974).
This leads to enlarged terminal airspaces, attenuated alveolar walls, and functional characteristics typical of
human emphysema (Fisk and Kuhn, 1976). Although the condition is not age related, this model may be useful for
certain studies of emphysema.

Experimentally Induced Emphysema

Experimental induction of emphysematous lesions in animals
has been accomplished using a variety of agents and approaches (Chrzanowski and Turino, 1977; Karlinsky and
Snider, 1978). However, the term "emphysema" is used
loosely and probably often in error, since many investigators have not adequately demonstrated destruction of alveolar walls. Each study should be examined critically
to determine its relevance to human emphysema.

The most commonly used method to induce emphysematous
changes is intrapulmonary administration of proteolytic
enzymes of plant or animal origin. This is thought to
simulate the antiprotease deficiency pathogenesis of human
emphysema, and widespread lesions can be created with
less bronchitis and bronchiolitis than some other models.
Papain is frequently used, and elastase recently has received considerable attention. These agents have been administered by intratracheal instillation or by inhalation
of aerosol. Papain- or porcine pancreatic elastase-
induced emphysema has been reported in the Syrian hamster
(Niewoehner and Kleinerman, 1973; Martorana et al., 1977;
Ackerman et al., 1978; Hayes and Christensen, 1978; Karlinsky and Snider, 1978), rat (Giles et al., 1973; Johanson
and Pierce, 1973; Johanson et al., 1973; Herget et al.,
1974; Will and Kay, 1974; Gardiner and Schanker, 1975;
Karlinsky and Snider, 1978; Mauderly et al., 1979), and
dog (Takaro and White, 1973; Weinbaum et al., 1974; Karlinsky and Snider, 1978; Haddad et al., 1979). Proteolytic
enzyme-containing homogenates of canine and human polymor-
phonuclear leukocytes have also been given to dogs by instillation and inhalation to produce emphysema (Weinbaum
et al., 1974; Karlinsky and Snider, 1978).

Cadmium chloride-induced emphysema has been reported
in hamsters, rats, guinea pigs, and dogs (Karlinsky and
Snider, 1978). This model was originally developed to

study the evolution of cadmium-induced lung disease in industrial workers. The emphysematous changes that occur in animals using this method are accompanied by inflammation, granulomatous changes, and fibrosis.

Exposure of animals to relatively high concentrations of nitrogen dioxide results in acute edema and inflammation, bronchitis and bronchiolitis, and development of emphysematous lesions. In some studies, the inflammatory alterations resolve with time, leaving a residual emphysema. This method has been used to induce the disease in mice (Blair et al., 1969; Port et al., 1977; Karlinsky and Snider, 1978), hamsters (Kleinerman and Niewoehner, 1973), rats (Haydon et al., 1965; Freeman et al., 1968, 1972; Karlinsky and Snider, 1978), and rabbits (Haydon et al., 1967).

A variety of less commonly used agents will also produce experimental emphysema. Exposure of dogs to phosgene gas produces bronchitis and bronchiolitis, which progress to disrupt the alveolar septae (Karlinsky and Snider, 1978). Long-term exposure to cigarette smoke (Karlinsky and Snider, 1978) and to mixtures of gasoline engine exhaust and other air pollutants (Gillespie et al., 1976; Hyde et al., 1978) also has been used to induce changes in the lungs. Chlorine gas exposure is thought to cause emphysematous lesions in rats (Karlinsky and Snider, 1978).

Mice exposed to 80-100 percent oxygen develop inflammatory, necrotic, and metaplastic lung lesions. If the mice survive the initial stages, emphysema develops (Rosan et al., 1970). Mice also develop edema and epithelial hyperplasia, followed by emphysema, after prolonged exposure to ozone (Werthamer et al., 1970; Penha et al., 1972). Mice exposed by inhalation to fungal mycotoxins develop emphysema, among other pathological changes (Forgacs and Caril, 1966).

A recent report (O'Dell et al., 1978) describes the induction of developmental "emphysema" in rats by feeding a copper-deficient diet to pregnant and nursing females. Weanlings are continued on the diet and show signs of copper deficiency by 6-10 weeks of age. Enlarged distal airspaces, reduced lung elastin content, and altered elastin ultrastructure are observed in these rats. The mechanism is thought to be similar to the connective tissue cross-linking defect of the blotchy mouse (Rowe et al., 1974; Hunt, 1974). However, alveolar wall destruction has not been demonstrated yet in this model.

ATHEROSCLEROSIS

Definition

Atherosclerosis is a variable combination of changes of
the arterial intima, occurring most commonly in the aorta
and the coronary and cerebral arteries. The lesion consists of the focal accumulation of lipids, complex carbohydrates, blood and blood products, fibrous tissue, and
calcium deposits. The incidence and severity correlate
directly with age and are influenced by both genetic and
environmental factors. Medical complications include
heart disease and cerebrovascular accidents. Atherosclerosis is the greatest cause of morbidity and death in
the United States.

Clinical and Pathological Manifestations

The clinical manifestations of atherosclerosis depend
upon the arteries that are affected. The clinical ex-
pressions of coronary atherosclerosis are ischemic heart
disease, angina pectoris, and myocardial infarction.
Cerebrovascular atherosclerosis may result in cerebral
infarction with associated sensory, motor, cognitive, and
emotional changes. Atherosclerosis in the arteries of
the legs produces ischemic leg disease, with associated
intermittent claudication and, eventually, gangrene.
   The earliest lesion, appearing in childhood, is the
fatty streak, an accumulation of lipid in intimal smooth
muscle cells. Among people in the United States and certain other industrialized countries, the fatty streaks
progress to fibromuscular atherosclerotic plaques that
constitute the basic lesion of atherosclerosis. The
plaque consists of a core of intra- and extracellular
lipid, necrotic debris and usually contains crystals of
cholesterol, areas of mineralization, and increased collagen accumulation. The core is separated from the lumen
of the artery by a fibromuscular cap. It is the exten-
siveness of fibromuscular atherosclerotic plaques that
determines the severity of the clinical disease.

Etiology and Pathogenesis

The etiology of atherosclerosis is unknown, but is currently considered to be multifactorial. Although genetic

factors are involved, the mode of inheritance and the
extent to which genetic factors play a part in the development of the disease have not been determined. Certain
factors that increase the risk of developing atherosclerosis have been identified. These risk factors include a
high concentration of serum cholesterol, a reduced concentration of serum high-density lipoproteins (HDL),
arterial hypertension, cigarette smoking, diabetes mellitus, and male gender. Much of the variability in incidence cannot be accounted for by these factors however,
and it is thought that reactivity of the arterial wall
may play a role as well.

Animal Models

Nonhuman Primates

The nonhuman primates have been the most widely used and
accepted models for research on atherosclerosis. The
rationale for use of these animals is their phylogenetic
closeness to humans and the remarkable similarities in
lipoprotein metabolism and atherogenesis between the nonhuman and human primates. Characteristics of the various
nonhuman primate models of atherosclerosis have been described in detail in a recent monograph (Strong, 1976)
and will be reviewed only briefly here. Further, this
summary includes only species commonly used in research
on atherosclerosis.

Squirrel Monkeys Two different phenotypes of squirrel
monkey (Saimiri sciureus) have been used for research
on atherosclerosis: one originating from the Colombian-
Brazilian border along the Amazon River and the other
from the vicinity of Iquitos, Peru (Cooper, 1968). Peruvian and Brazilian squirrel monkeys have the same diploid
chromosome number (Clarkson et al., 1971; T. B. Jones
et al., 1973), but the numbers of achrocentric and submetacentric chromosomes are different (T. B. Jones et
al., 1973). Squirrel monkeys have been studied in more
detail as models for atherosclerosis than any other New
World species, with regard to both naturally occurring
and experimental forms of the disease (Clarkson et al.,
1976b).
     Field studies have established the prevalence and ex-
tent of atherosclerosis among free-ranging squirrel monkeys in the vicinity of Leticia, Colombia (Middleton et

al., 1967b). The mean total serum cholesterol concentration in these animals is about 100 mg/dl, and there is a significant correlation of plasma cholesterol concentration and extent of atherosclerosis. Fatty streaking is absent in juveniles, but is prevalent in adults and more common in females than in males. Ten percent of the adults have lipid-containing lesions in small arteries within the myocardium.

Experimental studies have shown that the addition of cholesterol to the diet of squirrel monkeys results in hypercholesterolemia and exacerbation of atherosclerosis (Middleton et al., 1967a). Some squirrel monkeys (hyper-responders) achieve serum cholesterol concentrations of about 1,000 mg/dl after 4 to 5 months on a cholesterol-containing diet, while others (hyporesponders) will have average serum cholesterol concentrations of about 300 mg/dl. Approximately 65 percent of this variability is attributable to genetic factors (Clarkson et al., 1971). Atherosclerosis of squirrel monkeys also has been shown to be exacerbated by psychic stress (Lang, 1967), carbon monoxide (Webster et al., 1968), hypothyroidism, hypertension, and alloxan diabetes (Lehner et al., 1971).

There are some constraints to the use of squirrel monkeys in research on atherosclerosis. Their small bodies (0.8 to 1.0 kg) and arterial sizes limit the amount of blood that may be obtained and the amount of arterial tissue available for study. Female squirrel monkeys have estrous cycles only during the spring and early summer, and during the breeding season even females on high cholesterol diets have a marked lowering of total serum cholesterol concentration.

Rhesus macaques Naturally occurring atherosclerosis is not frequent in the rhesus macaque (Macaca mulatta). One study of 150 recently trapped rhesus macaques has shown only four with fatty streaks and one with plaques (Chawla et al., 1967). Atherosclerosis can be induced in these animals, however, by feeding them a diet comparable to that consumed by the average North American human. Fatty streaks and plaques have been shown to cover 75 percent of the surface of the aortas of rhesus macaques fed an "average American diet" (40 percent fat) for 2 years, while only 10 to 15 percent of the surface is involved in animals fed a "prudent American diet" (30 percent fat) (Wissler et al., 1965). The characteristics of the lesions and angiochemical changes induced in rhesus macaques fed cholesterol-containing diets have been studied by

numerous investigators (Scott et al., 1967a,b; Armstrong
et al., 1969; Manning and Clarkson, 1972), as has the
progression and regression of fatty streaks in this species (Eggen et al., 1974; Stary, 1974; Strong et al.,
1976). The regression of more advanced atherosclerosis
has also been studied (Armstrong et al., 1970; Bullock
et al., 1976; Weber et al., 1977).

Myocardial infarction has been associated with coronary arterial atherosclerosis in rhesus macaques fed
atherogenic diets. Healed, healing, and acute infarcts
in association with severe coronary arterial atherosclerosis were seen in the heart of an 8-year-old female
that died suddenly (Taylor et al., 1963). Fatal myocardial infarction was diagnosed in 2 of 265 juvenile
male rhesus monkeys fed an atherogenic diet for 16 months
(Hamm et al., 1974). Both had severe coronary artery
atherosclerosis and signs of acute myocardial necrosis.
Areas of necrosis, fibrosis, and neovascularization were
found in the left ventricle and interventricular septum
of a third rhesus monkey.

Long-tailed Macaques   Naturally occurring atherosclerosis appears to be more common among long-tailed (Macaca
fascicularis) than among rhesus macaques. Sixty-six
aortas from 73 male long-tailed macaques from Malaya
have been found to have intimal fatty streaks covering
approximately 2 percent of the surface, mainly near
branch points (Prathap, 1973). There were six fibrous
plaques in four aortas, but no complicated plaques.

In the earliest study of diet-induced atherosclerosis
in the United States (Kramsch and Hollander, 1968), young
adult male long-tailed macaques, fed a diet containing
cholesterol in banana mash and commercial monkey chow,
developed total serum cholesterol concentrations of 350-
475 mg/dl. After 18 months, atherosclerotic lesions were
found in the aorta and coronary and other arteries. Animals with an average total serum cholesterol concentration
above 350 mg/dl developed severe raised atherosclerotic
lesions of the main coronary arteries. Another study compared diet-induced atherosclerosis among adult male long-
tailed and rhesus macaques (Armstrong and Megan, 1974).
Although serum cholesterol concentrations were higher in
the rhesus macaques, atherosclerosis was more extensive
in all arteries of the long-tailed macaques. In a study
in which long-tailed macaques were fed several different
diets with varying types of fat and amounts of cholesterol, the lesions of animals fed cottonseed or corn oil

consisted mainly of foam cells, whereas the lesions of those fed butter had more collagen and elastin (Kramsch et al., 1973).

A very important aspect of the long-tailed macaque model is that the adult females share with Caucasian females considerable protection against coronary atherosclerosis. Coronary artery lesions are about 3 times more extensive in males than in females. This protection seems to be related to plasma lipoprotein characteristics (Pitts et al., 1976); the females have higher concentrations of HDL and smaller low-density lipoprotein (LDL) particles than the males.

Myocardial infarction associated with coronary atherosclerosis is apparently more common in long-tailed than in rhesus macaques (Kramsch and Hollander, 1968). Two of twelve young adult male long-tailed macaques died suddenly after 12 months of being fed an atherogenic diet. One had histologic evidence suggestive of myocardial ischemia, and both had marked stenosis of the coronary arteries. Additionally, fatal myocardial infarction was found in 2 of 12 male adults fed an atherogenic diet for 33 months (Bond and Bullock, 1980). The posterior wall of both ventricles and the posterior third of the interventricular septum was thin and fibrotic, and the coronary arteries were enlarged and had severe atherosclerotic lesions throughout the extramural branches.

Stump-tailed Macaques Several studies of diet-induced atherosclerosis have been carried out in the stump-tailed macaque (Macaca arctoides). A comparison of simple and complex carbohydrate effects on the serum lipids and atherosclerosis of cholesterol-fed stump-tailed macaques has shown that the diets are equally atherogenic (Lang and Barthel, 1972). Both produce extensive atherosclerotic lesions of the coronary arteries, as well as lesions in arteries of the kidney, testes, spleen, urinary bladder, pancreas, lung, and brain. An average total serum cholesterol concentration of 735 ± 29 mg/dl (mean $\pm$ SEM) has been shown in four adult male stump-tailed macaques fed a diet containing 1 mg cholesterol/Cal and 45 percent of calories from lard for 42 months (Bullock et al., 1975). Cutaneous xanthomata and xanthelasma, as well as extensive and severe atherosclerosis in the aorta and the coronary, carotid, and femoral arteries, have been shown in all animals. This species has a striking preponderance of connective tissue elements compared to lipid in their lesions. The number of intracranial arterial lesions is

small compared to the number of lesions in other vascular
beds. A study of the effect of hypertension on the development of diet-induced atherosclerosis has shown the
most extensive lesions in the aorta of the hypertensive,
hypercholesterolemic animals (Pick et al., 1974).

Pig-tailed Macaques Pig-tailed macaques (Macaca
nemestrina) have not been widely used in atherosclerosis
research; however, these animals have species characteristics that may be useful in studying this disease. Like
some races of humans, these animals appear to lack a negative feedback control mechanism to reduce cholesterol
biosynthesis when cholesterol is ingested (Raymond, 1974).
Pig-tailed macaques fed cholesterol-containing diets for
long periods of time have a high incidence of hepatic
cirrhosis (Bullock et al., 1974).

Recently, investigators have shown that alcohol decreases the severity of atherosclerosis. Animals consuming a cholesterol-containing diet and fed 30 percent of
calories as ethanol show increased concentrations of low-
density lipoprotein and diminished coronary artery atherosclerosis. However, these macaques also develop fatty
livers (Clarkson and Rudel, In press).

Pig-tailed macaques also have been used to evaluate
the interaction between platelets and the arterial wall
in atherogenesis. Damaging the aortic endothelium with
a ballon catheter produces intimal thickenings of prolif-
erated smooth muscle cells (without stainable lipid) that
regress from about 15 layers of smooth muscle cells to
2 or 3 cell layers within 6 months in normolipoproteinemic
animals (Stemerman and Ross, 1972). When injury is induced in the same way in cholesterol-fed pig-tailed
macaques (plasma cholesterol concentrations of 250-400
mg/dl), the lesions do not regress and do accumulate
stainable lipid.

African Green Monkeys A study of naturally occurring
atherosclerosis in African green monkeys (Cercopithecus aethiops), in captivity for 8 or 9 weeks, revealed
that half of the mature monkeys had macroscopic sudano-
philic lesions of the aorta (Gresham et al., 1965),
principally small fatty streaks around the orifices of
branches. An average total serum cholesterol concentration of 450 mg/dl was found in four male green monkeys
from Kenya fed a diet containing 1 mg cholesterol/Cal
and 45 percent of calories as lard for 42 months (Bullock
et al., 1975). At necropsy, plaques were present in the

abdominal aorta, the major coronary arteries, the femoral
arteries, and at the carotid bifurcations. The distribution and microscopic appearance of the lesions were similar to lesions found in human arteries. None of these
monkeys had lesions in the intracranial arteries, and
they had little cholesterol accumulation in organs or in
tissues other than arteries. The chemical composition
of the plaques was quite similar to that of man (Wagner
and Clarkson, 1975).

A key advantage of the African green monkey as a model
of human atherosclerosis is the similarity of the hyperlipoproteinemias (Rudel and Lofland, 1976). The response
to dietary cholesterol in African green monkeys is different from that of most other species of nonhuman primate. The only lipoproteins that show an increased concentration are the LDL and, to a small extent, the
intermediate-sized lipoproteins. Concentrations of very
low-density lipoproteins (VLDL) and HDL do not change.

Baboons A study of the prevalence of atherosclerosis
in captured baboons (Papio spp.) from Kenya has revealed that approximately three-fourths of the adult animals have some fatty streaking that is visible after the
aortas are stained with Sudan IV (McGill et al., 1960).
The coronary arteries have numerous small musculoelastic
plaques that do not contain lipid. These monkeys are not
strikingly responsive to dietary cholesterol, as has been
shown in a study in which different groups were fed diets
with two levels of added cholesterol (0.50 and 0.01 percent), either high or low in protein, and containing
either saturated or unsaturated fat (Strong et al., 1966).
An elevation of serum cholesterol concentration was found
in 12 to 18 percent of the group fed 0.5 percent cholesterol. They developed only small fatty streaks in the
aorta, and coronary artery atherosclerosis was minimal
even after prolonged periods of cholesterol feeding
(Strong and McGill, 1967). This relative lack of response
may be useful in studying the interaction of other risk
factors, such as hypertension and cigarette smoking. Baboons have been trained to smoke cigarettes (McGill, In
press).

Baboons have also been used successfully in studies of
the roles of genetic regulation and infant nutrition in
determining plasma cholesterol concentration. Because of
a strong effect of the sire on the plasma cholesterol
concentrations of their progeny, it has been possible to

use hyperresponding sires to produce hyperresponding progeny.

Lagomorphs

Rabbits have been used as animal models for research on atherosclerosis since the early studies on the effect of dietary cholesterol by Anitschkow and Chalatow (1913). Rabbits are particularly sensitive to dietary cholesterol. Most investigators have fed relatively large quantities of cholesterol, inducing a general disease that more nearly resembles a lipid storage disease than atherosclerosis (Prior et al., 1961). Their use has been reviewed extensively (Kritchevsky, 1964; Clarkson et al., 1974). It recently has been found that modest hyperlipoproteinemia and atherosclerosis can be induced in rabbits by feeding them a diet high in saturated fat, but with minimal dietary cholesterol (Shore and Shore, 1976). In addition, it has been recognized that there are major strain (van Zutphen and Fox, 1977) and stock (van Zutphen et al., 1980) differences in serum cholesterol levels and in the frequency of plaque formation in response to dietary cholesterol. These differences appear to be related to genetic differences in esterase, which may play a role in cholesterol metabolism (van Zutphen and Fox, 1977). These two developments should markedly increase the value of the rabbit as a model of hypercholesterolemia and atherosclerosis.

Rodents

Rats While rats have had some use as animal models in research on atherosclerosis, most comparative pathologists have noted little or no similarity between arterial lesions induced in these animals and those of human atherosclerosis. Rats are resistant to both naturally occurring (Wexler and Judd, 1970; Hashimoto and Dayton, 1974; Villa et al., 1977; Lewis, 1978; Parke et al., 1978) and diet-induced atherosclerosis. Some arterial lesions have been produced when the diet is very high in cholesterol and, in addition, contains high quantities of bile salts (Philip and Kurup, 1977; Satakopan and Kurup, 1977; Zahor and Czabanova, 1977) or an antithyroid agent such as thiouracil (Lelorier et al., 1976). Generally, the lesions that are induced are fatty streaks or fatty dots in the intima that bear little resemblance to atherosclerosis. The resistance of these animals to atherosclerotic lesions relates to their ability to increase bile acid excretion when fed dietary cholesterol, to their high levels of HDL, and to certain metabolic characteristics of the arterial wall.

The most widely discussed rat model of arterial disease is the repeatedly bred male or female rat (Wexler et al., 1976). Repeatedly bred animals of several stocks and strains are reported to develop increases in plasma lipids, blood pressure, and degenerative arterial lesions. The lesions of these repeatedly bred rats are primarily focal accumulations of glycosaminoglycans in the intima of arteries, sometimes associated with mineralization and smooth muscle cell proliferation. They should not be confused with atherosclerosis in which lipid is, by definition, a major component. This rat model has been widely explored (Wexler and Greenberg, 1974, 1978; Wexler, 1975, 1976).

Recently, Koletsky and Puterman (1977) have described a rat model with considerable potential for atherosclerosis research. While the model has not been fully characterized, the rat is obese, has increased plasma concentrations of VLDL and LDL, and develops arterial lesions that more closely resemble atherosclerosis than those seen in other rat models.

Other Animal Models

Swine Pigs provide very good models of human atherosclerosis. The disease occurs naturally (Gottlieb and Lalich, 1954) and can be exacerbated by diet (Moreland, 1965). The changes in plasma lipoproteins in response to changes in diet closely resemble those occurring in humans, and the atherosclerotic lesions bear a striking resemblance to those of man in both gross appearance and histological characteristics. A rapid method for the induction of advanced coronary artery atherosclerosis associated with myocardial infarction and sudden death has been described (Lee et al., 1971; Nam et al., 1973). A particularly important feature of the pig model may be the susceptibility of these animals to cerebrovascular atherosclerosis, a striking finding among pigs fed leftover food from restaurants (Ratcliffe and Luginbuhl, 1971). This important observation has not yet been

thoroughly studied, and there are numerous unanswered
questions concerning whether the effect is due to the fat
or the salt in the diet or to some interaction between
these and other dietary variables.

Pigeons During the past 20 years, pigeons have become
widely used animal models for research on atherosclerosis. Spontaneous aortic and coronary artery atherosclerosis are common in White Carneau pigeons, but rare
in the Show Racer breed (Clarkson et al., 1959; Prichard
et al., 1964a,b). Lesions occur in nearly 100 percent
of White Carneau pigeons more than 3 years of age even
though they consume a diet that is free of cholesterol. The lesions are found very predictably in the lower
thoracic aorta near the origin of the celiac axis. The
development of atherosclerotic lesions is markedly exacerbated by feeding cholesterol (Clarkson and Lofland, 1967),
and plaque complications, such as mineralization and
ulceration, are seen more commonly in White Carneau pigeons than in other animal models. Recently, selected
strains of White Carneau pigeons have been developed with
characteristics that are particularly useful in research
on atherosclerosis (Wagner et al. 1973; Clarkson, 1975).
The most widely used of these, the WC_2 strain, develops
more extensive and severe atherosclerosis than the random-
bred population of White Carneau even in the absence of
measurable differences in the known risk factors (Wagner,
1978). It is presumed that the increased susceptibility
of WC_2 pigeons is related to some aspect of arterial
metabolism. The pigeon model of atherosclerosis has also
been used to study regression of lesions (Kottke et al.,
1974), sterol balance (Siekert et al., 1975; Flynn et
al., 1976), cellular pathogenesis (Lauper et al., 1975),
and the role of clotting phenomena in lesion development
(Fuster et al., 1977).

MATURITY-ONSET DIABETES MELLITUS

Definition

Maturity-onset (Type II) diabetes mellitus is a disorder
of carbohydrate, lipid, and protein metabolism due to a
disturbance of insulin metabolism. It is characterized
by obesity, hyperglycemia, glycosuria, and abnormal glucose tolerance (Renold et al., 1972; Williams, 1975).
Its incidence increases from 0.2 percent at age 25 to 7

percent at age 75. It is important in geriatric medicine, not only because it is the fifth greatest cause
of death, but also because of the morbidity imposed by
complications of the primary metabolic disturbance,
such as blindness, atherosclerosis, neuropathy, and
nephropathy.

Clinical and Pathological Manifestations

In the absence of any known interfering factors, such as
anxiety, illness, infection, delayed gut transit time,
and prior carbohydrate deprivation, some authorities consider an abnormal glucose tolerance test diagnostic for
diabetes (Cahill, 1975). Three tests presently are in
common use: two glucose tolerance tests, oral and intravenous, and an intravenous tolbutamide test. The oral
test is favored (Hausmann et al., 1975; Prout, 1975).
Hyperglycemia can be controlled by proper diet or by oral
hypoglycemic agents; however, there is neither prevention
nor cure for the underlying metabolic defect; current
therapy is directed at the abnormalities that result from
it (Metz, 1975).

Maturity-onset diabetes may be completely asymptomatic
or may involve one or multiple organs or systems. The
severity of damage to these organs and systems generally
correlates with the duration of the disease. In the
cells or capillaries of the pancreatic islets, hyaline or
amyloid accumulations can be seen. In diabetes of long
duration, the hyaline deposits may replace the islets
(Robbins, 1974a).

Micro- and macroangiopathy (atherosclerosis) are very
common in diabetic patients. Microangiopathy is characterized morphologically by a thickening of the circumfer-
ential basal lamina of the capillaries and, occasionally,
of other small vessels. For unknown reasons, retinal
and glomerular capillaries are particularly predisposed
to microangiopathic lesions (Robbins, 1974a; Lin et al.,
1975; Yodaikeu and Pardo, 1975). Diabetes is the second
leading cause of blindness in the United States, and diabetic retinopathy accounts for most blindness associated
with the disease (Robbins, 1974a). The rate of development of atherosclerosis and incidence of its sequelae,
including myocardial infarction and cerebral vascular
accidents, are increased in diabetics. Atherosclerotic
diabetics also suffer intermittent claudication, and

eventually gangrene of the lower extremities, more frequently than nondiabetics with atherosclerosis.

There are two kinds of diabetic neuropathy, somatic and visceral. Somatic, or peripheral, neuropathy is more common in the lower than the upper extremities and affects both motor and proprioceptive fibers. Segmental degeneration of the myelin can be seen microscopically, and direct injury of the axons may be present (Robbins, 1974a). Visceral neuropathy can involve the eyes, joints, gastrointestinal tract, genito-urinary tract, and autonomic nervous system generally (Ellenberg, 1975). Sequelae of visceral neuropathy are varied. Extensive sensory anesthesia of the joints, particularly the knee and ankle, can result in chronic trauma leading to Charcot's joint (arthropathy). Similarly, neuropathic skin ulcers may develop, particularly on the feet, and become infected. The most frequent clinical manifestation of autonomic neuropathy is "neurogenic bladder," an asymptomatic overdistention of the bladder with urine. This overdistention, coupled with incomplete voiding, increases the risk of urinary tract infection (Watkins, 1975).

The most severe manifestations of diabetes are the renal complications. Diabetic nephropathies may involve the tubules, arteries and arterioles, and, most frequently, the glomeruli. Hypertension, which is common in diabetics, can complicate the pathological processes. Three morphological categories of glomerulosclerosis can be distinguished: nodular, intercapillary or diffuse, and exudative (Kimmelstiel, 1966). Because of the predisposition of diabetics to infection, acute or chronic pyelonephritis resulting from bacterial urinary infections is fairly common and is of considerable concern because it can precipitate renal papillary necrosis, ketosis, and coma (Kimmelstiel, 1966).

Etiology and Pathogenesis

While the exact metabolic defect causing diabetes is not understood, the maturity-onset form of the disorder is clearly hereditary, with environment, particularly nutrition, playing an important role (Cahill, 1975). Both simple autosomal recessive and polygenic (multifactorial) modes of inheritance have been suggested, but evidence favoring the latter is accumulating rapidly. The

possibility remains that there are different forms of
the disease with different genetic bases.

Hypoxic (ischemic) injury is postulated to play a role
in diabetic neuropathy. Microangiopathy of the afferent
blood vessels supplying the nerves may account for the
chronic, progressive degeneration of the myelin sheaths
and, later, of the axons themselves. There is also evidence to suggest that the increased activity of the polyol
(or sorbitol) pathway, as a result of the hyperglycemia,
may account for the damage.

Animal Models

Nonhuman Primates

Spontaneous diabetes mellitus is not uncommon in nonhuman
primates. The literature contains many case reports of
monkeys, including pets, zoo specimens, and research animals, with diabetes. Howard (1975b) has extensively reviewed and evaluated early reports. Although many are
poorly documented, there is good reason to believe that
a systematic survey of nonhuman primate populations will
uncover a significant number of diabetic individuals. To
serve as useful animal models, they must be identified
in adequate numbers for meaningful research.

The Oregon Regional Primate Center maintains a closed
breeding colony of some Celebes black apes (Macaca nigra;
Fooden, 1969), approximately half of which have abnormal
values for intravenous glucose tolerance tests (IV-GTT).
There is an indication that glucose intolerance may be
a species characteristic, because there is a similar frequency in Celebes black apes from other sources (Howard,
1975b). The incidence of diabetes is independent of
obesity in these macaques. In the wild, these macaques
exist in a small geographic range in the Celebese Islands
of the Indonesian Archipelago, where the species may be
highly inbred. The incidence of glucose intolerance in
free-ranging Celebes black apes is unknown, and it may be
that its prevalence is increased in captive populations
because of stress or dietary change (Howard, 1975b).

Correlating with the increasing severity of glucose
intolerance in Celebes black apes in the Oregon colony
are increases in fasting glucose, serum triglycerides,
pre-β lipoprotein, and nonesterified fatty acids. There
is generally a decrease in immunoreactive insulin. A few

animals are hyperinsulinemic (Howard, 1975b). Serum cholesterol levels are the same in both glucose intolerant
and control animals; however, amyloid infiltration of the
pancreatic islets is 8 times greater in glucose intolerant
animals than in controls. This correlates well with the
above changes and is independent of a general increase in
amyloid seen with aging (Howard, 1978). An increase in
thickness of muscle capillary basement membranes and
aortic atherosclerosis also is seen in the diabetic animals (Howard, 1975a). Clinical signs appear at 4 to 5
years of age in the form of weight loss, lethargy, polydipsia, polyphagia, and polyuria. Cataracts have been
reported in one individual. Diabetic Celebes black apes
do not require insulin replacement. To date, a single
male has sired most of the diabetic animals in the Oregon
colony, and insufficient data have been accumulated to
postulate a mechanism of inheritance.

The Celebes black ape has several advantages for research on the relationship between aging and diabetes
mellitus. Chief among these is the fact that the disease
is associated with the same changes in lipoprotein distribution and composition seen in humans and the same
micro- and macrovascular complications develop as in human diabetics. Other advantages are the high incidence
of spontaneous disease and the convenience of size that
permit the collection of ample blood and tissue samples
from individual animals. Disadvantages are that the pathogenesis of diabetes in this species appears to resemble
human juvenile-onset (Type I) rather than maturity-onset
diabetes mellitus, and the dyslipoproteinemia seen in
diabetic animals is not as striking as it usually is in
humans.

Diabetes in a rhesus macaque (Macaca mulatta) with
hyperphagic obesity secondary to an experimental lesion
of the hypothalamus was reported in 1938 (Ranson et al.,
1938). More recently, three of seven similarly lesioned
male rhesus macaques have been reported to develop diabetes (Hamilton and Brobeck, 1963). Spontaneously obese
male rhesus macaques, 10 to 14 years of age, also have
a high incidence of diabetes (Hamilton and Lewis, 1975).
Observed over a period of years, these animals show a
progressive hyperinsulinemia followed by hypoinsulinem-
ia, a loss of insulin response to IV-GTT, hyperglycemia,
glycosuria, and dependence on exogenous insulin for survival (Hamilton and Ciaccia, 1978).

Diabetes mellitus in older, obese male rhesus macaques
appears to be an excellent model of human maturity-onset

diabetes mellitus. One advantage of the model is that it is apparently readily available in any large population of middle-aged to slightly older animals. In addition, the pathophysiology, on the basis of the limited number of reports, seems to resemble Type II diabetes of humans, or at least a hyperinsulinemic type of diabetes mellitus. A disadvantage is that, at present, the characterization of the model is not complete. For example, it is not known whether the diabetes is associated with a deficiency of insulin receptors and whether there is dyslipoproteinemia, exacerbated atherosclerosis, microvascular disease, and diabetic neuropathy.

The Department of Comparative Medicine of the Bowman Gray School of Medicine, Wake Forest University, Winston-Salem, North Carolina, has established a breeding colony of long-tailed macaques (Macaca fascicularis) centered around a single male with spontaneous, insulin-deficient diabetes mellitus to determine whether the condition has a genetic basis for which selection can be made. Eleven offspring have been born to date. The male has been hyperglycemic, glycosuric, and ketonuric since he arrived from the importer and relies on daily exogenous insulin to prevent ketonuria. When untreated, he shows glucose intolerance and negligible insulin levels even after glucose challenge. On a diet of low cholesterol content (0.164 mg chol/Kcal, less cholesterol than in the "average American" diet), his plasma cholesterol is 1,368 mg/dl, with only 34 mg/dl as α lipoprotein (HDL) cholesterol. The plasma triglyceride level is 4,104 mg/dl. Four insulin-dependent, diabetic long-tailed macaques (two males and two females) recently have been identified in the same colony. Approximately 500 members of the species have been screened to identify these five individuals.

Hyperinsulinemic diabetes mellitus has been reported in an 8-year-old pig-tailed macaque (Macaca nemestrina). Although only a single individual is described, this report is significant in that the syndrome includes not only hyperinsulinemia, but glucosuria, fasting hyperglycemia, hypertriglyceridemia, and marked pre-β hyperlipoproteinemia as well (Leathers and Schedewie, In press).

Carnivores

Diabetes mellitus in dogs and cats is a common spontaneous disorder resembling Type I, insulin-dependent diabetes of humans. Insulin deficiency is secondary to pancreatic disease. Microangiopathy of renal and retinal vessels, as well as renal glomerulosclerosis, is seen in dogs with long-standing diabetes mellitus, and cataracts are common. A condition resembling maturity-onset diabetes of humans has not been reported in dogs and cats (Capen et al., 1975). Canine (Rosenblum et al., 1979) and feline (Johnson and Hayden, 1979) diabetes have been reviewed recently.

Rodents

Mice The diabetic mouse (db/db) has a single gene mutation that appears as an autosomal recessive trait on Chromosome 4 (Coleman, 1978). Because homozygotes are infertile, it is maintained on a C57BL/KsJ background through mating of heterozygotes. Other alleles producing similar syndromes have been identified and maintained on the C57BL/6J background (db^{2J}) and on a 129/J background (db^{3J}). By using a linkage to the coat color gene, misty (m), two congenic strains (BL/6mdb) and BL/ksmdb) have been developed to aid in identifying potential homozygous diabetics and heterozygotes for breeding. The diabetic syndrome in db/db and db^{2J} mice includes hyperphagia, hypertrophy of adipose tissue, hyperglycemia, and hyperinsulinemia. In the early stages of the disease, there is hyperplasia and hypertrophy of pancreatic β cells, but eventually they atrophy. Life span is shortened markedly in db/db mice, but normal in the db^{2J} mutation that produces a much milder diabetic condition. In contrast, the db^{3J} trait is associated with hypoglycemia, hyperinsulinemia, and hypertrophy of pancreatic islets (Coleman, 1978).

Rats Among rats that have been employed for aging studies, only one stock of male SD rat, the Crl:COBS® CD® (SD)[1] rat, has been sufficiently characterized under appropriately defined conditions to be evaluated as a possible model for maturity-onset diabetes in aging humans. There are remarkable similarities with regard to specific physiological correlates that are characteristic of the human disease. Pathological features are not identical

---

[1]COBS® and CD® are registered trademarks of the Charles River Breeding Laboratories, Wilmington, Massachusetts.

and are complicated by other chronic properties of this animal model; however, they are sufficiently related to the spectrum of relevant human pathology to warrant further investigation.

The relationships between aging and changes in metabolism that may contribute to the increased risk of diabetes in the elderly have been studied in more detail in the rat than in other animal models. Fasting blood sugar levels increase from 80 mg/100 ml of serum at 2 months of age to approximately 110 mg/100 ml at 12 and 24 months. Although a traditional glucose tolerance test at appropriate ages has not been reported, utilization, but not transportation into the circulation, of an administered load of glucose is slowed between 12 and 24 months of age (Gold et al., 1976).

Disturbances in the regulation of circulating levels of immunoreactive insulin (IRI) are seen during aging (Gold et al., 1976; Kitahara and Adelman, 1979). When rats are fasted for 72 hours and then administered glucose intragastrically, two distinct differences in the pattern of IRI response are evident during aging. First, the instantaneous increase in the concentration of IRI in serum collected from portal vein blood is twice as great and occurs over a longer period of time in 12- and 24-month-old rats than in 2-month-old rats. Second, a later rise in the levels of IRI is progressively delayed in time of onset from 30 minutes at 2 months of age to 3-4 hours at 12 months and 6-7 hours at 24 months of age. This complex response apparently reflects an age-associated change in distribution and function of distinct populations of pancreatic islets of Langerhans.

The ability to suppress circulating levels of immunoreactive glucagon (IRG) by administration of glucose is also impaired during aging (Klug et al., 1979). When 2-month-old rats that have been fasted 72 hours are administered glucose intragastrically, the concentration of IRG in serum collected from portal vein blood is rapidly diminished. In contrast, the concentration of IRG is increased to a small degree at 12 months and dramatically at 24 months of age. Indeed, the molar ratio of IRG to IRI increases sufficiently during aging to warrant consideration as a primary factor contributing to glucose intolerance (Adelman, 1979), as well as to the reported delayed adaptation in hepatic glucokinase activity (Adelman, 1970).

The pathology profile that accompanies aging in the SD rat (Cohen et al., 1978) includes several observations

pertinent to its potential use in research on diabetes.
While arteriolarsclerosis and peripheral neuropathy are
not evident, inflammatory lesions are seen in the large
arteries, and spinal cord lesions resulting in hind limb
paralysis are detectable. Loss of eyesight is evident,
though this may relate to the light sensitivity of albino
rats in general. The continuous increase in body weight
and obesity that accompanies aging in this animal model
needs to be considered in interpreting both the physiological and pathological changes described above.

Gerbils Although several studies have documented
diabetic metabolic changes in the Mongolian gerbil
(Meriones unguiculatus), it is difficult to evaluate the
usefulness of the animal as a model of human diabetes.
Some animals exhibit spontaneous obesity and hyperglycemia, increased IRI, glucosuria, and islet hyperplasia.
Other pancreatic changes, including islet cell adenomas
and "islet exhaustion," also have been documented (Boquist, 1972). Nakama (1977) has suggested that the gerbil might represent a model of β insulinoma. Degenerative
changes secondary to nonlipoid angiopathy appear in the
pancreas, kidneys, and heart, but these may be secondary
to hyperadrenocorticism (Wexler et al., 1971), and vascular lesions appear to precede the metabolic derangements
(Nakama, 1977). There appear to be no data on genetic
bases of these components or on their effects upon longevity of the gerbil.

Guinea pigs Spontaneous diabetes mellitus has been reported to occur in a colony of guinea pigs (Munger and
Lang, 1973; Lang and Munger, 1976; Lang et al., 1977).
Although this model has an infectious etiology, it has
many characteristics that make it suitable for studying
the interrelationships between diabetes mellitus and
aging. Features of the disease that are similar to human
diabetes include abnormal glucose tolerance, changes in
fat catabolism, exocrine pancreatic dysfunction, and histopathology. In general, animals with the most severe
glucose intolerance have the most distinctive islet pathology. The lesion consists of degranulation of islet
cells, cytoplasmic β cell inclusions, cytoplasmic masses
of rough endoplasmic reticulum, and scarring and fibrosis
in the vascular stroma of the islet. Some cases show
spontaneous recovery associated with β cell hyperplasia in
existing islets and formation of new islets composed entirely of β cells. Spontaneous remission of the clinical

syndrome is associated with residual pathognomonic scarring in the pancreatic islet vascular stroma, <u>viz</u>., tightly packed bundles of parallel collagen fibrils in islets containing both α and β cells. Hyperglycemia is regarded by some as a stimulus for β cell replication (Logothetopoulos <u>et al</u>., 1970), and some human diabetics show hyperplasia of β cells (Evans, 1972).

Renal lesions first appear 10 to 12 weeks after the islet lesions, indicating that they are probably secondary to the primary process. There is a diffuse thickening of the glomerular basal lamina that is often duplicated and contains electron-opaque material. The mesangial core of glomerular tufts is focally expanded with occasional droplets of periodic acid-Schiff positive material in Bowman's capsule that resembles the glomerular sclerosis seen in human diabetics. In some animals, fibrosis and scarring of Bowman's capsule, as well as diffuse peritubular scarring, are prominent. The glomerular lesions are similar to, but less severe than, those seen in human diabetics; this may simply reflect the fact that diabetic guinea pigs have not been studied beyond 3 years of age.

The pathological changes seen in the capillaries of diabetic guinea pigs also resemble those of human diabetics. The basal lamina of capillaries in normal animals is a thin, unilaminar, moderately opaque structure, about as thick as a muscle cell. In diabetic animals, the basal laminae are considerably thicker. In many sections, they appear as multilaminar structures in which bands of electron-opaque, filamentous material alternate with electron-lucent zones. In some cases, the electron-opaque material is similar to that seen in basal laminae from the capillaries of human diabetics.

As in the human patient, the concentration of bicarbonate and pancreatic enzyme activity (trypsin, lipase, amylase) is significantly reduced (Balk <u>et al</u>., 1975). Thus, the model can be used to study normal changes with age in exocrine pancreatic function, their alteration in diabetes mellitus, and whether such changes predispose the individual to other metabolic alterations.

In human diabetics, the abnormally high levels of glucose in the blood lead to abnormalities of lipid metabolism, which in turn increase the blood levels of acetoacetic and β-hydroxbutyric acids (Beyer <u>et al</u>., 1962; Roldan <u>et al</u>., 1971; Harano <u>et al</u>., 1972). Formation of these ketone bodies is a major complication of diabetes mellitus. Because of unexplained differences in fat catabolism, less than 10 percent of the diabetic guinea pigs have any evidence of ketonuria, and ketonemia has not been detected in any. The guinea pig is capable of developing ketonuria under other conditions, e.g., toxemia of pregnancy (Assali et al., 1972); therefore, this model affords the opportunity to determine whether ketonemia is an inevitable characteristic of uncontrolled diabetes mellitus or a preventable consequence of hyperglycemia.

Increased fatty-acid oxidation indicates a decrease in the utilization of carbohydrates and an increase in the oxidation of fat and free fatty acids as a primary source of energy for oxidative phosphorylation. It is not known whether this is a factor in normal aging, as well as an aspect of diabetes mellitus. The increased activity of β-hydroxybutyrate dehydrogenase suggests an increased potential for ketone body formation in peripheral tissue. The diabetic guinea pig, like man, has increased β-hydroxyybutyrate dehydrogenase activity, but unlike man, does not develop marked ketoacidosis, a difference that allows study of the two phenomena separately (Nevalainen et al., 1978).

The research potential of this model is enhanced by the absence of other factors that complicate the analysis of diabetes in man and closely similar models, such as failure to develop ketoacidosis, ability to survive without exogenous insulin, and spontaneous remission of islet cells. Disadvantages of the model include apparent differences in genetic predisposition among guinea pigs to develop the disease; lack of identification of the etiologic agent; incomplete characterization of the metabolic changes; and scarcity of affected animals for study.

Other rodents   Obesity and diabetes have been observed in wild species of mice adapted to the laboratory. When introduced to standard laboratory diets, many spiny mice (Acomys cahirinus), small rodents of semiarid natural habitats, develop obesity, characterized by hyperinsulinemia, glucose intolerance, and glycosuria (Gonet et al., 1965). Others develop diabetes, characterized by hyperglycemia and glycosuria without ketosis but with profound shortening of life span (Gonet et al., 1965). While substantial variation exists in these symptoms, all animals show hyperplasia of pancreatic β cells. This syndrome is suggested to be evidence of the "thrifty gene" hypothesis, which contends that diabetes and obesity can exist in a balanced polymorphism as an adaptive mechanism in animal populations faced with fluctuating food resources (Neel, 1962). Being prone to these conditions promotes more efficient storage and retrieval of energy stores in such an environment. The phenotypic expression of this genotype occurs in the laboratory, where food is plentiful and continuously available. Laboratory stocks of these animals presently are showing a decreasing incidence of the condition, suggesting that there is a selection against individuals prone to the extremes of the disease (Coleman, 1978).

OBESITY

Definition

Obesity is a chronic condition manifested as an excess accumulation of fat or adipose tissue. The definition of obesity is a statistical one. The prevalence, based on measurements of skinfold thickness, is estimated to be 17 percent of all adults (Bray, 1975), 13 percent among adult males and 23 percent among adult females.

Obesity is considered to be a pathological condition because it is associated with increased risks of morbidity and mortality, e.g., diabetes mellitus and hypertension (National Commission on Diabetes, 1975). Interest in obesity relative to aging stems from two considerations. First, although obesity usually occurs before old age, i.e., from childhood to middle age, the pathological consequences may be manifested most forcefully in old age. Second, adipose tissue mass increases until late middle age, but may actually decline as the individual becomes old (Masoro et al., 1979).

Clinical and Pathological Manifestations

The obese patient has been characterized psychologically as a person who eats more during a meal, eats more rapidly during a meal, is more responsive to the stimulus qualities of food (e.g., palatability and prominence), and is less willing to expend energy to obtain food dependent upon its stimulus qualities than normal people (Schacter and Rodin, 1974; Leon and Roth, 1977). It is not known whether obese people are less responsive than normal people to internal signals of hunger and satiety (Leon and Roth, 1977; Pudel, 1978; Rodin, 1978).

Obesity is viewed as a dysfunction in the regulation of energy storage. Triglycerides, the major energy reservoir of the body, are stored in adipocytes. Excess deposition of triglycerides causes adipocyte hyperplasia or hypertrophy. This has led to the classification of obesity into hyperplastic and hypertrophic types (Greenwood et al., 1978); however, since some hypertrophy of adipocytes always occurs in obesity, this classification cannot be rigidly applied.

Obese patients may have hyperinsulinemia, hyperglycemia, hypertriglyceridemia, hypercholesterolemia, and hypertension, either singly or in combination (Greenwood et al., 1978). Insulin antagonists of unknown origin result in hyperinsulinemia and increased synthesis of triglycerides and cholesterol. Hyperinsulinemia plus hyperglycemia can result in overstimulation and destruction of the pancreas. Hypercholesterolemia can result in lipid deposition in the arteries, producing atherosclerosis and other cardiovascular complications.

Etiology and Pathogenesis

Research into the pathogenesis of obesity has progressed along several lines. One line has been an attempt to determine whether obesity is related to abnormalities in neurophysiological functioning. However, these studies have been hindered by a lack of basic knowledge on the brain mechanisms involved in hunger motivation, specifically how satiety is communicated to the central nervous system (Marshall, 1978).

Environmental influences are important in obesity; the eating habits of individuals are profoundly affected by cultural factors (LeMagnen, 1978). For example, obesity is more prevalent among poor women than among those above the poverty level (Bray, 1975).

The genetics of obesity are difficult to evaluate. There is speculation that maturity-onset diabetes and the concomitant obesity may exist in human gene pools as a balanced polymorphism similar to the sickle cell trait (Cahill, 1978). This may have provided a selective advantage in past, hunter-gatherer cultures. From this perspective, obesity is a genotypic condition that has only recently been manifested phenotypically as human populations have become more sedentary (Cahill, 1978; Hirsch, 1978).

Animal Models

Nonhuman Primates

The nonhuman primate has not been extensively utilized as
a model for the study of obesity. The following summarizes the limited amount of work done in this area.

Rhesus Macaque Obesity has been produced in the rhesus
macaque (Macaca mulatta) by means of appropriately placed
hypothalamic lesions (Hamilton et al., 1972). Obesity
also appears spontaneously in this species when the animals reach 12-14 years of age (Hamilton and Rabinowitz,
1976; Hamilton and Ciaccia, 1978). This obesity often
involves hyperinsulinemia that can be reversed by weight
reduction, a blunted rise in serum insulin in response
to a glucose load, decreased ability to remove glucose
from the plasma, and elevated levels of low and very low
density lipoproteins. In some animals, these problems
progress to the point where they appear to represent overt
diabetes mellitus. In most instances, obesity in the
hypothalamic-lesioned rhesus macaques relates to hyperphagia, but in some instances it relates to increased
feeding-efficiency ratios (Hamilton et al., 1976).
    Recently, insulin and glucagon binding by partially
purified plasma membranes prepared from livers of normal,
spontaneously obese, and hypothalamic-lesion-induced obese
monkeys has been studied (Lockwood et al., 1979). Insulin binding is reduced in the membranes of obese rhesus
macaques because of a decreased number of available receptor sites. Glucagon binding is not significantly reduced in membranes prepared from spontaneously obese,
nondiabetic animals, but is reduced in those with diabetes and in those with hypothalamic obesity.

Pig-tailed Macaque Obesity occurs spontaneously in
some female pig-tailed macaques (Macaca nemistrina); the
adipose mass is about 40 percent of the total body mass
(Walike et al., 1977). All obese animals are estimated
to be at least 8 years old. Spontaneous obesity has
not been seen in the males. All of the obese animals
have elevated plasma insulin levels, but normal glucose
disappearance rates. It is not known presently whether
a sufficient number of spontaneously obese pig-tailed
macaques exists to make it an available model.

Carnivores

There is little information available on carnivores as
models of obesity. Casual observation indicates that
both dogs and cats may be good models; however, the model
must first be characterized before its relevance can be
determined.

Lagomorphs

The rabbit has not been well characterized as an obesity
model. Certain strains of rabbits at The Jackson Laboratory, Bar Harbor, Maine, tend to accumulate excessive body
fat, particularly in the peritoneal cavity, unless kept on
a restricted dietary intake. Strain OS/J is a good example. This strain is a very docile strain of Dutch
origin (Fox, 1975) with low blood pressure (Fox et al.,
1969). When fed a given amount of cholesterol in the
diet, this strain responds maximally as measured by serum
cholesterol levels and atherosclerotic plaques (van Zutphen and Fox, 1977). Since rabbits are herbivorous animals with gut fermentation playing an important role in
their metabolism, it seems unlikely that they are good
models for human obesity.

Rodents

Rats Before considering specific rat models that have
been used to study obesity, the age-related changes in
adipose mass of a normal rat population allowed to eat
ad libitum should be considered. A lifelong longitudinal study on the changes in adipose tissue mass has been
carried out on 14 male F344 rats (Masoro et al., 1979).
The data show that adipose mass increases until late,
middle age (18 months) after which it decreases. Similar data have been obtained for the mass of the epididymal and perirenal depots in a cross-sectional study
of another group of animals from the same rat population. The median life span of the population is 23.5
months.

The mass of an adipose depot can change either because
of changes in the number of adipocytes, mean volume of
adipocytes, or both. It is currently believed that the
number of adipocytes in the depots of adult mammals is
fixed, a concept based primarily on research using rats.

These studies involve only a small fraction of the life span (Masoro et al., 1979). In a recently published study (Bertrand et al., 1978), changes in epididymal and perirenal depot mass, mean adipocyte volume, and adipocyte number have been measured in male F344 rats from 6 to 18 months of age. Both depots increase in mass--the epididymal depot solely by adipocyte hypertrophy, the perirenal depot solely by adipocyte hyperplasia. Since similar information is not available for humans, it is not known whether increases in adipose mass are similar to those in rats.

There have been four general types of rat models that have been used to study obesity. These may be classified as follows: (1) obesity induced by lesions in the hypothalamus, (2) obesity of genetic origin, (3) obesity induced by nutritional manipulation, and (4) obesity caused by the limitation of physical activity.

Destruction of the ventromedial region of the hypothalamus induces obesity in rats (Morrison, 1977). This obesity does not progress indefinitely. Immediately after destruction of the ventromedial area, the rat becomes hyperphagic; however, at a certain stage of obesity, food intake falls to a level not appreciably above the preoperation level.

This obesity model shows the following clinical and pathological characteristics: "finickiness" of appetite, decreased spontaneous activity, hypometabolism, abnormal estrous behavior, atrophy of the gonads, enlargement of the pancreatic islets, increased concentration of insulin in the plasma, enhanced lipogenesis, aggressive behavior when aroused, and hypertriglyceridemia (Brobeck, 1946; Bray and York, 1971; Bernardis and Goldman, 1976; Inoue et al., 1977). Evidence has been presented that the rise in serum insulin in these lesioned animals is neurally mediated via the vagus nerves (Inoue et al., 1978). It also has been suggested that the high plasma insulin levels are the primary mechanism for the development of this obesity (Bray and Gallagher, 1975), but this hypothesis is far from established. On the basis of our limited knowledge of human obesity, it seems unlikely that this induced rat model closely resembles the common human obesities. Whether it relates to the relatively rare instances of hypothalamic obesity in man produced by traumatic injury or neoplasia remains to be explored.

The Zucker fatty rat (mutant symbol, fa) has been the major genetic rat model used for the study of obesity. This rat mutation is due to a single recessive gene

(Zucker and Zucker, 1961). The rats are hyperphagic, hyperlipidemic, and hyperinsulinemic with normal blood sugar levels (Bray and York, 1971; Bray, 1977; Martin and Gahagan, 1977). Hyperphagia appears to be the important characteristic leading to obesity in these animals, since in the early weeks of life there is little evidence of any significant decrease in physical activity. The fatty rat has an increase in both size and number of adipocytes. Glucose intolerance is not a characteristic of the fatty rat (Renold, 1968); moreover, the binding of insulin to the hepatocyte is not defective in this rat, as is the case with many models of obesity (Broer et al., 1977).

When given food ad libitum, fatty rats show identical rates of protein deposition, but greater rates of lipid and caloric deposition than their lean littermates. Of course, food intake is much greater in fatty rats. The conclusions drawn from this are: (1) food intake in the ad libitum fed fatty rat is precisely regulated with regard to the need for protein deposition and (2) the obesity is not entirely due to hyperphagia (Radcliffe and Webster, 1976). It is believed that the obesity in fatty rats relates to hypothalamic dysfunction (Bray and York, 1971), but this is far from established. Indeed, in response to the dilution of caloric value of the diet with cellulose or adulteration of the food with quinine, the fatty rat behaves more like normal rats than like rats in which the ventro-medial nuclei of the hypothalamus have been destroyed (Bray and York, 1972; Cruce et al., 1974).

An obese, spontaneously hypertensive rat has been described whose obesity results from an autosomal recessive mutation in rats originally derived from a cross between spontaneously hypertensive (SHR) and normotensive SD rats (Koletsky, 1973). This mutant has become known as the Koletsky obese or corpulent rat (gene symbol, cp). The corpulent rat has some characteristics that are similar to those manifested by the Zucker fatty rat, but it is distinct in other ways that may or may not be due to the hypertension.

The corpulent rat has the following characteristics: hyperphagia, hypertension, hypertriglyceridemia, hypercholesterolemia, proteinuria, and fasting plasma immunoreactive insulin levels 4 to 7 times that of the lean littermates (O'Dea and Koletsky, 1977). This model has been studied much less extensively than the Zucker fatty rat.

The relevance of these genetically obese rat models to the study of human obesity is difficult to assess. They do have some characteristics in common with most human obesity, but they differ with regard to others. Moreover, human obesity is rarely the result of single-gene inheritance.

It has long been known that a high fat diet will produce obesity in rats (Peckham et al., 1962). At 1 year of age, grain-fed Osborne-Mendel (OM) male rats contain 16 percent fat and the females 18 percent fat, while OM male rats fed a high fat diet had 49 percent fat and females 53 percent fat (Schemmel et al., 1969). The strain of rats has been shown to have a marked influence on the effects obtained with high fat diets; OM rats show the greatest development of obesity, S5B/Pl show the least (Schemmel et al., 1970).

Obesity can also be produced in rats by feeding highly palatable diets (Kanarek and Hirsch, 1977), such as Purina Chow plus fat enriched chow powder, sweetened condensed milk, chocolate chip cookies, salami, cheese, banana, marshmallows, milk chocolate, and peanut butter (Sclafani and Springer, 1976). Access to activity wheels reduces the extent of, but does not prevent, obesity. These rats generally are less willing to eat quinine-adulterated diets and work less for food than nonobese rats fed a Purina Chow diet. Rats with obesity induced by a high fat diet also show this "finickiness" in regard to the quality of food they are willing to ingest (Maller, 1964).

The mechanism of obesity in rats fed a high fat diet is not clear (Inoue et al., 1977). These rats do not show an increase in serum insulin or triglyceride levels, and there is no support for a peripheral endocrine or metabolic mechanism for this obesity. However, some changes in response to insulin have been observed (Susini and Lavau, 1978). This form of obesity seems to resemble the human obesity so prevalent in affluent nations; however, much more research is needed, both on the characteristics of this obese model and of human obesities, before a firm decision can be made with regard to the model's relevance.

Obesity can be produced in male SD rats by restriction of their activity (Ingle, 1949). Control rats, not restricted in physical activity and fed the same diet do not become obese. This model may well relate to the low level of physical activity that often accompanies human obesity. Unfortunately, it has been the subject of little or no further study.

Mice The mutation, yellow, is one of the oldest known single-gene mutations producing obesity in the mouse (Danforth, 1927). The mode of inheritance is well defined (Coleman, 1978). Linked to coat color, the trait is autosomal through the agouti locus of Chromosome 2. In the dominant, homozygous form (A^y/A^y), the gene is lethal in utero. The homozygous conditions of viable yellow (A^{vy}) and intermediate yellow (A^{iy}) are not lethal but produce a degree of obesity that is correlated with the degree of yellow coat coloration. These mutants are maintained on a variety of genetic backgrounds; the degree of obesity and metabolic disturbance is dependent upon the strain involved. In general, when compared to normal siblings, the metabolic and morphological aspects of the syndrome include moderate hyperphagia, hypertrophy of adipocytes, low-to-moderate levels of hyperglycemia and hyperinsulinemia, and some hypertrophy and hyperplasia of pancreatic islets (Coleman, 1978).

The mutation, obese (ob/ob), is a single-gene mutation that appears in its homozygous condition as an autosomal recessive trait on Chromosome 6 (Coleman, 1978). The mutation has been maintained on the C57BL/6J strain by inbreeding of heterozygotes because the homozygotes are infertile. Compared to normal, lean mice of this strain and to the yellow mouse, this syndrome produces marked hyperplasia and hypertrophy of adipose tissue, moderate hyperphagia and polydipsia, transient hyperglycemia and hyperinsulinemia, and hypertrophy and hyperplasia of pancreatic β cells (Coleman, 1978). The increased adiposity is observed even when the diet is strictly controlled (Alonzo and Maren, 1955).

The New Zealand obese (NZO) mouse is a product of selective breeding for obesity from heterogeneous stock (Bielschowsky and Bielschowsky, 1953). While the mode of inheritance is considered to be polygenic, it has not been mapped conclusively. The NZO mouse displays a slowly developing obesity manifested as hypertrophy of adipocytes, particularly in the abdomen, with less severe hyperglycemia but a definite age-related hyperinsulinemia perhaps resulting from the extreme hypertrophy and hyperplasia of the pancreatic islets (Coleman, 1978). The level of obesity in this model is extremely sensitive to dietary manipulations (Herberg et al., 1972).

The KK mouse is a product of selective breeding for large body size (Nakamura and Yamada, 1967). Several different lines of this mouse exist. The mode of inheritance is not known, although it is thought to be polygenic. Obesity in this strain is characteristically slow in development with moderate hyperphagia, polyuria, hyperglycemia, hyperinsulinemia, and hypertrophy and hyperplasia of pancreatic islets (Coleman, 1978).

There are other mice, such as the adipose mouse (Ad) (Falconer and Isaacson, 1959) and the PBB/Ld mouse (Hunt et al., 1976), that reportedly display symptoms of obesity, but these have not been studied as thoroughly as the aforementioned models. Such is the case with strains of hybrid mice including the C3IF$_1$ and the LAF$_1$ hybrids (Cahill et al., 1967; Dickie, 1969). In addition, new mutants are being discovered, such as the fat mouse (fat), that await further characterization (Coleman, 1978).

Gerbils Spontaneous diabetes and obesity occur in Mongolian gerbils maintained on a standard laboratory diet (Wexler et al., 1971; Wexler and Kittinger, 1963). The prevalence of obesity is about 10 percent; it begins early in life, may be temporary or lifelong, and shows a male preponderance of about 4:1. The median age of onset of obesity is 8 months and the median length of life is 24 months. It is frequently observed when these rodents are placed on unnatural diets (Burr, 1970). Obese animals may show decreased glucose tolerance, elevated serum insulin, hyperplasia of the endocrine pancreas, and cell degeneration. Glycosuria and hyperglycemia occur in only a few obese animals, however, suggesting that the endocrine pancreas has an adequate functional reserve (Burr, 1970; Nakama, 1977).

Other Animals

The use of the chicken and the pig as models for the study of obesity has recently been reviewed (Hunt, 1979).

REPRODUCTIVE DECLINE AND MENOPAUSE

Definition

Menopause, the cessation of menstruation, is the most salient event of the female climacteric, i.e., it marks

the normal end of the transition from the reproductive
to the nonreproductive stage of life. Menopause in women
is a phenomenon that generally occurs between the ages
of 40 and 55. Associated changes include:

- major decreases in plasma levels of the sex hormones, estrogen and progesterone;
- atrophic changes in target organs of the sex
hormones;
- increased plasma levels of follicle-stimulating hormone (FSH) and luteinizing hormone (LH); and
- a decrease in both the number of primordial follicles
in the ovary and their responsiveness to gonadotrophins.

Clinical and Pathological Manifestations

Cessation of menstruation, while a key sign of change in
the basic hormonal mechanisms that mediate reproduction,
does not ordinarily represent a clinical problem. Other
effects of the hormonal changes, however, are associated
with significant symptoms and changes in risk factors that
are of profound clinical importance. In the last decade
before menopause, chromosome anomalies of the newborn increase dramatically. Approximately 75 percent of menopausal women suffer from "hot flashes," and the accompanying sleep disturbance (Erlik et al., 1980) may have
secondary effects on affective and cognitive function.
In the years following the cessation of menstruation,
there is an increased incidence of a number of disorders
that are thought to be related in various degrees to the
changed hormonal status, particularly, genitourinary problems, osteoporosis, and atherosclerosis (See also the sections entitled "Atherosclerosis" and "Osteoporosis.")

Etiology and Pathogenesis

Menopause is a genetically determined event that occurs
in all women who reach sufficient age. The immediate cause
is a loss of the ovary's ability to respond to pituitary
FSH and LH stimulation with follicle growth, ovulation,
and the production of estrogen and progesterone. The underlying mechanism of this change is unknown.

There is a gradual decrease in cycle length that is related to a progressive shortening of the follicular phase,

a more rapid follicular development with regard to estrogen secretion, and an earlier occurrence of ovulation (Sherman and Korenman, 1975). In women aged 46 to 50, an elevation of FSH is noted in association with these shortened cycles. The steady depletion of oocytes (Block, 1952) occurring prior to menopause may result in a lowered secretion of inhibin with a diminished negative feedback on FSH secretion. Since the role of inhibin in the human female is not defined, the cause of these endocrine changes prior to the menopause has not been satisfactorily explained.

Immediately prior to the cessation of menses, long periods of anovulation may occur, during which both FSH and LH may be elevated. Episodes of bleeding follow intermittent declines of circulating estradiol and occasional subnormal luteal activity signaled by minor elevations of circulating progesterone. The final and most specific endocrine change accompanying cessation of menstruation is a fall of estradiol concentrations to the postmenopausal range. Both FSH and LH are then consistently elevated.

Isolated follicles are present in the ovary following menopause (Costoff and Mahesh, 1975); therefore, it is reasonable to assume that at least some of the last remaining oocytes are resistant to gonadotropin stimulation. The presence of less receptive oocytes could account for the periods of anovulation preceding menopause, since follicular maturation does not seem to occur in spite of elevated levels of gonadotropins. However, this would not be a satisfactory explanation for the earlier elevation of FSH accompanied by an apparent acceleration of estrogen synthesis by the ovary. The relationship of oocyte depletion, whether cause or effect, to these endocrine alterations is poorly understood.

The decline of negative feedback of sex steriods on hypothalamic-pituitary function results in increased pulsatile secretion of gonadotropins, most likely due to increased secretion of hypothalamic gonadotropin-releasing hormone (GnRH) (Bourguignon et al., 1979). Closely accompanying the pulsatile secretion of LH are profound changes in the peripheral control of perspiration and vascular tone that may be objectively measured in women complaining of postmenopausal "hot flashes" (Meldrum et al., 1979b). The occurrence of the subjective symptoms before any detectable peripheral changes and the physiological nature of the flushing and perspiration suggest a central hypothalamic origin of the hot flash. It has been postulated that the hot flash represents an inappropriate triggering of the normal mechanisms of heat dissipation, possibly related to changes of neurotransmitters associated with GnRH release, since some of the GnRH neurons lie in the same hypothalamic area (preoptic/ anterior) as the temperature regulation center (Tataryn et al., 1980).

Although changes involving many hormones occur, most efforts to establish a link to the clinical problems have centered on the decline in the anabolic sex steroid, estrogen. The pathogenesis of the genitourinary problems is clearly related to estrogen withdrawal, which results in atrophic changes in the vulva, vagina, and supportive structures for the bladder, rectum, and urethra. Thinning of the vaginal and vulvar epithelium, for example, may lead to a lessened resistance to irritation and discomfort during intercourse, or to infection, with resulting vaginitis. In some women, the extragonadal production of estrogen from adrenal androgen may prevent these atrophic changes; however, if the secretion is excessive, it may cause neoplastic evolution of the endometrium. This effect is enhanced by the loss of the cyclic secretion of progesterone, with its protective effect against excess estrogen stimulation. The major factor influencing the extent of peripheral aromatization of androgens appears to be obesity (Meldrum et al., 1980).

The most important health hazard of the menopause is the effect of lowered circulating estrogen on bone metabolism and secondarily on the incidence and severity of osteoporosis. Since estrogen receptors have not been found in bone, and other sex steroids affect bone resorption (Davidson et al., 1980), the effect of estrogen appears to be indirect. There are no current theories that are sufficient to explain entirely the alterations of calcium homeostasis accompanying the menopause and the therapeutic effect of exogenous estrogen, although it has been suggested that estrogen decreases the sensitivity of bone to parathyroid hormone (Atkins and Peacock, 1975). The relationship of changes in reproductive hormone levels to the risk of atherosclerosis also is unclear.

Animal Models

Although only a limited number of nonhuman primate species share the kind of menstrual cycle seen in the human female, all mammalian species exhibit a reproductive cycle mediated by hormones similar or identical to the gonadotropins and sex steroids involved in the menstrual cycle. Many of the species studied into old age undergo a failure of the reproductive cycle, which in nonmenstruating species is referred to as anestrus. Data regarding the age of onset of reproductive senescence in comparison to life span of the species are given in Table 27.

Nonhuman Primates

A number of characteristics of human menopause, such as the alterations in fertility, menstrual cyclicity, and plasma hormone levels, as well as degenerative and pathological changes in the genitourinary system, have also been observed and studied in several nonhuman primate species. The three species that have been studied most extensively--the rhesus (Macaca mulatta) and pig-tailed (Macaca nemestrina) macaques and the baboons (Papio sp.)-- all exhibit a general decline in female reproductive function with age. Manifestations of reproductive senescence

TABLE 27   Age at Reproductive Senescence

Species	Age Range Reproductive Senescence (yr)	Life Span (yr)
Rat	1.5 - 3.0[a]	3[b]
Mouse	1.0 - 2.5[a]	2.5[b]
Hamster	1.0 - 2.0[c]	3
Bushbaby	10.5 - 12.3[a]	14
Rhesus Macaque	25 - 30	33
Baboon	mid-20's	31
Chimpanzee	no record of menopause	50-60

[a]Age of anestrus
[b]Average life span
[c]Age when no more young are born

in these species include decreased conception rates in aged rhesus and baboon females (Sade et al., 1977; Lapin et al., 1979) and an increased incidence of stillbirths in aged pig-tailed macaques (Graham et al., 1979).

The perimenopausal age range in rhesus macaques that have a life span of 33 years (Bowden and Jones, 1979b) is the mid- and late 20's (van Wagenen, 1970, 1972). It is estimated that baboons, with a life span of 31 years (Bowden and Jones, 1979b), experience menopause in the mid-20's (Lapin et al., 1979). There is no corresponding age information for the pig-tailed macaque. If current estimates of maximal life span in these species are accurate, menopause occurs proportionally later in the life span than it does in the human female.

The increased variation in menstrual length and intermenstrual interval that precedes complete cessation of menses in the human female, has been observed in these three primate species (Hodgen et al., 1976, 1977; Graham et al., 1979; Lapin et al., 1979). Associated changes in sex hormone patterns, consisting of elevated levels of the gonadotropins (LH and FSH) and concomitant low serum levels of estradiol and progesterone, also have been documented in the two macaque species (Hodgen et al., 1976, 1977; Graham et al., 1979). A single menopausal pig-tailed macaque has been reported to exhibit an elevated LH level, hypertrophied anterior pituitary gonadotrophs, and a low estrone:estradiol ratio due to a low level of estradiol-17β (Graham et al., 1979). The hormonal profile of one rhesus macaque studied through the transition into menopause indicates that FSH levels are elevated, although LH, basal estrogen, and progesterone levels are normal toward the end of the last luteal phase. This suggests that regulation of FSH secretion may depend upon some factor other than these sex steroid hormones. A similar pattern has been reported as characteristic of the human female approaching menopause (Hodgen et al., 1977). These findings suggest that rhesus and pig-tailed macaques may be particularly relevant models for investigating hormonal changes that precede the menopause in primates.

Several morphological changes in the genitourinary tract related to abnormal sex hormone levels, particularly estrogen deficiency, have been reported in these primate species (Hisaw and Hisaw, 1958; van Wagenen and Simpson, 1973; Graham et al., 1979; Lapin et al., 1979). Uterine cellular atrophy has been identified in all three; the macaques also exhibit uterine glandular changes and hyalinization with vascular changes in the myometrium. Sclerosis of uterine tissue has been observed in the rhesus macaque and baboon, and adenomyosis has been reported in the pig-tailed macaque. Ovarian changes associated with the perimenopausal period, including follicular depletion, fibrosis, and vascular changes (thick-walled and convoluted blood vessels), occur in aged rhesus and pig-tailed macaques; the rhesus macaque also exhibits general ovarian atrophy with a dense stroma and inactive epithelium. Ovarian cysts have been reported in rhesus macaques and baboons (Hisaw and Hisaw, 1958; van Wagenen and Simpson, 1973; Graham et al., 1979; Lapin et al., 1979).

Clinical reports on these species provide information regarding pathological changes observed in the reproductive organs of aged females. Metastic cervical carcinoma, mammary fibroadenoma, and cervical polyps in aged rhesus females (Hisaw and Hisaw, 1958; Lapin et al., 1979); ovarian metastatic reticulosarcoma in an aged baboon; and a case of cervical polyps in an old pig-tailed macaque (Lapin et al., 1979) have been reported.

Information on reproductive senescence in other primate species is limited. Reproductive failure manifested as irregularities in the estrous cycle (i.e., variable cycle lengths, prolongation of metestrus and proestrus, and shortening of the estrus period), in addition to reduced copulation and fertility, have been reported in the greater bushbaby (Galago crassicaudatus panganiensis) females (Hendrickx and Newman, 1978). The age at onset of irregularities in the estrous cycle of this species (life span of 14 years [Cutler, 1976a; Bowden and Jones, 1979b]) is 10.5 to 12.5 years of age (Hendrickx and Newman, 1978). Although several age-related changes in reproductive capacity (Graham and McClure, 1977; Graham et al., 1979) and reproductive organ morphology (Bourne, 1975; Graham and Bradley, 1972; Graham and McClure, 1977) have been reported for the chimpanzee (Pan troglodytes), there is no record of menopause in this species (Keeling and Roberts, 1972; Bourne, 1975). Regular menstrual cyclicity and fertility continues in female chimpanzees to advanced age, i.e., 40-45 years of age; the maximum recorded life span in this species is in the early 50's. Thus, if menopause occurs at all in this species, it will appear, as in the macaque and baboon species, very late in life. It should be remembered, however, that current estimates of the maximal life span of all nonhuman primate species are based on small numbers of animals and may be unrealistically low.

The nonhuman primate also may be useful as a model for studying hot flashes. It is possible to monitor objectively the occurrence of hot flashes in women (Meldrum et al., 1979a). The similarity of heat regulation of the rhesus macaque (Johnson and Elizondo, 1979) to that of the human and the documentation of menopause in that species suggest that such an effort may be successful and will potentially allow the necessary pharmacological and neuroendocrine investigation to define this disturbance more precisely.

Although the complex interactions of the hormonal changes that occur at menopause and associated disease processes, such as atherogenesis and osteoporosis, are not understood, it has been speculated that estrogen deficiency may contribute to these and other pathological conditions of the postmenopausal female (Pelkonen, 1971; Gordon, 1977). Alteration of lipid and carbohydrate metabolism due to estrogen deficiency may be critical factors in the increased incidence of coronary heart disease observed in postmenopausal women (Pelkonen, 1971). Since estrogen deficiency and degenerative vascular changes in uterine and ovarian tissue have been reported in aged females of several nonhuman primate species, these may be relevant models for studying postmenopausal atherosclerosis.

Rodents

Rats   There are obvious differences between the estrous cycle of the rat and the menstrual cycle of primates; however, the control exerted by the hypothalamus and pituitary on ovarian function and the feedback by the ovarian hormones on hypothalamic and pituitary function appear to be very similar in these species (Talbert, 1977). For example, the hypothalamic decapeptide, LHRH, that regulates LH and FSH secretion, is the same molecule in all mammalian species tested thus far. LH and FSH have the same actions on the gonads of all mammals, inducing growth of follicles, ovulation, and formation of corpora lutea. One difference is that the hormone, prolactin, is important for maintaining progesterone secretion by the corpora lutea of rats (and mice), whereas it appears to be of relatively minor importance in maintaining progesterone secretion by the ovaries of primates. The positive feedback of estrogen (or estrogen and progesterone) on the release of LH, which normally occurs prior to ovulation, was first demonstrated in the female rat and has since been confirmed in primates and other mammals. Also, the negative feedback by estrogen and progesterone on LH and FSH secretion appears to be similar in rats and primates.

Female SD and LE rats first show irregularities in their estrous cycles at 8 to 15 months of age (Huang and Meites, 1975; Meites et al., 1978). These irregularities are characterized by lengthening of the cycle (usually the estrous phase) and, eventually, a constant estrous syndrome, with many well-developed and some cystic follicles, no corpora lutea, and estrogen secretion similar to that of the cycling rat. This constant estrous syndrome, which may last for many months, appears in the majority of aging female rats and often is followed by prolonged, repeated periods of pseudopregnancy with many corpora lutea secreting high levels of progesterone. It is not known whether ovulation occurs. In rats 2-3 years of age, the ovaries become atrophic and the uterus is infantile in appearance. These anestrous rats secrete very little estrogen or progesterone, and pituitary tumors are frequently present. The relative occurrence of constant estrus, pseudopregnancy, and anestrus may vary extensively from colony to colony (Meites et al., 1978).

There are two major differences between the anestrous female rat and the postmenopausal woman. In the rat, the ovaries appear to be capable of normal or near normal function throughout the life span, whereas the ovaries of women cease to function around midlife. Even the atrophic ovaries in rats 24 months or older can be made to function normally or near normally under appropriate gonadotropic stimulation (Meites et al., 1978). In addition, the hypothalamo-pituitary system of the rat shows a reduced capacity to secrete gonadotropins, whereas gonadotropin levels in postmenopausal women are increased. Thus, the changes in hypothalamic function in aging female rats appear to be primarily responsible for failure of the ovaries of old rats to function normally.

Many of the approaches and methods developed for studying reproductive aging changes in the female rat appear to be applicable to studies on other mammals. A principal approach has been to challenge the hypothalamus, pituitary, and ovaries by various stimuli to study their functional capacity. By use of appropriate central acting drugs (L-dopa, iproniazid), hormones (LHRH, estrogen, progesterone, ACTH), or environmental stimuli (diet, stress), it is possible to test the functional capacity of the hypothalamus and pituitary to respond by releasing LH and FSH and

of the ovaries to show follicular growth, ovulation, and
formation of corpora lutea. Such studies demonstrate important differences in the capacity of the hypothalamo-
pituitary system of old and young rats to respond to the
same stimuli and prolong or reinitiate cycling in old female rats (Meites et al., 1978).

Mice In mice and most, if not all, other mammals the de
novo formation of primordial oocytes is terminated during
fetal life and the ovary ages irreversibly thereafter
(Talbert, 1977). Mouse strains differ in their endowment
of oocytes, ranging from 9,800 to 15,300 at birth (Jones
and Krohn, 1961a). Early in postnatal life, follicular
development begins to draw on the limited stock of primary
oocytes. A major reduction of oocytes (50 percent) usually
occurs by puberty in both mice (Jones and Krohn, 1961a)
and humans (Block, 1952). This early phase of oocyte loss
is greatly attentuated by hypophysectomy (Jones and Krohn,
1961b; Edwards et al., 1977), indicating that extraovarian
endocrine factors, presumably pituitary gonadotropins, are
involved. Functional and morphological changes that occur
with aging in female mice are summarized in Table 28.

Most inbred strains maintain regular (4-5 days) ovulatory cycles and have maximum litter sizes between 4 and
8 months of age. Thereafter, litter size and cycle regu-
larity begin to decrease because of a variety of poorly
understood factors. In C57BL/6J mice, the number of implantation sites is only slightly (15 percent) lower by
11 to 12 months of age (Talbert, 1971; Holinka et al.,
1979a), with larger deficits occurring after 13 months
of age (Talbert, 1971; Parkening et al., 1978). These
data indicate that the major loss of fertility by 12 months
of age occurs despite production of nearly normal numbers
of ova at the beginning of gestation. Longitudinal studies
of the estrous cycles of C57BL/6J mice also show that cycle
length becomes progressively longer after 10 months (Nelson
et al., In press). In CBA mice, relatively larger age-
related decreases of ova, implantation sites, and corpora
lutea of pregnancy (CLP) occur by 10 months of age (Gosden,
1975; Gosden and Fowler, 1978). The cessation of cycling
follows the loss of fertility by more than 2 months (Thung
et al., 1956; Holinka et al., 1979a). In only two excep-
tional cases does the loss of fertility coincide with near
exhaustion of oocytes and developing follicles; W^x/w^v female mice have as few as 50 oocytes at birth and are rarely
fertile (Murphy, 1972), and CBA-related strains show oocyte

TABLE 28 Phenomena of Human Reproductive Aging That Occur in Inbred Mouse Strains[a]

Phenomenon	Strains
Fertility	
Fertility decreases before loss of cycles	Probably all strains
Increased stillbirths	C57BL/6J
Increased resorptions	C57BL/6J and CBA, and other strains
Increased fetal aneuploidy	CBA, C57BL/6J, NZB/J, A/J, C3H/HeJ, CF
Ovary	
Reduced number of growing follicles toward end of reproductive period	All strains
Reduced progesterone while cycles persist	C57BL/6J
Ovarian cysts	CBA
Cessation of cycles despite retention of some apparently normal primary oocytes	Most strains
Ovarian tumors	CBA
Hyperplasia of germinal epithelium or rete ovarii	$(O_{20}\text{xDBA}_f)F_1$
Uterus	
Uterine atrophy	BALB/c, C57BL/6J, A
Uterine cystic hyperplasia	DBAxCE hybrids (virgin) BALB/c
Leiomyosarcoma	BALB/c
Pituitary	
Increased tumors (probably prolactin secreting)	C57BL/6J, NZY, $(O_{20}\text{xDBA}_f)F_1$

Relatively few strains have been studied in detail; the generality of these observations is therefore unclear.

[a]Designation of mouse strains, based on recently updated, standardized nomenclature; strains cited in literature before 1950, though probably similar in most respects, cannot be assumed genetically identical with their present-day descendents (Staats, 1976). See text for citation of sources.

depletion to less than 100 oocytes when fertility and ovulatory cycles cease. The CBA mouse has been used recently
as a model for steroid replacement therapy of menopause because of its nearly complete exhaustion of oocytes (Papadaki et al., 1979). It is of interest that ovarian tumors
are frequent in both strains. In most strains, 1,000 or
more oocytes remain after the last litter (Jones and Krohn,
1961a,b), and while fertility begins to decline by 8 to
12 months of age, sporadic estrous cycles may persist for
many months (Thung et al., 1956; Nelson et al., In press).

Ovarian exchange experiments between young and old (noncycling) hosts suggest that age-related changes outside
the ovary may dicate the loss of fertility in rodents
(Jones and Krohn, 1961a, Aschheim, 1964/1965; Peng and
Huang, 1972). Old hosts fail to support regular estrous
cycles in young ovarian grafts, whereas young hosts do
support cycles in old ovaries. Further evidence for the
potential of the "postreproductive" ovary for continued
function is given by the reactivation of ovulatory cycles
by L-dopa and other adrenergic drugs, progesterone, or
stress (Finch, 1978a). Age-related deficiencies of hypothalamic catecholamine metabolism may be a factor in the
loss of regular cycles in a variety of mammals (Finch,
1972, 1978a; Quadri et al., 1973).

Reproductive senescence is evident in parameters other
than litter size and cyclicity. Fetal aneuploidy increases
strikingly with maternal age in a number of mouse strains,
particularly the CBA strain (Table 28; Gosden, 1973; Fabrikant and Schneider, 1978; Yamamoto et al., 1973). A
spectrum of aneuploidy occurs, including trisomies and
mosaics, with a 2 to 3 times increase in incidence to 60
percent by 11 to 13 months of age. Abnormal fetal morphology also can occur without evidence of aneuploidy (Fabrikant and Schneider, 1978). Stillbirths occur with an incidence of 25 percent in 11- to 12-month-old C57BL/6J mice,
compared with less than 0.5 percent at 3 to 7 months of
age (Holinka et al., 1978). A major cause of increased
stillbirths is the prolongation of gestation in aging
mothers. Prolonged gestation is associated with a delayed
preparturitional drop of progesterone (Holinka et al.,
1978) and delayed elevation of estradiol (Holinka et al.,
1979b) levels. Development of the postmature, stillborn
fetus appears normal (Holinka et al., 1979a). The inbred
mouse is, thus, a very useful model for study of the factors leading to increased birth defects and stillbirths
with increasing maternal age.

Most C57BL/6J mice, up to 12 months of age, mate successfully (Holinka et al., 1979a). Between 9 and 13 months
of age, however, ovulation and mating may desynchronize,
i.e., a larger fraction mate early, as judged by the corpus
luteum of pregnancy (CLP) morphology (Harman and Talbert,
1974). No age changes occur in the rate of ova transport
to the uterus (Harman and Talbert, 1974) or the time when
decidual swellings are first detected over this time span
(Holinka et al., 1979a). A few C57BL/6J mice, 12-15 months
of age, retain ova in their oviducts (Parkening, 1976).

Age-related changes in the hormonal stages of gestation
have been described in mice. Before day 12 of gestation,
the ovary is dependent on the pituitary hormones (Pencharz
and Long, 1933; Choudary and Greenwald, 1969). In 11- to
15-month-old C57BL/6J mice, plasma progesterone is 10-40
percent less than in younger mothers (Parkening et al.,
1978; Holinka et al., 1979a). Between days 12 and 15,
plasma P levels increase sharply to their maximum as the
CLP comes under placental control (Pencharz and Long, 1933;
Choudary and Greenwald, 1969). No age differences in the
number of CLP or in plasma progesterone or estrogen have
been found during this period in aged C57BL/6J mice (Parkening et al., 1978; Holinka et al., 1979a). These results
concur with the relative amounts of ovarian Δ^5, 3 β-steroid
dehydrogenase evaluated histochemically in pregnant C57BL/
6J mice up to 14 months of age (Albrecht et al., 1975).
After day 16, progesterone drops sharply and estradiol
rises in young, pregnant mice (McCormack and Greenwald,
1974); these changes are considered to be involved in
the normal onset of parturition at gestation day 18-19
(Goldman and Zarrow, 1973). In 11- to 12-month-old C57BL/
6J mice, the changes in progesterone and estradiol are
delayed about 2 days (Holinka et al., 1979a,b). Since
this delay corresponds to the prolongation of gestation,
and since experimental elevations of progesterone are known
to prolong gestation in young rats (Holinka et al., 1978),
delayed parturition in aging mice may result from the abnormal regulation of progesterone and estradiol.

Although estrous cycles tend to lengthen in mice at the
time fertility is dropping sharply, in most strains irregular cycles persist for months (Thung et al., 1956; Nelson
et al., In press). Significant interstrain differences
exist in the types of irregularities and final state of
the vaginal smear (Table 29). Most noncycling aging mice
have metestrous vaginal smears, i.e., cornified vaginal
epithelial cells, with varying numbers of leukocytes. This
vaginal state often is associated with polyfollicular

TABLE 29   Patterns of Vaginal Smears in Noncycling Aging
Mice

Strain	Last Age of Irregular Cycles	Major Smear Type in Noncycling Mice
C57BL[a]	20 mo	Metestrus
C57BL/6J[b]	15 mo	Metestrus
CBA[c]	12 mo	Metestrus
DBA$_f$[a]	15 mo	Diestrus
O$_{20}$[a]	20 mo	Metestrus and diestrus
(O$_{20}$xDBA$_f$)F$_1$[a]	22 mo	Metestrus and diestrus

[a]From Thung et al. (1956).
[b]From Nelson et al. (In press).
[c]From C. E. Finch, Andrus Gerontology Center, University of
Southern California, Los Angeles, Unpublished.

(polycystic) ovaries, as has been documented thoroughly
in constant metestrous rats. The trend toward longer estrous cycles is similar in some respects to the lengthening
of menstrual cycles seen as menopause approaches; the very
short cycles seen before menopause, are not seen in mice
(Collett et al., 1954; Treloar et al., 1967). It is important to be aware that occasional normal estrous cycles
may occur long after regular cycles have ceased, i.e., in
25 percent of C57BL/6J mice, 19-22 months of age (Nelson
et al., In press). Such occasional bursts of ovarian
activity may correspond to the occasional ovulations found
in menopausal women. Additionally, the patterns of cycle
loss during aging are not notably different between virgin
and repeatedly bred mice (Thung et al., 1956).

    Little is known about hormonal patterns during the phase
of irregular estrous cycles in the mouse. The preovulatory
LH surge may be delayed by 1 to 2 hours in aging rats (van
der Schoot, 1976). At proestrus, in 11- to 12-month-old
C57BL/6J mice, there are significant deficits (30 percent)
in the peak values of plasma LH and progesterone (K. F.
Flurkey, D. Gee, and C. E. Finch, Andrus Gerontology Center,
University of Southern California, Los Angeles, Unpublished). This is consistent with the age-related deficits
in progestrone observed during early gestation (see above).

In 12-month-old C57BL/6J mice with extended cycles, plasma estradiol levels are markedly lower at metestrus than the levels of young controls. Elevations in plasma estradiol at proestrus are similar in both age groups (Nelson et al., In press). Since deficits of progesterone and estradiol occur in premenopausal, still cycling women (Sherman et al., 1976), aging rodents may be useful models for altered ovarian functions in menopausal transitions.

In C57BL/6J mice, vaginal smears in 15-month-old mice (after cessation of regular cycling) typically show constant metestrus; in such mice, the plasma estradiol level is comparable to that at estrus or metestrus (10-15 pg/ml) and considerably above that in ovariectomized mice (3 pg/ml) (Felicio et al., In press). Gonadotropin levels have not been extensively studied in female mice during reproductive aging. On day 1 of gestation, (equivalent to estrous) in 12- to 15-month-old C57BL/6J mice, both LH and FSH are slightly, but not significantly, higher than in 3- to 5-month-old mice (Parkening et al., 1978). There is a slight downward trend of LH from 10 to 30 months of age in CBA and C57 mice (Gosden et al., 1978). These results concur with substantial data from aging rats, showing little change of plasma gonadotropins after cessation of cycling (Shaar et al., 1975; Huang et al., 1976a, 1978). In contrast, major increases of LH and FSH almost always occur after human menopause.

The ovaries of aging mice in constant metestrus (Table 28) show a marked decrease in the number of follicles and corpora lutea (Thung et al., 1956; Gosden et al., 1978). In DBA and C57BL mice, corpora lutea (CL) are found at ages up to 25 months, although newly formed CL are not found after 19 months of age. Ovarian cysts have been observed in some aging mice of both strains (Fekete, 1946). Extensive calcification and hyalinization of the CL is a peculiarity of DBA mice (Fekete, 1946; Thung et al., 1956); a tendency for ectopic calcification, e.g., of the myocardium, is also observed in related strains (Nabors and Ball, 1969; Rings and Waagner, 1972). Proliferative lesions, apparently deriving from the germinal epithelium or rete ovarii, occur prominantly among (O_{20} x DBA_f)F_1 hybrid mice, but are less common in other strains (Thung et al., 1956). Such proliferations are also reported in postmenopausal ovaries (Suarmo, 1952, cited by Thung et al., 1956). Massive ovarian cysts deriving from the rete ovarii tubules occur in DBA_f mice (Thung et al., 1956).

A degree of uterine atrophy involving the endometrium is common in some strains of aging mice (Table 28; Malinin and Malinin, 1972; Frantz and Kirschbaum, 1949). Similar changes in postmenopausal women are related to the major loss of sex steroids, but there are no data to support such a relationship in aging rodents. C57BL/6J mice in the constant metestrous state (14 months of age or older) have plasma estradiol levels that are definitely elevated above castrate levels, but are less than half the average level in younger mice (Felicio et al., In press).

Substantial strain differences in the uterine response to estrogens and castration (Fishman and Farmelant, 1953; Drasher, 1955) and in the vaginal response to exogenous estrogen (Muhlbock, 1947; Trentin, 1950) may reflect strain differences in extraovarian steroids or target cell function. Such variants could be useful models of human variations in vaginal atrophy after menopause (Masukawa, 1960; Lin and So-Bosita, 1972).

Hyperplastic uterine lesions also occur in some mouse genotypes during aging. In these strains, cystic hyperplasia of endometrial glands (Christie et al., 1951; Atkinson and Dickie, 1953) are apparently caused by ovarian hyperactivity (Atkinson et al., 1954). Hyperproduction of steroids is inferred, but no direct measurements are available. The vaginal epithelium and myometrium show pronounced hyperplasia. An apparently similar adenomatous, cystic hyperplasia, also is concurrent with endometrial atrophy in old BALB/c mice (Malinin and Malinin, 1972). These abnormalities, involving various types of persistent ovarian hyperactivity, could be useful models for studying the effects of some postmenopausal steroid replacement regimens, as well as for polycystic ovarian disease, which involves persistent (noncyclic) plasma levels of sex steroids with probable atypical ratios of estrogens and progesterone. Additionally, leiomyosarcomas and leiomyomas occur in 5-10 percent of 30-month-old BALB/c mice (Malinin and Malinin, 1972).

Investigators planning to use long-term ovariectomized mice should note that estrogen secreting adrenal cortical tumors are very common in some strains, e.g., DBA (Fekete et al., 1941), (CE x DBA)F_1 hybrids (Christie et al., 1951), and BALB/c, CBA, and C3H mice (Frantz and Kirschbaum, 1949). The C57BL mouse apparently does not develop such tumors (Fekete et al., 1941; Thung et al., 1956). Pituitary tumors occur spontaneously in some mouse strains during aging (Table 28; Bielschowsky et al., 1956; Thung et al., 1956; Nelson et al., In press), but have not been well characterized. Most 20- to 30-month-old C57BL/6J females have grossly enlarged pituitaries that contain hyperplastic mammatrophs (Felicio et al., In press). Such tumors are not present in male C57BL/6J mice (Finch, 1973a).

A variety of age-related changes in reproductive function occur in inbred mice during aging and offer models for investigating the spectrum of normal and pathological changes observed at menopause (summarized in Table 28). The possibility of genetic influences on human variations of menopause is readily apparent from differences between inbred mouse strains.

Hamsters   Reproductive function in Syrian hamsters declines between 13 and 17 months of age. Most females beyond this age have lost the ability to bear litters. Unilateral ovariectomy accelerates reproductive decline (Blaha, 1964a). Syrian hamsters continue to have regular estrous cycles up to at least 23 months of age, throughout the period of declining reproduction, and beyond the time of total loss of litter-bearing ability. Exceptions are females that cycle irregularly or become acyclic secondary to disease; these are comparable to the sick, anestrous rats noted by Aschheim (1976). Syrian hamsters do not manifest constant estrus or repetitive pseudopregnancies, as reported for aging female rats and mice. Mean plasma progesterone levels during various phases of the estrous cycle and pregnancy do not differ significantly between young and old female hamsters, but the variance increases (Blaha and Leavitt, 1974).

The stages of reproductive decline in female Syrian hamsters can be defined in terms of the outcome of matings (Blaha, 1964a). Pregnancies of females in the earliest stage generally proceed to full term but end in resorption of the fetuses or stillbirths. In old females with delayed delivery, there is a continuation of luteal progesterone secretion (Blaha and Leavitt, 1974) instead of the luteolysis that normally occurs at day 15. After 15 months of age, a more common outcome of mating is pseudopregnancy or resorption of conceptuses before 12 days of gestation. There are multiple problems at this stage involving almost every step of the reproductive process including ovulation, fertilization, ovum transport, implantation, and uterine accommodation. Perhaps most important is a delay of 2-5 hours in the time before 60 percent of ova are fertilized in old (14-17 months) as opposed to young hamsters (Parkening and Soderwall, 1975). This does not result from delayed ovulation, but rather from a prolonged time for penetration of the zona pellucida and vitellus by the spermatozoon. Also, about 40 percent of ova in females of this age group are infertile, abnormal, or degenerating at the time of implantation. Studies on experimentally delayed fertilization in young Syrian hamsters have shown that delay can lead to ovum degeneration or abnormality (Yanagimachi and Chang, 1961) and chromosomal anomalies (Yamamoto and Ingalls, 1972).

Morulae have been transferred from the uteri of young to those of old Syrian hamsters and vice versa. Both uteri and ova from old females show significant deficiency compared to those of young controls (Blaha, 1964b). Blastocyst development and uterine reaction are delayed by 12 hours in 14- to 15-month-old females compared to females 3 to 5 months of age (Parkening and Soderwall, 1973). Decidual cells and glycogen first appear at 96 hours postovulation in young pregnant hamsters, but are not found until 108 to 120 hours in older animals (Thorpe and Conners, 1975). Delay of the complete response by a full day may be detrimental to the conceptus.

The capacity of uteri in young and old hamsters to develop progesterone receptors has been compared in estradiol-treated, ovariectomized animals. Uteri of old animals develop progesterone receptor activity comparable to that seen in young ones (Blaha and Leavitt, 1978). The heavier old uteri have significantly lower progesterone receptor activity, however, on a per unit weight basis.

There are a number of ways that the aging Syrian hamster may serve as a model in studies of reproductive decline and menopause. It may be relevant for the study of ovarian abnormalities, delayed fertilization, and delayed delivery. Although it is not clear if the latter two are prevalent in aging human females, it has been suggested that delayed fertilization increases with age because of the reduced frequency of intercourse. This delayed fertilization is postulated to increase the risk of Down's Syndrome and other karyotypic abnormalities (German, 1968). Studies on the regulation of uterine steroid hormone receptors are easily performed on this animal, and it also may be useful for studying the problems encountered in steroid hormone replacement therapy.

BENIGN PROSTATIC HYPERPLASIA

Definition and Clinical Manifestations

Benign prostatic hyperplasia (BPH) is the proliferation
of stromal and/or glandular prostatic elements into mul-
tifocal nodules, which results in increased size of the
prostate gland. This enlargement compresses the urethra
resulting in urinary obstruction, secondary infection,
and renal failure. Five different histological types of
benign prostatic hyperplasia have been categorized
(Franks, 1954): stromal, fibromuscular, muscular, fibro-
adenomatous, and fibromyoadenomatous. Adenomatous nodules
also occur. The relative frequencies of the different
types are unknown, although there is general agreement
that the most common lesions are those of the fibroadeno-
matous type.
   The condition is one of the most frequent disorders
of aging men. Over 60 percent of men between the ages
of 40 and 49, and virtually all men over the age of 70,
have histopathological signs of the disorder (Harbitz and
Haugen, 1972); about 50 percent show symptoms. The usual
symptoms are dysuria, incontinence, and urinary tract obstruction with acute and/or chronic urinary retention.
About 10 percent of men with BPH require surgery for relief of obstruction.

Etiology and Pathogenesis

The etiology of BPH is presently unclear. It is age-
related and does not occur in the absence of testes.
Age-related changes in testicular steroidogenic function
include reduced plasma testosterone concentration, elevated plasma estradiol-testosterone ratio, increased
plasma gonadotrophin concentration, and elevated plasma
testosterone-binding globulin concentration. However, the
specific role of the testis in the development of BPH is
unknown.

Animal Models

Nonhuman Primates

The prostate gland of nonhuman primates (Hill, 1960) consists of two distinct lobes: the cranial and caudal lobes.

The cranial lobe lies at the neck of the bladder, surrounding the ductus deferens and ducts of the seminal vesicles. The caudal lobe is smooth and only partially surrounds the urethra. It has been suggested (Blacklock and Bouskill, 1977) that the cranial and caudal prostate lobes of the rhesus macaque (Macaca mulatta) are homologous, respectively, to the central and peripheral zones of man. The rhesus cranial lobe resembles the human central zone histologically, consisting of large, irregularly branching tubules with a prominent, dense fibromuscular stroma. The acini of the caudal lobe like those of the human peripheral zone are smaller and consist of simple straight tubules with a more regular appearance. The stroma of the caudal lobe is more delicate and loose compared to that of the cranial lobe. The ultrastructure of the prostate of the immature and mature rhesus macaque is homologous to that of man (Battersby et al., 1977), as is the androgen responsiveness (Ghanadian et al., 1977a,b,c). Similarities in metabolism and certain histochemical parameters of humans and nonhuman primates also have been described (Müntzing et al., 1975, 1976; Sufrin et al., 1975).

Although the incidence of BPH in nonhuman primates is not known, there have been case reports documenting the occurrence of prostatic adenomas in a lemur (Lemur sp.) and a dusky titi (Callicebus moloch) (Roberts, 1972); cystic prostatic hyperplasia in feral baboons (Papio sp.) (McConnell et al., 1974); and BPH in a rhesus macaque (Roberts, 1972), a squirrel monkey (Saimiri sciureus) (Adams and Bond, 1979), and a patas monkey (Erythrocebus patas) (M. R. Adams, Department of Comparative Medicine, Bowman Gray School of Medicine, Winston-Salem, North Carolina, Unpublished). In the squirrel monkey, diagnosis was based on the presence of a diffusely enlarged prostate gland containing numerous nodules, consisting of epithelial and stromal elements, located primarily in the periphery of both cranial and caudal lobes. Some nodules in the cranial lobe adjacent to the periurethral area were characterized by dilation of some acini and reduction in the height of acinar epithelium.

Although they virtually have been unevaluated in this area, the nonhuman primates with their close phylogenetic and anatomic relationships to man are potentially relevant as models of BPH. Systematic studies in large populations of aging nonhuman primates are now possible and are needed to determine their usefulness.

Carnivores

Prostatic hyperplasia is a common disease of adult and
aged dogs. No reports of the disease in cats have been
found. Some investigators (Schlotthauer, 1932; Bloom,
1954b) believe that essentially all male dogs over 5
years of age have some degree of prostatic hyperplasia.
The mean age of those presented for treatment is 9 years.
As in man, the first sign of the disorder is often difficult urination, but also the dog frequently exhibits
signs of difficult defecation. Complicated prostatic
hyperplasia appears to be more common in the dog than in
man; dogs frequently develop prostatitis and/or abscesses
(Campbell and Lawson, 1963; Borthwick and MacKenzie, 1971;
Hornbuckle et al., 1978).

In uncomplicated hyperplasia, the prostate gland of
the dog usually is symmetrically enlarged. On cut surfaces, the parenchyma is whitish to yellow in color with
a soft to moderately firm consistency. Most glands contain cysts that vary in size from less than 1 mm to over
1 cm in diameter. In contrast to the nodular lesions in
man (Mostofi and Price, 1973d), those of the dog are generally diffuse, although in mild cases, the hyperplasia
may be focal at the microscopic level. There is one report (Koltman, 1935) that prostatic hyperplasia in the
dog begins in the periurethral portion of the gland, the
most frequent site of the characteristic nodular lesion
in man; however, this has not been confirmed (Berg,
1958b).

Microscopically, the prostatic lesion in the dog is
characterized by papillary proliferation of the glandular
epithelium and cystic dilation of adjacent alveoli (Huggins and Clark, 1940; Berg, 1958b; Leav and Cavazos,
1975). The epithelium of the hyperplastic alveoli generally is composed of a single cell layer of well-differen-
tiated, columnar cells; however, in cystic areas, atrophic
and flattened epithelial cells are common. The alveoli
and small cysts contain abundant proteinaceous secretory
material and, occasionally, sloughed epithelial cells and
macrophages. The fibromuscular stroma may be hyperplastic.
In dogs, glandular hyperplasia usually predominates; in
man, stromal hyperplasia usually is present (Mostofi and
Price, 1973d). In addition, in dog prostates there are
infiltrates of lymphocytes, plasma cells, and a small number of histiocytes in the alveolar interstitium and stroma.
Neutrophils, when present, are associated with secondary
prostatitis (Jubb and Kennedy, 1963).

The etiology of prostatic hyperplasia in the dog is not known, but testicular hormones are considered important in its development. Castration is curative (Hornbuckle et al., 1978), and estrogen causes regression of the lesion (Berg, 1958b). Hyperplastic prostates from both men and dogs have been shown to contain up to 5 times more dihydrotestosterone than normal glands (Gloyna et al., 1970; Siiteri and Wilson, 1970; Lloyd et al., 1975), and the rate of conversion of testosterone to dihydrotestosterone is accelerated.

Attempts have been made to induce BPH in the dog. Prostatic weight is increased by the administration of dihydrotestosterone to castrated dogs (Gloya et al., 1970; Walsh and Wilson, 1976); however, the histological features and enlargement of the gland are not characteristic of the spontaneous disease. Administration of both dihydrotestosterone and estradiol also fails to produce typical lesions. Typical BPH can be induced in all dogs within one year using a combination of androstanediol (a testicular androgen) and estradiol. Using androstanediol alone produces changes characteristic of BPH in approximately 50 percent of dogs (Walsh and Wilson, 1976).

Prostatic hyperplasia of the dog represents a useful, but not an identical model of BPH in man. The lesion is diffuse rather than focal or nodular, and glandular hyperplasia is more common than stromal hyperplasia. From the standpoint of etiology and pathogenesis, however, the lesions are very similar in man and dog. Elevated concentrations of dihydrotestosterone and increased rates of conversion of testosterone to dihydrotestosterone are found in diseased glands of both species. The extremely high frequency of spontaneous disease and the ability to induce the condition in the dog provides a readily available source of case materials and an opportunity for studies under controlled experimental conditions.

Rodents

The prostate of the male mouse or rat is a compound tubuloacinar gland consisting of three pairs of anatomically distinct lobes. The collecting ducts of a discrete pair of ventral lobes enter the ventral surface of the urethra at the base of the bladder. A pair of anterior lobes (coagulating glands) are bound to the seminal vesicles and their ducts enter the urethra posteriorly. A complex group of tubuloacinar glands surround the urethra at the base of the bladder to form the dorsolateral prostate, the ducts of which enter the urethra laterally at the common junction of dorsal and lateral prostatic ducts. Embryological similarities have been indicated for the dorsal and lateral lobes of the male rat and human prostate (Price, 1963). However, recent studies suggest these similarities may be more apparent than real (McNeal, 1972), and it appears that morphological homologies are limited to the male rat anterior prostate and the human prostate central zone (McNeal, 1976). Well-developed prostate glands are present in immature and adult female Arvicanthis cinereus (Rauther, 1909), Rattus norvegicus (Marx, 1931), Praomys (Mastomys) natalensis (Mastomys erythroleucus Temm; Brambell and Davis, 1941), Apodemus sylvaemus sylvaticus (Raynaud, 1942), and Microtus arvalis P. (Delost, 1953).

Obstructive benign prostatic hyperplasia has not been reported to occur in mouse or rat prostate. Nonobstructive papillary hyperplasia has been observed in prostates of aged (16- to 33-month-old) female mastomys (Snell and Stewart, 1965). In these lesions, branching papillomas composed of columnar to cuboidal epithelium with basally polar nuclei occluded many acini. The hyperplasias were frequently associated with spontaneous prostatic adenocarcinomas. Nonobstructive atypical hyperplasia has been observed in the ventral prostates of aged (33- to 46-month-old) male AXC rats (Shain et al., 1979). The glandular epithelium of the atypical hyperplasias was irregularly thickened by increased numbers of epithelial cells with slightly enlarged pleomorphic nuclei. Many cells with swollen, foamy, intensely PAS-positive cytoplasm and condensed eccentric nuclei were interspersed throughout the atypical epithelium. Basilar nuclear polarity, typical of normal prostate acinar epithelium, was absent in atypical epithelium. Atypical hyperplasia was frequently found in close association with spontaneous adenocarcinoma of the ventral prostate of the AXC rat (Shain et al., 1979). Stromal hyperplasia was not a component of the hyperplastic lesions in the prostates of either female mastomys (Snell and Stewart, 1965) or male AXC rats (Shain et al., 1979).

Chronic estrogenization of male mice has been employed as an experimental approach to the induction of BPH in the rodent (Lacassagne, 1933; Burrows and Kennaway, 1934; Fingerhut and Veenema, 1966; Caine and Superstine, 1973).

The treatment produces hyperplasia of the posterior urethra and bladder neck with resultant urinary retention,
hydroureter, and hydronephrosis. Histological changes
include stromal hyperplasia, cystic dilation of prostatic acini, and squamation of glandular epithelium (Burrows and Kennaway, 1934; Fingerhut and Veenema, 1966).
Chronic androgenization of male rats with 5 α-dihydrotes-
tosterone or testosterone causes marked prostatic enlargement and papillary hyperplasia (Gloyna and Wilson, 1969;
McGuire et al., 1973). Treatment with 5 α-dihydrotestos-
terone caused infrequent increases in connective tissue
in one study (Gloyna and Wilson, 1969), but not in a second study (McGuire et al., 1973).

Morphologically, the prostate of the mouse and rat is
not similar to that of man. Nonobstructive hyperplasia
is found in prostates of aged mice and rats; however, the
lesions do not involve proliferation of stromal components, are frequently associated with prostatic adenocarcinomas, and may be a type of preneoplastic transformation. To date, hormonal manipulations have failed to
produce stromal hyperplasia in mouse or rat prostate that
is reminiscent of human BPH. The rodent does not appear
to be a useful model for studies of benign prostatic
hyperplasia.

References

Aaron, J.E., J.C. Gallagher, and B.E.C. Nordin. 1974. Seasonal variations of histological osteomalacia in femoral neck fractures. Lancet 2:84-85.

Abercrombie, M. 1946. Estimation of nuclear population from microtome sections. Anat. Rec. 94:238-248.

Ackerman, N.R., R. Corkey, and D. Perkins. 1978. Pathogenesis of papain-induced emphysema in the hamster. Inflammation 3:49-58.

Adams, M.R., and M.G. Bond. 1979. Benign prostatic hyperplasia in a squirrel monkey (Saimiri sciureus). Lab. Anim. Sci. 29(5):674-676.

Adams, P.H., and J. Jowsey. 1965. Sodium fluoride in the treatment of osteoporosis and other bone diseases. Ann. Intern. Med. 63:1151-1155.

Adams, R.A., H.A. Zander, and A.M. Polson. 1979. Cell populations in the transseptal fiber region before, during and after experimental periodontitis in squirrel monkeys. J. Periodontol. 50:7-12.

Adelman, R.C. 1970. An age-dependent modification of enzyme regulation. J. Biol. Chem. 245:1032-1035.

Adelman, R.C. 1975. Disruptions in enzyme regulation during aging. Basic Life Sci. 6:304-311.

Adelman, R.C. 1976. Age-dependent functional capacities of the mammalian cell. Interdiscip. Top. Gerontol. 9:2-7.

Adelman, R.C. 1979. Loss of adaptive mechanisms during aging. Fed. Proc. 38:1968-1971.

Adelman, R.C., G. Stein, G.S. Roth, and D. Englander. 1972. Age-dependent regulation of mammalian DNA synthesis and cell proliferation in vivo. Mech. Ageing Dev. 1:49-59.

Adelman, R.C., G.W. Britton, S. Rotenberg, L. Ceci, and K. Karoly. 1978. Endocrine regulation of enzyme

activity in aging animals of different genotypes.
Pages 355-364 in D. Bergsma and D.E. Harrison, eds.
Genetic effects on aging. Birth defects original ar-
ticle series. Vol. 14, No. 1. A.R. Liss, Inc., New
York.

Adler, W.H. 1975. Aging and immune function. Bioscience.
25:652-657.

Agress, C.M., M.J. Rosenberg, H.I. Jacobs, M.J. Binder, A.
Schneiderman, and W.G. Clark. 1952. Protracted shock
in the closed-chest dog following coronary embolization
with graded microspheres. Am. J. Physiol. 170:536-549.

Aguirre, G.D. 1976. Inherited retinal degenerations in
the dog. Trans. Am. Acad. Ophthalmol. Otolaryngol.
81:OP 667-676.

Aguirre, G.D., and A. Laties. 1976. Pigment epithelial
dystrophy in the dog. Exp. Eye Res. 23:247-256.

Ahlstedt, S., and H. Rylander. 1975. Immunoradiometric
assay for quantification of serum antibodies to dental
plaque in immunized dogs. J. Periodontal Res.
10:224-229.

Akiskal, H.S., and W.T. McKinney. 1975. Overview of recent research on depression. Arch. Gen. Psychiat.
32:285-305.

Albrecht, E.D., R.D. Koos, and W.B. Wehrenberg. 1975.
Ovarian Δ^5-3β-hydroxysteroid dehydrogenase and cholesterol in the aged mouse during pregnancy. Biol. Reprod.
13:158-162.

Alexander, N.J., and T.B. Clarkson. 1978. Vasectomy increases the severity of diet-induced atherosclerosis
in Macaca fascicularis. Science 201:538-541.

Aleksandrovskaia, M.M., and G.I. Shirkova. 1960. Histological and functional changes in the central nervous
system of an old monkey (M. mulatta). Trudy Instituta
Vyeshei Nervoi Deiatel'nostri: Seria Fiziolog.
5:238-249.

Alffram, P.H. 1964. An epidemiologic study of cervical
and intertrochanteric fractures of the femur in an urban
population. Acta Orthop. Scand. Suppl. 65:1-109.

Allanson, M. 1970. Gerbils. Pages 237-243 in E.S.S.
Hafez, ed. Reproduction and breeding techniques in
laboratory animals. Lea and Febiger, Philadelphia.

Allen, G.M. 1940. The mammals of China and Mongolia.
Vol. 11, Part 2. American Museum of Natural History,
New York. 1350 p.

Alonzo, L.G., and T.H. Maren. 1955. Effect of food restriction on body composition of hereditary obese mice.
Am. J. Physiol. 183:284-290.

Alspauth, M.A., and G.L. Van Hoosier. 1973. Naturally
occurring and experimentally-induced arthritides in rodents: A review of the literature. Lab. Anim. Sci.
23:724-742.

Altman, N.A., and D.G. Goodman. 1979. Neoplastic dis-
eases. Pages 333-376 in H.J. Baker, J.R. Lindsey, and
S.H. Weisbroth, eds. The laboratory rat. Vol. 1.
Biology and diseases. Academic Press, New York.

Altmann, J., S.A. Altmann, G. Hausfater, and S.A. McCuskey.
1977. Life history of yellow baboons: Physical development, reproductive parameters and infant mortality.
Primates 18:315-330.

Alvord, E., L. Forno, J. Kusske, R.J. Kauffman, J.S.
Rhoades, and C.R. Goetowski. 1974. The pathology of
parkinsonism: A comparison of degenerations in cerebral
cortex and brainstem. Adv. Neurol. 5:175-193.

American College of Chest Physicians--American Thoracic
Society Joint Committee on Pulmonary Nomenclature. 1975.
Pulmonary terms and symbols. Chest 67:583-593.

American Thoracic Society. 1962. Chronic bronchitis,
asthma, and pulmonary emphysema: A statement by the
Committee on Diagnostic Standards for Non-tuberculous
Respiratory Diseases. Am. Rev. Respir. Dis. 85:762-768.

American Thoracic Society. 1978. Health effects of air
pollution. Am. Thorac. Soc. News 4:22-63.

Ammons, W.F., L.R. Schectman, and R.C. Page. 1972. Host
tissue response in chronic periodontal disease. I. The
normal periodontium and clinical manifestations and
periodontal disease in the marmoset. J. Periodontal
Res. 7:131-143.

Andersen, A.C. 1957. Puppy production to the weanling
age. J. Am. Vet. Med. Assoc. 130:151-158.

Andersen, A.C. 1958. A comparison of Beagles released
for private ownership with those maintained under kennel
conditions. J. Am. Vet. Med. Assoc. 132:95-96.

Andersen, A.C. 1965. Reproduction ability of female
Beagles in relationship to advancing age. Exp. Gerontol.
1:189-192.

Andersen, A.C. [ed.] 1970. The Beagle as an experimental
dog. Iowa State University Press, Ames, Iowa. 616 p.

Andersen, A.C., and L.S. Rosenblatt. 1965. Survival of
dogs under natural and laboratory conditions. Exp.
Gerontol. 1:193-199.

Andersen, A.C., and L.S. Rosenblatt. 1969. The effects
of whole-body x-irradiation on the median life span
of female dogs (Beagles). Radiat. Res. 39:177-220.

Andersen, A.C., and F.T. Shultz. 1958. Inherited (congenital) cataract in the dog. Am. J. Pathol. 34:965-975.

Andersen, A.C., and M.E. Simpson. 1973. The ovary and reproductive cycle of the dog (Beagle). Geron-X, Inc., Los Altos, California. 290 p.

Anderson, C., and K.D. Danylchuk. 1979a. Studies on bone remodeling rates on the Beagle: A comparison between similar biopsy sites on different ribs. Am. J. Vet. Res. 40:294-296.

Anderson, C., and K.D. Danylchuk. 1979b. Age-related variations in cortical bone-remodeling measurements in male beagles 10 to 26 months of age. Am. J. Vet. Res. 40:869-873.

Anderson, K.V., and W.K. O'Steen. 1972. Black-white and pattern discrimination in rats without photoreceptors. Exp. Neurol. 34(3):446-454.

Anderson, K.V., and W.K. O'Steen. 1974. Altered response latencies on visual discrimination tasks in rats with damaged retinas. Physiol. Behav. 12:633-637.

Andrew, W. 1961. Aging changes in the alimentary tract. Pages 63-69 in G.H. Bourne and E.M.H. Wilson, eds. Structural aspects of aging. Hafner Publishing Company, New York.

Andrews, E.J., B.C. Ward, and N.H. Altman [eds.] 1979. Spontaneous animal models of human disease. Vols. I and II. Academic Press, New York. 646 p.

Antischkow, N., and S. Chalatow. 1913. Über experimentelle Cholesterinsteatose und ihre Bedeutung für die Entstehung einiger pathologischer Prozesse. Zentrabl. Allg. Pathol. 24:1-9.

Anver, M.R., and B.J. Cohen. 1976. Ulcerative colitis induced in guinea pigs with degraded carrageenan. Am. J. Pathol. 84(2):431-434.

Anver, M.R., and B.J. Cohen. 1979. Lesions associated with aging. Pages 377-399 in H.J. Baker, J.R. Lindsey, and S.H. Weisbroth, eds. The laboratory rat. Vol. 1. Biology and diseases. Academic Press, New York.

Aoi, W., and M.H. Weinberger. 1976. The effect of age and norepinephrine on renin release by rat kidney slices in vitro. Proc. Soc. Exp. Biol. Med. 151(1): 47-52.

Appel, S.H. 1974. Brain macromolecular synthesis and aging. Pages 93-102 in G.J. Maletta, ed. Survey report on the aging nervous system. DHEW Pub. No. (NIH) 74-296. U.S. Department of Health, Education, and Welfare, Washington, D.C.

Archibald, J. [ed.] 1974. Canine surgery. 2nd ed. American Veterinary Publications, Inc., Santa Barbara, California. 1172 p.

Arenberg, D., and E.A. Robertson-Tchabo. 1977. Learning and aging. Pages 421-449 in J.E. Birren and K.W. Schaie, eds. Handbook of the psychology of aging. Van Nostrand Reinhold, New York.

Armstrong, M.L., and M.B. Megan. 1974. Responses of two macaque species to atherogenic diet and its withdrawal. Pages 336-338 in G. Schettler and A. Weizel, eds. Atherosclerosis III. Springer-Verlag, Berlin.

Armstrong, M.L., W.E. Connor, and E.D. Warner. 1969. Tissue cholesterol concentration in the hypercholesterolemic rhesus monkey. Arch. Pathol. 87:87-92.

Armstrong, M.L., E.D. Warner, and W.E. Connor. 1970. Regression of coronary atheromatosis in rhesus monkeys. Circ. Res. 27:59-67.

Arnold, L., and P. Baram. 1973. Periodontal disease in chimpanzees. J. Periodontol. 44:437-442.

Arrington, L.R., T.C. Beaty, Jr., and K.C. Kelly. 1973. Growth, longevity and reproductive life of the Mongolian gerbil. Lab. Anim. Sci. 23:262-265.

Asaro, J.P., R. Nisengard, E.H. Beutner, and M. Neiders. 1978. Experimental periodontal disease: Reverse passive arthus reactions. Clin. Immunol. 9:398-407.

Aschheim, P. 1964/1965. Résultats fournis par la greffe hétérochrone des ovaires dans l'étude de la régulation hypothalamo-hypophyso-ovarienne de la ratte sénile. Gerontologia 10:65-75.

Aschheim, P. 1976. Aging in the hypothalamic-hypophyseal-ovarian axis in the rat. Pages 376-418 in A.V. Everitt and J.A. Burgess, eds. Hypothalamus, pituitary, and aging. Charles C. Thomas, Springfield, Illinois.

Aslan, A., A. Vrabiescu, C. Domilescu, L. Câmpeanu, M. Costiniu, and S. Stanescu. 1965. Long-term treatment with procaine. (Gerovital H_3) in albino rats. J. Gerontol. 20:1-8.

Assali, N.S., L.D. Longo, and L. Holm. 1960. Toxemia-like syndromes in animals, spontaneous and experimental. Obstet. Gynecol. Surv. 15:151-181.

Astle, C.M., and D.E. Harrison. 1976. Mitogen synergism in low-responding CBA/CaJ mice. Cell. Immunol. 21:192-197.

Atkins, D., and M. Peacock. 1975. A comparison of the effects of the calcitonins, steroid hormones and thyroid hormones on the response of bone to parathyroid hormone in tissue culture. J. Endocrinol. 64:573-583.

Atkinson, W.B., and M.M. Dickie. 1953. Further studies on the pathogenesis of uterine lesions in DBA x CE and reciprocal hybrid mice. Cancer Res. 13:165-167.

Atkinson, W.B., M.M. Dickie, and E. Fekete. 1954. Effects of breeding on the development of ovarian, adrenal, and uterine lesions in DBA x CE and reciprocal hybrid mice. Endocrinology 55:316-326.

Attström, R. 1970. Presence of leukocytes in crevices of healthy and chronically inflamed gingivae. J. Periodontal Res. 5:42-47.

Attström, R., and U. Larsson. 1974. Effect of decomplementation by carragheenan on the emigration of neutrophils and monocytes into dog gingival crevices. J. Periodontal Res. 9:165-175.

Attström, R., and H.E. Schroeder. 1979. Effect of experimental neutropenia on initial gingivitis in dogs. Scand. J. Dent. Res. 87:7-23.

Attström, R., A.-B. Laurell, U. Larsson, and A. Sjoholm. 1975. Complement factors in gingival crevice material from healthy and inflamed gingiva in humans. J. Periodontal Res. 10:19-27.

Auskaps, A.M., O.P. Gupta, and J.H. Shaw. 1957. Periodontal disease in the rice rat. III. Survey of dietary influences. J. Nutr. 63:325-343.

Autrup, H., L.A. Barrett, F.E. Jackson, M.L. Jesudason, G. Stoner, P. Phelps, B.F. Trump, and C.C. Harris. 1977. Explant culture of human colon. Gastroenterology 74:1248-1257.

Avery, B.E., and D.M. Simpson. 1973. The baboon as a model system for the study of periodontal disease; clinical and light microscopic observations. J. Periodontol. 44:675-686.

Avioli, L.V. 1977. Osteoporosis: Pathogenesis and therapy. Pages 307-388 in L.V. Avioli and S.M. Krane, eds. Metabolic bone disease. Vol. 1. Academic Press, New York.

Axelsson, A. 1968. The vascular anatomy of the cochlea in the guinea pig and in man. Acta Otolaryngol. Suppl. 243:1-134.

Baer, P.N., and J.E. Lieberman. 1959. Observation on some genetic characteristics of the periodontium in three strains of inbred mice. Oral Surg. Oral Med. Oral Pathol. 12:820-829.

Baer, P.N., and J.E. Lieberman. 1960. Periodontal disease in six strains of inbred mice. J. Dent. Res. 39:215-225.

Baer, P.N., and C.L. White. 1960. Studies on periodontal disease in the mouse. 1. Effect of age, sex, cage factor, diet. J. Periodontol. 31:27-30.

Baer, P.N., L.B. Crittenden, G.E. Jay, Jr., and J.E. Lieberman. 1961. Studies on periodontal disease in the mouse. II. Genetic and maternal effects. J. Dent. Res. 40:23-33.

Bailey, D.W. 1978. Sources of subline divergence and their relative importance for sublines of six inbred strains of mice. Pages 197-215 in H.C. Morse III, ed. Origins of inbred mice. Academic Press, New York.

Bailey, D.W. 1979. Definition of inbred strains. Pages 4-7 in P.L. Altman and D.D. Katz, eds. Inbred and genetically defined strains of laboratory animals. Part 1. Mouse and rat. Federation of American Societies for Experimental Biology, Bethesda, Maryland.

Bailey, I., L.S.C. Griffith, J. Rouleau, H. W. Strauss, and B. Pitt. 1977. Thallium-201 myocardial perfusion imaging at rest and during exercise: Comparative sensitivity to electrocardiography in coronary artery disease. Circulation 55:79-87.

Baird, M.B., J.A. Zimmerman, H.R. Massie, and H.V. Samis. 1974. Response of liver and kidney catalase to clofibrate in C57BL/6J male mice of different ages. Gerontologia 20:169-178.

Baird, M.B., R.J. Nicolosi, H.R. Massie, and H.V. Samis. 1975. Microsomal mixed-function oxidase activity and senescense. I. Hexobarbital sleep time and induction of components of the hepatic microsomal enzyme system in rats of different ages. Exp. Gerontol. 10(2):89-99.

Baker, H.J., J.R. Lindsey, and S.H. Weisbroth [eds.] 1979. The laboratory rat. Vol. I. Biology and diseases. Academic Press, New York. 435 p.

Balazs, T., and L. Rubin. 1971. A note on the lens in aging Sprague-Dawley rats. Lab. Anim. Sci. 21:267-268.

Balazs, T., S. Ohtake, and J.F. Noble. 1970. Spontaneous lenticular changes in the rat. Lab. Anim. Care 20:215-219.

Balk, M.W., C.M. Lang, W.J. White, and B.L. Munger. 1975. Exocrine pancreatic dysfunction in guinea pigs with diabetes mellitus. Lab. Invest. 32:28-32.

Ball, M.J. 1977. Neuronal loss, neurofibrillary tangles and granuovacuolar degeneration in the hippocampus with aging and dementia. Acta Neuropathol. 37:111-112.

Ball, M.J. 1978. Histotopography of cellular changes in Alzheimer's disease. Pages 89-104 in K. Nandy, ed. Senile dementia: A biomedical approach. Vol. 3.

Developments in neuroscience. Elsevier North-Holland
Biomedical Press, New York.

Ball, M.J., and P. Lo. 1977. Granulovacuolar degeneration in the ageing brain and in dementia. J. Neuropathol. Exp. Neurol. 36:474-487.

Balls, M., D. Brown, and N. Fleming. 1976. Long-term
amphibian organ culture. Meth. Cell Biol. 13:213-238.

Barden, H. 1975. The histochemical relationships and the
nature of neuromelanism. Pages 79-117 in H. Brody,
D. Harman, and J.M. Ordy, eds. Clinical, morphologic,
and neurochemical aspects in the aging central nervous
system. Vol. 1. Aging series. Raven Press, New York.

Barlow, C.H., and B. Chance. 1976. Ischemic areas in per-
fused rat hearts: Measurement by NADH fluorescence photography. Science 193:909-910.

Barlow, C.H., A.H. Harken, and B. Chance. 1977. Evaluation of cardiac ischemia by NADH fluorescence photography. Ann. Surg. 186:737-740.

Barnes, C.A. 1979. Memory deficits associated with senescence: A neurophysiological and behavioral study
in the rat. J. Comp. Physiol. Psychol. 93:74-104.

Barnett, K.C. 1978. Hereditary cataract in the dog.
J. Small Anim. Pract. 19:109-120.

Barnett, T.B. 1972. Chronic bronchitis and pulmonary emphysema. Pages 632-664 in C.W. Holman and C. Muschen-
heim, eds. Bronchopulmonary diseases and related disorders. Vol. 2. Harper and Row, New York.

Baroldi, G., O. Mantero, and G. Scomazzoni. 1956. The
collaterals of the coronary arteries in normal and
pathologic hearts. Circ. Res. 4:223-229.

Barrows, C.H., Jr., and G. Kokkonen. 1975. Protein synthesis, development, growth and life span. Growth
39:525-533.

Barrows, C.H., Jr., and G.C. Kokkonen. 1977. Relationship
between nutrition and aging. Pages 253-335 in H.H.
Draper, ed. Advances in nutritional research. Vol. I.
Plenum Publishing Corp., New York.

Barrows, C.H., Jr., and L.M. Roeder. 1965. The effect of
reduced dietary intake on enzymatic activities and life
span. J. Gerontol. 20:69-71.

Barrows, C.H., Jr., and L.M. Roeder. 1977. Nutrition.
Pages 561-581 in C.E. Finch and L. Hayflick, eds. Hand-
book of the biology of aging. Van Nostrand Reinhold,
New York.

Bartus, R.T. 1978. Short-term memory in the rhesus monkey: Effects of dopamine blockade via acute halopendol
administration. Pharmacol. Biochem. Behav. 9:353-357.

Bartus, R.T., D. Fleming, and H.R. Johnson. 1978. Aging
in the rhesus monkey: Debilitating effects on short-
term memory. J. Gerontol. 33:858-871.

Barzel, U.S., and J. Jowsey. 1969. The effects of chronic
acid and alkali administration on bone turnover in adult
rats. Clin. Sci. 36:517-524.

Baskin, G.B., and A. DePaoli. 1977. Primary renal neoplasms of the dog. Vet. Pathol. 14:591-605.

Bates, D.V., P.T. Macklem, and R.V. Christie. 1971a.
Chronic bronchitis and chronic infective asthma. Pages
133-155 in Respiratory function in disease. 2nd ed.
W. B. Saunders Co., Philadelphia.

Bates, D.V., P.T. Macklem, and R.V. Christie. 1971b.
Pulmonary emphysema. Pages 156-218 in Respiratory
function in disease. 2nd ed. W. B. Saunders Co.,
Philadelphia.

Battersby, S., J.A. Chandler, M.E. Harper, and N.J. Blacklock. 1977. The ultrastructure of rhesus monkey prostate. Urol. Res. 5:175-183.

Battista, A.F., M. Goldstein, S. Nakatani, and B. Anagnoste. 1969. Ventrolateral thalamic lesions. Arch.
Neurol. 21:611-614.

Bauer, G.C.H., A. Carlsson, and B. Lindquist. 1957. Bone
salt metabolism in humans studied by means of radiocal-
cium. Acta Med. Scand. 158:143-150.

Baumstark, A.E., D.C. Levin, and M.C. Fishbein. 1978.
Experimental myocardial infarction in dogs with normal
coronary arteries: Angiographic resolution of coronary
arterial emboli. Radiology 128:31-36.

Beadman, R., R.N. Smith, and A.S. King. 1964. Vertebral
osteophytes in the cat. Vet. Rec. 76:1005-1007.

Beasley, A.B. 1963. Inheritance and development of a lens
abnormality in the mouse. J. Morphol. 112:1-7.

Beatty, R.A., and D.P. Mukherjee. 1963. Spermatozoan
characteristics in mice of different ages. J. Reprod.
Fertil. 6:261-268.

Beauchene, R.R., L.M. Roeder, and C.H. Barrows, Jr. 1967.
The effects of age and of ethionine feeding on the
ribonucleic acid and protein synthesis of rats. J.
Gerontol. 22:318-324.

Becci, P.J., E.M. McDowell, and B.F. Trump. 1978a. The
respiratory epithelium. IV. Histogenesis of epidermoid
metaplasia and carcinoma in situ in the hamster. J.
Natl. Cancer Inst. 61:577-586.

Becci, P.J., E.M. McDowell, and B.F. Trump. 1978b. The
respiratory epithelium. VI. Histogenesis of lung

tumors induced by benzo[a]pyrene-ferric oxide in the hamster. J. Natl. Cancer Inst. 61:607-618.

Bedard, P., J. Delean, J. Lafleur, and L. Larochelle. 1977. Haloperidol-induced dyskinesias in the monkey. Can. J. Neurol. Sci. 4(3):197-201.

Beddoe, A.A. 1977. Measurements of microscopic structure of cortical bone. Phys. Med. Biol. 22:298-308.

Beddoe, A.A. 1978. A quantitative study of the structure of trabecular bone in man, rhesus monkey and miniature pig. Calcif. Tissue Res. 25:273-282.

Beecher, M.D. 1974. Pure-tone thresholds of the squirrel monkey (Saimiri sciureus). J. Acoust. Soc. Am. 55: 196-198.

Bell, D.P., O.L. Wade, and T. Williams. 1974. Emphysema in pathogen-free and bronchitic rats. An electronic lung scanning technique. Am. Rev. Respir. Dis. 109: 297-300.

Bell, J., and G.B.D. Scott. 1977. A qualitative and quantitative comparison of the fat in human, feline and canine kidneys. Br. J. Exp. Pathol. 58:13-18.

Bell, R.R., D.T. Engelmann, T.-L. Sie, and H.H. Draper. 1975. Effect of a high protein intake on calcium metabolism in the rat. J. Nutr. 105:475-483.

Bell, R.R., H.H. Draper, D.Y.M. Tzeng, H.K. Shin, and G.R. Schmidt. 1977. Physiological responses of human adults to foods containing phosphate additives. J. Nutr. 107:42-50.

Bellhorn, R.W., and C.A. Fisher. 1970. Feline central retinal degeneration. J. Am. Vet. Med. Assoc. 157: 842-849.

Bellhorn, R.W., M. Bellhorn, A.H. Friedman, and P. Henkind. 1973. Urethan-induced retinopathy in pigmented rats. Invest. Ophthalmol. 12:65-76.

Bellhorn, R.W., G.D. Aguirre, and M.B. Bellhorn. 1974. Feline central retinal degeneration. Invest. Ophthalmol. 13:608-616.

Bellhorn, R.W., C.D. King, G.E. Aguirre, H. Ripps, I.M. Siegel, and H. Tsai. 1980. Pigmentary abnormalities of the macula in rhesus monkeys: Clinical observation. Unpublished paper. Available from R. W. Bellhorn, Department of Ophthalmology, Albert Einstein College of Medicine, Montefiore Hospital and Medical Center, Bronx, New York.

Bellhorn, R.W., M.S. Burns, and J.V. Benjamin. In press. Retinal vessel abnormalities of phototoxic retinopathy in rats. Invest. Ophthalmol. Vis. Sci.

Bender, A.D. 1964. Pharmacologic aspects of aging: A survey of the effect of increasing age on drug activity in adults. J. Am. Geriatr. Soc. 12:114-134.

Bender, A.D. 1965. The effect of increasing age on the distribution of peripheral blood flow in man. J. Am. Geriatr. Soc. 13:192-198.

Bender, A.D. 1967. Pharmacologic aspects of aging: Additional literature. J. Am. Geriatr. Soc. 15(1):68-74.

Bender, A.D., C.G. Kormendy, and P. Powell. 1970. Pharmacological control of aging. Exp. Gerontol. 5:97-129.

Bengelloun, W.A., R.G. Burright, and P.J. Donovick. 1977. Septal lesions, cue availability, and passive avoidance acquisition by hooded male rats of two ages. Physiol. Behav. 18:1033-1037.

Benirschke, K. 1978. Cytogenetics. Pages 1698-1747 in K. Benirschke, F.M. Garner, and T.C. Jones, eds. Pathology of laboratory animals. Vol. II. Springer-Verlag, New York.

Benirschke, K., F.M. Garner, and T.C. Jones. 1978. Pathology of laboratory animals. Vols. I and II. Springer-Verlag, New York. 2171 + 108 p.

Benitz, K.F., and A.W. Kramer, Jr. 1965. Spontaneous tumors in the Mongolian gerbil. Lab. Anim. Care 15: 281-294.

Benjamin, M.M., and D.H. McKelvie. 1978. Clinical biochemistry. Pages 1749-1815 in K. Benirschke, F.M. Garner, and T.C. Jones, eds. Pathology of laboratory animals. Vol. II. Springer-Verlag, New York.

Benjamin, S.A., and A.L. Brooks. 1977. Spontaneous lesions in Chinese hamsters. Vet. Pathol. 14:449-462.

Benjamin, S.A., A.L. Brooks, and R.O. McClellan. 1976. The biological effectiveness of ^{239}Pu, ^{144}Ce and ^{90}Sr citrate in producing chromosome damage, bone-related tumors, liver tumors and life shortening in the Chinese hamster. Pages 143-152 in Biological and environmental effects of low level radiation. Vol. II. International Atomic Energy Agency, Vienna, Austria.

Bennington, J.L., and J.B. Beckwith. 1975. Tumors of the kidney, renal pelvis, and ureter. Atlas of tumor pathology. Section 2, Fascicle 12. Armed Forces Institute of Pathology, Washington, D.C. 353 p.

Benten, C., K. Stounkel, and K. Petzoldt. 1977. Thymectomy in the gerbil (Meriones unguiculatus). Techniques in newborn and 17- and 34-day-old animals. Zentralbl. Veterinaermed. (A)24:210-219.

Bentinck-Smith, J. 1969. Hematology. Pages 205-246 in W. Medway, J.E. Prier, and J.S. Wilkinson, eds.

Textbook of veterinary clinical pathology. The Williams and Wilkins Company, Baltimore.

Berg, A., and I.D. Zimmerman. 1975. Effects of electrical stimulation and norepinephrine on cyclic-AMP levels in the cerebral cortex of the aging rat. Mech. Ageing Develop. 4:377-383.

Berg, B.N. 1960. Nutrition and longevity in the rat. I. Food intake in relation to size, health and fertility. J. Nutr. 71:242-254.

Berg, B.N. 1967. Longevity studies in rats. II. Pathology of aging rats. Pages 749-786 in E. Cotchin and F.J.C. Roe, eds. Pathology of rats and mice. Blackwell Scientific Publications, Oxford; F.A. Davis Company, Philadelphia.

Berg, B.N., and H.S. Simms. 1960. Nutrition and longevity. II. Longevity and onset of disease with different levels of food intake. J. Nutr. 71:255-263.

Berg, B.N., A. Wolf, and H.S. Simms. 1962. Degenerative lesions of spinal roots and peripheral nerves in aging rats. Gerontologia 6:72-80.

Berg, O.A. 1958a. The normal prostate gland of the dog. Acta Endocrinol. 27:129-139.

Berg, O.A. 1958b. Parenchymatous hypertrophy of the canine prostate gland. Acta Endocrinol. 27:140-154.

Berger, M., J. Chazand, Ch. Jean-Faucher, M. de Turckheim, G. Veyssieve, and Cl. Jean. 1976. Developmental patterns of plasma and testicular testosterone in rabbits from birth to 90 days of age. Biol. Reprod. 15: 561-564.

Bermant, G., and D.G. Lindburg [eds.] 1975. Primate utilization and conservation. John Wiley and Sons, Inc., New York. 196 p.

Bernardis, L.L., and J.K. Goldman. 1976. Origin of endocrine-metabolic changes in the weanling rat ventromedial syndrome. J. Neurosci. Res. 2:91-116.

Bernfeld, P. 1979. Longevity of the Syrian hamster. Pages 118-126 in F. Homburger, ed. Symposium on the Syrian hamster in toxicology and carcinogenesis research. Proceedings of a symposium held November 30-December 2, 1977 in Boston, Massachusetts. Bio-Research Institute, Cambridge, Massachusetts.

Bernheimer, H., W. Birkmayer, O. Hornykiewicz, K. Jellinger, and F. Seitelberger. 1973. Brain dopamine and the syndromes of Parkinson and Huntington. Clinical, morphological and neurochemical correlations. J. Neurol. Sci. 20:415-455.

Bernstein, I.S., R.M. Rose, and T.P. Gordon. 1974. Behavioral and environmental events influencing primate testosterone levels. J. Hum. Evol. 3:517-526.

Berson, E.L., K.C. Hayes, A.R. Rabin, S.Y. Schmidt, and G. Watson. 1976. Retinal degeneration in cats fed casein. II. Supplementation with methionine, cysteine or taurine. Invest. Ophthalmol. 15:52-58.

Bertrand, H.A., E.J. Masoro, and B.P. Yu. 1978. Increasing adipocyte number as the basis for perirenal depot growth in adult rats. Science 201:1234-1235.

Bevans, M., B.C. Seegal, and R. Kaplan. 1955. Glomerulonephritis produced in dogs by specific antisera. II. Pathologic sequences following the injection of rabbit serum or rabbit antidog-kidney serum. J. Exp. Med. 102:807-821.

Beveridge, W.I.B. 1972. Frontiers in comparative medicine. University of Minnesota Press, Minneapolis. 104 p.

Beyer, R.E., C.A. Shamoian, and M.N. Abend. 1962. Effect of the diabetic state on selected mitochondrial reactions. Metabolism 11:394-403.

Bielfelt, S.W., A.J. Wilson, H.C. Redman, R.O. McClellan, and L.S. Rosenblatt. 1969. A breeding program for the establishment and maintenance of a stable gene pool in a Beagle dog colony to be utilized for long-term experiments. Am. J. Vet. Res. 30:2221-2229.

Bielschowsky, M., and F. Bielschowsky. 1953. A new strain of mice with hereditary obesity. Proc. Univ. Otago Med. Sch. 31(4):29-31.

Bielschowsky, M., F. Bielschowsky, and D. Lindsay. 1956. A new strain of mice with a high incidence of mammary cancers and enlargement of the pituitary. Brit. J. Cancer 10:688-699.

Bierman, E.L. 1978. The effect of donor age on the in vitro life span of cultured human arterial smooth-muscle cells. In Vitro 14:951-955.

Billingham, R.E., and W.H. Hildemann. 1958. Studies on the immunological responses of hamsters to skin homografts. Proc. R. Soc. London Ser. B 149:216-233.

Bindra, D., and W.R. Thompson. 1953. An evaluation of defecation and urination as measures of fearfulness. J. Comp. Physiol. Psychol. 46:43-45.

Binns, R. 1975. Animal inhalation studies with tobacco smoke: A review. Rev. Environ. Health 2:81-116.

Birren, J.E. 1955. Age differences in startle reaction time of the rat to noise and electric shock. J. Gerontol. 10:437-440.

Birren, J.E. 1962. Age differences in learning a two-choice water maze by rats. J. Gerontol. 17:207-213.

Birren, J.E., and H. Kay. 1958. Swimming speed of the albino rat. I. Age and sex differences. J. Gerontol. 13:374-377.

Birren, J.E., and R.D. Wall. 1956. Age changes in conduction velocity refractory period, number of fibers, connective tissue space and blood vessels in sciatic nerve of rats. J. Comp. Neurol. 104:1-16.

Bissett, J.K., J.W. Watson, J.A. Scovil, N. Schmidt, J.R. McConnell, and J. Kane. 1979. Changes in myocardial refractory periods following ischemia in the porcine heart. J. Electrocardiol. 12:35-40.

Bivin, W.S., and E.H. Timmons. 1974. Basic biomethodology. Pages 73-90 in S.H. Weisbroth, R.E. Flatt, and A.L. Kraus, eds. The biology of the laboratory rabbit. Academic Press, New York.

Blacklock, N.J., and K. Bouskill. 1977. The zonal anatomy of the prostate in man and in the rhesus monkey (Macaca mulatta). Urol. Res. 5:163-167.

Blaha, G.C. 1964a. Reproductive senescence in the golden hamster. Anat. Rec. 150:405-412.

Blaha, G.C. 1964b. Effect of age of the donor and recipient on the development of transferred golden hamster ova. Anat. Rec. 150:413-416.

Blaha, G.C., and W.W. Leavitt. 1974. Ovarian steroid dehydrogenase histochemistry and circulating progesterone in aged golden hamsters during the estrous cycle and pregnancy. Biol. Reprod. 11:153-161.

Blaha, G.C., and W.W. Leavitt. 1978. Uterine progesterone receptors in the aged golden hamster. J. Gerontol. 33:810-814.

Blair, W.H., M.C. Henry, and R. Erlich. 1969. Chronic toxicity of nitrogen dioxide. Arch. Environ. Health 18:186-192.

Blake, R., and R.W. Bellhorn. 1978. Visual acuity in cats with central retinal lesion. Vision Res. 18:15-18.

Bland, J.H., B. Chir, and E. Lowenstein. 1976. Halothane-induced decrease in experimental myocardial ischemia in the non-failing canine heart. Anesthesiology 45:287-293.

Blankwater, M.-J. 1978. Survival data and age-related pathology of CBA, C57BL/Ka and NZB mice. Pages 61-73 in Ageing and the humoral immune response in mice. Institute for Experimental Gerontology of the Organization for Health Research TNO, Rijswijk, The Netherlands.

Blau, J.N. 1972. DNA synthesis in the adult and ageing guinea pig thymus. Clin. Exp. Immunol. 11(3):461-468.

Block, E. 1952. Quantitative morphological investigations of the follicular system in women. Variations at different ages. Acta Anat. 14:108-123.

Bloom, F. 1954a. Mammary glands. Pages 403-446 in Pathology of the dog and cat: The genitourinary system, with clinical considerations. American Veterinary Publications, Inc., Evanston, Illinois.

Bloom, F. 1954b. Pathology of the dog and cat: The genitourinary system, with clinical considerations. American Veterinary Publications, Inc., Evanston, Illinois. 463 p.

Blumenthal, H.T. 1975. Athero-arteriosclerosis as an aging phenomenon. Pages 123-147 in R. Goldman and M. Rockstein, eds. The physiology and pathology of human aging. Academic Press, New York.

Board on Agriculture and Renewable Resources (BARR) Subcommittee on Dog Nutrition, Committee on Animal Nutrition. 1974. Nutrient requirements of dogs. Vol. No. 8. Rev. ed. Nutrient requirements of domestic animals series. National Academy of Sciences, Washington, D.C. 71 p.

Board on Agriculture and Renewable Resouces (BARR) Subcommittee on Rabbit Nutrition, Committee on Animal Nutrition. 1977. Nutrient requirements of rabbits. Vol. No. 9. 2nd rev. ed. Nutrient requirements of domestic animals series. National Academy of Sciences, Washington, D.C. 30 p.

Board on Agriculture and Renewable Resources (BARR) Panel on Cat Nutrition, Subcommittee on Laboratory Animal Nutrition, Committee on Animal Nutrition. 1978a. Nutrient requirements of cats. Vol. No. 13. Rev. ed. Nutrient requirements of domestic animals series. National Academy of Sciences, Washington, D.C. 49 p.

Board on Agriculture and Renewable Resources (BARR) Panel on Nonhuman Primate Nutrition, Subcommittee on Laboratory Animal Nutrition, Committee on Animal Nutrition. 1978b. Nutrient requirements of nonhuman primates. Vol. No. 14. Nutrient requirements of domestic animals series. National Academy of Sciences, Washington, D.C. 83 p.

Board on Agriculture and Renewable Resources (BARR) Subcommittee on Animal Nutrition, Committee on Animal Nutrition. 1978c. Nutrient requirements of laboratory animals. Vol. No. 10. 3rd rev. ed. Nutrient requirements of domestic animals series. National Academy of Sciences, Washington, D.C. 96 p.

Boatman, E.S., and H.B. Martin. 1965. Electron microscopy of pulmonary emphysema of rabbits. Am. Rev. Respir. Dis. 91:197-199.

Boatman, E.S., P. Arce, D. Luchtel, K.K. Pump, and C.J. Martin. 1979. Pulmonary function, morphology, and morphometrics. Pages 292-313 in D.M. Bowden, ed. Aging in nonhuman primates. Van Nostrand Reinhold, New York.

Bojrab, M.J. [ed.] 1975. Current techniques in small animal surgery. Lea and Febiger, Philadelphia. 585 p.

Bolton, C.F., R.K. Winkelmann, and P.J. Dyck. 1966. A quantitative study of Meissner's corpuscles in man. Neurology 16(1):1-17.

Bond, E., and H.D. Dorfman. 1969. Squamous cell carcinoma of the tongue in cats. J. Am. Vet. Med. Assoc. 154: 786-789.

Bond, M.G., and B.C. Bullock. 1980. Myocardial infarction among macaques fed atherogenic diets. Abstract No. 2667. Fed. Proc. 39(3):773.

Bondareff, W., and R. Narotzky. 1972. Age changes in the neuronal environment. Science 176:1135-1136.

Bonte, F.J., R.W. Parkey, K.D. Graham, J. Moore, and E.M. Stokely. 1974. A new method for radionuclide imaging of myocardial infarcts. Radiology 110:473-474.

Book, S.A., C. Crisp, and M. Goldman. 1979. Comparative toxicity of 90Sr and 226Ra: Experimental design and current status. Pages 200-237 in Annual Report 1978-1979. UCD 472-125. DOE Research and Development Report UC-48. Biomedical and Environmental Research. University of California, Davis, California.

Boorman, G.A., and C.F. Hollander. 1973. Spontaneous lesions in the female WAG/Rij (Wistar) rat. J. Gerontol. 28:152-159.

Booth, B.H., R. Patterson, and C.H. Talbot. 1970. Immediate-type hypersensitivity in dogs: Cutaneous, anaphylactic, and respiratory responses to Ascaris. J. Lab. Clin. Med. 76:181-189.

Boquist, L. 1972. Obesity and pancreatic islet hyperplasia in the Mongolian gerbil. Diabetologia 8: 274-282.

Borthwick, R., and C.P. MacKenzie. 1971. The signs and results of treatment of prostatic disease in dogs. Vet. Rec. 89:374-384.

Botwinick, J. 1959. Drives, expectancies and emotions. Pages 739-768 in J.E. Birren, ed. Handbook of aging and the individual. University of Chicago Press, Chicago.

Botwinick, J., J.F. Brinley, and J.S. Robbin. 1963. Learning and reversing a four-choice multiple Y-maze by rats of three ages. J. Gerontol. 18:279-282.

Bourguignon, J.-P., C. Hoyoux, A. Reuter, and P. Franchimont. 1979. Urinary excretion of immunoreactive luteinizing hormone-releasing hormone-like material and gonadotropins at different stages of life. J. Clin. Endocrinol. Metab. 48:78-84.

Bourne, G.H. 1975. The aging process. Yerkes Newsletter 12(1):6-11. Available from Yerkes Regional Primate Research Center, Emory University, Atlanta, Georgia.

Bourne, M.C., D.A. Campbell, and K. Tansley. 1938. Hereditary degeneration of the rat retina. Brit. J. Ophthalmol. 22:613-623.

Bowden, D.M. [ed.] 1979. Aging in nonhuman primates. Van Nostrand Reinhold, New York. 393 p.

Bowden, D.M., and M.E. Jones. 1979. Aging research in nonhuman primates. Pages 1-13 in D.M. Bowden, ed. Aging in nonhuman primates. Van Nostrand Reinhold, New York.

Bowden, D.M., and W.T. McKinney, Jr. 1974. Effects of selective frontal lobe lesions on response to separation in adolescent rhesus monkeys. Brain Res. 75: 167-171.

Bowden, D.M., J.A. Spillane, G. Curzon, W. Meier-Ruge, P. White, M.J. Goodhart, P. Iwangoft, and A.N. Davison. 1979a. Accelerated ageing or selective neuronal loss as an important cause of dementia? Lancet 1:11-14.

Bowden, D.M., C. Teets, J. Witkin, and D.M. Young. 1979b. Long bone calcification and morphology. Pages 335-347 in D.M. Bowden, ed. Aging in nonhuman primates. Van Nostrand Reinhold, New York.

Bowen, D.M., C.B. Smith, P. White, and A.N. Davison. 1976. Neurotransmitter-related enzymes and indices of hypoxia in senile dementia and other abiotrophies. Brain 99:459-496.

Bowen, D.M., J.A. Spillane, G. Curzon, W. Meier-Ruge, P. White, M.J. Goodhart, P. Iwangoft, and A.N. Davison. 1979. Accelerated ageing or selective neuronal loss as an important cause of dementia? Lancet 1:11-14.

Bowen, W.H., and G. Koch. 1970. Determination of age in monkeys Macaca irus on the basis of dental development. Lab. Anim. 4:113-123.

Bowlby, J. 1960. Separation anxiety. Int. J. Psychoanal. 41:89-113.

Boyce, B.F., D. Courpron, and P.J. Meunier. 1978. Amount
of bone in osteoporosis and physiological senile osteopenia. Comparison of two histomorphometric parameters.
Metab. Bone Dis. Relat. Res. 1:35-38.

Brachfeld, N. 1976. Metabolic evaluation of agents designed to protect the ischemic myocardium and to reduce
infarct size. Amer. J. Cardiol. 37:528-532.

Brambell, F.W.R., and D.H.S. Davis. 1941. The normal occurrence, structure and homology of prostate glands
in adult female Mastomys erythroleucus Temm. J. Anat.
75:64-74.

Bramblett, C.A. 1969. Non-metric skeletal age changes
in the Darajani baboon. Amer. J. Phys. Anthropol.
30(2):161-172.

Brandfonbrener, M., M. Landowne, and N.W. Shock. 1955.
Changes in cardiac output with age. Circulation
12:557-566.

Bras, G., and M.H. Ross. 1964. Kidney disease and nutrition in the rat. Toxicol. Appl. Pharmacol. 6:247-262.

Braunlich, H. 1966. Age-dependent effects of codeine and
morphine in the rat. Acta Biol. Med. Ger. 16(2):
178-186.

Braunwald, E., and P.R. Maroko. 1976. Effects of hyaluronidase and hydrocortisone on myocardial necrosis
after coronary occlusion. Am. J. Cardiol. 37:550-556.

Bray, G.A. [ed.] 1975. Obesity in perspective. Fogarty
International Center Series on preventive medicine.
Vol. 2, Part 1. DHEW Pub. No. (NIH) 75-708. U.S.
Department of Health, Education, and Welfare, Wash-
ington, D.C. 107 pp.

Bray, G.A. 1977. The Zucker-fatty rat: A review. Fed.
Proc. 26:148-153.

Bray, G.A., and T.F. Gallagher, Jr. 1975. Manifestations
of hypothalamic obesity in man: A comprehensive investigation of eight patients and a review of the literature. Medicine 54:301-330.

Bray, G.A., and D.A. York. 1971 Genetically transmitted
obesity in rodents. Physiol. Rev. 51(3):598-646.

Bray, G.A., and D.A. York. 1972. Studies on food intake
of genetically obese rats. Am. J. Physiol. 223:
176-179.

Breazile, J.E., and E.M. Brown. 1976. Anatomy. Pages
53-62 in J.E. Wagner and P.J. Manning, eds. The biology
of the guinea pig. Academic Press, New York.

Bredberg, G. 1967. The human cochlea during development
and ageing. J. Laryngol. Otol. 81:739-758.

Bredberg, G. 1968. Cellular pattern and nerve supply of the human organ of Corti. Acta Otolaryngol. Suppl. 236:1-135.

Breeze, R.G., and E.B. Wheeldon. 1977. The cells of the pulmonary airways. Am. Rev. Resp. Dis. 116:705-777.

Breeze, R.G., and E.B. Wheeldon. 1979. Emphysema. Pages 185-187 in E.J. Andrews, B.C. Ward, and N.H. Altman, eds. Spontaneous animal models of human disease. Vol. II. Academic Press, New York.

Bressot, C., P. Courpron, C. Edouard, and P. Meunier. 1976. Histomorphometric des osteopathies endocriniennes. Travail de la Clinique de Rhumatologie du C.H.U. de Lyon (Dr. G. Vignon) effective au Laboratorie des Recherches sur l'Histodynamique Osseuse (Dr. P. Meunier). Doctoral dissertation available from the Laboratorie des Recherches sur l'Histodynamique Osseuse, Rue Guillaume-Paradin, 69008 Lyon, France.

Briner, W.W., and J.A. Wunder. 1977. Sensitivity of dog plaque microorganisms to chlorhexidine during longitudinal studies. J. Periodontal Res. 12:135-139.

Britton, G.W., and F.G. Sherman. 1975. Altered regulation of protein synthesis during aging as determined by in vitro ribosomal assays. Exp. Gerontol. 10:67-77.

Britton, G.W., S. Rotenberg, C. Freeman, V.J. Britton, K. Karoly, L. Ceci, T.L. Klug, A.G. Lacko, and R.C. Adelman. 1975. Regulation of corticosterone levels and liver enzyme activity in aging rats. Pages 209-228 in V.J. Cristofalo, J. Roberts, and R.C. Adelman, eds. Explorations in aging. Plenum Publishing Corp., New York.

Brizzee, K.R. 1973. Quantitative histological studies on aging changes in cerebral cortex of rhesus monkey and albino rat with notes on effects of prolonged low-dose ionizing irradiation in the rat. Prog. Brain Res. 40:141-160.

Brizzee, K.R. 1975. Gross morphometric analyses and quantitative histology of the aging brain. Pages 401-423 in J.M. Ordy and K.R. Brizzee, eds. Neurobiology of aging. Plenum Publishing Corp., New York.

Brizzee, K.R., N. Sherwood, and P.S. Timiras. 1968. A comparison of cell populations at various depth levels in cerebral cortex of young adult and aged Long-Evans rats. J. Gerontol. 23:289-297.

Brizzee, K.R., P.S. Cancilla, N. Sherwood, and P.S. Timiras. 1969. The amount and distribution of pigments in neurons and glia of the cerebral cortex. J. Gerontol. 24:127-135.

Brizzee, K.R., J.M. Ordy, and B. Kaack. 1974. Early appearance and regional differences in intraneuronal and
extraneuronal lipofuscin accumulation with age in the
brain of a nonhuman primate, Macaca mulatta. J.
Gerontol. 29:366-381.

Brizzee, K.R., J.M. Ordy, J. Hansche, B. Kaack. 1976.
Quantitative assessment of changes in neuron and glial
cell packing density and lipofuscin accumulation with
age in the cerebral cortex of a nonhuman primate, Macaca
mulatta. Pages 229-261 in R.D. Terry and S. Gershon,
eds. Neurobiology of aging. Vol. 3. Aging series.
Raven Press, New York.

Brizzee, K.R., J.M. Ordy, H. Hofer, and B. Kaack. 1978.
Animal models for the study of senile brain disease
and aging changes in the brain. Pages 515-553 in R.
Katzman, R.D. Terry, and K.L. Bick, eds. Alzheimer's
disease: Senile dementia and related disorders.
Vol. 7. Aging series. Raven Press, New York.

Brobeck, J.R. 1946. Mechanism of the development of
obesity in animals with hypothalamic lesions. Physiol.
Rev. 26:541-559.

Broderson, J.R., J.R. Lindsey, and J.E. Crawford. 1976.
The role of environmental ammonia in respiratory mycoplasmosis of rats. Am. J. Pathol. 85:115-127.

Brodey, R.S. 1960. A clinical and pathologic study of
130 neoplasms of the mouth and pharynx in the dog.
Am. J. Vet. Res. 21:787-812.

Brodey, R.S. 1966. Alimentary tract neoplasms in the
cat. A clinicopathologic survey of 46 cases. Am. J.
Vet. Res. 27:74-80.

Brodey, R.S. 1970. Canine and feline neoplasia. Pages
309-354 in C.A. Brandy and C.E. Cornelius, eds. Advances in veterinary science and comparative medicine.
Vol. 14. Academic Press, New York.

Brodey, R.S., and D. Cohen. 1964. A epizootiologic and
clinicopathologic study of AS cases of gastrointestinal neoplasms in the dogs. Pages 167-179 in
Scientific Proceedings of the 101st Annual Meeting of
the American Veterinary Medical Association. American Veterinary Medical Association, Schaumburg,
Illinois.

Brodey, R.S., I.J. Fidler, and A.E. Howson. 1966.
The relationship of estrous irregularity, pseudopregnancy and pregnancy to development of canine mammary
neoplasms. J. Am. Vet. Med. Assoc. 149:1047-1049.

Brody, H. 1973. Aging in the vertebrate brain. Pages 121-133 in M. Rockstein and M. Sussman, eds. Development and aging in the central nervous system. Academic Press, New York.

Brody, H. 1976. An examination of cerebral cortex and brainstem aging. Pages 177-181 in R.D. Terry and S. Gershon, eds. Neurobiology of aging. Vol. 3. Aging series. Raven Press, New York.

Brody, H., and N. Vijayashankar. 1977. Anatomical changes in the nervous system. Pages 241-261 in C.E. Finch and L. Hayflick, eds. Handbook of the biology of aging. Van Nostrand Reinhold, New York.

Broekhuyse, R.M. 1971. Lipids in tissues of the eye. Part 5. Phospholipid metabolism in normal eyes and cataractous lens. Biochem. Biophys. Acta 231:360-369.

Broer, Y., P. Freychet, and G. Rosselin. 1977. Insulin and glucagonreceptor interactions in the genetically obese Zucker rat: Studies of hormone binding and glucagon-stimulated cyclic AMP levels in isolated hepatocytes. Endocrinology 101:236-249.

Bromley, R.G., N.L. Dockum, J.S. Arnold, and W.S.S. Jee. 1966. Quantitative histological study of human lumbar vertebrae. J. Gerontol. 21:537-543.

Bronson, F.H., and C. DesJardins. 1977. Reproductive failure in aged CBF male mice: Interrelationships between pituitary gonadotropic hormones, testicular function, and mating success. Endocrinology 101:939-945.

Brooks, A.L., S.A. Benjamin, and R.O. McClellan. 1974. Toxicity of $^{90}Sr-^{90}Y$ in Chinese hamsters. Radiat. Res. 57:471-481.

Brown, D., and N. Fleming. 1976. Long-term amphibian organ culture. Methods Cell Biol. 13:213-238.

Brown, E.R., K. Nakano, and G.L. Vankin. 1970. Early development of an inherited cataract in mice. Exp. Anim. 19:95-100.

Brown, N.O., M.L. Helphrey, and R.G. Prata. 1977. Thoracolumbar disk disease in the dog: A retrospective analysis of 187 cases. J. Am. Anim. Hosp. Assoc. 13:655-672.

Bruni, J.F., H.-H. Huang,, S. Marshall, and J. Meites. 1977. Effects of single and multiple injections of synthetic GnRH on serum LH, FSH, and testosterone in young and old male rats. Biol. Reprod. 17:309-312.

Bruno, F.P., F.R. Cobb, F. Rivas, and J.K. Goodrich. 1976. Evaluation of ^{99m}technetium stannous pyrophosphate as an imaging agent in acute myocardial infarction. Circulation 54:71-78.

Buell, S.J., and P.D. Coleman. 1979. Dendritic growth in the aged human brain and failure of growth in senile dementia. Science 206:854-856.

Buja, L.M., R.W. Parkey, E.M. Stokely, F.J. Bonte, and J.T. Willerson. 1976. Pathophysiology of technetium-99m stannous pyrophosphate and thallium-201 scintigraphy of acute anterior myocardial infarcts in dogs. J. Clin. Invest. 57:1508-1522.

Buja, L.M., R.W. Parkey, F.J. Bonte, and J.T. Willerson. 1979. Pathophysiology of "cold spot" and "hot spot" myocardial imaging agents used to detect ischemia or infarction. Cardiovasc. Clin. 10:105-123.

Bull, R.W., R. Schirmer, and A.J. Bowdler. 1971. Auto-immune hemolytic disease in the dog. J. Am. Vet. Med. Assoc. 159:880-884.

Bullock, B.C., R. Paula, and L.L. Rudel. 1974. Dietary-induced cirrhosis in the pig-tailed macaque (Macaca nemestrina). Abstract No. 2352. Fed. Proc. 33:626.

Bullock, B.C., N.D.M. Lehner, T.B. Clarkson, M.A. Feldner, W.D. Wagner, and H.B. Lofland. 1975. Comparative primate atherosclerosis. I. Tissue cholesterol concentration and pathologic anatomy. Exp. Mol. Pathol. 22:151-175.

Bullock, B.C., M.G. Bond, N.D.M. Lehner, and T.B. Clarkson. 1976. Effect of plasma cholesterol concentration (220 vs 300 mg/dl) on preexisting coronary atherosclerosis in rhesus monkeys. Abstract No. 0549. Circulation Suppl. 54:II-139.

Bunch, C.C., and T.S. Raiford. 1931. Race and sex variation in auditory acuity. Arch. Otolaryngol. 13:423-434.

Burdeaux, G.C., and W.J. Hutchinson. 1953. Etiology of traumatic osteoporosis. J. Bone Joint Surg. 35A:479-488.

Burek, J.D. 1978. Pathology of aging rats. CRC Press, West Palm Beach, Florida. 230 p.

Burek, J.D., and C.F. Hollander. 1980. Experimental gerontology. Pages 149-159 in H.J. Baker, J.R. Lindsey, and S.H. Weisbroth, eds. The laboratory rat. Vol. II. Research applications. Academic Press, New York.

Burek, J.D., A.J. Van der Kogel, and C.F. Hollander. 1976. Degenerative myelopathy in three strains of aging rats. Vet. Pathol. 13:321-331.

Burek, J.D., B. Goldberg, G. Hutchins, and J.D. Strandberg. 1979. The pregnant Syrian hamster as a model
to study intravascular trophoblasts and associated
maternal blood vessel changes. Vet. Pathol.
16:553-566.

Burich, R.L. 1975. Effects of age on renal function
and enzyme activity in male C57BL/6J mice. J. Gerontol. 30:539-545.

Burkhart, J.M., and J. Jowsey. 1967. Parathyroid and
thyroid hormones in the development of immobilization
osteoporosis. Endocrinology 81:1053-1062.

Burleigh, I.G., and R.T. Schimke. 1969. The activities
of some enzymes concerned with energy metabolism in
mammalian muscles of differing pigmentation. Biochem.
J. 113:157-166.

Burns, R.P., and L. Feeney. 1975. Hereditary cataracts
in deermice (Peromyscus maniculatus). Am. J. Ophthalmol. 80:370-378.

Burr, I. 1970. The pathogenesis of diabetes mellitus.
Possible usefulness of spontaneous hyperglycemic syndromes in animals. Calif. Med. 112:23-34.

Burrows, H., and N.M. Kennaway. 1934. On some effects
produced by applying oestrin to the skin of mice. Am.
J. Cancer 20:48-57.

Burzynski, N.J. 1967a. Relationship between age and
palatal tissue and gingival tissue in the guinea pig.
J. Dent. Res. 46(3):539-543.

Burzynski, N.J. 1967b. Variations in oral tissues as
associated with ageing. Arch. Oral Biol.
12(2):307-309.

Burzynski, N.J. 1971. Phospholipid content and aging
in the submandibular salivary gland. J. Dent. Res.
50(1):164.

Burzynski, N.J., and K.R. Goljan. 1967. Effects of age
on the concentration of DNA and RNA in the guinea pig
palate. J. Dent. Res. 46(1):311.

Burzynski, N.J., and J.B. Rogers. 1965. Effects of ageing on palatal tissue of the guinea pig. J. Gerontol.
20(3):420-422.

Busuttil, R.W., W.J. George, and R.L. Hewitt. 1975.
Protective effect of methylprednisolone on the heart
during ischemic arrest. J. Thorac. Cardiovasc. Surg.
70:955-965.

Buxton, R.S. 1966. Guinea-pig mast cells and age. Nature 211(53):1103-1104.

Cadwallader, J.A., B.E. Goulden, R.S. Wejburn, and R.D. Jolly. 1973. Renal haemangiomas in a dog. N. Z. Vet. J. 21:48-51.

Caffesse, R.G., and C.D. Nasjleti. 1976. Enzymatic penetration through intact sulcular epithelium. J. Periodontol. 47:391-397.

Cahill, G.F., Jr. 1975. Diabetes mellitus. Pages 1599-1619 in P.B. Beeson and W. McDermott, eds. Textbook of medicine. 14th ed. W.B. Saunders Co., Philadelphia.

Cahill, G.F., Jr. 1978. Obesity and diabetes. Pages 101-110 in G.A. Bray, ed. Recent advances in obesity research: II. Proceedings of the 2nd International Congress on Obesity, held October 23-26, 1977 in Washington, D.C. Newman Publishing, Ltd., London.

Cahill, G.F., Jr., E.E. Jones, V. Lauris, J. Steinke, and J.S. Soeldner. 1967. Studies on experimental diabetes in the Wellesley hybrid mouse. 2. Serum insulin levels and response of peripheral tissues. Diabetologia 3:171-174.

Caine, M., and E. Superstine. 1973. Effect of hydroxy-progesterone caproate on experimental benign prostatic obstruction in the mouse. Isr. J. Med. Sci. 9:1559-1564.

Callingham, B.A., and L. Della Corte. 1972. The influence of growth and of adrenalectomy upon some rat heart enzymes. Br. J. Pharmacol. 46:530P-531P.

Callingham, B.A., and R. Laverty. 1973. Studies on the nature of the increased monoamine oxidase activity in the rat heart after adrenalectomy. J. Pharm. Pharmacol. 25:940-947.

Calloway, N.O. 1971. A critical ratio of aging: Water loss--heat production. J. Am. Geriatr. Soc. 19(5):386-390.

Calloway, N.O. 1974. Heat production and senescence. J. Am. Geriatr. Soc. 22(4):149-150.

Cameron, A.M., and L.J. Faulkin, Jr. 1971. Hyperplastic and inflammatory nodules in the canine mammary gland. J. Natl. Cancer Inst. 47:1277-1287.

Caminiti, B. 1979. The aged nonhuman primate: A bibliography. Primate Information Center, Regional Primate Research Center, University of Washington, Seattle, Washington. 12 p.

Campbell, J.R., and D.D. Lawson. 1963. The signs of prostatic disease in dog. Vet. Rec. 75:4-7.

Cannon, D.J., and P.F. Davison. 1977. Aging and cross-
linking in mammalian collagen. Exp. Aging Res.
3(2):87-105.

Capen, C.C., B.E. Belshaw, and S.L. Martin. 1975. Endocrine disorders. Pages 1351-1452 in S.J. Ettinger,
ed. Textbook of veterinary internal medicine. Diseases of the dog and cat. Vol. 2. W. B. Saunders
Company, Philadelphia.

Carbrey, E.A., L.N. Brown, T.L. Chow, R.F. Kahrs, D.G.
McKercher, L.K. Smithies, and T.W. Tamoglia. 1971.
Recommended standard laboratory technique for diagnos-
ing infectious bovine rhinotracheitis, bovine virus
diarrhea, and shipping fever (Parainfluenza 3). Proc.
U.S. Anim. Health Assoc. 75:629-648.

Carlsson, A. 1978. Age-dependent changes in brain mono-
amines. Adv. Exp. Med. Biol. 113:1-14.

Carlsson, A., and B. Winblad. 1976. Influence of age and
time interval between death and autopsy on dopamine
and 3-methoxytyramine levels in human basal ganglia.
J. Neural Transm. 38:271-276.

Carrel, A., and A.H. Ebeling. 1923. Antagonistic growth
principles of seruum and their relation to old age.
J. Exp. Med. 38:419-425.

Carroll, K.K. 1975. Experimental evidence of dietary
factors and hormone-dependent cancers. Cancer Res.
35:3374-3383.

Carter, G.R., D.L. Whitenack, and L.A. Julius. 1969.
Natural Tyzzer's disease in Mongolian gerbils
(Meriones unguiculatus). Lab. Anim. Care 19:648-651.

Casarett, G.W. 1953. Obstructive pulmonary emphysema
and bronchial obstruction by lymphatic tissue in aging rats. J. Gerontol. 8:146-149.

Casey, H.W., K.M. Ayers, and F.R. Robinson. 1978. The
urinary system. Pages 115-173 in K. Benirschke, F.M.
Garner, and T.C. Jones, eds. Pathology of laboratory
animals. Vol. I. Springer-Verlag, New York.

Casey, H.W., R.C. Giles, and R.P. Kwapien. 1979. Mammary neoplasia in animals: Pathologic aspects and the
effect of contraceptive steroids. Recent Results Cancer Res. 66:129-160.

Castleberry, M.W., J.F. Ferell, L.D. Jones, and C.H.
Gravin. 1965. Mucoid impaction of the canine bronchi.
J. Am. Vet. Med. Assoc. 146:607-610.

Castleman, W.L., D.L. Dungworth, and W.S. Tyler. 1975.
Intrapulmonary airway morphology in three species of
monkeys: A correlated scanning and transmission electron microscopic study. Am. J. Anat. 142:107-121.

Catcott, E.J., C.J. McCammon, and P. Kotin. 1958. Pulmonary pathology in dogs due to air pollution. J. Am. Vet. Med. Assoc. 133:331-335.

Ceremużyński, L., J. Staszewska-Barczak, and K. Herbaczynska-Cedro. 1969. Cardiac rhythm disturbances and the release of catecholamines after acute coronary occlusion in dogs. Cardiovasc. Res. 3:190-197.

Chaffee, J., M. Nassef, and S. Bobin. 1978. Cytotoxic auto-antibody to the brain. Pages 61-72 in K. Nandy, ed. Senile dementia: A biomedical approach. Vol. 3. Developments in neuroscience. Elsevier North-Holland Biomedical Press, New York.

Chakrin. L.W., and L.Z. Saunders. 1974. Experimental chronic bronchitis: Pathology in the dog. Lab. Invest. 30:145-154.

Chan, P.C., J.F. Head, L.A. Cohen, and E.L. Wynder. 1977. Influence of dietary fat on the induction of mammary tumors by N-nitrosomethylurea: Associated hormone changes and differences between Sprague-Dawley and F344 rats. J. Natl. Cancer Inst. 59(4):1279-1284.

Chapman, W.L., Jr. 1968. Neoplasia in nonhuman primates. J. Am. Vet. Med. Assoc. 153:872-878.

Chapman, W.L., Jr. 1975. Diseases of the lymph nodes and spleen. Pages 1664-1678 in S.J. Ettinger, ed. Textbook of veterinary internal medicine. Diseases of the dog and cat. Vol. 2. W.B. Saunders Company, Philadelphia.

Chapman, W.L., W.J. Bopp, A.S. Brightwell, H. Cohen, A.H. Nielsen, C.R. Gravelle, and A.A. Werder. 1967. Preliminary report on virus-like particles in canine leukemia and derived cell cultures. Cancer Res. 27:18-25.

Chawla, K.K., C.D.S. Murthy, R.N. Chakravarti, and P.N. Chhuttani. 1967. Arteriosclerosis and thrombosis in wild rhesus monkeys. Am. Heart J. 73:85-91.

Chen, J.C., J.B. Warshaw, and D.R. Sanadi. 1972. Regulation of mitochondrial respiration in senescence. J. Cell. Physiol. 80:141-148.

Cheraskin, E., and W.M. Ringsdorf. 1971. Younger at heart: A study of the P-R interval. J. Am. Geriatr. Soc. 19:271-275.

Chesky, J.A., and M. Rockstein. 1976. Life span characteristics in male Fischer rat. Exp. Aging Res. 2:399-401.

Cheville, N.F. 1968. Amyloidosis associated with cyclic neutropenia in the dog. Blood 31:111-114.

Chino, F., T. Makinodan, W.E. Lever, and W.J. Peterson. 1971. The immune systems of mice reared in clean and in dirty conventional farms. I. Life expectancy and pathology of mice with long lifespans. J. Gerontol. 26:497-507.

Choudary, J.B., and G.S. Greenwald. 1969. Luteotropic complex of the mouse. Anat. Rec. 163:373-388.

Christensen, T.G., A. Korthy, G.L. Snider, and J.A. Hayes. 1977. Irreversible bronchial goblet cell metaplasia in hamsters with elastase induced emphysema. J. Clin. Invest. 59:397-404.

Christie, B.A. 1971. Incidence and etiology of vesicoureteral reflux in dogs. Invest. Urol. 8:184-194.

Christie, N.P., M.M. Dickie, W.B. Atkinson, and G.W. Woolley. 1951. The pathogenesis of uterine lesions in virgin mice and in gonadectomized mice bearing adrenal cortical and pituitary tumors. Cancer Res. 11:413-425.

Chrzanowski, P.J., and G.M. Turino. 1977. Experimental emphysema: Concepts and questions. Bull. Europ. Physiopath. Respir. 13:471-477.

Ciaranello, R.D., H.J. Hoffman, J.G.M. Shire, and J. Axelrod. 1974. Genetic regulation of the catecholamine biosynthetic enzymes. II. Inheritance of tyrosine hydroxylase, dopamine-β-hydroxylase, and phenylethanolamine $\underline{N}$-methyltransferase. J. Biol. Chem. 249:4528-4536.

Clark, W.E.L. 1959. The antecedents of man. Edinburgh University Press, Edinburgh. 374 p.

Clarkson, T.B. 1975. Genetic studies of atherosclerosis in animals. Pages 123-142 in Report by the Task Force on Genetic Factors in Atherosclerotic Disease. National Heart and Lung Institute. DHEW Pub. No. (NIH) 76-922. U.S. Department of Health, Education, and Welfare, Washington, D.C.

Clarkson, T.B., and H.B. Lofland, Jr. 1967. Response of pigeon arteries to cholesterol as a function of time. Arch. Pathol. 84:513-516.

Clarkson, T.B., and L.L. Rudel. In press. Nonhuman primate models for research on alcohol-lipoprotein-atherosclerosis relationships. Circulation.

Clarkson, T.B., R.W. Prichard, M.G. Netsky, and H.B. Lofland. 1959. Atherosclerosis in pigeons: Its spontaneous occurrence and resemblance to human atherosclerosis. Arch. Pathol. 68:143-147.

Clarkson, T.B., H.B. Lofland, B.C. Bullock, and H.O.
Goodman. 1971. Genetic control of plasma cholesterol.
Arch. Pathol. 92:37-45.

Clarkson, T.B., N.D.M. Lehner, and B.C. Bullock. 1974.
Specialized research applications: I. Arteriosc(lero)-
sis research. Pages 155-165 in S.H. Weisbroth, R.E.
Flatt, and A.L. Kraus, eds. The biology of the laboratory rabbit. Academic Press, New York.

Clarkson, T.B., T. Hamm, B.C. Bullock and N.D.M. Lehner.
1976a. Atherosclerosis in Old World monkeys. Primates Med. 9:66-89.

Clarkson, T.B., N.D.M. Lehner, B.C. Bullock, H.B. Lofland, and W.D. Wagner. 1976b. Atherosclerosis in New
World monkeys. Primates Med. 9:90-144.

Clemens, J.A., Y. Amenomori, T. Jenkins, and J. Meites.
1969. Effects of hypothalamic stimulation, hormones
and drugs on ovarian function in old female rats.
Proc. Exp. Biol. Med. 132:561-563.

Clemens, J.A., and D.R. Bennett. 1977. Do aging changes
in the preoptic area contribute to loss of cyclic
endocrine function? J. Gerontol. 32:19-24.

Clifford, D.H., and F. Gyorkey. 1967. Myenteric gan-
glial cells in dogs with and without achalasia of the
esophagus. J. Am. Vet. Med. Assoc. 150:205-211.

Cock, D.J., and W.H. Bowen. 1967. Occurrence of Bacte-
rionema matruchotii and Bacteroides melaninogenicus in
gingival plaque from monkeys. J. Periodontal Res.
2:36-39.

Cockrell, B., and Y. Krehbiel. 1972. Ultrastructural
changes in histiocytic ulcerative colitis in a Boxer.
Am. J. Vet. Res. 33:453-459.

Code of Federal Regulations (CFR). Title 9. Animal and
Animal Products. Chapter 1.1-4. Animal and Plant
Health Inspection Service, Department of Agriculture.
U.S. Government Printing Office, Washington, D.C.

Cohen, B.J. 1968. Effects of environment on longevity
in rats and mice. Pages 21-29 in The laboratory animal in gerontological research. Proceedings of a symposium organized by the Institute of Laboratory Animal
Resources (ILAR) Committee on Animal Research in Gerontology, held November 10, 1967 in St. Petersburg,
Florida. National Academy of Sciences, Washington,
D.C.

Cohen B.J. 1979. Dietary factors affecting rats used
in aging research. J. Gerontol. 34:803-807.

Cohen, B.J., and M.R. Anver. 1976. Pathologic changes
during aging in the rat. Pages 379-403 in M.F. Elias,

B.E. Eleftheriou, and P.K. Elias, eds. Special review of experimental aging research: Progress in biology. EAR, Inc., Bar Harbor, Maine; Beech Hill Company, Mount Desert, Maine.

Cohen B.J., M.R. Anver, D.H. Ringler, and R.C. Adelman. 1978. Age-associated pathological changes in male rats. Fed. Proc. 37:2848-2850.

Cohen, C. 1955. A method for bleeding rabbits. Am. J. Clin. Pathol. 25:604.

Cohen, D., and D. Dunner. In press. Assessment of cognitive dysfunction in dementing illness. In J.O. Cole and J. Barrett, eds. Psychopathology in the aged. Raven Press, New York.

Cohen, D., and C. Eisdorfer. 1980. Serum immunoglobulins and cognitive status in the elderly: A population study. Br. J. Psychiat. 136: 33-39.

Cohen, D., C. Eisdorfer, and D.M. Bowden. 1979. Cognition. Pages 4855 in D.M. Bowden, ed. Aging in nonhuman primates. Van Nostrand Reinhold, New York.

Cohen, D.W., and H.M. Goldman. 1960. Oral disease in primates. Ann. N.Y. Acad. Sci. 85:889-909.

Cohen, M.M. 1970. The somatic karyotype of Meriones unguiculatus: A morphologic and autoradiographic study. J. Hered. 61:158-160.

Cohen, M.M., S. Shusterman, and G. Shklar. 1969. The effect of stressor agents on the grey lethal mouse strain periodontium. J. Periodontol. 40:462-466.

Cohn, M.A., H. Baier, and A. Wanner. 1978. Failure of hypoxic pulmonary vasoconstriction in the canine asthma model. J. Clin. Invest. 61: 1463-1470.

Cohnheim, J., and A. von Schultess-Rechberg. 1881. Über die Folgen der Kranzarterienschliessung für das Herz. Virchows Arch. Pathol. Anat. 85:503.

Coleman, D.L. 1978. Genetics of obesity in rodents. Pages 142-152 in G.A. Bray, ed. Recent advances in obesity research: II. Proceedings of the 2nd International Congress on Obesity, held October 23-26, 1977 in Washington, D.C. Newman Publishing, Ltd., London.

Coleman. G.L., S.W. Barthold, G.W. Osbaldistan, S.J. Foster, and A.M. Jonas. 1977. Pathological changes during aging in barrier-reared Fischer 344 male rats. J. Gerontol. 32:258-278.

Coleman, J.W. 1976. Hair cell loss as a function of age in the normal cochlea of the guinea pig. Acta Otolaryngol. 82(1-2):33-40.

Coles, E.H. 1967. Veterinary clinical pathology. W.B. Saunders Company, Philadelphia. 455 p.

Collett, M.E., G.E. Wertenberger, and V.M. Fiske. 1954.
The effect of age upon the pattern of the menstrual
cycle. Fertil. Steril. 5:437-448.

Collins, E.J., E.R. Garrett, and R.L. Johnston. 1962.
Effect of adrenal steroids on radio-calcium metabolism
in dogs. Metabolism 11:716-726.

Collins, R.L. 1966. What else does the defecation score
measure? Proc. Ann. Meet. Am. Psychol. Assoc.
2:147-148.

Comfort, A. 1956. Maximum ages reached by domestic cats.
J. Mammal. 37:118-119.

Comfort, A. 1964. Ageing. The biology of senescence.
Rev. ed. Routledge and Kegan Paul, London; Holt,
Rinehart, Winston, New York. 365 p.

Comfort, A. 1969. Test-battery to measure ageing-rate
in man. Lancet 2:1411-1414.

Constantinidis, J. 1978. Is Alzheimer's disease a major form of senile dementia? Clinical, anatomical,
and genetic data. Pages 15-25 in R. Katzman, R.D.
Terry, and K.L. Bick, eds. Alzheimer's disease: Senile dementia and related disorders. Vol. 7. Aging
series. Raven Press, New York.

Cooper, A. 1824. Treatment of dislocations and fractures of the joints. 4th ed. Longmans, London.

Cooper, J.T., and S. Goldstein. 1977. Comparative studies on human fibroblasts: Life span and lipid metabolism in medium containing fetal bovine or human serum.
In vitro 13:473-476.

Cooper, R.W. 1968. Squirrel monkey taxonomy and supply.
Pages 1-29 in L.A. Rosenblum and R.W. Cooper, eds.
The squirrel monkey. Academic Press, New York.

Corday, E., M.K. Heng, S. Meerbaum, T.-W. Lang, J.-C.
Farcot, J. Osher, and K. Hashimoto. 1977. Derangements of myocardial metabolism preceding onset of
ventricular fibrillation after coronary occlusion.
Am. J. Cardiol. 39:880-889.

Cordeau, J.P., J. Gybels, H. Jasper, and L.J. Poirier.
1960. Microelectric studies of unit discharges in
the sensorimotor cortex. Neurology 10:591-600.

Cornelius, L.M., and W.E. Wingfield. 1975. Diseases of
the stomach. Pages 1125-1149 in S.J. Ettinger, ed.
Textbook of veterinary internal medicine. W.B.
Saunders Co., Philadelphia.

Cornwell, G.G., G. Heisby, P. Westermark, J.G. Natvig,
T.E. Michaelsen, and B. Skogen. 1977. Identification
and charaterization of different amyloid fibrils

proteins in tissue sections. Scand. J. Immunol. 6:1071-1080.

Corsellis, J.A.N. 1962. Mental illness and the aging brain. Oxford University Press, London. 76 p.

Cosgrove, G.E., L.C. Satterfield, N.D. Bowles, and W.C. Klima. 1978. Diseases of aging untreated virgin female RFM and BALB/c mice. J. Gerontol. 33:178-183.

Costantin, L. 1963. Extracardiac factors contributing to hypotension during coronary occlusion. Amer. J. Cardiol. 11:205-217.

Costoff, A., and V.B. Mahesh. 1975. Primordial follicles with normal oocytes in the ovaries of postmenopausal women. J. Am. Geriatr. Soc. 23:193-196.

Cotchin, E. 1954. Further observations on neoplasms in dogs with particular reference to site of origin and malignancy. Part I. Cutaneous, female genital and alimentary systems. Br. Vet. J. 110:218-230.

Cotchin, E. 1958. Mammary neoplasms of the bitch. J. Comp. Pathol. 68:1-21.

Cotchin, E., and F.J.C. Roe [eds.] 1967. Pathology of rats and mice. Blackwell Scientific Publications, Oxford; F.A. Davis Company, Philadelphia. 848 p.

Cotton, D.J., E.R. Bleecker, S.P. Fisher, P.D. Grof, W.M. Gold, and J.A. Nadel. 1977. Rapid shallow breathing after Ascaris suum antigen inhalation: Role of vagus nerves. J. Appl. Physiol. 42:101-106.

Cotzias, G.C., S.T. Miller, L.C. Tang, P.S. Papavasiliou, and Y.Y. Wang. 1977. Levodopa, fertility and longevity. Science 196:549-551.

Courant, D.R., S.R. Saxe, L. Nash, and S. Roddy. 1968. Sulcular bacteria in the Beagle dog. Periodontics 6:250-252.

Cramlet, S.H., J.D. Toft II, and N.W. Olsen. 1974. Malignant melanoma in a black gerbil (Meriones unguiculatus). Lab. Anim. Sci. 24:545-547.

Crary, D.D., and P.B. Sawin. 1960. Genetic differences in growth rate and maturation of rabbits. Growth 24:111-130.

Crawford, A., S.S. Socransky, and G. Brathal. 1975. Predominant cultivable microbiota of advanced periodontis. J. Dent. Res. 54:209.

Crispens, C.G., Jr. 1975. Tables 30-33, Pages 143-155 in Handbook on the laboratory mouse. Charles C. Thomas, Springfield, Illinois.

Cristofalo, V.J. 1972. Animal cell cultures and aging. Adv. Gerontol. Res. 4:45-79.

Crowley, D.E. 1975. Conference on animal models of aging in the auditory system. Ann. Otol. Rhinol. Laryngol. 84:560-561.

Crowley, D.E., V.L. Schramm, R.E. Swain, R.H. Maisel, E. Rauchbach, and S.N. Swanson. 1972a. An animal model for presbycusis. Laryngoscope 82:2079-2091.

Crowley, D.E., V.L. Schramm, R.E. Swain, and S.N. Swanson. 1972b. Analysis of age-related changes in electrical responses from the inner ear of rats. Ann. Otol. Rhinol. Laryngol. 81:739-746.

Crowley, D.E., V.L. Schramm, R.E. Swain, and S.N. Swanson. 1973. Age-related wave-form changes of VIIIth nerve action potentials in rats. Laryngoscope 83:264-275.

Cruce, J.A.F., M.R.C. Greenwood, P.R. Johnson, and D. Quartermain. 1974. Genetic versus hypothalamic obesity: Studies of intake and dietary manipulations in rats. J. Comp. Physiol. Psychol. 87(2): 295-301.

Csallany, A.S., K.L. Ayaz, and L.C. Su. 1977. Effect of dietary vitamin E and aging on tissue lipofuscin pigment concentration in mice. J. Nutr. 107:1792-1799.

Cummings, J.F., and H. DeLahunta. 1977. An adult case of canine neuronal ceroid-lipofuscinosis. Acta Neuropathol. 39:43-51.

Curtis, H.J., and K. Miller. 1971. Chromosome aberrations in liver cells of guinea pigs. J. Gerontol. 26(3):292-293.

Cutler, G.J., and F. Ederer. 1958. Maximum utilization of the life table method in analyzing survival. J. Chronic Dis. 8:699-712.

Cutler, R.G. 1976a. Evolution of longevity in primates. J. Hum. Evol. 5:169-202.

Cutler, R.G. 1976b. Nature of aging and life maintenance processes. Interdiscip. Top. Gerontol. 9:83-133.

Dahme, E. 1962. Pathologische Befunde an den Hirngefässen bei Tieren. Die Veränderungen der Hirngefässe beim alten Hund. Acta Neuropathol. Suppl. I:54-60.

Danforth, C.H. 1927. Heredity adiposity in mice. J. Hered. 18:153-162.

Das, L.N., and J.H. Magilton. 1971. Age changes in the relationship among endocrine glands of the Beagle. Exp. Gerontol. 6:313-324.

Davidorf, F., and D. Egilitis. 1966. A study of a hereditary cataract in the mouse. J. Morphol. 119:89-93.

Davidson, B.J., L.J. Deftos, D.R. Meldrum, and H.L. Judd. 1980. Effect of medroxyprogesterone acetate (MPA) on bone metabolism of postmenopausal women. Abstract No. 279, Page 166 in Society for Gynecologic Investigation scientific abstracts. Abstracts of the 27th annual meeting, held March 19-22, 1980 in Denver, Colorado. Society for Gynecologic Investigation, c/o Dr. W. Anne Reynolds, Office of Academic Affairs, Ohio State University, Columbus, Ohio.

Davies, J.E., P.M. Ellery, and R.E. Hughes. 1977. Dietary ascorbic acid and life span of guinea pigs. Exp. Gerontol. 12(5-6):215-216.

Davies, P. 1978. Studies on the neurochemistry of central cholinergic systems in Alzheimer's disease. Pages 453-459 in R. Katzman, R.D. Terry, and K.L. Bick, eds. Alzheimer's disease: Senile dementia and related disorders. Vol. 7. Aging series. Raven Press, New York.

Davies, P., and A.J.F. Maloney. 1976. Selective loss of central cholinergic neurons in Alzheimer's disease. Lancet 2:1403.

Davies, P., and A.H. Veith. 1978. Regional distribution of muscarinic acetylcholine receptor in normal and Alzheimer's type-dementia brains. Brain Res. 138: 385-392.

Davis, D.H.S. 1965. Classification problems of African Muridae. Zool. Afr. 1:121-145.

Davis, K.L., and H.I. Yamamura. 1978. Cholinergic underactivity in human memory disorder. Life Sci. 23: 1729-1734.

Davis, R.K., G.T. Stevenson, and K.A. Busch. 1956. Tumor incidence in normal Sprague-Dawley female rats. Cancer Res. 16:194-197.

Davis, R.T. 1978. Old monkey behavior. Exp. Gerontol. 13:237-250.

Dayan, A.D. 1970a. Quantitative histological studies on the aged human brain. I. Senile plaques and neurofibrillary tangles in "normal" patients. Acta Neuropathol. 16:85-94.

Dayan, A.D. 1970b. Quantitative histological studies on the aged human brain. II. Senile plaques and neurofibrillary tangles in senile dementia. Acta Neuropathol. 16:95-102.

Dayan, A.D. 1971. Comparative neuropathology of ageing. Studies on the brains of 47 species of vertebrates. Brain 94:31-42.

DeLahunta, A., and J.N. Shively. 1975. Neurofibrillary accumulation in a puppy. Cornell Vet. 65:240-247.

Dellenback, R.J., and D.A. Ringle. 1963. Age changes in
the plasma glycoproteins of the Mongolian gerbil. Proc.
Soc. Exp. Biol. Med. 114:783-786.

Delost, P. 1953. Existence de glandes prostatiques chez
le campagnol des champs (Microtus arvalis P.) de sexe
femelle. Compt. Rend. Soc. Biol. 47:758-760.

Demartini, J.C., D.E. Green, and T.P. Monath. 1975. Lassa
virus infection in Mastomys natalensis in Sierra Leone.
Bull. W.H.O. 52:651-663.

DeNayer, D. 1969. Les effets de la resection du tendon
d'Achille sur la structure des os chez l'animal en
fin de croissance. Acta Orthop. Belg. 35:947-967.

Denckla, D. 1974. Role of the pituitary and thyroid
glands in the decline of the minimal O_2 consumption
with age. J. Clin. Invest. 53:572-581.

Dennis, M.O., R. C. Nealeigh, R.L. Pyle, S.H. Gilbert,
A.C. Lee, and C.W. Miller. 1978. Echocadiographic
assessment of normal and abnormal valvular function
in Beagle dogs. Am. J. Vet. Res. 39:1591-1598.

Dent, N.J. 1976. The use of the Syrian hamster to estab-
lish its clinical chemistry and haematology profile.
Pages 321-323 in W.A. Duncan and B.J. Leonard, eds.
The prediction of chronic toxicity from short-term
studies. International Congress Series No. 376.
Elsevier, Amsterdam.

DeOme, K.B., L.J. Faulkin, Jr., H.A. Bern, and P.B. Blair.
1959. Development of mammary tumors from hyperplastic
alveolar nodules transplanted into gland-free mammary
fat pads of female C3H mice. Cancer Res. 19:515-520.

Dequeker, J. 1975. Bone and aging. Ann. Rheum. Dis.
34:100-115.

Dermer, G.B. 1978. Basal cell proliferation in benign
prostatic hyperplasia. Cancer 41:1857-1862.

Detweiler, D.K., and D.F. Patterson. 1965. The prevalence and types of cardiovascular disease in dogs. Ann.
N.Y. Acad. Sci. 127:481-516.

Detweiler, D.K., D.F. Patterson, and H. Luginbuhl. 1972.
Observations on naturally occurring myocardial fibrosis
and necrosis in dogs. Pages 574-578 in E. Bajusz and
G. Rona, eds. Recent advances in studies on cardiac
structure and metabolism. University Park Press,
Baltimore.

Dewey, J.R., G.J. Armelagos, and M.H. Bartley. 1969.
Femoral cortical involution in three Nubian archaeolog-
ical populations. Hum. Biol. 41:13-28.

Dewson, J.H., and A.C. Burlingame. 1975. Auditory discrimination and recall in monkeys. Science 187:267-268.

Diamant, N., M. Szczepanski, and H. Mui. 1973. Manometric characteristics of idiopathic megaesophagus in the dog: An unsuitable animal model for achalasia in man. Gastroenterology 65:216-223.

Diamond, M.C., R.E. Johnson, and C. Ingham. 1975. The development, adult and aging patterns of the cerebral cortex, hippocampus and diencephalon. Behav. Biol. 14:163-174.

Dickie, M.M. 1969. Mutations at the agouti locus in the mouse. J. Hered. 60:20-25.

Dickie, M.M., W.B. Atkinson, and E. Fekete. 1957. The ovary, estrous cycle and fecundity of DBA x CE and reciprocal hybrid mice in relation to age and the hyperovarian syndrome. Anat. Rec. 127:187-199.

Dillon, W.G., and C.A. Glomski. 1975. The Mongolian gerbil: Qualitative and quantitative aspects of the cellular blood picture. Lab. Anim. 9:283-287.

Dittus, W.P.J. 1975. Population dynamics of the Toque monkey, Macaca sinica. Pages 125-151 in R. Tuttle, ed. Socioecology and psychology of primates. Mouton, The Hague.

Dittus, W.P.J. 1977. The social regulation of population density and age-sex distribution in the Toque monkey. Behaviour 63:281-322.

Divry, P. 1934. De la nature de l'alteration fibrillaire d'Alzheimer. J. Belge Neurol. Psychiatr. 34:197-201.

Dixon, F.J., and R.A. Moore. 1953. Testicular tumors. A clinicopathological study. Cancer 6:427-454.

Dodds, W.J., S.L. Raymond, A.C. Moynihan, and D.N. McMartin. 1977. Spontaneous atrial thrombosis in aged Syrian hamsters. II. Hemostasis. Thromb. Haemost. 38:457-464.

Doherty, P.C. 1977. Diminished surveillance of T cell function in old mice infected with lymphocytic choriomeningitis virus. Immunology 32:751-754.

Dorn, C.R., and W.A. Priester. 1976. Epidemiologic analysis of oral and pharyngeal cancer in dogs, cats, horses, and cattle. J. Am. Vet. Med. Assoc. 169:1202-1206.

Dorn, C.R., D.O.N. Taylor, and H.H. Hibbard. 1967. Epizootiologic characteristics of canine and feline leukemia and lymphoma. Am. J. Vet. Res. 28:993-1001.

Dorn, C.R., D.O.N. Taylor, F.L. Frye, and H.H. Hibbard. 1968a. Survey of animal neoplasms in Alameda and Contra

Costa Counties, California. I. Methodology and description of cases. J. Natl. Cancer Inst. 40:295-305.

Dorn, C.R., D.O.N. Taylor, R. Schneider, H.H. Hibbard, and M.R. Klauber. 1968b. Survey of animal neoplasms in Alameda and Contra Costa Counties, California. II. Cancer morbidity in dogs and cats from Alameda County. J. Natl. Cancer Inst. 40:307-318.

Doty, B.A., and R. Dalman. 1969. Diphenylhydantoin effects on avoidance conditioning as a function of age and problem difficulty. Psychon. Sci. 14:109-111.

Dowling, J.E., and R.L. Sidman. 1962. Inherited retinal dystrophy in the rat. J. Cell. Biol. 14:73-109.

Draper, H.H. 1964. Physiological aspects of aging. V. Calcium and magnesium metabolism. J. Nutr. 83:65-72.

Draper, H.H., C.T. Liu, and A. Saari Csallany. 1970. Composition of mouse adipose tissue as a function of adult age. Pages 274-277 in J. Mašek, K. Ošancová, and D.P. Cuthbertson, eds. Nutrition. International Congress Series No. 213. Excerpta Medica, Amsterdam.

Drasher, M.L. 1955. Strain differences in the response of the mouse uterus to estrogens. J. Hered. 46:190-192.

Dreizen, S., and B.M. Levy. 1977. Monkey models in dental research. J. Med. Primatol. 6:133-144.

Dreyfuss, J., B. Beer, D.D. Devine, B.F. Roberts, and E.C. Schreiber. 1972. Fluphenazine-induced parkinsonism in the baboon: Pharmacological and metabolic studies. Neuropharmacology 11:223-230.

Duchen, L.W., and P.H. Schurr. 1976. The pathology of the pituitary gland in old age. Pages 137-156 in A.V. Everitt and J.A. Burgess, eds. Hypothalamus, pituitary, and aging. Charles C. Thomas, Springfield, Illinois.

Duffy, P.H., and G.A. Sacher. 1976. Age-dependence of body weight and linear dimensions in adult Mus and Peromyscus. Growth 40:19-31.

Durbin, P.W., M.H. Williams, N. Jeung, and J.S. Arnold. 1966. Development of spontaneous mammary tumors over the life span of the female Charles River (Sprague-Dawley) rat: The influence of ovariectomy, thyroidectomy, and adrenalectomy-ovariectomy. Cancer Res. 26:400-411.

Duvoisin, R.C. 1976. Parkinsonism: Animal analogues of the human disorder. Pages 293-303 in M.D. Yahr, ed. The basal ganglia. Research Publications, Association for Research in Nervous and Mental Disease. Vol. 55. Raven Press, New York.

Ebbesen, P. 1972. Long survival time of isolated Balb/c
and DBA/2 male mice. Acta Pathol. Microbiol. Scand.
80:149-150.

Eddy, T.P. 1972. Deaths from domestic falls and fractures. Br. J. Prev. Soc. Med. 26:173-179.

Ediger, R.E. 1976. Care and management. Pages 5-12 in
J.E. Wagner and P.J. Manning, eds. The biology of the
guinea pig. Academic Press, New York.

Edington, D.W., and A.C. Cosmas. 1972. Effect of maturation and training on mitochondrial size distribution
in rat hearts. J. Appl. Physiol. 33(6):715-718.

Edwards, G.A., V.B. Bernardino, Jr., V.I. Babcock, and
C.M. Southam. 1975. Cataracts in bleomycin-treated
rats. Am. J. Ophthalmol. 80:538-542.

Edwards, R.G., R.E. Fowler, R.E. Gore-Langton, R.G. Gosden,
E.C. Jones, C. Readhead, and P.C. Steptoe. 1977. Normal and abnormal follicular growth in mouse, rat, and
human ovaries. J. Reprod. Fertil. 51:237-263.

Effron, M., L. Griner, and K. Benirschke. 1977. Nature
and rate of neoplasia found in captive wild mammals,
birds, and reptiles at necropsy. J. Natl. Cancer Inst.
59:185-198.

Egelberg, J. 1964. Gingival exudate measurements for
evaluation of inflammatory changes of the gingivae.
Odontol. Revy 15:381-398.

Egelberg, J. 1965a. Local effect of diet on plaque formation and development of gingivitis in dogs. I. Effect
of hard and soft diets. Odontol. Revy 16:31-34.

Egelberg, J. 1965b. Local effect of diet on plaque forma-
tion and development of gingivitis in dogs. III.
Effect of frequency of meals and tube feeding. Odontol.
Revy 16:50-60.

Egelberg, J. 1967. The topography and permeability of
vessels at the dentino-gingival junction in dogs. J.
Periodontal Res. 2: Suppl. 1.

Eggen, D.A., J.P. Strong, W.P. Newman III, C. Catsulis,
G.T. Malcolm, and M.G. Kokatnur. 1974. Regression of
diet-induced fatty streaks in rhesus monkeys. Lab.
Invest. 31:294-301.

Ehling, U. 1957. Untersuchungen zur Kausalen Genese
erblicher Katarakte beim Kaninchen. Z. Menschl. Vererb.
Konstitutionsl. 34:77-104.

Ehret, G. 1974. Age-dependent hearing loss in normal
hearing mice. Naturwissenschaften 61:506-507.

Eisdorfer, C., and D. Cohen. 1978. The cognitively impaired elderly: Differential diagnosis. Pages 7-42
in M. Storandt, I. Siegler and M. F. Elias, eds. The

clinical psychology of aging. Plenum Publishing Corp.,
New York.

Eisdorfer, C., and D. Cohen. In press. Research diagnostic criteria for primary neuronal degeneration of the
Alzheimer type. J. Family Med.

Eisdorfer, C., D. Cohen, and C.E. Buckley, III. 1978.
Serum immunoglobulins and cognition in the impaired
elderly. Pages 401-408 in R. Katzman, R.D. Terry,
and K.L. Bick, eds. Alzheimer's disease: Senile
dementia and related disorders. Vol. 7. Aging series.
Raven Press, New York.

Eleftheriou, B.E. 1975. Changes with age in protein-
bound iodine and body temperature in the mouse. J.
Gerontol. 30:417-421.

Eleftheriou, B.E., and L.A. Lucas. 1974. Age-related
changes in testes, seminal vesicles and plasma testosterone levels in male mice. Gerontologia 20:231-238.

Eleftheriou, B.E., A.J. Zolovick, and M.F. Elias. 1975.
Electroencephalographic changes with age in male mice.
Gerontologia 21:21-30.

Elias, J.W., M.F. Elias, and G. Schlager. 1975. Aggressive social interaction in mice genetically selected
for blood pressure extremes. Behav. Biol. 13:155-166.

Elias, M.F. 1979. Aging studies of behavior with Fischer
344 and Long Evans rats. Pages 253-297 in D.C. Gibson,
R.C. Adelman, and C. Finch, eds. Development of the
rodent as a model system of aging. Book II. DHEW Pub.
No. (NIH) 79-161. U.S. Department of Health, Education,
and Welfare, Washington, D.C.

Elias, M.F., and P.K. Elias. 1975. Hormones, aging and
behavior. Pages 395-439 in B.E. Eleftheriou and R.L.
Sprott, eds. Hormonal correlates of behavior. Vol. I.
A lifespan view. Plenum Publishing Corp., New York.

Elias, M.F., and P.K. Elias. 1977. Drive, motivation,
and activity. Pages 357-383 in J.E. Birren and K.W.
Schaie, eds. Handbook of the psychology of aging.
Van Nostrand Reinhold, New York.

Elias, P.K., and M.F. Elias. 1976. Effects of age on
learning ability; contribution from the animal literature. Exp. Aging Res. 2:165-186.

Elias, P.K., and E.S. Redgate. 1975. Effects of immobilization stress on open field behavior and corticosterone
response of aging C57BL/6J mice. Exp. Aging Res.
1:127-137.

Elias, P.K., M.F. Elias, and B.E. Eleftheriou. 1975.
Emotionality, exploratory behavior and locomotion in
aging inbred strains of mice. Gerontologia 21:46-55.

Ellegaard, B., T. Karring, M. Listgarten, and H. Loe.
1973. New attachment after treatment of interradicular
lesions. J. Periodontol. 44:209-217.

Ellenberg, M. 1975. Diabetic neuropathy. Pages 201-205
in K.E. Sussman and R.J.S. Metz, eds. Diabetes mellitus. 4th ed. American Diabetes Association Inc., New
York.

Ellerman, J.R. 1940-1949. Families and genera of living
rodents. Vols. I-III. British Museum of Natural History, London. 1589 p.

Ellis, F.R., S. Holesh, and T.A.B. Sanders. 1974. Osteoporosis in British vegetarians and omnivores. Am. J.
Clin. Nutr. 27:769-770.

Ellsasser, J.C., C.F. Moyer, P.A. Lesker, and D.J. Simmons.
1973. Effect of low doses of disodium ethane-1-
hydroxy-1, 1-diphosphonate on disuse osteoporosis in
the denervated cat tail. Clin. Orthop. Relat. Res.
91:235-242.

Elmes, P.C., and D.P. Bell. 1963. The effects of chlorine
gas on the lungs of rats with spontaneous pulmonary
disease. J. Pathol. Bacteriol. 86:317-326.

El-Mofty, A., P. Gouras, G. Eisen, and E. Balazs. 1978.
Macular degeneration in rhesus monkey (Macaca mulatta).
Exp. Eye Res. 27:499-502.

Emminger, A., G. Reznik, H. Reznik-Schuller, and U. Mohr.
1975. Differences in blood values depending on age
in laboratory-bred European hamsters (Cricetus cricetus
L.). Lab. Anim. 9:33-42.

Epstein, L.J. 1976. Depression in the elderly. J.
Gerontol. 31:278-282.

Erlik, Y., I.V. Tataryn, P. Lomax, D.R. Meldrum, J.G.
Bajorek, and H.L. Judd. 1980. Association of hot
flashes (HF) with waking episodes in postmenopausal
women. Abstract No. 83, Page 52 in Society for Gynecologic Investigation scientific abstracts. Abstracts
of the 27th annual meeting held March 19-22, 1980 in
Denver, Colorado. Society for Gynecologic Investigation, c/o Dr. W. Anne Reynolds, Office of Academic
Affairs, Ohio State University, Columbus, Ohio.

Estes, P.C., C.B. Richter, and J.A. Franklin. 1971. De-
modectic mange in the golden hamster. Lab. Anim. Sci.
21:825-828.

Ettinger, S.J. [ed.] 1975. Textbook of veterinary internal medicine: Diseases of the dog and cat. Vols. I
and II. W.B. Saunders, Philadelphia. 1767 p.

Ettinger, S.J., and P.F. Suter. 1970. Canine cardiology.
W.B. Saunders Co., Philadelphia. 616 p.

Evans, D.J. 1972. Generalized islet hypertrophy and beta-cell hyperplasia in a case of long-term juvenile diabetes. Diabetes 21:114-116.

Ewing, G.O., and J.A. Gomez. 1973. Canine ulcerative colitis. J. Am. Anim. Hosp. Assoc. 9:395-406.

Fabrikant, J.D., and E.L. Schneider. 1978. Studies of the genetic and immunologic compounds of the maternal age defect. Dev. Biol. 66:337-343.

Falconer, D.S., and J.H. Isaacson. 1959. Adipose, a new inherited obesity of the mouse. J. Hered. 50:290-292.

Farner, D., and F. Verzar. 1961. The age parameter of pharmacological activity. Experientia 17:421-422.

Feinberg, I., R.L. Loresko, and N. Heller. 1967. EEG sleep patterns as a function of normal and pathological aging in man. J. Psychiat. Res. 5:107-144.

Fekete, E. 1946. A comparative study of the ovaries of virgin mice of the dba and C57 Black strains. Cancer Res. 6:263-269.

Fekete, E., G.W. Woolley, and C.C. Little. 1941. Histological changes following ovariectomy in mice. I/dba high tumor strain. J. Exp. Med. 74:1-8.

Feldman, M.L. 1976. Aging changes in the morphology of cortical dendrites. Pages 211-227 in R.D. Terry and S. Gershon, eds. Neurobiology of aging. Vol. 3. Aging series. Raven Press, New York.

Feldman, M.L., and A. Peters. 1974. Morphological changes in the aging brain. Pages 5-22 in G.J. Maletta, ed. Survey report on the aging nervous system. DHEW Pub. No. (NIH) 74-296. U.S. Department of Health, Education, and Welfare, Washington, D.C.

Feldman, M.L., and D.W. Vaughan. 1979. Changes in the auditory pathway with age. Pages 143-162 in Special senses in aging. A current biological assessment. Proceedings of a symposium held October 10-11, 1977 at the University of Michigan, Ann Arbor. Institute of Gerontology, University of Michigan, Ann Arbor, Michigan.

Felicio, L.S., J.F. Nelson, and C.E. Finch. In press. Spontaneous pituitary tumorigenesis in aging female C57BL/6J mice. Exp. Gerontol.

Ferencz, C. 1969. Pulmonary arterial design in mammals. Johns Hopkins Med. J. 125:207-224.

Ferguson, H.W., and R.L. Hartles. 1970. The combined effects of calcium deficiency and ovariectomy on the bones of young adult cats. Calcif. Tissue Res. Suppl. 4:140-141.

Fernandes, G., E.J. Yunis, and R.A. Good. 1976. Influence of diet on survival of mice. Proc. Natl. Acad. Sci. U.S.A. 73:1279-1283.

Festing, M.F.W. [ed.] 1980. International index of laboratory animals. 4th ed. Medical Research Council, Laboratory Animal Centre, Carshalton, Surrey, England. 141 p.

Festing, M.F.W. 1976. Genetics. Pages 99-120 in J.E. Wagner and P.J. Manning, eds. The biology of the guinea pig. Academic Press, New York.

Festing, M.F.W., and D.K. Blackmore. 1971. Life span of specified-pathogen-free (MRC category 4) mice and rats. Lab. Anim. 5:179-192.

Festing, M.F.W., and J. Bleby. 1970. Breeding performance and growth of SPF cats (Felis catus). J. Small Anim. Pract. 11:533-542.

Field, T.M., C. Dabiri, and H.H. Shuman. 1977. Developmental effects of prolonged pregnancy and the postmaturity syndrome. J. Pediatr. 90:836-839.

Finch, C.E. 1972. Cellular pacemakers of ageing in mammals. Pages 123-126 in R. Harris and D. Viza, eds. Proc. 1st European conference on cell differentiation (Nice, 1971). Munksgaard, Copenhagen.

Finch, C.E. 1973a. Catecholamine metabolism in the brains of aging male mice. Brain Res. 52:261-276.

Finch, C.E. 1973b. Retardation of hair regrowth, a phenomenon of senescence in C57BL/6J male mice. J. Gerontol. 28:13-17.

Finch, C.E. 1977. Neuroendocrine and autonomic aspects of aging. Pages 262-280 in C.E. Finch and L. Hayflick, eds. Handbook of the biology of aging. Van Nostrand Reinhold, New York.

Finch, C.E. 1978a. Age-related changes in brain catecholamines: A synopsis of findings in C57BL/6J mice and other rodent models. Adv. Exp. Med. Biol. 113:15-41.

Finch, C.E. 1978b. Genotype influences on female reproductive senescence in rodents. Pages 335-354 in D. Bergsma and D.E. Harrison, eds. Genetic effects on aging. Birth defects original article series. Vol. 14, No. 1. A.R. Liss, Inc., New York.

Finch, C.E., and F.G. Girgis. 1974. Enlarged seminal vesicles of senescent C57BL/6J mice. J. Gerontol. 29:134-138.

Finch, C.E., and L. Hayflick [eds.] 1977. Handbook of the biology of aging. Van Nostrand Reinhold, New York. 771 p.

Finch, C.E., J.R. Foster, and A.E. Mirksy. 1969. Ageing
and the regulation of cell activities during exposure
to cold. J. Gen. Physiol. 54:690-712.

Finch, C.E., V. Jonec, J.R. Wisner, Jr., Y.N. Sinha, H.S.
de Vellis, and R.S. Swerdloff. 1977. Hormone production by the pituitary and testes of male C57BL/6J mice
during aging. Endocrinology 101:1310-1318.

Fine, B.S., and R.D. Kwapien. 1978. Pigment epithelial
windows and drusen: An animal model. Invest. Ophthalmol. Vis. Sci. 17:1059-1068.

Fingerhut, B., and R.J. Veenema. 1966. Histology and
radioautography of induced benign enlargement of the
mouse prostate. Invest. Urol. 4:112-124.

Finkel, M.P., and G.M. Scribner. 1955. Mouse cages and
spontaneous tumors. Br. J. Cancer 9:464-472.

Finkiewicz-Murawiejska, L. 1972. Cytochemical evaluation
of the aging process in nerve cells of the spiral ganglion of the cochlea in guinea pigs. Folia Morphol.
Warsaw 31(2):155-167.

Fisk, D.E., and C. Kuhn. 1976. Emphysema-like changes
in the lungs of the blotchy mouse. Am. Rev. Resp. Dis.
113:787-797.

Fishman, W.H., and M.H. Farmelant. 1953. Effects of androgens and estrogens in β-glucuronidase in inbred mice.
Endocrinology 52:536-545.

Flatt, R.E., S.H. Weisbroth, and A.L. Kraus. 1974. Metabolic, traumatic, mycotic, and miscellaneous diseases
of rabbits. Pages 435-451 in S.H. Weisbroth, R.E.
Flatt, and A.L. Kraus, eds. The biology of the laboratory rabbit. Academic Press, New York.

Flir, K. 1952. Die primaren Nierengeschwulste der
Haustiere. Wiss. Z. Humboldt-Univ. Berlin Math.
Naturwiss. Reihe 93-119 p.

Florini, J.R. 1975. Differences in enzyme levels and
physiological processes in mice of different ages. Exp.
Aging Res. 1:137-144.

Florini, J.R., and R.N. Sorrentino. 1976. Protein metabolism during aging. Annu. Rev. Exp. Aging Res. 1:
181-197.

Florini, J.R., Y. Saito, and E.J. Manowitz. 1973. Effect
of age on thyroxine-induced cardiac hypertrophy in mice.
J. Gerontol. 28:293-297.

Flower, S.S. 1931. Contributions to our knowledge of the
duration of life in vertebrate animals. Part V. Mammals. Proc. Zool. Soc. London 1:145-234.

Flynn, K.J., J.F. Schumacher, and M.T.R. Subbiah. 1976.
The effect of ilial bypass on sterol balance and plasma

cholesterol in the White Carneau pigeon. Atherosclerosis 24:75-80.

Flynn, R.J. [ed.] 1963. Conference on Pseudomonas aeruginosa infection and its effects on biological and medical research. Lab. Anim. Care 13:1-69.

Flynn, R.J. 1973. Parasites of laboratory animals. Iowa State University Press, Ames, Iowa. 884 p.

Foley, W.A., D.C.L. Jones, G.K. Osborn, and D.J. Kimeldorf. 1964. A renal lesion associated with diuresis in the aging Sprague-Dawley rats. Lab. Invest. 13:439-450.

Fooden, J. 1969. Taxonomy and evolution of the monkeys of Celebes. Bibliotheca primatologica. Fasc. 10. S. Karger, Basel, Switzerland. 148 p.

Ford, O.H., and R.L. Rhines. 1969. ^{3}H-lysine accumulation in motor neurons in rats of different ages compared with accumulation in other tissues. Acta Neurol. Scand. 45:41-52.

Fore, F.N., G.T. Smith, and J.J. McNamara. 1978. Prediction of infarct size with baboons. A proposed model for accurately determining the efficacy of therapeutic interventions. Circ. Res. 43:455-465.

Forgacs, J., and W.T. Caril. 1966. Mycotoxicoses: Toxic fungi in tobacco. Science 152:1634-1635.

Forno, L.S. 1978. The locus caeruleus in Alzheimer's disease. J. Neuropathol. Exp. Neurol. 37:614.

Fowler, E.H., G.P. Wilson, and A. Koestner. 1974. Biologic behavior of canine mammary neoplasms based on a histogenetic classification. Vet. Pathol. 11(3): 212-229.

Fox, R.R. 1974. Taxonomy and genetics. Pages 1-22 in S.H. Weisbroth, R.E. Flatt, and A.L. Kraus, eds. The biology of the laboratory rabbit. Academic Press, New York.

Fox, R.R. 1975. Handbook of genetically standardized JAX rabbits. 1st ed. The Jackson Laboratory, Bar Harbor, Maine. 28 p.

Fox, R.R., and M. Cherry. 1978. Effect of rabbit strain on activity level and cytotoxicity of serum complement. II. Comparison of five murine target cells. J. Hered. 69:331-336.

Fox, R.R., G. Schlager, and C.W. Laird. 1969. Blood pressure in thirteen strains of rabbits. J. Hered. 60: 312-314.

Fox, R.R., M. Cherry, and K.L. Shultz. 1978. Effect of rabbit strain on activity level and cytotoxicity of serum complement. J. Hered. 69:107-112.

Frangipane, G., and F. Aporti. 1969. Improved indirect method for the measurement of systolic blood pressure in the rat. J. Lab. Clin. Med. 73:872-876.

Frank, D.W. 1976. Physiological data of laboratory animals. Pages 23-64 in E.C. Melby, Jr. and N.H. Altman, eds. Handbook of laboratory animal science. Vol. III. CRC Press, Inc., Cleveland, Ohio.

Franks, L.M. 1954. Benign nodular hyperplasia of the prostate: A review. Ann. R. Coll. Surg. Engl. 14: 92-106.

Franks, L.M., P.D. Wilson, and R.D. Whelan. 1974. The effects of age on total DNA and cell number in the mouse brain. Gerontologia 20:21-26.

Frantz, M.J., and A. Kirschbaum. 1949. Sex hormone secretion by tumors of the adrenal cortex of mice. Cancer Res. 9:257-266.

Fraser, F.C., and M.L. Herer. 1950. The inheritance and expression of the "lens rupture" gene. J. Hered. 41:3-7.

Fraser, F.C., and G. Schabtach. 1962. "Shrivelled": A hereditary degeneration of the lens in the house mouse. Genet. Res. 3:383-387.

Fraser, H., and A.G. Dickinson. 1973. Scrapie in mice. Agent-strain differences in the distribution and intensity of grey matter vacuolation. J. Comp. Pathol. 83:29-40.

Frazer, J., and W.K. Yang. 1972. Isoaccepting transfer ribonucleic acids in liver and brain of young and old BC3F mice. Arch. Biochem. Biophys. 153:610-618.

Freeman, G., S.C. Crane, R.J. Stephens, and N.J. Furiosi. 1968. Pathogenesis of the nitrogen dioxide-induced lesion in the rat lung: A review and presentation of new observations. Am. Rev. Respir. Dis. 98:429-443.

Freeman, G., R.J. Stephens, D.L. Coffin, and J.F. Stara. 1973. Changes in dog's lungs after long-term exposure to ozone. Arch. Environ. Health 26:209-216.

Frenkel, J.K., P. Rasmussen, and O.D. Smith. 1959. Synergism of cortisol (F) and desoxycorticosterone (DOC) in the production of dissecting aortic aneurysms in hamsters. Abstract No. 1879. Fed. Proc. 18:477.

Friede, R.L., and M. Knoller. 1964. Proximo-distal increase of enzymic activity in the dorsal spinal tracts. J. Neurochem. 11:679-686.

Friedhoff, A.J., K. Bonnet, and H. Rosengarten. 1977. Reversal of two manifestations of dopamine receptor supersensitivity by administration of l-dopa. Res. Commun. Chem. Pathol. Pharmacol. 16:411-423.

Friedman, S.M., M. Nakashima, and C.L. Friedman. 1965.
Prolongation of lifespan in the old rat by adrenal
and neurohypophyseal hormones. Gerontologia 11(3):
129-149.

Frol'kis, V.V., and L.N. Bogatskaya. 1967. Age-specific
peculiarities of the energy balance in the heart.
Kardiologiya 7:66-71. (in Russian)

Frol'kis, V.V., S.A. Bezhanyan, V.V. Bezrukov, N.S.
Verkhratsky, V.P. Zamostyan, S.M. Karpova, V.G. Shevchuk, and I.V. Schegoleva. 1968. Age-specific peculiarities of the organism's reaction to the introduction of catecholamines. Farmakol. Toksikol. 31:
222-226. (in Russian)

Frol'kis, V.V., V.V. Bezrukov, and V.G. Shevchuk. 1974.
Control of haemodynamics in the old age. Kardiologiya
14:51-59. (in Russian)

Frol'kis, V.V., S.F. Golovchenko, and B.V. Pugach. 1976.
Vasopressin concentration in the blood and sensitivity
of the cardiovascular system to it during aging.
Fiziol. Zh. SSSR 62:586-593. (in Russian)

Frol'kis, V.V., L.N. Bogatskaya, A.S. Stupina, and V.G.
Shevchuk. 1977. Experimental analysis of development
of cardiac insufficiency in old age. Am. Heart J.
93:334-348.

Frost, H.M. 1969. Tetracycline-based histological analysis of bone remodeling. Calcif. Tissue Res. 3:211-
237.

Frye, C.R., D.O.N. Taylor, H.H. Hibbard, and M.R. Klauber.
1967. Characteristics of canine mammary gland tumor
cases. Anim. Hosp. 3:1-12.

Fujisawa, K. 1976. Some observations on the skeletal
musculature of aged rats. III. Abnormalities of terminal axons found in motor endplates. Exp. Gerontol.
11:43-47.

Fukuchi, Y. 1972a. Aging of the bronchial tree and the
bronchial vascular system. 1. Changes in bronchial
muscular tone due to aging. Jpn. J. Geriatr. 9:1-9.
(in Japanese)

Fukuchi, Y. 1972b. Aging of the bronchial tree and the
bronchial vascular system. 2. Changes in the bronchial
vascular system tone due to aging. Jpn. J. Geriatr.
9:10-18. (in Japanese)

Fuster, V., J.C. Lewis, B.A. Kottke, C.E. Ruiz, and E.J.W.
Bowie. 1977. Platelet factor 4-like activity in the
initial stages of atherosclerosis in pigeons. Thromb.
Res. 10:169-172.

Gad, T. 1968. Periodontal disease in dogs. I. Clinical investigation. J. Periodontal Res. 3:268-272.

Gage, E. 1975. Incidence of clinical disc disease in the dog. J. Am. Anim. Hosp. Assoc. 11:135-138.

Gage, A.A., K.C. Olson, and W.H. Chardack. 1956. Experimental coronary thrombosis in dog; description of method. Ann. Surg. 143:535-543.

Gajdusek, D.C. 1972. Slow virus infection and activation of latent virus infections in aging. Adv. Gerontol. Res. 4:201-218.

Gajdusek, D.C. 1977. Unconventional viruses and the origin and disappearance of kuru. Science 197:943-960.

Galloway, J.H., D. Glover, and W.C. Fox. 1964. Relationship of diet and age to metastatic calcification in guinea pigs. Lab. Anim. Care 14:6-12.

Ganaway, J.R. 1976. Bacterial, mycoplasma, and rickettsial diseases. Pages 121-135 in J.E. Wagner and P.J. Manning, eds. The biology of the guinea pig. Academic Press, New York.

Gandalovičová, D. 1974. Enterochromaffin cells in the guinea pig digestive tube in relation to aging. Folia Morphol. Praha 22(1):102-108.

Gardiner, T.H., and L.S. Schanker. 1975. Effect of papain-induced emphysema on permeability of rat lung to drugs. Proc. Soc. Exp. Biol. Med. 149:972-977.

Garn, S.M. 1970. The earlier gain and later loss of cortical bone. Charles C. Thomas, Springfield, Illinois. 146 p.

Garn, S.M. 1975. Bone-loss and aging. Pages 39-57 in R. Goldman and M. Rockstein, eds. The physiology and pathology of human aging. Academic Press, New York.

Garant, P.R., and J.E. Mulvihill. 1972. The fine structure of gingivitis in the Beagle. J. Periodontal Res. 7:161-172.

Gass, J.D.M. 1967. Pathogenesis of disciform detachment of the neuroepithelium. Am. J. Ophthalmol. 63:573-585.

Gasset, A.R., M. Itoi, and Y. Ishii. 1975. Experimental BUdR congenital cataracts. Invest. Ophthalmol. 14:145-146.

Gaulin, S.J.C., and M. Konner. 1977. On the natural diet of primates, including humans. Pages 1-86 in R.J. Wurtman and J.J. Wurtman, eds. Nutrition and the brain. Raven Press, New York.

Gavan, J.A. 1967. Eruption of primate deciduous dentition: A comparative study. J. Dent. Res. 40:984-988.

Gavan, J.A., and T.C. Huchinson. 1973. The problem of age estimation: A study using rhesus monkeys (Macaca mulatta). Am. J. Phys. Anthropol. 38:69-81.

Geinisman, 1979. Loss of axosomatic synapses in the dentate gyrus of aged rats. Brian Res. 168:485-492.

Geinisman, Y., W. Bondareff, and J.T. Dodge. 1977. Partial deafferentation of neurons in the dentate gyrus of the senescent rat. Brain Res. 134:541-545.

Geinisman, Y., W. Bondareff, and J.T. Dodge. 1978a. Dendritic atrophy in the dentate gyrus of the senescent rat. Am. J. Anat. 152:321-330.

Geinisman, Y., W. Bondareff and J.T. Dodge. 1978b. Hypertrophy of astroglial processes in the dentate gyrus of the senescent rat. Am. J. Anat. 153:537-544.

Gelatt, K.N. 1972. Cataracts in the Golden Retriever dog. Vet. Med. Small Anim. Clin. 67:1113-1115.

Gelatt, K.N., R.D. Whitley, and J.D. Lavach. 1979. Familial cataracts in the Chesapeake Bay Retriever. J. Am. Vet. Med. Assoc. 175:1176-1178.

Georgi, J.R., L.F. LeJambre, and L.H. Ratcliffe. 1969. Ancylostoma canium burden in relationship to erythrocyte loss in dogs. J. Parasitol. 55:1205-1211.

Gerbase-DeLima, M., R.K. Liu, K.E. Cheney, R. Mickey, and R.L. Walford. 1975. Immune function and survival in a long-lived mouse strain subjected to undernutrition. Gerontologia 21:184-202.

German, J. 1968. Mongolism, delayed fertilization, and human sexual behavior. Nature 217:516-518.

Gershon, H., and D. Gershon. 1973. Inactive enzyme molecules in aging mice: Liver aldolase. Proc. Natl. Acad. Sci. USA 70:909-913.

Gertz, E.W. 1973. Animal model of human disease. Myocardial failure, muscular dystrophy. Am. J. Pathol. 70:151-154.

Getty, R., and C.R. Ellenport. 1974. Laboratory animals in aging studies. Pages 41-179 in W.I. Gay, ed. Methods of animal experimentation. Vol. 5. Academic Press, New York.

Ghanadian. R., G. Auf, C.B. Smith, G.D. Chisholm, and N.J. Blacklock. 1977a. Androgen receptors in the prostate of the rhesus monkey. Urol. Res. 5:169-173.

Ghanadian, R., G. Auf, C.B. Smith, P.J. Chaloner, G.D. Chisholm, and N.J. Blacklock. 1977b. Characterization and measurement of an androgen receptor protein in the cytosol of rhesus monkey prostate. J. Endocrinol. 75:26P.

Ghanadian, R., C.B. Smith, G.D. Chisholm, and N.J. Blacklock. 1977c. Differential androgen uptake by the lobes
of the rhesus monkey prostate. Br. J. Urol. 49:701-
704.

Gibbs, C.T., Jr., D.C. Gajdusek, and C.L. Masters. 1978.
Considerations of transmissible subacute and chronic
infections, with a summary of the clinical, pathological
and virological characteristics of kuru, Creutzfeldt-
Jakob disease and scrapie. Pages 115-130 in K. Nandy,
ed. Senile dementia: A biomedical approach. Developments in neuroscience. Vol. 3. Elsevier North-Holland
Biomedical Press, New York.

Giddens, W.E., Jr., K.K. Keahey, C.R. Carter, and C.K.
Whitehair. 1968. Pneumonia in rats due to infection
with Corynebacterium kutscheri. Pathol. Vet. 5:227-
237.

Giles, R.C., R.P. Kwapien, R.G. Geil, and H.W. Casey.
1977. Mammary nodules in Beagle dogs administered investigational oral contraceptive steroids. J. Natl.
Cancer Inst. 60:1351-1364.

Giles, R.E., J.C. Williams, and M.P. Finkel. 1973. Progesterone antagonism of papain emphysema: Role of sex,
estrogens and serum antitrypsin. Proc. Soc. Exp. Biol.
Med. 144:487-491.

Gillespie, J.R., J.D. Berry, Y.-Y. Yang, L.L. White, D.M.
Hyde, and J.F. Stara. 1976. Abnormal pulmonary function values of Beagles two years after exposure to
auto exhaust and other pollutant mixtures. Abstract
No. 2351. Fed. Proc. 35:632.

Gillis, R.A. 1971. Role of the nervous system in the
arrhythmias produced by coronary occlusion in the cat.
Am. Heart J. 81:677-681.

Gillis, R.A., F.H. Levine, H. Thibodeaux, A. Raines, and
F.G. Standaert. 1973. Comparison of methyllidocaine
and lidocaine on arrhythmias produced by coronary occlusion in the dog. Circulation 47:697-703.

Gillis, R.A., P.B. Corr, D.G. Pace, D.E. Evans, J. DiMicco,
and D.L. Pearle. 1976. Role of the nervous system in
experimentally induced arrhythmias. Cardiology 61:
37-49.

Gilmore, C.E., V.H. Gilmore, and T.C. Jones. 1964a. Bone
marrow and peripheral blood of cats: Techniques and
normal values. Pathol. Vet. 1:18-40.

Gilmore, C.E., V.H. Gilmore, and T.C. Jones. 1964b. Re-
ticuloendotheliosis; a myeloproliferative disorder of
cats: A comparison with lymphocytic leukemia. Pathol.
Vet. 1:161-183.

Gilmore, S.A. 1972. Spinal nerve root degeneration in aging laboratory rats: A light microscopic study. Anat. Rec. 147:251-257.

Gladilov, V.V., and L.I. Irzhak. 1975. Age related changes in the affinity of hemoglobin to oxygen in rabbits. Zh. Evol. Biokhim. Fiziol. 11:310-311. (in Russian)

Gleiser, C.A., G.L. Van Hoosier, W.G. Sheldon, and W.K. Read. 1971. Amyloidosis and renal paramyloid in a closed hamster colony. Lab. Anim. Sci. 21:197-202.

Glende, E.A., Jr., and W.E. Cornatzer. 1966. The phospholipid fatty acid composition of liver, kidney, heart and spleen mitochondria from rats of various age groups. Biochem. Biophys. Acta 125:310-318.

Glenner, G.G., and D.L. Page. 1976. Amyloid, amyloidosis and amyloidogenesis. Int. Rev. Exp. Pathol. 15:1-92.

Glenner, G.G., D. Ein, and W.D. Terry. 1972. The immunoglobulin origin of amyloid. Am. J. Med. 52:141-147.

Glenner, G.G., W.D. Terry, and C. Isersky. 1973. Amyloidosis: Its nature and pathogenesis. Semin. Hematol. 10:65-86.

Glickman, I., and J. Quintarelli. 1960. Further observations regarding the effects of ovariectomy upon the tissues of the periodontium. J. Periodontol. 31:31-37.

Glickman, I., I.C. Stone, and T.N. Chawla. 1953. The effect of the systemic administration of cortisone upon the periodontium of white mice. J. Periodontol. 24:161-166.

Gloyna, R.E., and J.D. Wilson. 1969. Evidence that dihydrotestosterone formation may be involved in prostatic growth. Clin. Res. 17:284.

Gloyna, R.E., P.K. Siiteri, and J.D. Wilson. 1970. Dihydrotestosterone in prostatic hypertrophy. II. The formation and content of dihydrotestosterone in the hypertrophic canine prostate and the effect of dihydrotestosterone on prostate growth in the dog. J. Clin. Invest. 49:1746-1753.

Goco, R.W., M.B. Kress, and O.C. Brantigan. 1963. Comparison of mucous glands in the tracheobronchial tree of man and animals. Ann. N.Y. Acad. Sci. 106:555-571.

Gold, G., K. Karoly, C. Freeman, and R.C. Adelman. 1976. A possible role for insulin in the altered capability for hepatic enzyme adaptation during aging. Biochem. Biophys. Res. Comm. 73:1003-1010.

Gold, P.E., and J.L. McGaugh. 1975. Changes in learning and memory during aging. Pages 145-158 in J.M. Ordy and K.R. Brizzee, eds. Neurobiology of aging. Plenum Publishing Corp., New York.

Gold, P.H., M.V. Gee, and B.L. Strehler. 1968. Effect of age on oxidative phosphorylation in the rat. J. Gerontol. 23:509-512.

Gold, W.M., G.F. Kessler, D.Y.C. Yu, and O.L. Frick. 1972. Pulmonary physiologic abnormalities in experimental asthma in dogs. J. Appl. Physiol. 33:496-501.

Goldberg, P.B. 1978. Cardiac function of Fischer 344 rats in relation to age. Pages 87-100 in G. Kaldor and W.J. DeBattista, eds. Aging in muscle. Vol. 6. Aging series. Raven Press, New York.

Goldberg, P.B., and J. Roberts. 1976. Influences of age on the pharmacology and physiology of the cardiovascular system. Pages 71-103 in M.F. Elias, B.E. Eleftheriou, and P.K. Elias, eds. Special review of experimental aging research: Progress in biology. EAR, Inc., Bar Harbor, Maine; Beech Hill Company, Mount Desert, Maine.

Goldberg, P.B., and J. Roberts. 1978. Effects of age on cardiac contractility at various Ca^{++} concentrations. Page 88 in Abstracts for Sectional Sessions of the XI International Congress of Gerontology, held August 20-25, 1978 at Tokyo, Japan. Exerpta Medica, Amsterdam.

Goldberg, P.B., S.I. Baskin, and J. Roberts, Jr. 1975. Effects of aging on ionic movements of atrial muscle. Fed. Proc. 34(2):188-190.

Golden, G.S. and L.H. Golden. 1974. The "nona" electrocardiogram: Findings in 100 patients of the 90+ age group. J. Am. Geriatr. Soc. 22(7):329-332.

Goldman, B.D., and M.X. Zarrow. 1973. The physiology of progestins. Pages 547-572 in R.O. Greep, and E.B. Astwood, eds. Handbook of physiology. Section 7: Endocrinology, Vol. II. The female reproductive system, Part 1. American Physiological Society, Bethesda, Maryland.

Goldstein, M., B. Anagnoste, A.F. Battista, and M. Ogawa. 1976. Monkeys with nigrostriatal lesions: Effects of monoaminergic drugs. Pharmacol. Ther. B2:97-103.

Gonet, A.E., W. Stauffacher, R. Pictet, and A.E. Renold. 1965. Obesity and diabetes mellitus with striking hyperplasia of the islets of Langerhans in spiny mice (Acomys cahirinus). I. Histological findings and preliminary metabolis observations. Diabetologia. 1:162-171.

Good, R.A., and E. Yunis. 1974. Association of autoimmunity, immunodeficiency and aging in man, rabbits and mice. Fed. Proc. 33:2040-2050.

Goodman, M. 1976. Toward a genealogical description of primates. Pages 321-353 in M. Goodman and R.E. Tashian, eds. Molecular anthropology. Plenum Publishing Corp., New York.

Goodman, M., and R.E. Tashian [eds.] 1976. Molecular anthropology. Plenum Publishing Corp., New York. 466 p.

Goodrick, C.L. 1975. Life-span and the inheritance of longevity of inbred mice. J. Gerontol. 30:257-263.

Gordon, G.S. 1977. Postmenopausal osteoporosis: Cause, prevention and treatment. Clinics in Obstetrics and Gynaecology, The Menopause. 4(1):169-179.

Gordon, H.A., and B.S. Wostmann. 1959. Responses of the animal host to changes in the bacterial environment: Transition of the albino rat from germfree to the conventional state. Pages 336-339 in G. Tunevall, ed. Recent progress in microbiology. Almquist and Wiksell, Stockholm.

Gordon, H.A., E. Bruckner-Kardoss, and B.S. Wostmann. 1966. Aging in germ-free mice: Life tables and lesions observed at natural death. J. Gerontol. 21:380-387.

Gordon, W.C., S.R. Scobie, and S.E. Frankl. 1978. Age-related differences in electric shock detection and escape thresholds in Sprague-Dawley albino rats. Exp. Aging Res. 4:23-35.

Gorev, N.N., and L.P. Cherkasski'i. 1976. Age-specific characteristics of functional disorders of the cardiovascular system and respiration in experimental atherosclerosis. Kardiologiya. 16:12-19. (in Russian)

Gorev, N.N., and A.S. Stupina. 1973. Age factor in the development of experimental atherosclerosis. Arkh. Patol. 35:3-12. (in Russian)

Gorlin, R.J., and W.C. Peterson. 1967. Oral disease in man and animals. Arch. Dermatol. 96:390-403.

Gorlin, R.J., C.N. Barron, A.P. Chaudry, and J.J. Clar. 1959. The oral and pharyngeal pathology of domestic animals. A study of 487 cases. Am. J. Vet. Res. 20:1032-1061.

Gorthy, W.C. 1977. Cataracts in the aging rat lens. Ophthalmol. Res. 9:329-342.

Gorthy, W.C. 1978. Cataracts in the aging rat lens. Morphology and acid phosphatase histochemistry of incipient forms. Exp. Eye. Res. 27:301-322.

Gorthy, W.C., and Y.Z. Abdelbaki. 1974. Morphology of a hereditary cataract in the rat. Exp. Eye Res. 19:147-156.

Gosden, R.G. 1973. Chromosomal anomalies of preimplantation mouse embryos in relation to maternal age. J. Reprod. Fertil. 35:351-354.

Gosden, R.G. 1975. Ovarian support of pregnancy in aging inbred mice. J. Reprod. Fertil. 42:423-430.

Gosden, R.G. 1976. Uptake and metabolism in vivo of ^{3}H-estradiol-17 tissues of aging female mice. J. Endocrinol. 68:153-157.

Gosden, R.G., and R.E. Fowler. 1978. Corpus luteum function in ageing inbred mice. Experientia 35:128-129.

Gosden, R.G., E.C. Jones, and F. Jacks. 1978. Pituitary-ovarian relationships during the post-reproductive phase of inbred mice. Exp. Gerontol. 13:159-166.

Gottfries, C.G., I. Gottfries, and B.E. Roos. 1969. Homovanillic acid and 5-hydroxyindoleacetic acid in cerebrospinal fluid of patients with senile dementia, presenile dementia and parkinsonism. J. Neurochem. 16:1341-1345.

Gottfries, C.G., I. Gottfries, and B.E. Roos. 1970. Homovanillic acid and 5-hydroxyindoleacetic acid in cerebrospinal fluid related to rated mental and motor impairment in senile and presenile dementia. Acta Psychiatr. Scand. 46:99-105.

Gottlieb, H., and J.J. Lalich. 1954. The occurence of arteriosclerosis in the aorta of swine. Am. J. Pathol. 30:851-855.

Gough, J. 1952. Discussion on the diagnosis of pulmonary emphysema. Proc. R. Soc. Med. 45:576-577.

Gourevitch, G. 1970. Detectability of tones in quiet and in noise by rats and monkeys. Pages 67-97 in W.C. Stebbins, ed. Animal psychophysics: The design and conduct of sensory experiments. Appleton, New York.

Govoni, S., P. Loddo, P.T. Spano, and M. Trabuccho. 1977. Dopamine receptor sensitivity in brain and retina of rats during aging. Brain Res. 138:565-570.

Grad, B., and V.A. Kral. 1957. The effect of senescence on resistance to stress. I. Response of young and old mice to cold. J. Gerontol. 12:172-181.

Graham, C.E. 1979. Reproductive function in aged female chimpanzees. Am. J. Phys. Anthropol. 50(3):291-300.

Graham, C.E., and C.F. Bradley. 1972. Microanatomy of the chimpanzee genital system. Chimpanzee 5:77-126.

Graham, C.E., and H.M. McClure. 1977. Ovarian tumors and related lesions in aged chimpanzees. Vet. Pathol. 14:380-386.

Graham, C.E., O.R. Kling, and R.A. Steiner. 1979. Reproductive senescence in female nonhuman primates. Pages

183-202 in D.M. Bowden, ed. Aging in nonhuman primates. Van Nostrand Reinhold, New York.

Grahn, D. 1972. Data collection and genetic analysis in the selection and study of rodent model systems in aging. Pages 55-65 in D.C. Gibson, ed. Development of the rodent as a model system of aging. DHEW Publ. No. (NIH) 72-121. U.S. Department of Health, Education, and Welfare, Washington, D.C.

Granados, H. 1968. Nutrition. Pages 157-170 in R.A. Hoffman, P.F. Robinson, and H. Magalhaes, eds. The golden hamster. Its biology and use in medical research. Iowa State University Press, Ames, Iowa.

Grant, D.A., J. Chase, and S. Bermick. 1973. Biology of the periodontium in primates of the Galago species. J. Periodontol. 44:540-550.

Gray, J.E. 1977. Chronic progressive nephrosis in the albino rat. CRC Crit. Rev. Toxicol. 5(2):115-144.

Gray, W.R. 1979. Computed tomography: Imaging the heart. Cardiovasc. Clin. 10:239-242.

Grebenskaya, N.I. 1966. Age changes in the intrapulmonary arteries in rabbits. Arkh. Anat. Gistol. Embriol. 50:55-60. (in Russian)

Green, E.L. [ed.] 1966. Biology of the laboratory mouse, 2nd ed. McGraw-Hill, Inc. New York. 706 p.

Green, P.D., and P.B. Little. 1974. Neuronal ceroid lipofuscin storage in Siamese cats. Can. J. Comp. Med. 38:207-212.

Greenberg, L.H. and B. Weiss. 1978. Beta-adrenergic receptors in aged rat brain: Reduced number and capacity of pineal gland to develop supersensitivity. Science 201:61-62.

Greenwood, M.R.C., R. Gruen, and M.P. Cleary. 1978. Adipose tissue growth and development of fat cells. Pages 169-182 in G.A. Bray, ed. Recent advances in obesity research: II. Proceedings of the 2nd International Congress on Obesity, held October 23-26, 1977 in Washington, D.C. Newman Publishing, Ltd., London.

Gresham, G.A., A.N. Howard, J. McQueen, and D.E. Bowyer. 1965. Atherosclerosis in primates. Br. J. Exp. Pathol. 46:94-103.

Grindle, C.F.J., and J. Marshall. 1978. Aging changes in Bruch's membrane and their functional implications. Trans. Ophthalmol. Soc. U.K. 98:172-175.

Grinna, L.S., and A.A. Barber. 1972. Age-related changes in membrane lipid content and enzyme activities. Biochim. Biophys. Acta. 288:347-353.

Guffy, M.M. 1975. Esophageal disorders. Pages 1098-1124 in S.J. Ettinger, ed. Textbook of veterinary internal medicine. Vol. 2. W.B. Saunders Co., Philadelphia.

Gupta, O.P., and J.H. Shaw. 1956. Periodontal disease in rice rat. I. Anatomic and histopathologic finds. Oral Surg. Oral Med. Oral Pathol. 9:592-603.

Gupta, O.P., and J.H. Shaw. 1960. Dental anatomy and characteristics of peridontal lesions in the Mongolian gerbil. J. Dent. Res. 39:1014-1022.

Gurland, B.J. 1976. The comparative frequency of depression in various adult age groups. J. Gerontol. 31: 283-292.

Gusel', V.A., and O.N. Grigor'eva. 1975. Age peculiarities of trace discharges of after-effect and of the activity of epileptogenic zone in the hippocampus of rabbits. Zh. Evol. Biokhim. Fiziol. 11:410-418. (in Russian)

Guttman, P.H., and A.C. Andersen. 1968. Progressive intercapillary glomerulosclerosis in aging and irradiated Beagles. Radiat. Res. 35:45-60.

Guzman, S.V., E. Swenson, and M. Jones. 1962. Intercoronary reflex. Demonstration by coronary angiography. Circ. Res. 10:739-745.

Hachek, D.B., E. Mikat, H.E. Lebovitz, K. Schmidt-Nielsen, E.S. Horton, and T.D. Kinney. 1967. The sand rat (Psammomys obesus) as an experimental animal in studies of diabetes mellitus. Diabetologia 3:130-134.

Haddad, A.G., R.L. Pimmel, D.D. Scaperoth, and P.A. Bromberg. 1979. Forced oscillatory respiratory parameters following papain exposure in dogs. J. Appl. Physiol.: Respir. Environ. Exercise Physiol. 46:61-66.

Hadorn, E. 1965. Problems of determination and transdetermination. Brookhaven Symp. Biol. 18:148-161.

Hafez, E.S.E. 1970. Rabbits. Pages 273-298 in E.S.E Hafez, ed. Reproduction and breeding techniques of laboratory animals. Lea and Febiger, Philadelphia.

Hagen, K.W. 1974. Colony husbandry. Pages 23-47 in S.H. Weisbroth, R.E. Flatt, and A.L. Kraus, eds. The biology of the laboratory rabbit. Academic Press, New York.

Haining, J.L., M.D. Turner, and R.M. Pantall. 1970. Local cerebral blood flow in young and old rats during hypoxia and hypercapnia. Am. J. Physiol. 218:1020-1024.

Hall, E.R., and K.R. Kelson. 1959. The mammals of North America. Ronald Press, New York. 1162 p.

Hall, M.C. 1964. Articular changes in the knee of the adult rat after prolonged immobilization in extension. Clin. Orthop. 34:184-195.

Hall, W.B., H.E. Grupe, and C.K. Claycomb. 1967. The periodontium and periodontal pathology in the howler monkey. Arch. Oral Biol. 12:359-365.

Hallgrimsson, J., W. Friberg, and J.F. Burke. 1970. Changes with age in the metabolism of sulfated glycosaminoglycans in guinea pig cardiac valves. Exp. Mol. Pathol. 12(1):70-83.

Ham, R.G., and W.L. McKeehan. 1978. Development of improved media and culture conditions for clonal growth of normal diploid cells. In Vitro 14:11-22.

Hamai, Y., and T. Kuwabara. 1975. Early cytologic changes in Fraser cataract. An electron microscopic study. Invest. Ophthalmol. 14:517-527.

Hamilton, C.L., and J.R. Brobeck. 1963. Diabetes mellitus in hyperphagic monkeys. Endocrinology 73:512-555.

Hamilton, C.L., and P. Ciaccia. 1978. The course of development of glucose intolerance in the monkey. (Macaca mulatta). J. Med. Primatol. 7:165-173.

Hamilton, C.L., and D. Lewis. 1975. Feeding behavior in monkeys with spontaneous diabetes mellitus. J. Med. Primatol. 4:145-153.

Hamilton, C.L., and J.L. Rabinowitz. 1976. Weight reduction and serum insulin levels in hypothalamic obese monkeys. J. Med. Primatol. 5:276-283.

Hamilton, C.L., P.I. Kuo, and L.Y. Feng. 1972. Experimental production of syndrome of obesity, hyperinsulinemia and hyperlipidemia in monkeys. Proc. Soc. Exper. Biol. Med. 140:1005-1008.

Hamilton, C.L., P.J. Ciaccio, and D.O. Lewis. 1976. Feeding behavior in monkeys with and without lesions of the hypothalamus. Am. J. Physiol. 230:818-830.

Hamilton, J.B., R.S. Hamilton, and M.E. Mestler. 1969. Duration of life and causes of death in domestic cats: Influence of sex, gonadectomy, and inbreeding. J. Gerontol. 24:427-437.

Hamilton, J.M. 1974. Comparative aspects of mammary tumors. Adv. Cancer Res. 19:1-45.

Hamlin, C.R., and R.R. Kohn. 1972. Determination of human chronological age by study of a collagen sample. Exp. Gerontol. 7:377-379.

Hamm, T.E., C.R. Abee, T.A. Riggs, and T.B. Clarkson. 1974. Myocardial infarction in three rhesus monkeys (Macaca mulatta) fed atherogenic diets. Abstract No. 188. Fed. Proc. 33:236.

Hammond, E.C., O. Auerbach, D. Kirman, and L. Garfinkel. 1970. Effects of cigarette smoking on dogs. Arch. Environ. Health 21:740-753.

Hamp, S.E, and C.G. Emilson. 1974. Some effects of chlorhexidine on the plaque flora of the Beagle dog. J. Periodontal Res. Suppl. 12:28-40.

Hamp, S.E., and R. Lindberg. 1977. Histopathology of spontaneous periodontitis in dogs. J. Periodontal Res. 12:46-54.

Hamp, S.E., J. Lindhe, and G. Heyden. 1972. Experimental gingivitis in the dog. An enzyme-histochemical study. Arch. Oral Biol. 17: 329-337.

Hampe, J.F., and W. Misdorp. 1974. IX. Tumours and dysplasias of the mammary gland. Bull. WHO 50:111-133.

Hancox, N.M. 1972. Biology of bone. Cambridge University Press, London. 199 p.

Handler, A.H. 1965. Spontaneous lesions of the hamster. Pages 210-240 in W.E. Ribelin and J.R. McCoy, eds. The pathology of laboratory animals. Charles C. Thomas, Springfield, Illinois.

Handler, A.H., S.I. Magalini, and D. Pav. 1966. Oncogenic studies on the Mongolian gerbil. Cancer Res. 26:844-847.

Hansard, S.L., and H.M. Crowder. 1957. The physiological behavior of calcium in the rat. J. Nutr. 62:325-339.

Hansen, H.J. 1952. A pathologic-anatomical study on disc degeneration in the dog, with special reference to the so-called enchondrosis intervertebralis. Acta Orthop. Scand. Suppl. 11:1-117.

Harano, Y., R.G. DePalma, L. Lavine, and M. Miller. 1972. Fatty acid oxidation, oxidative phosphorylation and ultrastructure of mitochondria in the diabetic rat liver. Hepatic factors in diabetic ketosis. Diabetes 21: 257-270.

Harbitz, T.B., and O.A. Haugen. 1972. Histology of the prostate in elderly men. Acta Pathol. Microbiol. Scand. Sect. A 80:756-768.

Hardy, W.D. 1974. Feline leukemia virus-related diseases. Pages 154-157 in Scientific presentations and seminar symposia of the 41st Annual American Animal Hospital Association meeting. American Animal Hospital Association, South Bend, Indiana.

Harken, A.H., C.H. Barlow, W.R. Harden, III, and B. Chance. 1978. Two and three-dimensional display of myocardial ischemic "border zone" in dogs. Am. J. Cardiol. 42: 954-959.

Harman, S.M., and G.B. Talbert. 1974. Effect of maternal age on synchronization of ovulation and mating and on tubal transport of ova in mice. J. Gerontol. 5:493-498.

Harris, A.S. 1950. Delayed development of ventricular ectopic rhythms following experimental coronary occlusion. Circulation 1:1318-1328.

Harris, A.S., H. Otero, and A.J. Bocage. 1971. The induction of arrhythmias by sympathetic activity before and after occlusion of a coronary artery in the canine heart. J. Electrocardiol. 4:34-43.

Harris, J.W., and R.W. Kellermeyer. 1970. The red cell. Harvard University press, Cambridge, Massachusetts. 795 p.

Harris. R. 1975. Cardiac changes with age. Pages 109-122 in R. Goldman and R. Rockstein, eds. Physiology and pathology of human aging. Academic Press, New York.

Harris, R.S. [ed.] 1970. Feeding and nutrition of non-human primates. Academic Press, New York. 310 p.

Harrison, D.E. 1975. Defective erythropoietic responses of aged mice not improved by young marrow. J. Gerontol. 30:286-288.

Harrison, D.E. 1978. Genetically defined animals valuable in testing aging of erythroid and lymphoid stem cells and microenvironments. Pages 187-196 in D. Bergsma and D.E. Harrison, eds. Genetic effects on aging. Birth defects original article series. Vol. 14, No. 1. A.R. Liss, Inc., New York.

Harrison, D.E. 1979. Proliferative capacity of erythropoietic stem cell lines and aging: An overview. Mech. Ageing Dev. 9:409-426.

Harrison, D.E, and J.R. Archer. 1978. Measurement of changes in mouse tail tendon collagen with age: Temperature dependence and procedural details. Exp. Gerontol. 13:75-82.

Hart, R.W., and R.B. Setlow. 1974. Correlation between deoxyribonucleic acid excision-repair and life-span in a number of mammalian species. Proc. Natl. Acad. Sci. USA 71:2169-2173.

Hart, R.W., G.A. Sacher, and T.L. Koskins. 1979. DNA repair in a short- and a long-lived rodent species. J. Gerontol. 34:808-817.

Hasan, M., and P. Glees. 1973. Ultrastructural age changes in hippocampal neurons, synapses and neuroglia. Exp. Gerontol. 8:75-83.

Hasan, M., P. Glees, and E. ElGhazzawi. 1974. Age-associated changes in the hypothalamus of the guinea

pig: Effect of dimethylaminoethyl p-chlorophenoxyace-
tate. An electron microscopic and histochemical study.
Exp. Gerontol. 9(4):153-159.

Hashimoto, K., T. Tsukada, H. Matsuda, Y. Nakagawa, and
S. Imai. 1979. Antiarrhythmic effects of bupuranolol
against canine ventricular arrhythmias induced by
halothane-adrenaline or two-stage coronary ligation.
J. Cardiovasc. Pharmacol. 1:205-217.

Hashimoto, S., and S. Dayton. 1974. Cholesterol-esteri-
fying activity of aortas from atherosclerosis-resistant
and atherosclerosis-susceptible species. Proc. Soc.
Exp. Biol. Med. 145:89-92.

Hasleton, S. 1972. The internal surface area of the
adult human lung. J. Anat. 112:391-400.

Hauschka, S.D. 1977. Cultivation of muscle tissue. Pages
67-130 in G.H. Rothblat and V.J. Cristofalo, eds.
Growth, nutrition, and metabolism of cells in culture.
Vol. III. Academic Press, New York.

Hausmann, L., P. Zofel, R. Schubotz, and H. Kaffarnik.
1975. A statistical comparison between different tests
for the diagnosis of latent diabetes and their clinical
relevance. Acta Diabetol. Lat. 12:160-170.

Haverland, L.H., C.H. Yoon, and F. Homburger. 1972.
Studies on the aging of inbred Syrian golden hamsters:
Effect of age on organ weight. Prog. Exp. Tumor Res.
16:120-141.

Hawkins, J.E., and L. Johnsson. 1968. Light microscopic
observation of the inner ear in man and monkey. Ann.
Otol. Rhinol. Laryngol. 77:608-629.

Hay, R.J. 1970. Cell strain senescence in vitro: Cell
culture anomaly or an expression of a fundamental in-
ability of normal cells to survive and proliferate.
Pages 7-24 in E. Holeckova and V.J. Cristofalo, eds.
Aging in cell and tissue culture. Plenum Publishing
Corp., New York.

Haydon, G.B., G. Freeman, and N.J. Furiosi. 1965. Covert
pathogenesis of NO_2-induced emphysema in the rat. Arch.
Environ. Health 11:776-783.

Haydon, G.B., J.T. Davidson, G.R. Lillington, and K. Wasserman. 1967. Nitrogen dioxide-induced emphysema in
rabbits. Am. Rev. Resp. Dis. 95:797-805.

Hayes, H.M., and T.W. Pendergrass. 1976. Canine testicular tumors: Epidemiologic features of 410 dogs. Int.
J. Cancer 18(4):482-487.

Hayes, J.A., and T.G. Christensen. 1978. Bronchial mucus
hypersecretion induced by elastase in hamsters: Ultrastructural appearances. J. Pathol. 125:25-31.

Hayes, J.A., T.G. Christensen, and G.L. Snider. 1977. The hamster as a model of chronic bronchitis and emphysema in man. Lab. Anim. Sci. 27:762-770.

Hayes, K.C., A.R. Rabin, and E.L. Berson. 1975. An ultrastructural study of nutritionally induced and reversed retinal degeneration in cats. Am. J. Pathol. 78:505-516.

Hayflick, L. 1977. The cellular basis for biological aging. Pages 159-168 in C.E. Finch and L. Hayflick, eds. Handbook of the biology of aging. Von Nostrand Reinhold, New York.

Hayflick, L., and P. Moorhead. 1961. The serial cultivation of human diploid cell strains. Exp. Cell Res. 25:585-621.

Head, J.R., P.F. Suter, and S.J. Ettinger. 1975. Lower respiratory tract diseases. Pages 661-723 in S.J. Ettinger, ed. Textbook of veterinary internal medicine. Diseases of the dog and cat. Vol. 1. W.B. Saunders Co., Philadelphia.

Head, K.W. 1976. Tumors of the upper alimentary tract. Bull. WHO 53:145-166.

Healy, G.R., A. Spielman, and N. Gleason. 1976. Human babesiosis: Reservoir of infection on Nantucket Island. Science 192:479-480.

Heaney, R.P. 1974. Pathophysiology of osteoporosis: Implications for treatment. Tex. Med. 70:37-45.

Heaney, R.P. 1976. Estrogens and postmenopausal osteoporosis. Clin. Obstet. Gynecol. 19:791-803.

Heffley, J.D., and R.J. Williams. 1974. The nutritional teamwork approach: Prevention and regression of cataracts in rats. Proc. Natl. Acad. Sci. USA 71:4164-4168.

Hegsted, M., and H.M. Linkswiler. 1980. The long term effect of level of protein intake on calcium balance in young adult women. Abstract No. 3334. Fed. Proc. 39(3):901.

Heijl, L., B.R. Rifkin, and H.A. Zander. 1976. Conversion of chronic gingivitis to periodontitis in squirrel monkeys. J. Periodontol. 47:710-716.

Heiniger, H.J., and J.L. Dorey [eds.] 1980. Handbook on genetically standardized Jax mice. 3rd ed. The Jackson Laboratory, Bar Harbor, Maine.

Heitmann, H.H. 1971. Die morphologie der knochenmarkund blutzellen von Mastomys natalensis. Die Blauen Hefte für den Tierarzt 46:260-271.

Helfman, P.M., and J.L. Bada. 1976. Aspartic acid race-
misation in dentine as a measure of ageing. Nature
262:279-281.

Helldén, L., and J. Lindhe. 1973. Enhanced emigration
of crevicular leukocytes mediated by factors in human
dental plaque. Scand. J. Dent. Res. 81:123-129.

Heller, L.J., and W.V. Whitehorn. 1972. Age-associated
alterations in myocardial contractile properties. Am.
J. Physiol. 222:1613-1619.

Henderson, R.F., J.H. Diel, and B.S. Martinex [eds.]
1978. Inhalation Toxicology Research Institute annual
report 1977-1978, DOE research and development report
LF-60. Inhalation Toxicology Research Institute, Albuquerque, New Mexico. 542 p.

Heng, M.K., R.M. Norris, T. Peter, H.D. Nisbet, and B.N.
Singh. 1978. The effects of glucose-insulin-potassium
on experimental myocardial infarction in the dog. Cardiovasc. Res. 12:429-435.

Hendrickx, A.G., and L.M. Newman. 1978. Reproduction of
the greater bushbaby (Galago crassicaudatus panganiensis) under laboratory conditions. J. Med. Primatol.
7:26-43.

Henrikson, P.A. 1968. Periodontal disease and calcium
deficiency. An experimental study in the dog. Acta
Odontol. Scand. 26 (Suppl. 50):1-132.

Heppleston, A.G., and J.G. Leopold. 1961. Chronic pulmonary emphysema: Anatomy and pathogenesis. Am. J.
Med. 31:279-291.

Herberg, L., M. Bergmann, U. Hemmings, E. Major, and F.A.
Gries. 1972. Influence of diet on the metabolic syndrome of obesity. Israel J. Med. Sci. 8:822-823.

Herget, J., R. Holusa, and F. Paleck. 1974. Pulmonary
hypertension in rats with experimental emphysema.
Physiol. Bohemoslov. 23:55-65.

Hernandez, J.A., A.E. Anderson, W.L. Holmes, N. Morroen,
and A.G. Foraker. 1965. The bronchial glands in aging.
J. Am. Geriatr. Soc. 13:799-804.

Hernandez, J.A., A.E. Anderson, W.L. Holmes, and A.G.
Foraker. 1966. Pulmonary parenchymal defects in dogs
following prolonged cigarette smoke exposure. Am. Rev.
Resp. Dis. 93:78-82.

Heston, L.L. 1977. Alzheimer's disease, trisomy 21, and
myeloproliferative disorders: Associations suggesting
a genetic diathesis. Science 196:322-323.

Heston, L.L., and A.R. Mastri. 1977. The genetics of Alzheimer's disease: Associations with myeloproliferative

disorders and Down's Syndrome. Arch. Gen. Psychiatry. 34:976-981.

Heywood, R. 1971. Juvenile cataracts in the Beagle dog. J. Small Anim. Pract. 12:171-177.

Higgins, C.B., M. Savak, W. Schmidt, and P.T. Siemers. 1979. Differential accumulation of radiopaque contrast material in acute myocardial infarction. Am. J. Cardiol. 43:47-51.

Hill, B.T. 1976. Influence of age on chromatin transcription in murine tissues using an heterologous and an homologous RNA polymerase. Gerontology 22:111-123.

Hill, B.T., and R.D.H. Whelan. 1978. Studies on the degradation of ageing chromatin DNA by nuclear and cytoplasmic factors and deoxyribonucleases. Gerontology 24:326-336.

Hill, F.G., and D.F. Kelly. 1974. Naturally occurring intestinal malabsorption in the dog. Dig. Dis. 19:649-665.

Hill, J.L. 1974. Peromyscus. Effect of early pairing on reproduction. Science 186:1042-1044.

Hill, M.J. 1977. The etiology of colonic cancer. Pages 124-132 in J.H. Yardley, B.C. Morson, and M.R. Abell, eds. The gastrointestinal tract. International Academy of Pathology. Monographs in pathology, No. 18. The Williams and Wilkins Co., Baltimore.

Hill, W.C. 1960. Cebidae: A monograph. Volume 4. Primates, comparative anatomy and taxonomy. The Edinburgh University Press, Edinburgh. 523 p.

Hinds, J.W., and N.A. McNelly. 1977. Aging of the rat olfactory bulb: Growth and atrophy of constituent layers and changes in size and number of mitral cells. J. Comp. Neurol. 171:345-368.

Hirano, A., and H.M. Zimmerman. 1962. Alzheimer's neurofibrillary changes: A topographic study. Arch. Neurol. 7:227-242.

Hirokawa, H. 1975. Characterization of age associated kidney disease in Wistar rats. Mech. Ageing Dev. 4:301-316.

Hirsch, J. 1978. Obesity: A perspective. Pages 1-5 in G.A. Bray, ed. Recent advances in obesity research: II. Proceedings of the 2nd International Congress on Obesity, held October 23-26, 1977 in Washington, D.C. Newman Publishing, Ltd., London.

Hirth, R.S., E.T. Greenstein, and R.L. Peer. 1974. Anterior opacities (spurious cataracts) in Beagle dogs. Vet. Pathol. 11:181-194.

Hisaw, F.L., and F.L. Hisaw, Jr. 1958. Spontaneous carcinoma of the cervix uteri in a monkey (Macaca mulatta). Cancer 11:810-816.

Hjarre, A. 1933. The occurrence of amyloid degeneration in animals. Acta Pathol. Microbiol. Scand. 16:132-162.

Hoar, R.M. 1976. Biomethodology. Pages 13-20 in J.E. Wagner and P.J. Manning, eds. The biology of the guinea pig. Academic Press, New York.

Hodgen, G.D., A.L. Goodman, A. O'Conner, and D.K. Johnson. 1976. Menopause in rhesus monkeys: Hormonal and menstrual patterns. Am. Assoc. Lab. Anim. Sci. 76:99 (Abstract).

Hodgen, G.D., A.L. Goodman, A. O'Connor, and D.K. Johnson. 1977. Menopause in rhesus monkeys: Model for study of disorders in the human climateric. Am. J. Obstet. Gynecol. 127:581-584.

Hodosh, M., M. Povar, and G. Shklar. 1971. Periodontitis in the baboon (Papio anubis). J. Periodontol. 42: 594-596.

Hoel, D.B., and H.E. Walburg. 1972. Statistical analysis of survival experiments. J. Natl. Cancer Inst. 49: 361-372.

Hoerlein, B.F. 1956. Further evaluation of the treatment of disc protrusion paraplegia in the dog. J. Am. Vet. Med. Assoc. 129:495-501.

Hoffman, H.J. 1979. Survival distributions for selected laboratory rat strains and stocks. Pages 19-34 in D.C. Gibson, R.C. Adelman, and C. Finch, eds. Development of the rodent as a model system of aging. Book II. DHEW Pub. No. (NIH) 79-161. U.S. Department of Health, Education, and Welfare, Washington, D.C.

Hoffman, J.L., and M.T. McCoy. 1974. Stability of the nucleoside composition of tRNA during biological aging of mice and mosquitoes. Nature 249:558-559.

Hoffman, R.A., P.F. Robinson, and H. Magalhaes [eds.] 1968. The golden hamster. Its biology and use in medical research. Iowa State University Press, Ames, Iowa. 545 p.

Holinka, C.F., Y.-C. Tseng, and C.E. Finch. 1978. Prolonged gestation, elevated preparturitional progesterone, and reproductive aging in C57BL/6J mice. Bio. Reprod. 19:807-816.

Holinka, C.F., Y.-C. Tseng, and C.E. Finch. 1979a. Reproductive aging in C57BL/6J mice: Plasma progesterone, viable embryos, and resorption frequency throughout pregnancy. Biol. Reprod. 20:1201-1211.

Holinka, C.F., Y.-C. Tseng, and C.E. Finch. 1979b. Impaired preparturitional rise of plasma estradiol in aging C57BL/6J mice. Biol. Reprod. 21:1009-1013.

Holland, J.M., and T.J. Mitchell. 1976. The relationship of strain, sex, and body weight to survival following sublethal whole-body x-irradiation. Radiat. Res. 66: 363-372.

Holland, J.M., T.J. Mitchell, and H.E. Walburg. 1977. Effects of prepubertal ovariectomy on survival and specific disease in female RFM mice given 300 r of x-rays. Radiat. Res. 69:317-327.

Holland, J.M., T.J. Mitchell, L.C. Gipson, and M.S. Whitaker. 1978. Survival and cause of death in aging germfree athymic nude and normal inbred C3Hf/He mice. J. Natl. Cancer Inst. 61:1357-1361.

Hollander, C.F. 1976. Current experience using the laboratory rat in aging studies. Lab. Anim. Sci. 26:320-328.

Hollander, C.F. 1979. The proper use of laboratory rats and mice in gerontological research. Pages 223-227 in A. Cherkin, C.E. Finch, H. Kharasch, T. Makinodan, F.L. Scott, and B.L. Strehler, eds. Physiology and cell biology of aging. Vol. 8. Aging series. Raven Press, New York.

Hollander, J., and C.H. Barrows, Jr. 1968. Enzymatic studies in senescent rodent brains. J. Gerontol. 23:174-179.

Holman, B., T.T. Toshiyuki, and M. Lesch. 1976. Evaluation of radiopharmaceuticals for the detection of acute myocardial infarction in man. Nucl. Med. 121:427-430.

Holzworth, J. 1960. Leukemia and related neoplasms in the cat. I. Lymphoid malignancies. J. Am. Vet. Med. Assoc. 136:47-69.

Homburger, F. [ed.] 1972. Pathology of the Syrian hamster. Prog. Exp. Tumor Res. 16:1-637.

Homburger, F., and C.W. Nixon. 1970. Cystic prostatic hypertrophy in two inbred lines of Syrian hamsters. Proc. Soc. Exp. Biol. Med. 134:284-286.

Homburger, F., C.W. Nixon, J.R. Baker, and R. Whitney. 1964. Some anatomical characteristics of eight inbred strains of Mesocricetus auratus auratus. J. Genet. 59:1-6.

Hooper, M.W., and F.S. Vogel. 1976. The limbic system in Alzheimer's disease. Am. J. Pathol. 85:1-13.

Hoover, E.A., G.J. Kociba, W.D. Hardy, Jr., and D.S. Yohn. 1974. Erythroid hypoplasia in cats inoculated with feline leukemia virus. J. Natl. Cancer Inst. 53:1271-1276.

Hooykass, J.A.P., J.R. Benfield, S.F. Wolfe, S.W. French, and A.B. Crummy. 1969. A physiologic and anatomic study after pulmonary irradiation in dogs. Dis. Chest 55:123-126.

Hoppe, P.C., C.W. Laird, and R.R. Fox. 1969. A simple technique for bleeding the rabbit ear vein. Lab. Anim. Care 19:524-525.

Hopps, R.M., and N.W. Johnson. 1974. Relationship between histological degree of inflammation and epithelial proliferation in macaque gingiva. J. Periodontal Res. 9:273-283.

Hori, Y., E.H. Perkins, and M.K. Halsall. 1973. Decline in phytohemagglutinin responsiveness of spleen cells from aging mice. Proc. Soc. Exp. Biol. Med. 144:48-52.

Horita, A. 1968. The influence of age on the recovery of cardiac monoamine oxidase after irreversible inhibition. Biochem. Pharmacol. 17:2091-2096.

Hornbuckle, W.E., D.M. MacCoy, G.S. Allan, and R. Gunther. 1978. Prostatic disease in a dog. Cornell Vet. 68(7): 284-305.

Horneffer, P.J., and M. Weksler. 1976. A method to study in vitro proliferation of lymphocytes from individual mice on repeated occasions. J. Immunol. Methods 11:99-105.

Hornsby, P.J., and G.N. Gill. 1978. Characterization of adult bovine adrenocortical cells throughout their life span in tissue culture. Endocrinology 102:926-936.

Hornykiewicz, O. 1972. Neurochemistry of parkinsonism. Pages 465-501 in A. Lajtha, ed. Handbook of neurochemistry. Vol. VII. Pathological chemistry of the nervous system. Plenum Press, New York.

Hornykiewics, O. 1975. Parkinsonism induced by dopaminergic antagonists. Adv. Neurol. 9:155-164.

Horrocks, L.A., G.Y. Sun, and R.A. D'Amato. 1975. Changes in brain lipids in aging. Pages 359-366 in J.M. Ordy and K.R. Brizzee, eds. Neurobiology of aging. Plenum Publishing Corp., New York.

Horton, D.L., and H.J. Whiteley. 1969. The effect of age on hair growth in the CBA mouse. Observations on repeated plucking. J. Gerontol. 24:324-329.

Host, R., and S. Sveinson. 1936. Aruelig katarakt hos hunder. Nor. Vet. Tidsskr. 48:244-247.

Hottendorf, G.H., and R.S. Hirth. 1974. Lesions of spontaneous subclinical disease in Beagle dogs. Vet. Pathol. 11:240-258.

Howard, C.F. 1975a. Basement membrane thickness in muscle capillaries of normal and spontaneously diabetic Macaca nigra. Diabetes 24:201-206.

Howard, C.F. 1975b. Diabetes and lipid metabolism in nonhuman primates. Adv. Lipid Res. 13:91-134.

Howard, C.F. 1978. Insular amyloidosis and diabetes mellitus in Macaca nigra. Diabetes 27:357-364.

Hrachovec. J.P. 1971. The effect of age on tissue protein synthesis. I. Age changes in amino acid incorporation by rat liver purified microsomes. Gerontologia 17: 75-86.

Hrdy, S.B. 1974. Male-male competition and infanticide among langurs (Presbytis entellus) of Abu, Rajasthan. Folia Primatol. 22:19-58.

Hruza, Z. 1973. Catabolism of epinephrine and histamine during aging in rats. Exp. Gerontol. 8(6):333-336.

Huang, H.-H., and J. Meites. 1975. Reproductive capacity of aging female rats. Neuroendocrinology. 17:289-295.

Huang, H.-H., S. Marshall, and J. Meites. 1976a. Capacity of old versus young female rats to secrete LH, FSH, and prolactin. Biol. Reprod. 14:538-543.

Huang, H.-H., S. Marshall, and J. Meites. 1976b. Induction of estrous cycles in old non-cyclic rats by progesterone, ACTH, ether stress or l-dopa. Neuroendocrinology. 20:21-34.

Huang, H.-H., R.W. Steger, J.F. Bruni, and J. Meites. 1978. Patterns of sex steroid and gonadotropin secretion in aging female rats. Endocrinology 103:1855-1859.

Huggins, C., and P.J. Clark. 1940. Quantitative studies of prostatic secretion. II. The effect of castration and of estrogen injection on the normal and on the hyperplastic prostate glands of dogs. J. Exp. Med. 72:747-762.

Huggins, C., M.H. Marina, L. Eichelberger, and J.D. Wharton. 1940. Quantitative studies of prostatic secretion. I. Characteristics of the normal secretion; the influence of thyroid, suprarenal, and testis extirpation and androgen substitution on the prostatic output. J. Exp. Med. 72:543-556.

Hull, P.S., J.V. Soames, and R.M. Davis. 1974. Periodontal disease in a Beagle dog colony. J. Comp. Pathol. Ther. 84:143-150.

Hunt, C.E. 1979. Obesity. Pages 76-79 in E.J. Andrews, B.C. Ward, and N.H. Altman, eds. Spontaneous animal models of human disease. Vol. II. Academic Press, New York.

Hunt, C.E., and D.D. Harrington. 1974. Nutrition and nutritional diseases of the rabbit. Pages 403-433 in S.H. Weisbroth, R.E. Flatt, and A.L. Kraus, eds. The biology of the laboratory rabbit. Academic Press, New York.

Hunt, C.E., J.R. Lindsey, and S.U. Walkley. 1976. Animal models of diabetes and obesity including the PBB/Ld mouse. Fed. Proc. 35:1206-1217.

Hunt, D.M. 1974. Primary defect in copper transport underlies mottled mutants in the mouse. Nature 249: 852-854.

Hunt, H.F., and L.S. Otis. 1953. Conditioned and unconditioned emotional defecation in the rat. J. Comp. Physiol. Psychol. 461:378-382.

Hurme, V.O. 1961. Basic data on the emergence of permanent teeth of the rhesus monkey Macaca mulatta. Proc. Am. Philos. Soc. 105:105-140.

Hurvitz, A.I. 1975. Immunology. Pages 1701-1712 in S.J. Ettinger, ed. Textbook of veterinary internal medicine. Diseases of the dog and cat. Vol. 2. W.B. Saunders Company, Philadelphia.

Huxley, T.H. 1863. Evidence as to man's place in nature. Williams and Norgate, London. 159 p.

Hyde, D.M., N.E. Robinson, J.R. Gillespie, and W.S. Tyler. 1977. Morphometry of the distal air spaces in lungs of aging dogs. J. Appl. Physiol. 43:86-91.

Hyde, D., J. Gillespie, R. Carter, and J. Ortheofer. 1978. Correlations of pulmonary structural and functional changes in dogs after long-term exposure to auto exhaust and other air pollutants. Am. Rev. Respir. Dis. Suppl. 117(4):243.

Hyttel, J. 1978. Dopamine-receptor binding and adenylate-cyclase activity in mouse striatal tissue in the supersensitivity phase after neuroleptic treatment. Psychopharmacology 59:211-216.

Ingle, D.J. 1949. A simple means of producing obesity in the rat. Proc. Soc. Exp. Biol. Med. 72:604-605.

Ingvar, D.H., J. Risberg, and M.S. Schwartz. 1975. Evidence of subnormal function of association cortex in presenile dementia. Neurology 25:964-974.

Innes, J.R.M., W. Zeman, J.K. Frenkel, and G. Borner. 1962. Occult endemic encephalitozoonoses of the central nervous system of mice. J. Neuropathol. 21: 519-533.

Inoue, S., L.A. Campfield, and G.A. Bray. 1977. Comparison of metabolic alterations in hypothalamic and high fat diet-induced obesity. Am. J. Physiol. 233:R162-R168.

Inoue, S., G.A. Bray, and Y.S. Mullen. 1978. Transplantation of pancreatic β-cells prevents development of hypothalamic obesity in rats. Am. J. Physiol. 235:E266-E271.

Institute of Laboratory Animal Resources (ILAR) Committee on Standards. 1960. Standards for the breeding, care, and management of Syrian hamsters. National Academy of Sciences, Washington, D.C. 15 p.

Institute of Laboratory Animal Resources (ILAR) Committee on Laboratory Animal Diseases. 1971. A guide to infectious diseases of mice and rats. National Academy of Sciences, Washington, D.C. 41 p.

Institute of Laboratory Animal Resources (ILAR) Committee on Standards, Subcommittee on Dog and Cat Standards. 1973. Dogs. Standards and guidelines for the breeding, care, and management of laboratory animals. National Academy of Sciences, Washington, D.C. 48 p.

Institute of Laboratory Animal Resources (ILAR) Committee on Animal Models for Thrombosis and Hemorrhagic Diseases. 1976a. Animal models of thrombosis and hemorrhagic diseases. Proceedings of a workshop held March 12-13, 1975 at the National Academy of Sciences, Washington, D.C. DHEW Pub. No. (NIH) 76-982. U.S. Department of Health, Education, and Welfare, Washington, D.C.

Institute of Laboratory Animal Resources (ILAR) Committee on Conservation of Nonhuman Primates. 1976b. Nonhuman primates: Usage and availability for biomedical programs. DHEW Pub. No. (NIH) 76-892. U.S. Department of Health, Education, and Welfare, Washington, D.C. 122 p.

Institute of Laboratory Animal Resources (ILAR) Committee on Long-Term Holding of Laboratory Rodents. 1976c. Long-term holding of laboratory rodents. ILAR News 19:L1-L25.

Institute of Laboratory Animal Resources (ILAR) Committee on Rodents. 1977. Laboratory animal management: Rodents. ILAR News 20:L1-L15.

Institute of Laboratory Animal Resources (ILAR) Committee on Care and Use of Laboratory Animals. 1978a. Guide for the care and use of laboratory animals. Rev. ed. DHEW Pub. No. (NIH) 78-23. U.S. Department of Health, Education, and Welfare, Washington, D.C. 70 p.

Institute of Laboratory Animal Resources (ILAR) Committee on Cats. 1978b. Laboratory animal management-cats. ILAR News 21(3):C1-C19.

Institute of Laboratory Animal Resources (ILAR) Committee on Laboratory Animal Diets. 1978c. Control of diets in laboratory animal experimentation. ILAR News 21:A3-A12.

Institute of Laboratory Animal Resources (ILAR). 1979a. Animals for research - A directory of sources. 10th ed. National Academy of Sciences, Washington, D.C. 141 p.

Institute of Laboratory Animal Resources (ILAR) Committee on Education. 1979b. Laboratory animal medicine: Guidelines for education and training. ILAR News 22(2):M1-M26.

Institute of Laboratory Animal Resources (ILAR) Committee on Laboratory Animal Records. 1979c. Laboratory animal records. DHEW Pub. No. (NIH) 80-2064. U.S. Department of Health, Education, and Welfare, Washington, D.C. 45 + 22 p.

Institute of Laboratory Animal Resources (ILAR) Subcommittee on Care and Use, Committee on Nonhuman Primates. 1980. Laboratory animal management: Nonhuman primates. ILAR News 23(2-3):P1-P44.

Interagency Primate Steering Committee. 1980. National primate plan. DHEW Pub. No. (NIH) 80-1520. U.S. Department of Health, Education, and Welfare, Washington, D.C. 81 p.

Iravani, J., and A. van As. 1972. Mucus transport in the tracheobronchial tree of normal and bronchitic rats. J. Pathol. 106:81-93.

Irving, J.T., S.S. Socransky, and J.D. Heely. 1974. Histological changes in experimental periodontal disease in gnotobiotic rats and conventional hamsters. J. Periodontal Res. 9:73-80.

Irving, J.T., M.G. Newman, S.S. Socransky, and J.D. Heeley. 1975. Histological changes in experimental periodontal disease in rats monoinfected with a gram-negative organism. Arch. Oral Biol. 20:219-220.

Isaacson, M. 1975. The ecology of Praomys (Mastomys) natalensis in southern Africa. Bull. WHO 52:629-636.

Isaacson, R.L. Limbic System. Plenum Publishing Company, New York.

Iwata, S., and J.H. Kinoshita. 1971. Mechanism of development of hereditary cataract in mice. Invest. Ophthalmol. 10:504-512.

Jacobs, B.B., and R.A. Huseby. 1967. Neoplasms occurring in aged Fischer rats with special reference to testicular, uterine, and thyroid tumors. J. Natl. Cancer Inst. 39:303-309.

Jakoubek, B., E. Gutmann, J. Fischer, and A. Babicky. 1968. Rate of protein renewal in spinal motor neurons of adolescent and old rats. J. Neurochem. 15:633-641.

Jakubczak, L.F. 1966. Behavioral thermoregulation in young and old rats. J. Appl. Physiol. 21:19-21.

Jakubczak, L.F. 1967. Age, endocrines and behavior. Pages 231-245 in L. Gitman, ed. Endocrines and aging. Charles C. Thomas, Springfield, Illinois.

Jakubczak, L.F. 1973. Age and animal behavior. Pages 98-111 in C. Eisdorfer and M.P. Lawton, eds. The psychology of adult development and aging. American Psychological Association, Washington, D.C.

Jakubczak, L.F. 1977. Age differences in the effects of palatability of diet on regulation of calorie intake and body weight of rats. J. Gerontol. 32:49-57.

Jarrett, O. 1970. Evidence for the viral etiology of leukemia in domestic animals. Adv. Cancer Res. 13: 39-42.

Jaworski, Z.F.G. 1971. Some morphologic and dynamic aspects of remodeling on the endosteal-cortical and trabecular surface. Proc. Eur. Symp. Calcif. Tissue 8:159-169.

Jaworski, Z.F.G., and E. Lok. 1972. The rate of osteoclastic bone erosion in haversian remodeling sites of adult dogs. Calcif. Tissue Res. 10:103-112.

Jee, W.S.S. 1976. The health effects of plutonium and radium. J.W. Press, Salt Lake City, Utah. 802 p.

Jee, W.S.S. 1978. Relationship of trabecular bone surface areas, bone turnover rates, and initial uptake of Pu and Ra to sites of occurrence of osteosarcoma in Beagles. Pages 220-223 in Research in radiobiology. University of Utah Radiobiology Laboratory report, COO-119253. University of Utah, Salt Lake City, Utah.

Jee, W.S.S., D.B. Kimmel, E.G. Hashimoto, R.B. Dell, and L.A. Woodbury. 1976. Quantitative studies of Beagle lumbar vertebral bodies. Pages 110-117 in Z.F.G. Jaworski, ed. Bone morphometry. University of Ottawa Press, Ottawa, Ontario, Canada.

Jee, W.S.S., J.M. Smith, D.B. Kimmel, S.C. Miller, C. VanDura, C. Smith, and R. Dell. 1978. Preliminary surface/volume ratios and bone turnover rates of trabecular bone in young adult Beagles. Pages 224-230 in Research in radiobiology. University of Utah

Radiobiology Laboratory report, COO-119-253. University of Utah, Salt Lake City, Utah.

Jelínková, M., E. Struchlíková, and M. Sorzu. 1970. The effect of theophylline and adrenaline on the lipolytic response of rats of different age. Exp. Gerontol. 5(3):257-260.

Jellinger, K. 1976. Neuropathological aspects of dementias resulting from abnormal blood and cerebrospinal fluid dynamics. Acta Neurol. Belg. 76:83-102.

Jennings, A.R. 1949. Plasma-cell myelomatosis in the dog. J. Comp. Pathol. Ther. 59:113-118.

Jerome, E.A. 1959. Age and learning--experimental studies. Pages 655-699 in J.E. Birren, ed. Handbook of aging and the individual. University of Chicago Press, Chicago.

Jett, S., K. Wu, H. Duncan, and H.M. Frost. 1970. Adrenalcorticosteroid and salicylate actions on human and canine haversian bone formation and resorption. Clin. Orthop. Relat. Res. 68:301-315.

Jick, H., and O.S. Miettinen. 1976. Regular aspirin use and myocardial infarction. Br. Med. J. 1:1057.

Jobe, C.L. 1968. Selection and development of animal models of myocardial infarction. Pages 101-108 in Animal models for biomedical reresearch. Proceedings of a symposium sponsored jointly by the Institute of Laboratory Animal Resources and the American College of Laboratory Animal Medicine, held July 10, 1967 in Dallas, Texas. National Academy of Sciences, Washington, D.C.

Johanson, W.G., Jr., and A.K. Pierce. 1973. Lung structure and function with age in normal rats and rats with papain emphysema. J. Clin. Invest. 52:2921-2927.

Johanson, W.G., Jr., R.C. Reynolds, T. Scott, and A.K. Pierce. 1973. Connective tissue damage in emphysema: An electron microscopy study of papain-induced emphysema in rats. Am. Rev. Respir. Dis. 107:589-595.

Johnson, G.S., and R.S. Elizondo. 1979. Thermoregulation in Macaca mulatta: A thermal balance study. J. Appl. Physiol: Respir. Environ. Exercise Physiol. 46(2):268.

Johnson, K.H., and D.W. Hayden. 1979. Diabetes mellitus in cats with amyloidosis of pancreatic islets. Pages 118-121 in E.J. Andrews, B.C. Ward, and N.H. Altman, eds. Spontaneous animal models of human disease. Vol. I. Academic Press, New York.

Johnson, N.W., and R.M. Hopps. 1974. Epithelial cell proliferation in gingiva of macaque monkeys studied

by local injections of tritiated thymidine. Arch. Oral
Biol. 19:265-268.

Johnsson, L.-G., and J.E. Hawkins, Jr. 1972. Sensory and
neural degeneration with aging as seen in microdissec-
tions of the human inner ear. Ann. Otol. Rhinol. Laryngol. 81:179-193.

Johnsson, L.-G., and J.E. Hawkins, Jr. 1979. Age-related
degeneration of the inner ear. Pages 119-135 in Special
senses in aging. A current biological assessment.
Proceedings of a Symposium held October 10-11, 1977
at the University of Michigan, Ann Arbor. Institute
of Gerontology, University of Michigan, Ann Arbor,
Michigan.

Jonas, A.M., D.H. Percy, and J. Craft. 1970. Tyzzer's
disease in the rat. Its possible relationship with
megaloileitis. Arch. Pathol. 90:516-528.

Jonec, V., and C.E. Finch. 1975. Ageing and dopamine uptake by subcellular fractions of the C57BL/6J male mouse
brain. Brain Res. 91:197-215.

Jones, D.C., D.J. Kimeldorf, D.O. Rubadeau, and T.J. Cas-
tanera. 1953. Relationships between volitional activity and age in the male rat. Am. J. Physiol. 172:
109-114.

Jones, E.C., and P.L. Krohn. 1961a. The relationships
between age, numbers of oocytes, and fertility in virgin
and multiparous mice. J. Endocrinol. 21:469-495.

Jones, E.C., and P.L. Krohn. 1961b. The effect of hypophysectomy on age changes in the ovaries of mice. J.
Endocrinol. 21:497-509.

Jones, R., P. Bolduc, and L. Reid. 1973. Goblet cell
glycoprotein and tracheal gland hypertrophy in rat airways: The effect of tobacco smoke with or without
the anti-inflammatory agent phenylmethyloxadiazole.
Br. J. Exp. Pathol. 54:229-239.

Jones, T.B., R.W. Thorington, M.M. Hu, E. Adams, and R.W.
Cooper. 1973. Karotypes of squirrel monkeys (Saimiri
sciureus) from different geographic regions. Am. J.
Anthrop. 38:269-278.

Jones, T.C., and C.E. Gilmore. 1968. Pathological findings in aged dogs and cats. Pages 83-97 in The laboratory animal in gerontological research. National
Academy of Sciences, Washington, D.C.

Jones, T.C., and B.C. Zook. 1965. Aging changes in the
vascular system of animals. Ann. N.Y. Acad. Sci.
127:671-684.

Jönsson, L. 1972. Coronary arterial lesions and myocardial infarcts in the dog. A pathologic and microangiographic study. Acta Vet. Scand. Suppl. 38:1-80.

Jordan, H.V. 1971. Rodent model systems in periodontal disease research. J. Dent. Res. 50:236-242.

Jordan, H.V., R.J. Fitzgerald, and H.R. Stanley. 1965. Plaque formation and periodontal pathology in gnotobiotic rats infected with an oral actinomycete. Am. J. Pathol. 47:1157-1163.

Jordan, H.V., P.H. Keyes, and S. Bellack. 1972. Periodontal lesions in hamsters and gnotobiotic rats infected with Actinomyces of human origin. J. Periodontal Res. 7:21-28.

Joseph, J.A., R.E. Berger, B.T. Engel, and G.S. Roth. 1978. Age-related changes in the nigrostriatum: A behavioral and biochemical analysis. J. Gerontol. 33:643-649.

Jowsey, J. 1960. Age changes in human bone. Clin. Orthop. 17:210-217.

Jowsey, J. 1969. Effect of long-term administration of porcine calcitonin in the development of dietary osteoporosis in cats. Endocrinology 85:1196-1201.

Jowsey, J., and J. Gershon-Cohen. 1964. Effect of dietary calcium levels on production and reversal of experimental osteoporosis in cats. Proc. Soc. Exp. Biol. Med. 116:437-441.

Jowsey, J., and L.G. Raisz. 1968. Experimental osteoporosis and parathyroid activity. Endocrinology 82:384-396.

Jowsey, J., E. Reiss, and J.M. Canterbury. 1974. Long-term effects of high phosphate intake on parathyroid hormone levels and bone metabolism. Acta Orthop. Scand. 45:801-808.

Jubb, K.V.F., and P.C. Kennedy. 1963. The male genital system. Pages 355-387 in Pathology of domestic animals. Vol. 1. Academic Press, New York.

Jubb, K.V.F., and P.C. Kennedy. 1971a. The upper alimentary system. Pages 1-45 in Pathology of domestic animals. Vol. 2. 2nd ed. Academic Press, New York.

Jubb, K.V.F., and P.C. Kennedy. 1971b. The urinary system. Pages 247-289 in Pathology of domestic animals. Vol. 2. 2nd ed. Academic Press, New York.

Jugdutt, B.I., L.C. Becker, and G.M. Hutchins. 1979. Early changes in collateral blood flow during myocardial infarction in conscious dogs. Am. J. Physiol. 237(3):H371-H380.

Kahnberg, K.-E., J. Lindhe, and R. Attstrom. 1977. The
effect of decomplementation by carragheenan on experimental initial gingivitis in hyperimmune dogs. J.
Periodontal Res. 12:479-490.

Kakehashi, S., P.N. Baer, and C.L. White. 1963. Comparative pathology of periodontal disease. I. Gorilla.
Oral Surg. Oral Med. Oral Pathol. 16:397-406.

Kakuk, T.J., R.W. Hinz, R.F. Langham, and G.H. Conner.
1968. Experimental transmission of canine malignant
lymphoma to the Beagle neonate. Cancer Res. 28:716-
723.

Kalish, M.I., M.S. Katz, M.A. Pineyro, and R.I. Gregerman.
1977. Epinephrine- and glucagon-sensitive adenylate
cyclases of rat liver during aging. Evidence for membrane instability associated with increased enzymatic
activity. Biochem. Biophys. Acta 483(2): 452-466.

Kalser, M.H. 1976a. Classification of malassimilation
syndromes and diagnosis of malabsorption. Pages 231-243
in H. Bockus, ed. Gastroenterology II. W.B. Saunders
Co., Philadelphia.

Kalser, M.H. 1976b. Celiac sprue (gluten-induced enter-
opathy, nontropical sprue, idiopathic steatorrhea).
Pages 244-284 in H. Bockus, ed. Gastroenterology II.
W.B. Saunders Co., Philadelphia.

Kanarek, R.B., and E. Hirsch. 1977. Dietary-induced over-
eating in experimental animals. Fed. Proc. 36:154-158.

Kaneko, J.J., J.E. Moulton, R.S. Brodey, and V.D. Perryman.
1965. Malabsorption syndrome resembling nontropical
sprue in dogs. J. Am. Vet. Med. Assoc. 146:463-473.

Kaplan, M.L., D.A. Garcia, P. Goldhaber, M.A. Davis, and
S.J. Adelstein. 1975. Uptake of ^{99m}Tc-Sn-EHDP in
Beagles with advanced periodontal disease. Calcif.
Tissue Res. 19:91-98.

Kaplan, M.L., M.A. Davis, P.H. Aschaffenburg, S.J. Adelstein, and P. Goldhaber. 1978a. Clinical, radiographic
and scintigraphic findings in experimental periodontal
disease in dogs. Arch. Oral Biol. 23:273-280.

Kaplan, M.L., M.A. Davis, and P. Goldhaber. 1978b. Blood
flow measurements in selected oral tissues in dogs using
radiolabelled microspheres and rubidium-86. Arch. Oral
Biol. 23:281-284.

Kaplan, M.L., M.K. Jeffcoat, and P. Goldhaber. 1978c.
Radiolabeled microsphere measurements of alveolar bone
blood flow in dogs. J. Periodontal Res. 13:304-308.

Kapur, Y.P., and P. Patt. 1967. Hearing in Todas of
South India. Arch. Otolaryngol. 85:400-406.

Karakasis, D., and A. Tsaknakis. 1976. Aging changes in the articular disk of the temporomandibular joint in the guinea pig. J. Dent. Res. 55(2):262-265.

Karavodin, L.M., and L.R. Ash. 1977a. Weak mixed lymphocyte culture response in the Mongolian gerbil (Meriones unguiculatus). Lab. Anim. Sci. 27:195-203.

Karavodin, L.M., and L.R. Ash. 1977b. Weak graft-vs-host response in the Mongolian gerbil (Meriones unguiculatus). Lab. Anim. Sci. 27:1035-1036.

Karlinsky, J.B., and G.L. Snider. 1978. Animal models of emphysema. Am. Rev. Respir. Dis. 117:1109-1133.

Kato, R., and A. Takanaka. 1968. Metabolism of drugs in old rats. II. Metabolism in vivo and effect of drug in old rats. Jap. J. Pharmacol. 18(4):389-396.

Katosova, L.K. 1977. Enzymatic characteristics of blood lymphocytes in postnatal ontogenesis of rabbit. Zh. Evol. Biokhim. Fiziol. 13:403-404. (in Russian)

Kay, D.W.K. 1972. Epidemiological aspects of organic brain disease in the aged. Pages 15-28 in C.M. Gaitz, ed. Aging and the brain. Plenum Publishing Corp., New York.

Kay, H., and M.E. Sime. 1962. Discrimination learning with old and young rats. J. Gerontol. 17:75-80.

Kay, M.M.B. 1978a. Immunological aging patterns: Effects of parainfluenza type I virus infection on aging mice of eight strains and hybrids. Pages 213-240 in D. Bergsma and D.E. Harrison, eds. Genetic effects on aging. Birth defects original article series. Vol. 14, No. 1. A.R. Liss, Inc., New York.

Kay, M.M.B. 1978b. Long term subclinical effects of parainfluenza (Sendai) infection on immune cells of aging mice. Proc. Soc. Exp. Biol. Med. 158:326-331.

Kayser, C. 1961. The physiology of natural hibernation. Pergamon Press, Elmsford, New York. 325 p.

Kebabian, J.W., and D.B. Calne. 1979. Multiple receptors for dopamine. Nature 277:93-96.

Kebabian, J.W., G.L. Petzold, and P. Greengard. 1972. Dopamine-sensitive adenylate cyclase in caudate nucleus of rat brain, and its similarity to the "dopamine receptor." Proc. Natl. Acad. Sci. USA 69:2145-2149.

Keeling, M.E., and J.R. Roberts. 1972. Breeding and reproduction of chimpanzees. Pages 127-152 in G.H. Bourne, ed. The chimpanzee. Vol. 5. Karger, Basel and University Park Press, Baltimore.

Kelliher, G.J., and J. Roberts. 1974. A study of the antiarrhythmic action of certain beta-blocking agents. Am. Heart J. 87(4):458-467.

Kelly, S.S. 1978. The effect of age on neuromuscular transmission. J. Physiol. 274:51-62.

Kendrick, Z.V., F.J. Uricchio, and S.I. Baskin. 1978. Effect of age on Na, K, Mg-dependent ATPase activity and the regional distribution of Ca and Mg in the hearts of the Fischer 344 rat. Abstract No. 3502. Fed. Proc. 37:881.

Kennedy, J.E., and A.M. Polson. 1973. Experimental marginal periodontitis in squirrel monkeys. J. Periodontol. 44:140-144.

Kennett, F.F., and W.B. Weglicki. 1978. Lack of effect of methylprednisolone on lysosomal and microsomal enzymes after two hours of well-defined canine myocardial ischemia. Circ. Res. 43(5):759-768.

Kent, G.C., Jr. 1968. Physiology of reproduction. Pages 119-138 in R.A. Hoffman, P.F. Robinson, and H. Magalhaes, eds. The golden hamster. Its biology and use in medical research. Iowa State University Press, Ames, Iowa.

Kepron, W., J.M. James, B. Kirk, A.H. Sehon, and K.S. Tse. 1977. A canine model for reaginic hypersensitivity and allergic bronchoconstriction. J. Allergy Clin. Immunol. 59:64-69.

Kerley, E.R. 1965. The microscopic determination of age in human bone. Am. J. Anthropol. 23:141-164.

Kerr, G.R. 1972. Nutrient requirements of subhuman primates. Physiol. Rev. 52:415-467.

Keyes, P.H. 1968. Odontopathic infections. Pages 253-284 in R.A. Hoffman, P.F. Robinson, and H. Magalhaes, eds. The golden hamster. Its biology and use in medical research. Iowa State University Press, Ames, Iowa.

Khaw, B.A., G.A. Beller, and E. Haber. 1978a. Experimental myocardial infarct imaging following intravenous administration of iodine-131 labeled antibody (Fab')$_2$ fragments specific for cardiac myosin. Circulation 57:743-750.

Khaw, B.A., H.K. Gold, R.C. Leinbach, J.T. Fallon, W. Strauss, G.M. Pohost, and E. Haber. 1978b. Early imaging of experimental myocardial infarction by intracoronary administration of ^{131}I-labelled anticardiac myosin (Fab')$_2$ fragments. Circulation 58:1137-1142.

Kimmel, D.B., and W.S.S. Jee. 1978a. Quantitative studies of bone cells in Beagles. Pages 231-233 in Research in radiobiology. University of Utah Radiobiology Laboratory report, COO-119-253. University of Utah, Salt Lake City, Utah.

Kimmel, D.B., and W.S.S. Jee. 1978b. Comparison of biologic activity of young adult human and Beagle trabecular bone. Pages 237-242 in Research in radiobiology. University of Utah Radiobiology Laboratory report, COO-119-253. University of Utah, Salt Lake City, Utah.

Kimmelstiel, P. 1966. Diabetic nephropathy. Pages 226-252 in F.K. Mostofi and D.E. Smith, eds. The kidney. International Academy of Pathology. Monographs in pathology, No. 6. Williams and Wilkins Co., Baltimore.

King, J.A. 1965. Body, brain, and lens weights of Peromyscus. Zool. Jb. Anat. Bd. 82:177-188.

King, J.A. 1968. Biology of Peromyscus (Rodentia). Oklahoma State University Press, Stillwater, Oklahoma. 593 p.

Kirk, R.W. [ed.] 1977. Current veterinary therapy VI. W.B. Saunders Co., Philadelphia. 1481 p.

Kirkman, H., and F.T. Algard. 1968. Spontaneous and nonviral-induced neoplasms. Pages 227-240 in R.A. Hoffman, P.F. Robinson, and H. Magalhaes, eds. The golden hamster. Its biology and use in medical research. Iowa State University Press, Ames, Iowa.

Kitahara, A., and R.C. Adelman. 1979. Altered regulation of insulin secretion in isolated islets of different sizes in aging rats. Biochem. Biophys. Res. Comm. 87:1207-1213.

Kleinerman, J., and D. Niewoehner. 1973. Physiological, pathological and morphometric studies of long-term nitrogen dioxide exposures and recovery in hamsters. Am. Rev. Respir. Dis. 107:1081.

Kleinerman, J., D. Rynbrandt, and J. Sorensen. 1976. Chronic obstructive airways disease in cats produced by NO_2. Am. Rev. Resp. Dis. 113(4, part 2):107.

Klimenko, E.M. 1975. Catecholamine concentration in several structures of the cat and rabbit sympathetic nervous systems during postnatal ontogenesis. Zh. Evol. Biokhim. Fiziol. 11:65-69. (in Russian)

Klocke, R.A. 1977. Influence of aging on the lung. Pages 432-444 in C.E. Finch and L. Hayflick, eds. Handbook of the biology of aging. Van Nostrand Reinhold, New York.

Klug, T.L., K. Karoly, and R.C. Adelman. 1979. Regulation of glucagon levels in rats during aging. Biochem. Biophys. Res. Comm. 89:907-912.

Knapka, J.J., K.P. Smith, and F.J. Judge. 1974. Effect of open and closed formula rations on the performance of three strains of laboratory mice. Lab. Anim. Sci. 24:480-487.

Knecht, C.D. 1970. The effect of delayed hemilaminectomy in the treatment of intervertebral disc protrusions in dogs. J. Am. Anim. Hosp. Assoc. 6:71-77.

Knook, D.L., and E. Ch. Sleyster. 1976. Lysosomal enzyme activities in parenchymal and nonparenchymal liver cells isolated from young, adult and old rats. Mech. Ageing Dev. 5:389-397.

Koch, S.A. 1972. Cataracts in interrelated Old English Sheepdogs. J. Am. Vet. Med. Assoc. 160:299-301.

Koch, S.A., and L.F. Rubin. 1972. Distribution of cones in retina of the normal dog. Am. J. Vet. Res. 33:361-363.

Koch, S.A., and J.F. Skelley. 1967. Colitis in a dog resembling Whipple's disease in man. J. Am. Vet. Med. Assoc. 150:22-26.

Koestner, A., and L. Buerger. 1965. Primary neoplasms of the salivary glands in animals compared to similar tumors in man. Vet. Pathol. 2:201-226.

Kohn, D.F. 1971. Sequential pathogenicity of Mycoplasma pulmonis in laboratory rats. Lab. Anim. Sci. 21:849-855.

Koletsky, S. 1973. Obese spontaneously hypertensive rats--a model for study of atherosclerosis. Exp. Mol. Pathol. 19:53-60.

Koletsky, S., and D.I. Puterman. 1977. Reduction of atherosclerotic disease in genetically obese rats by low calorie diet. Exp. Mol. Pathol. 26:415-424.

Koltman, A. 1935. Histologische untersuchungen über das wesen der prostata-hypertrophie beim hunde. Diss. München.

Koppang, N. 1973. Canine ceroid-lipofuscinosis--a model for human neuronal ceroid-lipofuscinosis and aging. Mech. Ageing Dev. 2:421-445.

Korc, I., H.C. DeMate, M.I. Muse, and O.A. DeSirtori. 1970. Soluble lens proteins in rats on different sugar diets. Exp. Eye Res. 10:313-318.

Kottke, B.A., K.K. Unni, I.A. Carlo, and M.T.R. Subbiah. 1974. Regression of established natural atherosclerotic lesions by intestinal bypass surgery in pigeons: Structure and chemistry. Trans. Assoc. Am. Physician 87:263-270.

Kovalevsky, E.I., and L.F. Stebaeva. 1973. The role of age-specific peculiarities of the choroid ultrastructure in experimental uveitis. Vestn. Oftal'mol. 1:12-17. (in Russian)

Koyama, N., K. Norikoshi, and T. Mano. 1975. Population dynamics of Japanese monkeys at Arashiyama. Pages

411-417 in S. Kondo, ed. Contemporary primatology. Proceedings of the 5th International Congress of Primatology, held August 21-24, 1974 in Nagoya, Japan. Karger, Basel.

Kozhura, I.M. 1967a. Some features peculiar to the development of experimental atherosclerosis in rabbits in connection with age. Kardiologiya 7:86-90. (in Russian)

Kozhura, I.P. 1967b. Some features peculiar to vascular permeability in animals of various age. Pat. Fiziol. Eksp. Ter. 11:28-30. (in Russian)

Kozima, K. 1977. Immunological features of mastomys. Pages 19-30 in J. Soga and H. Sato, eds. Praomys (Mastomys) natalensis. The significance of their tumors and diseases for cancer research. The Daiichi Printing Co., Ltd, Niigata, Japan.

Kozma, C., L.M. Cummins, and S. Tekeli. 1973. The use of Long-Evans rats in long term toxicity studies. Pages 283-301 in Proceedings of the V International ICLA Symposium held in 1972 at Hannover, Germany. Gustav Fischer Verlag, Stuttgart, Germany.

Kozma, C., W. Macklin, L.M. Cummins, and R. Mauer. 1974. Anatomy, physiology and biochemistry of the rabbit. Pages 49-72 in S.H. Weisbroth, R.E. Flatt, and A.L. Kraus, eds. The biology of the laboratory rabbit. Academic Press, New York.

Kraemer, G.W., and W.T. McKinney. 1979. Interactions of pharmacological agents which alter biogenic amine metabolism and depression: An analysis of contributing factors within a primate model of depression. J. Affect. Disord. 1:33-54.

Kraemer, G.W., W.T. McKinney, G.R. Breene, and A.J. Prange. 1976. Behavioral and biochemical effects of micro injections of 6-hydroxydopamine into the substantia nigra of the rhesus monkey. Abstract No. 707, Page 494 in Neuroscience Abstracts. Vol. 2, Part 1. Society for Neuroscience, Bethesda, Maryland.

Kraft, G.H. 1968. Experimental allergic neuritis: Model of idiopathic (Guillain-Barre) polyneuritis. Arch. Phys. Med. 49:490-501.

Kraft, G.H. 1972. Effects of temperature and age on nerve conduction velocity in the guinea pig. Arch. Phys. Med. Rehabil. 53(7):328-332.

Kramer, A.W. 1964. Body and organ weights and linear measurements of the adult Mongolian gerbil. Anat. Rec. 150:343-348.

Kramsch, D.M., and W. Hollander. 1968. Occlusive atherosclerotic disease of the coronary arteries in monkey
(Macaca irus) induced by diet. Exp. Mol. Pathol. 9:
1-22.

Kramsch, D.M., W. Hollander, and S. Renaud. 1973. Induction of fibrous plaques versus foam cell lesions in
Macaca fascicularis by varying the composition of dietary fats. Circulation Suppl. 48:IV-41.

Krasse, B., and N. Brill. 1960. Effect of consistency
of diet on bacteria in gingival pockets in dogs.
Odontol. Revy 11:152-165.

Krishnarao, G.V.G., and H.H. Draper. 1969. Age-related
changes in the bones of adult mice. J. Gerontol.
24:149-151.

Kritchevsky, D. 1964. Experimental atherosclerosis.
Pages 63-130 in R. Paoletti, ed. Lipid pharmacology.
Academic Press, New York.

Krohn, K. 1968. Experimental gastritis in the dog. I.
Production of astrophic gastritis and antibodies to
parietal cells. Ann. Med. Exp. Fenn. 46:249-258.

Kronenberg, R.S., and C.W. Drage. 1973. Attenuation of
the ventilatory and heart rate responses to hypoxia
and hypercapnia with aging in normal men. J. Clin.
Invest. 52:1812-1819.

Krook, L., L. Lutwak, P.A. Henrikson, F. Kallfelz, C.
Hirsch, B. Romanus, L.F. Belanger, J.R. Marier, and
B.E. Sheffy. 1971. Reversibility of nutritional
osteoporosis: Physicochemical data on bones from an
experimental study in dogs. J. Nutr. 101:233-246.

Krygier, G., R.J. Genco, P.A. Mashimo, and E. Hausmann.
1973. Experimental gingivitis in Macaca speciosa monkeys: Clinical bacteriologic and histologic similarities to human gingivitis. J. Periodontol. 44:454-463.

Kulonen, E., and J. Pikkarainean. 1968. The reflection
of the age, tissue and solubility of the amberlite
CG-50 fractions of denatured collagens. Acta Physiol.
Scand. 74(1):10-15.

Kummer, H. 1971. Primate societies. Aldine Press,
Chicago. 160 p.

Kunstyr, I., and H.-G.W. Leuenberger. 1975. Gerontological data of C57BL/6J mice. I. Sex differences in
survival curves. J. Gerontol. 30:157-162.

Kupersmith, J. 1976. Antiarrhythmic drugs: Changing
concepts. Am. J. Cardiol. 38:119-121.

Kurtz, J.M., S.W. Russell, J.C. Lee, D.O. Slauson, and
R.D. Schechter. 1972. Naturally occurring canine
glomerulonephritis. Am. J. Pathol. 67:471-482.

Kuttner, R.E., and A.B. Lorincz. 1969. The effect of catecholamines on free amino acids in rat heart and other organs. Arch. Int. Pharmacodyn. Ther. 182:300-309.

Labelle, R.E., and E.M. Schaffer. 1966. The effects of cortisone and induced local factors on the periodontium of the albino rat. J. Periodontol. 37:483-489.

Lacassagné, A. 1933. Métaplasie épidermoïde de la prostate provoquée, chez la souris par des injections répétées de fortes doses de folliculine. C.R. Soc. Biol. 113:590-592.

Laflamme, G.H., and J. Jowsey. 1972. Bone and soft tissue changes with oral phosphate supplements. J. Clin. Invest. 51:2834-2840.

Lai, Y.L., R.O. Jacoby, A.M. Jonas, and D.S. Papermaster. 1975. A new form of hereditary retinal degeneration in WAG/Rij rats. Invest. Ophthalmol. 14:62-67.

Laird, C.W. 1974. Clinical pathology: Blood chemistry. Pages 347-436 in E.C. Melby and N.H. Altman, eds. The handbook of laboratory animal science. Vol. II. CRC Press, Cleveland, Ohio.

Lakatta, E.G. 1978. Perspectives on the aged myocardium. Adv. Exp. Med. Biol. 97:147-169.

Lakatta, E.G., G. Gerstenblith, C.S. Angell, N.W. Shock, and M.L. Weisfeldt. 1975. Prolonged contraction duration in aged myocardium. J. Clin. Invest. 55(1):61-68.

Lamarre, Y. 1975. Tremorgenic mechanisms in primates. Adv. Neurol. 10:23-34.

Lamb, D., and L. Reid. 1968. Mitotic rates, goblet cell increase and histochemical changes in mucus in rat bronchial epithelium during exposure to sulphur dioxide. J. Pathol. Bacteriol. 96:97-111.

Lamb, D., and L. Reid. 1969. Goblet cell increase in rat bronchial epithelium after exposure to cigarette and cigar tobacco smoke. Br. Med. J. 1:33-35.

Landfield, P.W. 1978. An endocrine hypothesis of brain aging and studies of brain-endocrine correlations and monosynaptic neurophysiology during aging. Adv. Exp. Med. Biol. 113:179-200.

Landfield, P.W. 1979. Neurobiological changes in hippocampus of aging rats: Quantitative correlations with behavioral deficits and with endocrine mechanisms. Pages 495-496 in H. Orimo, K. Shimada, M. Iriki, and D. Maeda. Recent advances in gerontology. Proceedings of the XIth International Congress of Gerontology.

August 20-25, 1978, Tokyo, Japan. Excerpta Medica, Amsterdam.

Landfield, P.W. In press. Correlative studies of brain neurophysiology and behavior during aging in D. Stein, ed. Psychobiology of aging. Elsevier North-Holland Biomedical Press, New York.

Landfield, P.W., and G. Lynch. 1977. Impaired monosynaptic potentiation in in vitro hippocampal slices from aged, memory-deficient rats. J. Gerontol. 32:523-533.

Landfield, P.W., G. Rose, L. Sandles, T. Wohlstadter, and G. Lynch. 1977. Patterns of astroglial hypertrophy and neuronal degeneration in the hippocampus of aged, memory-deficient rats. J. Gerontol. 32:3-12.

Landfield, P.W., J.C. Waymire, and G. Lynch. 1978a. Hippocampal aging and adrenocorticoids: Quantitative correlations. Science 202:1098-1102.

Landfield, P.W., J.L. McGaugh, and G. Lynch. 1978b. Impaired synaptic potentiation processes in the hippocampus of aged, memory-deficient rats. Brain Res. 150:85-101.

Landfield, P.W., J.D. Lindsey, L. Braun, C. Wurtz, M. Maxwell, and G. Lynch. 1978c. Quantitative E.M. and semithin studies of synaptic vesicles and degeneration, astrocyte reactivity, microglia, displaced nucleoli and lipofuscin in hippocampus of aging rats. Gerontologist 18:92.

Landfield, P.W., C. Wurtz, and J.D. Lindsey. 1979. Quantification of synaptic vesicles in hippocampus of aging rats and initial studies of possible relations to neurophysiology. Brain Res. Bull. 4:757-763.

Landowne, M., and J. Stanley. 1960. Aging of the cardiovascular system. Pages 159-187 in N.W. Shock, ed. Aging--Some social and biological aspects. American Association for the Advancement of Science, Washington, D.C.

Lane, P.W., and M.M. Dickie. 1958. The effect of restricted food intake on the life span of genetically obese mice. J. Nutr. 64:549-554.

Lang, C.M. 1967. Effects of psychic stress on atherosclerosis in the squirrel monkey (Saimiri sciureus). Proc. Soc. Exp. Biol. Med. 126:30-34.

Lang, C.M., and C.H. Barthel. 1972. Effects of simple and complex carbohydrates on serum lipids and atherosclerosis in nonhuman primates. Am. J. Clin. Nutr. 25:470-475.

Lang, C.M., and B.L. Munger. 1976. Diabetes mellitus in the guinea pig. Diabetes 25:434-443.

Lang, C.M., B.L. Munger, and F. Rapp. 1977. The guinea pig as an animal model of diabetes mellitus. Lab. Anim. Sci. 27:789-805.

Lapin, B.A. 1973. The importance of monkeys for the study of malignant tumors in man. Pages 213-224 in G.H. Bourne, ed. Nonhuman primates and medical research. Academic Press, New York.

Lapin, B.A., R.I. Krilova, G.M. Cherkovich, N.S. Asanov. 1979. Observation from Sukhumi. Pages 14-37 in D.M. Bowden, ed. Aging in nonhuman primates. Van Nostrand Reinhold, New York.

Larsson, T., T. Sjogren, and G. Jacobson. 1963. Senile dementia. A clinical, sociomedical and genetic study. Acta Psychiatr. Scand. Suppl. 39(167):1-259.

Lasagna, L. 1956. Drug effects as modified by aging. J. Chronic Dis. 3:567-574.

Lathers, C.M. 1975. Effect of practolol and sotalol on ouabain-induced nonuniform adrenergic nerve activity. Abstract No. 2978. Fed. Proc. 34:745.

Lathers, C.M. 1979. The effect of methylprednisolone on autonomic neural discharge associated with acute coronary occlusion in the cat. The Pharmacologist 21:201.

Lathers, C.M. 1980. The effect of metroprolol on coronary occlusion-induced arrythmia and autonomic neural discharge. Abstract No. 2655. Fed. Proc. 39:771.

Lathers, C.M., G.J. Kelliher, J. Roberts, A.J. Teres, and A.B. Beasley. 1976. Effect of practolol and coronary anatomy on occlusion-induced arrhythmia and the associated nonuniform neural discharge. Clin. Res. 24:617A.

Lathers, C.M., G.J. Kelliher, J. Roberts, and A.B. Beasley. 1977. Role of the adrenergic nervous system in arrhythmia produced by acute coronary artery occlusion. Pages 123-149 in A. Lefer, G.J. Kelliher, and M. Rovetto, eds. Pathophysiology and therapeutics of myocardial ischemia. Spectrum Publications, New York.

Lathers, C.M., G.J. Kelliher, J. Roberts, and A.B. Beasley. 1978. Nonuniform cardiac sympathetic nerve discharge: Mechanism for coronary occlusion and digitalis-induced arrythmia. Circulation 57(6):1058-1065.

Lauper, N.T., K.K. Unni, B.A. Kottke, and J.L. Titus. 1975. Anatomy and histology of aorta of White Carneau pigeon. Lab. Invest. 32:536-551.

Laurell, C.B., and S. Erickson. 1963. The electrophoretic alpha$_1$ globulin pattern in alpha$_1$ antitrypsin deficiency. Scand. J. Clin. Lab. Invest. 15:132-140.

Laver-Rudich, Z., E. Skutelsky, and D. Danon. 1978. Age-related changes in aortic intima of rats. J. Gerontol. 33(3):337-346.

Lawick-Goodall, J.V. 1971. In the shadow of man. Houghton Mifflin, Boston. 297 p.

Lawrence, M. 1979. Cochlear physiology and the aging process. Pages 136-142 in Special senses in aging. A current biological assessment. Proceedings of a symposium held October 10-11, 1977 at the University of Michigan, Ann Arbor. Institute of Gerontology, University of Michigan, Ann Arbor, Michigan.

Leathem, J.H., and E.D. Albrecht. 1974. Effect of age on testis Δ^5-3β-hydroxysteroid dehydrogenase in the rat. Proc. Soc. Exp. Biol. Med. 145:1212-1214.

Leathers, C.W., and B.C. Bullock. 1975. Naturally occurring neoplasms in a group of aged, non-breeding Mongolian gerbils. Abstract No. 3 in Abstracts of papers presented at the 26th Annual Session of the American Association for Laboratory Animal Science. Pub. No. 75-2. American Association for Laboratory Animal Science. Joliet, Illinois.

Leathers, C.W., and H.K. Schedewie. In press. Maturity onset diabetes mellitus in a pig-tailed macaque (Macaca nemestrina). J. Med. Primatol.

Leav, I., and L.F. Cavazos. 1975. Some morphologic features of normal and pathologic canine prostate. Pages 69-107 in M. Goland, ed. Normal and abnormal growth of the prostate. Charles C. Thomas, Springfield, Illinois.

LeBeau, A. 1953. L'âge du chien et celui de l'homme. Essai de statistique sur la mortalité canine. Bull. Acad. Vet. Fr. 26:229-232.

Lechner, J.F., K. Shankar Narayan, Y. Ohnuki, M.S. Babcock, L.W. Jones, and M.E. Kaighn. 1978. Replicative epithelial cell cultures from normal human prostate gland: Brief communication. J. Natl. Cancer Inst. 60:797-799.

Lee, J.C., L.M. Karpeles, and S.E. Downing. 1972. Age-related changes of cardiac performance in male rats. Amer. J. Physiol. 222:432-438.

Lee, K.T., J. Jarmolych, D.M. Kim, C. Grant, J.A. Krasney, W.A. Thomas, and A.M. Bruno. 1971. Production of advanced coronary atherosclerosis, myocardial infarction, and sudden death in swine. Exp. Mol. Pathol. 15(2):170-190.

Lee, T., P. Seeman, A. Rajput, I.J. Farley, and O. Hornykiewicz. 1978. Receptor basis for dopaminergic supersensitivity in Parkinson's disease. Nature 273:59-61.

LeGuilly, Y., M. Simon, P. Lenoir, and M. Bourel. 1973.
Long-term culture of human adult liver cells: Morphological changes related in vitro to senescence and
effect of donor's age on growth potential. Gerontologia 19:303-313.

Lehner, N.D.M., T.B. Clarkson, and H.B. Lofland. 1971.
The effect of insulin deficiency, hypothyroidism and
hypertension on atherosclerosis in the squirrel monkey.
Exp. Mol. Pathol. 15:230-244.

Lelorier, J., M. Tremblay, J. de Champlain, A. Gattereau,
and J. Davignan. 1976. Effects of 6-hydroxydopamine
on diet-induced hyperlipidemia and atherosclerosis in
rats. Can. J. Physiol. Pharmacol. 54:83-85.

LeMagnen, J. 1978. Metabolically driven and learned
feeding responses in man. Pages 45-53 in G.A. Bray,
ed. Recent advances in obesity research: II. Proceedings of the 2nd International Congress on Obesity,
held October 23-26, 1977 in Washington, D.C. Newman
Publishing, Ltd., London.

Leon, G.R., and L. Roth. 1977. Obesity: Psychological
causes, correlations, and speculations. Psychol.
Bull. 84(1):117-139.

Leonard, A., and G. Dekundt. 1970. The chromosomes of
gerbils (Meriones unguiculatus). Acta Zool. Pathol.
Antverp. 50:61-66.

Lepeschkin, E., and F.N. Wilson. 1951. Modern electrocardiography. Williams and Wilkins, Baltimore. 598 p.

Les, E.P. 1979. Effect of pasteurized feed on weight
gain, feed utilization and lifespan of inbred and hybrid laboratory mice. Unpublished paper available from
Dr. E.P. Les, The Jackson Laboratory, Bar Harbor, Maine.

Lesser, G.T., S. Deutsch, and J. Marofsky. 1973. Aging
in the rat: Longitudinal and cross-sectional studies
of body composition. Am. J. Physiol. 225:1472-1478.

Leto, S., G.C. Kokkonen, and C.H. Barrows. 1976. Dietary
proteins, lifespan and biochemical variables in female
mice. J. Gerontol. 31:144-148.

Leveille, G.A. 1972. The long-term effects of meal-
eating on lipogenesis, enzyme activity and longevity
in the rat. J. Nutr. 102:549-566.

Levine, S., and E.M. Hoenig. 1972. Amyloidosis in parabiotic gerbils. Arch. Pathol. 94:461-465.

Levitt, B., N. Cagin, J. Kleid, J. Somberg, and R. Gillis.
1976. Role of the nervous system in the genesis of

cardiac rhythm disorders. Am. J. Cardiol. 37:1111-1113.

Levkova, N.A., and V.I. Trunov. 1970. Features peculiar to the structure of mitochondria on the senile myocardium. Kardiologia 10(9): 94-97.

Levy, B.M. 1963. The marmoset as an experimental animal in periodontal research. Page 115, Abstract No. 318 in Abstracts of the 41st general meeting of the International Association for Dental Research, held in Pittsburgh, Pennsylvania. International Association for Dental Research, Washington, D.C.

Levy, B.M., S.H. Hampton, and J.K. Hampton, Jr. 1972. Some aspects of marmoset biology. Int. Zoo Yearb. 12:51-56.

Levy, B.M., P.B. Robertson, S. Dreizen, B.F. Mackler, and S. Bernick. 1976. Adjuvant induced destructive periodontitis in non-human primates: A comparative study. J. Periodontal Res. 11:54-60.

Lewis, L.A. 1978. Atherosclerosis-an epilogue. Cleveland Clinic Quart. 45:253-266.

Lewis, R.M. 1974. Spontaneous autoimmune diseases of domestic animals. Int. Rev. Exp. Pathol. 13:55-82.

Lewis, R.M., W. B. Henry, Jr., G.W. Thornton, and C.E. Gilmore. 1963. A syndrome of autoimmune hemolytic anemias and thrombocytopoiesis in dogs. Pages 140-163 in The American Veterinary Medical Association proceedings book. Scientific proceedings of the 100th annual meeting, held July 28-August 1, 1963, in New York, New York. American Veterinary Medical Association, Schaumberg, Illinois.

Lewis, R.M., R.S. Schwartz, and C.E. Gilmore. 1965. Autoimmune diseases in domestic animals. Ann. N.Y. Acad. Sci. 124:178-200.

Lewis, T.R., K.I. Campbell, and T.R. Vaughan, Jr. 1969. Effects on canine pulmonary function via induced NO_2 impairment, particulate interaction, and subsequent SO_x. Arch. Environ. Health 18:596-601.

Lewis, T.R., W.J. Moorman, Y.Y. Yang, and J.F. Stara. 1974. Long-term exposure to auto exhaust and other pollutant mixtures. Arch. Environ. Health 29:102-106.

Libby, P., P.R. Maroko, J.W. Covell, C.I. Malloch, J. Ross, Jr., and E. Braunwald. 1973a. Effect of practolol on the extent of myocardial ischaemic injury after experimental coronary occlusion and its effect on ventricular function in the normal and ischaemic heart. Cardiovasc. Res. 7:167-173.

Libby, P., P.R. Maroko, C.M. Bloor, B.E. Sobel, and E. Braunwald. 1973b. Reduction of experimental myocardial infarct size by corticosteroid administration. J. Clin. Invest. 52:599-607.

Liebow, A.A. 1964. Biochemical and structural changes in the aging lung. Pages 97-104 in L. Cander and J. Moyer, eds. Aging of the lung. Grune and Stratton, New York.

Lijinsky, W. 1978. Nitrosamines in animal feed. Science 202:1034.

Limas, C.J. 1975. Comparison of the handling of norepinephrine in the myocardium of adult and old rats. Cardiovasc. Res. 9(5):664-668.

Lin, J.H., J.L. Duffy, and M.S. Roginsky. 1975. Microcirculation in diabetes mellitus. Hum. Pathol. 6(1): 77-96.

Lin, K.H., Y.M. Peng, M.T. Peng, and T.M. Tseng. 1976. Changes in the nuclear volume of rat hypothalamic neurons in old age. Neuroendocrinology 21:247-254.

Lin, T.J., and J.L. So-Bosita. 1972. Pitfalls in the interpretation of estrogenic effect in postmenopausal women. Am. J. Obstet. Gynecol. 114:929-931.

Lindeman, R.D. 1975. Age changes in renal function. Pages 19-38 in R. Goldman and M. Rockstein, eds. The physiology and pathology of human aging. Academic Press, New York.

Lindhe, J., and H. Rylander. 1975. Experimental gingivitis in young dogs. Scand. J. Dent. Res. 83:314-326.

Lindhe, J., and G. Svanberg. 1974. Influence of trauma from occlusion on progression of experimental periodontitis in the Beagle dog. J. Clin. Periodontol. 1:3-14.

Lindhe, J., S.E. Hamp, and H. Loe. 1973. Experimental periodontitis in the Beagle dog. J. Periodontal Res. 8:1-10.

Lindhe, J., S.E. Hamp, and H. Loe. 1975. Plaque induced periodontal disease in Beagle dogs. J. Periodontal Res. 10:243-551.

Lindop, P.J., and J. Rotblat. 1961. Long-term effects of a single whole-body exposure of mice to ionizing radiations. II. Causes of death. Proc. R. Soc. London Ser. B 154:350-368.

Lindsey, J.D., P.W. Landfield, and G. Lynch. 1979. Early onset and topographical distribution of hypertrophied astrocytes in hippocampus of aging rats: A quantitative study. J. Gerontol. 34:661-671.

Lindsey, J.R., H.J. Baker, R.G. Overcash, G.H. Cassell, and C.E. Hunt. 1971. Murine chronic respiratory disease. Significance as a research complication and experimental production with Mycoplasma pulmonis. Am. J. Pathol. 64:675-716.

Lindsey, J.R., M.W. Conner, and H.J. Baker. 1978. Physical, chemical, and microbial factors affecting biologic responses. Pages 31-43 in Laboratory animal housing. Proceedings of a Symposium organized by the Institute of Laboratory Animal Resources (ILAR) Committee on Laboratory Housing, held at Hunt Valley, Maryland, Septemmber 22-23, 1976. National Academy of Sciences, Washington, D.C.

Ling, E.A., and C.P. LeBlond. 1973. Investigation of glial cells in semithin sections. II. Variation with age in the numbers of the various glial cell types in rat cortex and corpus callosum. J. Comp. Neurol. 149: 73-82.

Lingeman, C.H., F.M. Garner, and D.O.N. Taylor. 1971. Spontaneous gastric adenocarcinoma of dogs. A review. J. Natl. Cancer Inst. 47:137-153.

Lipowitz, A.J., A. Schwartz, G.P. Wilson, and J.W. Ebert. 1973. Testicular neoplasms and concomitant clinical changes in the dog. J. Am. Vet. Med. Assoc. 163:1364-1368.

Lips, P., P. Courpron, and P.J. Meunier. 1978. Mean wall thickness of trabecular bone packets in human iliac crest: Changes with age. Calcif. Tissue Res. 26:13-17.

Lipton, M.A. 1976. Age differentiation in depression: Biochemical aspects. J. Gerontol. 31:293-299.

Lithner, F., and J. Pontén. 1966. Bovine fibroblasts in long-term tissue culture: Chromosome studies. Int. J. Cancer 1:579-588.

Litvak, J., L.E. Siderides, and A.M. Vineberg. 1957. The experimental production of coronary artery insufficiency and occlusion. Am. Heart J. 53:505-518.

Lloyd, E., and D. Hodges. 1971. Quantitative characterization of bone: A computer analysis of microradiographs. Clin. Orthop. 78:230-250.

Lloyd, J.W., J.A. Thomas, and M.G. Mawhinney. 1975. Androgens and estrogens in the plasma and prostatic tissue of normal dogs and dogs with benign prostatic hypertrophy. Invest. Urol. 13(3):220-222.

Lloyd, K.G., L. Davidson, and O. Hornykiewicz. 1975. The neurochemistry of Parkinson's disease: Effect of L-dopa therapy. J. Pharmacol. Exp. Ther. 195:453-464.

Lockwood, D.H., C.H. Hamilton, and J. Livingston. 1979.
The influence of obesity and diabetes in the monkey
on insulin and glucagon binding to liver membranes.
Endocrinology 104:76-81.

Löe, H., and M.A. Listgarten. 1973. Periodontium. Pages
1-56 in H.M. Goldman and D.W. Cohen, eds. Periodontal
therapy. 5th ed. C.V. Mosby Co., St. Louis.

Löe, H., E. Theilade, and S.B. Jensen. 1965. Experimental gingivitis in man. J. Periodontol. 36:177-187.

Loew, F.M. 1968. The management and diseases of gerbils.
Pages 416-418 in R.W. Kirk, ed. Current veterinary
therapy III. Small animal practice. W.B. Saunders,
Philadelphia.

Loewi, G., and P. Stasny. 1974. Animal models of arthritis. Prog. Immunol. 5:293-296.

Logothetopoulos, J., G. Brosky, H.F. Kern. 1970. Islet
cell proliferation in experimental and genetic diabetes. Pages 15-23 in S. Falkmer, B. Hellman, and
I.-B. Täljedal, eds. The structure and metabolism of
the pancreatic islets. Pergamon Press, Elmsford,
New York.

Long, J.O., and R.W. Cooper. 1968. Physical growth and
dental eruption in captive-bred squirrel monkeys Saimiri sciureus Leticia Colombia. Pages 193-205 in L.A.
Rosenblum and R.W. Cooper, eds. The squirrel monkey.
Academic Press, New York.

Lorenz, K. 1963. Rats. Pages 157-164 in On aggression.
Translated by M.K. Wilson. Harcourt, Brace, and World,
Inc., New York.

Loskota, W.J. 1974. The Mongolian gerbil (Meriones unguiculatus) for the study of the epilepsies and anti-
convulsants. Doctoral dissertation, Department of
Pharmacology, University of California at Los Angeles.
265 p.

Loskota, W.J., P. Lomax, and S.T. Rich. 1974. The gerbil
as a model for the study of the epilepsies. Seizure
patterns and ontogenesis. Epilepsia 15:109-119.

Lovdal, A., O. Schei, J. Waerhaug, and A. Arno. 1959.
Tooth mobility and alveolar bone resorption as a function of occlusal stress and oral hygiene. Acta Odontol. Scand. 17:61-77.

Lovelace, F., L. Will, G. Sperling, and C.M. McCay. 1958.
Teeth, bones and aging of Syrian hamsters. J. Gerontol. 13:27-31.

Lown, B., and M. Wolf. 1971. Approaches to sudden death
from coronary heart disease. Circulation 44:130-142.

Lown, B. R.L. Verrier, and S.H. Rabinowitz. 1977. Neural and psychologic mechanisms and the problem of sudden cardiac death. Am. J. Cardiol. 39:890-902.

Lucchesi, B.R., W.E. Burmeister, T.E. Lomas, and G.D. Abrams. 1976. Ischemic changes in the canine heart as affected by the demethyl quarternary analog of propranolol, UM-272 (SC-27761). J. Pharmacol. Exp. Ther. 199:310-328.

Lvovich, E.G., M.N. Ostroumova, A.S. Vishevsky, and V.M. Dilman. 1974. A study of physiological action of lipotropin and its derivatives on rabbits: The appearance of resistance, separation of the fat-mobilizing and hypocalcemic effects, its influence on carbohydrate metabolism. Probl. Endokrinol. 20:71-76. (in Russian)

Lyon, M.F. 1978. Standardized genetic nomenclature for mice: Past, present, and future. Pages 445-455 in H.C. Morse III, ed. Origins of inbred mice. Academic Press, New York.

Lyttkens, L., B. Larsson, H. Goller, S. Englesson, and J. Stahle. 1979. Melanin capacity to accumulate drugs in the internal ear. A study on lidocaine, bupivacaine and chlorpromazine. Acta Otolaryngol. 88:61-73.

Machado-Salas, J.P., and A.B. Scheibel. 1979. Limbic system of the aged mouse. Exp. Neurol. 63:347-355.

Machado-Salas, J., M.E. Scheibel, and A.B. Scheibel. 1977. Neuronal changes in the aging mouse: Spinal cord and lower brain stem. Exp. Neurol. 54:504-512.

Madden, D.L., R.E. Horton, and N.B. McCullough. 1970. Spontaneous infection in ex-germfree guinea pigs due to Clostridium perfringens. Lab. Anim. Care 20:454-455.

Madison, R.M., L.S. Rabstein, and W.R. Bryan. 1968. Mortality rate and spontaneous lesions found in 2,928 untreated BALB/cCr mice. J. Natl. Cancer Inst. 40:683-685.

Magalhaes, H. 1968. Gross anatomy. Pages 91-109 in R.A. Hoffman, P.F. Robinson, and H. Magalhaes, eds. The golden hamster. Its biology and use in medical research. Iowa State University Press, Ames, Iowa.

Mainwaring, W.I. 1969. Effect of age on protein synthesis in mouse liver. Biochem. J. 113:869-878.

Maisel, H. 1965. Phylogenetic properties of primate lens antigens. Protides Biol. Fluids Pro. Colloq. 12:146-148.

Maisel, H., and M. Goodman. 1964. Analysis of mammalian lens proteins by electrophonesis. Arch. Ophthalmol. 71:697-704.

Maisel, H., and M. Goodman. 1965. The antigen and speci-
ficities of human lens proteins. Invest. Ophthalmol.
4:129-137.

Majumdar, S.K., and M. Solomon. 1970. The somatic karyotype of the Mongolian gerbil (Meriones unguiculatus,
Rodentia, Gerbillinae). Mammalian Chromosomes Newsletter 11:129-131. Available from M.D. Anderson Hospital, University of Texas, Houston.

Makinodan, T. 1978. Mechanism, prevention and restoration of immunologic aging. Pages 197-212 in D.
Bergsma and D.E. Harrison, eds. Genetic effects on
aging. Birth defects original article series. Vol.
14, No. 1. A.R. Liss, Inc., New York.

Makinodan, T., and W.J. Peterson. 1962. Relative anti-
body-forming capacity of spleen cells as a function
of age. Proc. Natl. Acad. Sci. USA. 48:234-238.

Makman, M.H., H.S. Ahn, L.J. Thal, B. Dvorkin, S.G. Horo-
witz, N.S. Sharpless, and M. Rosenfeld. 1978. Biogenic amine-stimulated adenylate cyclase and spiro-
peridol-binding sites in rabbit brain: Evidence for
selective loss of receptors with aging. Adv. Exp. Med.
Biol. 113:211-230.

Malinin, G.I., and I.M. Malinin. 1972. Age-related spontaneous uterine lesions in mice. J. Gerontol. 27:193-
196.

Malinow, M.R., and A. Corcoran. 1966. Growth of the lens
in howler monkeys Alouatta caraya. J. Mammal. 47:58-
63.

Maller, O. 1964. The effect of hypothalamic and dietary
obesity on taste preference in rats. Life Sci.
3:1281-1291.

Malliani, A., P.J. Schwartz, and A. Zanchetti. 1969. A
sympathetic reflex elicited by experimental coronary
occlusion. Am. J. Physiol. 217:703-709.

Mankin, H.J., and A.Z. Thrasher. 1977. The effect of
age on glycosamino-glycan synthesis in rabbit articular
and costal cartilages. J. Rheumatol. 4:343-350.

Manning, P.J. 1976. Neoplastic diseases. Pages 211-225
in J.E. Wagner and P.J. Manning, eds. The biology of
the guinea pig. Academic Press, New York.

Manning, P.J., and T.B. Clarkson. 1972. Development,
distribution, and lipid concentration of diet-induced
atherosclerotic lesions of rhesus monkeys. Exp. Mol.
Pathol. 17:38-54.

Manski, W., S.P. Halbert, and T.P. Averbach. 1964. Immunochemical analysis of the phylogeny of lens proteins. Pages 454-554 in C.A. Leone, ed. Taxonomic biochemistry and serology. A Ronald Press, New York.

Marcus, R.E. 1968. Vestibular function and additional findings in Waardenburg's syndrome. Acta Otolaryngol. Suppl. 229:1-30.

Markham, C.H., L.J. Treciokas, and S.G. Diamond. 1974. Parkinson's disease and levodopa. A five year follow-up and review. West. J. Med. 121:188-206.

Maroko, P.R., P. Libby, C.M. Bloor, B.E. Sobel, and E. Braunwald. 1972. Reduction by hyaluronidase of myocardial necrosis following coronary artery occlusion. Circulation 46:430-437.

Marotti, G. 1973. Map of bone formation rate values recorded throughout the skeleton of the dog. Pages 202-207 in Z.F.G. Jaworski, ed. Proceedings of the first workshop on bone morphometry. University of Ottawa Press, Ottawa, Ontario, Canada.

Marshall, J.H., E.L. Lloyd, J. Rundo, J. Liniechi, G. Marotti, C.W. Mays, H.A. Sissons, and W.S. Snyder. 1973. Alkaline earth metabolism in adult man. Health Phys. 24:125-221.

Marshall, J.L. 1978. The role of central catecholamine-containing neurons in food intake. Pages 6-16 in G.A. Bray, ed. Recent advances in obesity research: II. Proceedings of the 2nd International Congress on Obesity, held October 23-26, 1977, in Washington, D.C. Newman Publishing, Ltd., London.

Marshall, R.J., and J.R. Parratt. 1974. The effects of practolol in the early stages of experimental myocardial infarction. Br. J. Pharmacol. 52:124P.

Marston, J.H., and M.C. Chang. 1965. The breeding management and reproductive physiology of the Mongolian gerbil (Meriones unguiculatus). Lab. Anim. Care 15:34-48.

Martin, C.J., and T. Sugihara. 1973. Simulation of tissue properties in irreversible diffuse obstructive pulmonary syndromes. J. Clin. Invest. 52:1918-1924.

Martin, G.M., C.A. Sprague, and C.J. Epstein. 1970. Replicative lifespan of cultivated human cells. Effect of donor's age, tissue, and genotype. Lab. Invest. 23:86-92.

Martin, H.B. 1963. The effect of aging on the alveolar pores of Kohn in the dog. Am. Rev. Respir. Dis. 88:773-778.

Martin, K., and D.A. Rutty. 1969. Haematological values of the multimammate mouse Praomys (Mastomys) natalensis. Lab. Anim. 3:27-33.

Martin, R.J., and J.H. Gahagan. 1977. The influence of age and fasting on serum hormones in the lean and obese Zucker rat. Proc. Soc. Exp. Biol. Med. 154:610-614.

Martorana, P.A., N.N. Share, and J.W. Richard. 1977. Free alveolar cells in papain-induced emphysema in the hamster. Am. Rev. Respir. Dis. 116:57-63.

Marx, L. 1931. Versuche über heterosexuelle Merkmale bei Ratten. Arch. Entwicklungsmech. Org. 124:584-612.

Mason, R.J., L.G. Dobbs, R.D. Greenleaf, and M.C. Williams. 1977. Alveolar type II cells. Fed. Proc. 36(13):2697-2702.

Mason, T.J., F.W. McKay, R. Hoover, W.J. Blot, and J.F. Fraumeni. 1975. Atlas of cancer mortality for U.S. counties: 1950-1969. DHEW Pub. No. (NIH) 75-780. U.S. Department of Health, Education, and Welfare, Washington, D.C. 103 p.

Masoro, E.J. 1980. Mortality and growth characteristics of rat strains commonly used in aging research. Exp. Aging Res.

Masoro, E.J., H. Bertrand, G. Liepa, and B.P. Yu. 1979. Analysis and exploration of age-related changes in mammalian structure and function. Fed. Proc. 38:1956-1961.

Master, A.M., and R.P. Lasser. 1961. Blood pressure elevation in the elderly. Pages 24-34 in A.M. Brest and J.H. Moyer, eds. Hypertension: Recent advances. Lea and Febiger, Philadelphia.

Master, A.M., R.P. Lasser, and H.L. Jaffe. 1958. Blood pressure in white people over 65 years of age. Ann. Intern. Med. 48:284-299.

Masters, T.N., N.B. Harbold, D.G. Hall, R.D. Jackson, D.C. Mullen, H.K. Daugherty, and F. Robiscek. 1976. Beneficial metabolic effects of methylprednisolone sodium succinate in acute myocardial ischemia. Am. J. Cardiol. 37:557-563.

Masukawa, T. 1960. Vaginal smears in women past 40 years of age, with emphasis on their remaining hormonal activity. Obstet. Gynecol. 16:407-414.

Mathies, M., L. Lipps, G.S. Smith, and R. Walford. 1973. Age-related decline in response to phytohemagglutinin and pokeweed mitogen by spleen cells from hamsters and a long-lived mouse strain. J. Gerontol. 28:425-430.

Matkovic, V., K. Kostial, I. Simonovic, R. Buzina, A. Broderac, and B.E.C. Nordin. 1979. Bone status and fracture rates in two regions of Yugoslavia. Am. J. Clin. Nutr. 32:540-549.

Mauderly, J.L. 1974. Influence of sex and age on the pulmonary function of the unanesthetized Beagle dog. J. Gerontol. 29:282-289.

Mauderly, J.L. 1977. A new technique for evaluating nitrogen washout efficiency. Am. J. Vet. Res. 38:69-74.

Mauderly, J.L. 1979. The effect of age on pulmonary structure and function of immature and adult animals and man. Fed. Proc. 28:173-177.

Mauderly, J.L. In press. Lung-thorax system in E.J. Masoro, ed. CRC handbook of physiology in aging. CRC Press, Boca Raton, Florida.

Mauderly, J.L., J.A. Pickrell, C.H. Hobbs, S.A. Benjamin, F.F. Hahn, R.K. Jones, and J.E. Barnes. 1973. The effects of inhaled ^{90}Y fused clay aerosol on pulmonary function and related parameters of the Beagle dog. Radiat. Res. 56:83-96.

Mauderly, J.L., E.G. Damon, and R.K. Jones. 1979. Effects of intratracheally-instilled elastase on lung function of Fischer-344 rats. Fed. Proc. 38:1325.

Maxim, P.E. 1979. Social behavior. Pages 56-70 in D.M. Bowden, ed. Aging in nonhuman primates. Van Nostrand Reinhold, New York.

Maxwell, L.C., J.A. Faulkner, and G.J. Hyatt. 1974. Estimation of number of fibers in guinea pig skeletal muscles. J. Appl. Physiol. 37(2):259-264.

Mazess, R.B., and W. Mather. 1974. Bone mineral content of Northern Alaskan Eskimos. Am. J. Clin. Nutr. 27:916-925.

Mays, A., Jr. 1969. Baseline hematological and blood biochemical parameters of the Mongolian gerbil (Meriones unguiculatus). Lab. Anim. Care 19:838-842.

McClellan, R.O., J.E. Barnes, B.B. Boecker, T.L. Chiffelle, C.H. Hobbs, R.K. Jones, J.L. Mauderly, J.A. Pickrell, and H.C. Redman. 1970. Toxicity of beta-emitting radionuclides inhaled in fused clay particles - An experimental approach. Pages 395-415 in P. Nettesheim, M. Hanna, and J. Deatherage, eds. Morphology of experimental respiratory carcinogenesis. U.S. Atomic Energy Commission, Division of Technical Information Services, Oak Ridge, Tennessee.

McClure, H.M. 1975. Neoplasia in rhesus monkeys. Pages 369-398 in G.H. Bourne, ed. The rhesus monkey. Vol. 2. Academic Press, New York.

McClure, H.M., W.L. Chapman, Jr., B.E. Hooper, F.G. Smith, and O.J. Fletcher. 1978. The digestive system. Pages 175-317 in K. Benirschke, F.M. Garner, and T.C. Jones, eds. Pathology of laboratory animals. Vol. I. Springer-Verlag, New York.

McConnell, E.E., P.A. Basson, V. de Vos, B.J. Myers, and R.E. Kuntz. 1974. A survey of diseases among 100 free-ranging baboons (Papio ursinus) from the Kruger National Park. Onderstepoort J. Vet. Res. 41(3):97-167.

McCormack, J.E., and A.L. Nutall. 1976. Auditory research. Pages 281-303 in J.E. Wagner and P.J. Manning, eds. The biology of the guinea pig. Academic Press, New York.

McCormack, J.T., and G.S. Greenwald. 1974. Progesterone and oestradiol 17 β concentrations in the peripheral plasma during pregnancy in the mouse. J. Endocrinol. 62:101-107.

McCormick, J.G., C.B. Hartley, I. Holleman, and J. Harrill. In press. Deafness and atherosclerosis. Laryngoscope.

McEntee, K., and S.W. Nielsen. 1976. Tumors of the female genital tract. Bull. WHO 53:217-226.

McGeer, P.L., and E.G. McGeer. 1978. Aging and neurotransmitter systems. Adv. Exp. Med. Biol. 113:41-58.

McGeer, E.G., H.C. Fibiger, P.L. McGeer, and V. Wickson. 1971. Aging and brain enzymes. Exp. Gerontol. 6:391-396.

McGeer, P.L., E.G. McGeer, and J.S. Suzuki. 1977. Aging and extrapyramidal function. Arch. Neurol. 34:33-35.

McGill, H.C., Jr. In press. Cigarette smoking. In Symposium on the use of nonhuman primates in cardiovascular diseases. Southwest Foundation. Texas Univ. Press.

McGill, H.C., Jr., J.P. Strong, R.L. Holman, and N.T. Werthessen. 1960. Arterial lesions in Kenya baboons. Circ. Res. 8:670-681.

McGovern, V.J. 1977. Lymphomas of the gastric intestinal tract. Pages 184-205 in J.H. Yardley, B.C. Morson, and M.R. Abell, eds. The gastrointestinal tract. International Academy of Pathology. Monographs in pathology, No. 18. Williams and Wilkins Co., Baltimore.

McGuire, J.L., C.D. Bariso, L.E. VanPetten, C.L. Washington, J.P. Da Vanzo, and D.A. Willigan. 1973. 5 α-Dihydrotestosterone-induced changes in the rat prostate. Invest. Urol. 11:101-105.

McKeown, F. 1965. Pathology of the aged. Butterworths, London. 361 p.

McKinney, W.T., Jr. 1977. Biobehavioral models of depression in monkeys. Pages 117-126 in I. Hanin and E. Usdin, eds. Animal models in psychiatry and neurology. Pergamon Press, Oxford.

McKinney, W.T., and W.E. Bunney, Jr. 1969. Animal model of depression, I. Review of evidence: Implications for research. Arch. Gen. Psychiat. 2:240-248.

McLaughlin, R.F., W.S. Tyler, and R.O. Canada. 1961. A study of the subgross pulmonary anatomy in various mammals. Am. J. Anat. 108:149-165.

McManus, J.J. 1972. Water relations and food consumption of the Mongolian gerbil, Meriones unguiculatus. Comp. Biochem. Physiol. 43A:959-967.

McMartin, D.N. 1977. Spontaneous atrial thrombosis in aged Syrian hamsters. I. Incidence and pathology. Thromb. Haemost. 38:447-456.

McNamara, M.C., V.A. Benignus, G. Benignus, and A.T. Miller, Jr. 1977. Active and passive avoidance in rats as a function of age. Exp. Aging Res. 3:3-16.

McNeal, J.E. 1972. The prostate and prostatic urethra: A morphologic synthesis. J. Urol. 107:1008-1016.

McNeal, J.E. 1974. Structure and pathology of the prostate. Pages 55-68 in M. Goland, ed. Normal and abnormal growth of the prostate. Charles C. Thomas, Springfield, Illinois.

McNeal, J.E. 1976. Developmental and comparative anatomy of the prostate. Pages 1-9 in J.T. Grayhack, J.D. Wilson, and M.J. Scherbenske, eds. Benign prostatic hyperplasia. DHEW Pub. No. (NIH) 76-1113. U.S. Department of Health, Education, and Welfare, Washington, D.C.

McNulty, W.P. 1973. Spontaneous cardiopulmonary disease in nonhuman primates: Potential models. Pages 829-839 in L.T. Harmison, ed. Research animals in medicine. DHEW Pub. No. (NIH) 72-333. U.S. Department of Health, Education, and Welfare, Washington, D.C.

McPhaul, J.J., G.J. Grey, D.F. Wagner, and W.F. MacKenzie. 1974. Nephrotoxic canine glomerulonephritis. Kidney Int. 6:123-127.

Medical Research Council on Aetiology of Chronic Bronchitis. 1965. Definition and classification of chronic bronchitis for clinical and epidemiological purposes. Lancet 1:775-779.

Medin, D.L., and R.T. Davis. 1974. Memory. Pages 2-49 in A.M. Schrier and R. Stollnitz, eds. Behavior of nonhuman primates. Vol. 5. Academic Press, New York.

Meek, R.L. 1978. Aging, transformation and tumorigenicity of cultured embryonic mouse and rat cells. Doctoral dissertation, Department of Biology, Thimann Labs., University of California at Santa Cruz, Santa Cruz, California.

Mehta, P.D., and H. Masel. 1967. Albuminoid of human and cynomolgus monkey lens. Am. J. Ophthalmol. 63:967-972.

Meier, H., and G.A. Yerganian. 1959. Spontaneous hereditary diabetes mellitus in the Chinese hamster (Cricetulus griseus). 1. Pathological findings. Proc. Soc. Exp. Biol. Med. 100:810-815.

Meites, J., H.-H. Huang, and G.D. Riegle. 1976. Relation of the hypothalamo-pituitary-gonadal system to decline of reproductive functions in aging female rats. Pages 3-20 in F. Labrie, J. Meites, and G. Pelletier, eds. Hypothalamus and endocrine functions. Plenum Publishing Co., New York.

Meites, J., H.-H. Huang, and J.W. Simpkins. 1978. Recent studies on neuoendocrine control of reproductive senescence in rats. Pages 213-235 in E.L. Schneider, ed. The aging reproductive system. Vol. 4. Aging series. Raven Press, New York.

Melby, E.C., Jr., and N.H. Altman [eds.] 1974a. Handbook of laboratory animal science. Vol. I. CRC Press, Inc., Cleveland. 451 p.

Melby, E.C., Jr., and N.H. Altman [eds.] 1974b. Handbook of laboratory animal science. Vol. II. CRC Press, Inc., Cleveland. 523 p.

Melby, E.C., Jr., and N.H. Altman [eds.] 1976. Handbook of laboratory animal science. Vol. III. CRC Press, Inc., Cleveland. 943 p.

Melcher, A.H., and W.H. Bowen. 1969. Biology of the periodontium. Academic Press, London, New York. 563 p.

Meldrum, D.R., I.M. Shamonki, A.M. Frumar, I.V. Tataryn, R.J. Chang, and H.L. Judd. 1979a. Elevations in skin temperature of the finger as an objective index of postmenopausal hot flashes: Standardization of the technique. Am. J. Obstet. Gynecol. 135:713-717.

Meldrum, D.R., I.V. Tataryn, A.M. Frumar, Y. Erlik, K.H. Lu, and H.L. Judd. 1979b. Physical and hormonal changes during the menopausal hot flash. Paper presented at the Conference on the Endocrine Aspects of Aging, Cosponsored by the National Institute on Aging, Endocrine Society, and Veterans Administration. Held

October 18-20, 1979 in Bethesda, Maryland. For information contact Dr. D.R. Meldrum, Department of Obstetrics and Gynecology, UCLA Medical Center, Los Angeles, California.

Meldrum, D.R., I.V. Tataryn, A.M. Frumar, Y. Erlik, K.H. Lu, and H.L. Judd. 1980. Gonadotropins, estrogens, and adrenal steroids during the menopausal hot flash. Clin. Endocrinol. Metab. 50:685-689.

Melsen, F., and L. Mosekilde. 1978. Tetracycline double-labeling of iliac trabecular bone in 41 normal adults. Calcif. Tissue Res. 26:99-102.

Meltzer, R.S., J.N. Woythaler, A.J. Buda, J.C. Griffin, W.D. Harrison, R.P. Martin, D.C. Harrison, and R.L. Popp. 1979. Two dimensional echocardiographic quantification of infarct size alteration by pharmacologic agents. Am. J. Cardiol. 44:257-262.

Mende, T.J., and L. Viamonte. 1967. Studies on chloral hydrate and camphor sensitivity in rats of different ages. Gerontologia 13(3):165-172.

Mervis, R. 1978. Structural alterations in neurons of aged canine neocortex: A Golgi study. Exp. Neurol. 62:417-432.

Merz, W.A., and R.K. Schenk. 1970. Quantitative structural analysis of human cancellous bone. Acta Anat. 75:54-66.

Metz, R.J.S. 1975. Objectives of therapy. Pages 69-75 in K.E. Sussman and R.J.S. Metz, eds. Diabetes mellitus. 4th ed. American Diabetes Association, Inc., New York.

Metzger-Freed, L. 1977. Haploid vertebrate cell cultures. Pages 57-79 in G.H. Rothblat and V.J. Cristofalo, eds. Growth, nutrition, and metabolism of cells in culture. Vol. III. Academic Press, New York.

Meunier, P., P. Courpron, C. Edouard, J. Bernard, J. Bringuier, and G. Vignon. 1973. Physiological senile involution and pathological rarefaction of bone. Quantitative and comparative histological data. Clin. Endocrinol. Metab. 2:239-256.

Meyer, M.W. 1969. Distribution of cardiac output to oral tissue in dogs. J. Dent. Res. 49:787-794.

Michalopoulos, G., and H.C. Pitot. 1975. Primary culture of parenchymal liver cells on collagen membrane. Exp. Cell Res. 94:70-78.

Michejda, M. 1978. The problem of age estimation and skeletal age. J. Med. Primatol. 7:257-263.

Middleton, C.C., T.B. Clarkson, H.B. Lofland, and R.W. Prichard. 1967a. Diet and atherosclerosis of squirrel monkeys. Arch. Pathol. 83:145-153.

Middleton, C.C., J. Rosal, T.B. Clarkson, W.P. Newman, and H.C. Mcgill, Jr. 1967b. Arterial lesions in squirrel monkeys. Arch. Pathol. 83:352-358.

Mikaelian, D.O., D. Warfield, and O. Norris. 1974. Genetic progressive hearing loss in the C57/BL6 mouse. Acta Otolaryngol. 77:327-334.

Mikhaylova, I.A., and T. Ya. Nadirova. 1977. Alterations in the activity of some enzymes of energy metabolism in rabbit aorta in ageing. Vopr. Med. Khim. 23:463-468. (in Russian)

Miles, A.E.W. 1963. The dentition in the assessment of individual age in skeletal material. Pages 191-201 in D.R. Brothwell, ed. Symposia of the study of human biology. Vol. 55. MacMillan Company, New York.

Milicic, M., and J. Jowsey. 1968. Effect of fluoride on disuse osteoporosis in the cat. J. Bone Joint Surg. 50-A:701-708.

Miller, A.E., and G.D. Riegle. 1975. Aging effects on hypothalamic catecholamine and testosterone secretion in the male rat. Fed. Proc. 34:303.

Miller, C.W., R.C. Nealeigh, and M.E. Crowder. 1976. Evaluation of the cardiovascular changes associated with aging in a colony of dogs. Biomed. Sci. Instrum. 12:107-110.

Miller, C.W., R.W. Norrdin, S.S. Sawyer, and R.C. Nealeigh. 1977. Renal function changes associated with aging and ionizing radiation. Pages 66-74 in CSU-FDA Collaborative Radiological Health Laboratory annual report 1977. DHEW Pub. No. (FDA) 77-8056. U.S. Department of Health, Education, and Welfare, Washington, D.C.

Miller, J.D. 1970. Audibility curve of the chinchilla. J. Acoust. Soc. Am. 48:513-523.

Miller, S.C., D.B. Kimmel, and W.S.S. Jee. 1978. Histological studies of trabecular bone of Beagle ribs. Pages 243-244 in Research in radiobiology. University of Utah Radiobiology Laboratory report, COO-119-253. University of Utah, Salt Lake City, Utah.

Miller, W.R., R.A. Rosellini, and M.E.P. Seligman. 1978. Learned helplessness and depression. Pages 104-130 in J.D. Maser and M.E.P. Seligman, eds. Psychopathology: Experimental models. Freeman, San Francisco.

Mills, C.A. 1945. Influence of environmental temperature on warm-blooded animals. Ann. N.Y. Acad. Sci. 46:97-105.

Mills, T.M., amd V.B. Mahesh. 1978. Pituitary function in the aged. Pages 1-11 in R.B. Greenblatt, ed. Geriatric endocrinology. Raven Press, New York.

Milne-Edwards, A. 1867. Observations sur quelques mammiferes du Nord de la Chine. Ann. Sci. Natl. Zool. Biol. Anim. 7:375-377.

Milner, B. 1970. Memory and the medial temporal regions of the brain. Pages 29-50 in K.H. Pribram and D.E. Broadbent, eds. Biology of memory. Academic Press, New York.

Minaire, P., P. Meunier, C. Edouard, J. Bernard, P. Courpron, and J. Bourret. 1974. Quantitative histological data on disuse osteoporosis. Comparison with biological data. Calcif. Tissue Res. 17:57-73.

Misdorp, W., E. Cotchin, J.F. Hampe, A.G. Jabara, and J. von Sandersleben. 1971. Canine malignant mammary tumors. I. Sarcomas. Vet. Pathol. 8:99-117.

Misdorp. W., E. Cotchin, J.F. Hampe, A.G. Jabara, and J. von Sandersleben. 1972. Canine malignant mammary tumors. II. Adenocarcinoma, solid carcinoma and spindle cell carcinoma. Vet. Pathol. 9:447-470.

Mitchell, H.S., and W.M. Dodge. 1935. Cataract in rats fed on high lactose rations. J. Nutr. 9:37-49.

Mitchell, R.S. 1974. Chronic airway obstruction. Pages 579-600 in G.L. Baum, ed. Textbook of pulmonary diseases. Little Brown, Boston.

Mohr, U., J. Althoff, and N. Page. 1972. Tumors of the respiratory system of the common European hamster (Cricetus criectus L) induced by N-diethylnitrosamine (DEN). J. Natl. Cancer Inst. 49:595-597.

Mohr, U., H. Schuller, G. Reznik, J. Althoff, and N. Page. 1973. Breeding of European hamsters. Lab. Anim. Sci. 23:799-802.

Monath, T.P. 1975. Biological hazards associated with Mastomys. WHO Chron. 29:241.

Monlux, A.W. 1953. The histopathology of nephritis of the dog. I. Introduction. II. Inflammatory Interstitial Disease. Am. J. Vet. Res. 14:425-439.

Monlux, A.W., J.F. Roszel, D.W. MacLean, and T.W. Palmer. 1977. Classification of epithelial canine mammary tumors in a defined population. Vet. Pathol. 14:194-217.

Montoye, H.J., P.W. Willis, III, G.E. Howard, and J.B. Keller. 1971. Cardiac pre-ejection period: Age and sex comparison. J. Gerontol. 26:208-216.

Moody, D.B., W.C. Stebbins, J.M. Miller. 1970. A primate restraint and handling system for auditory research. Behav. Res. Methods Instrum. 2:180-182.

Moore, R.A. 1936. The evolution and involution of the prostate gland. Am. J. Pathol. 12:599-624.

Moreland, A.F. 1965. Experimental atherosclerosis of swine. Pages 21-24 in J.C. Roberts, Jr. and R. Straus, eds. Comparative atherosclerosis. Harper and Row, New York.

Morgan, B. 1973a. Aging and osteoporosis, in particular spinal osteoporosis. Clin. Endocrinol. Metab. 2:187-201.

Morgan, B. 1973b. Osteomalacia, renal osteodystrophy and osteoporosis. Charles C. Thomas, Springfield, Illinois. 423 p.

Morgan, J.P. 1967. Spondylosis derformans in the dog. A morphologic study with some clinical and experimental observations. Acta Orthop. Scand. 96:1-88.

Mori, K., and J.P. Duruisseau. 1960. Water and electrolyte changes in aging process with special reference to calcium and magnesium in cardiac muscle. Can. J. Biochem. 38:919-928.

Morrison, A.S. 1976. Cryptorchidism, hernia and cancer of the testes. J. Natl. Cancer Inst. 56:731-733.

Morrison, S.D. 1977. The hypothalamic syndrome in rats. Fed. Proc. 36:139-142.

Morrison, W.I., and N.G. Wright. 1977. Viruses associated with renal disease of man and animals. Prog. Med. Virol. 23:22-50.

Moskow, B.S., B.H. Wasserman, and M.C. Rennert. 1968. Spontaneous periodontal disease in the Mongolian gerbil. J. Periodontal Res. 3:69-83.

Mostofi, F.K., and E.B. Price, Jr. 1973a. Tumors of the testes. Introduction. Pages 1-6 in Tumors of the male genital system. Atlas of tumor pathology. Second series, fascicle 8. Armed Forces Institute of Pathology, Washington, D.C.

Mostofi, F.K., and E.B. Price, Jr. 1973b. Tumors of the testes. Seminoma. Pages 21-39 in Tumors of the male genital system. Atlas of tumor pathology. Second series, fascicle 8. Armed Forces Institute of Pathology, Washington, D.C.

Mostofi, F.K., and E.B. Price, Jr. 1973c. Tumors of the prostate. Introduction. Pages 177-181 in Tumors of the male genital system. Atlas of tumor pathology. Second series, fascicle 8. Armed Forces Institute of Pathology, Washington, D.C.

Mostofi, F.K., and E.B. Price, Jr. 1973d. Tumors of the prostate. Pages 182-194 in Tumors of the male genital system. Atlas of tumor pathology. Second series, fascicle 8. Armed Forces Institute of Pathology, Washington, D.C.

Moudgil, V.K., and M.S. Kanugo. 1973. Effect of age on the circadian rhythm of acetylcholinesterase of the brain of the rat. Comp. Gen. Pharmacol. 4:127-130.

Moulton, J.E. 1978. Tumors of the genital system. Pages 330-336 in J.E. Moulton, ed. Tumors in domestic animals. 2nd ed. University of California Press, Berkeley, California.

Moulton, J.E., D.O.N. Taylor, C.R. Dorn, and A.C. Andersen. 1970. Canine mammary tumors. Pathol. Vet. 7:289-320.

Mueller, E., E. Rosen, and E. Levine. 1980. Cellular senescence in a cloned strain of bovine fetal aortic endothelial cells. Science 207:889-891.

Mueller, T.M., M.L. Marcus, J.C. Erhardt, T. Chaudhuri, and F.M. Abboud. 1976. Limitations of thalium-201 myocardial perfusion scintigrams. Circulation 54: 640-646.

Muhlbock, O. 1947. On the susceptibility of different inbred strains of mice for estrone. Acta Brevia Neerl. Physiol. Pharmacol. Microbiol. 15:18-20.

Muieson, G., C.A. Sorbine, and V. Grassi. 1971. Respiratory function in the aged. Bull. Physiopathol. Respir. 7:973-1007.

Müller, G.H., and R.W. Kirk. 1976. Small animal dermatology. 2nd ed. W.B. Saunders Co., Philadephia. 809 p.

Müller, H.F., and B. Grad. 1974. Clinical-psychological electroencephalographic and adrenocortical relationships in elderly psychiatric patients. J. Gerontol. 29:28-38.

Müller-Peddinghaus, R., and G. Trautwein. 1977a. Spontaneous glomerulonephritis in dogs. I. Classification and immunopathology. Vet. Pathol. 14:1-13.

Müller-Peddinghaus, R., and G. Trautwein. 1977b. Spontaneous glomerulonephritis in dogs. II. Correlation of glomerulonephritis with age, chronic interstitial nephritis and extrarenal lesions. Vet. Pathol. 14:121-127.

Mulligan, R.M. 1949. Neoplasms of the dog. The Williams & Wilkins Co., Baltimore. 135 p.

Mulligan, R.M. 1963. Comparative pathology of human and canine cancer. Ann. N.Y. Acad. Sci. 108:642-690.

Mulvihill, J.E., F.R. Susi, J.H. Shaw, and P. Goldhaber. 1967. Histological studies of the periodontal syndrome in rice rats and the effects of penicillin. Arch. Oral Biol. 12:733-744.

Munger, B.L., and C.M. Lang. 1973. Spontaneous diabetes mellitus in guinea pigs. The acute cytopathology of the islets of Langerhans. Lab. Invest. 29:685-702.

Müntzing, J., M.J. Varkarakis, J. Saroff, and G.P. Murphy. 1975. Comparison and significance of respiration and glycolysis of prostatic tissue from various species. J. Med. Primatol. 4:245-251.

Müntzing, J., H. Myhrberg, J. Saroff, A.A. Sandberg, and G.P. Murphy. 1976. Histochemical and ultrastructural study of prostatic tissue from baboons treated with antiprostatic drugs. Invest. Urol. 14:162-167.

Murphy, E.D. 1972. Hyperplastic and early neoplastic changes in the ovaries of mice after genic deletion of germ cells. J. Natl. Cancer Inst. 48:1283-1295.

Murray, M., and N.G. Wright. 1974. A morphologic study of canine glomerulonephritis. Lab. Invest. 30:213-221.

Myers, D.D. 1978. Review of disease patterns and life span in aging mice: Genetic and environmental interactions. Pages 41-53 in D. Bergsma and D.E. Harrison, eds. Genetic effects on aging. Birth defects original article series. Vol. 14, No. 1. A.R. Liss, Inc., New York.

Nabeya, D. 1923. A study in the comparative anatomy of the blood-vascular system of the internal ear in mammalia and in homo. Acta Sch. Med. Univ. Imp. Kioto. 6:1-132.

Nabors, C.E., and C.R. Ball. 1969. Spontaneous calcification in hearts of DBA mice. Anat. Rec. 164:153-162.

Nachlas, M.M., and T.K. Shnitka. 1963. Macroscopic identification of early myocardial infarcts by alterations in dehydrogenase activity. Am. J. Pathol. 42:379-405.

Nagatsu, T., T. Kanamuri, T. Kato, R. Iizuka, and H. Narabayaski. 1978. Dopamine-stimulated adenylate cyclase activity in the human brain: Changes in Parkinsonism. Biochem. Med. 19:360-365.

Najarian, H.H. 1961. Haemobartonella in the Mongolian gerbil. Tex. Rep. Biol. Med. 19:123-133.

Nakama, K. 1977. Studies on diabetic syndrome and influences of longterm tolbutamide administration in Mongolian gerbils (Meriones unguiculatus). Endocrinol. Jpn. 24:421-433.

Nakamura, M., and K. Yamada. 1967. Studies on a diabetic (KK) strain of mouse. Diabetologia 3:212.

Nakano, J., A.C. Gin, and T. Ishii. 1971. Effects of age on norepinephrine-, ACTH-, theophylline- and dibutryl cyclic AMP-induced lipolysis in isolated rat fat cells. J. Gerontol. 26(1):8-12.

Nakano, K., S. Yamamoto, G. Kutsukake, H. Ogawa, A. Nakajima, and E. Takano. 1960. Hereditary cataract in mice. Jap. J. Clin. Ophthalmol. 14:196.

Nam, S.C., W.M. Lee, J. Jarmolych, K.T. Lee, and W.A. Thomas. 1973. Rapid production of advanced atherosclerosis in swine by a combination of endothelial injury and cholesterol feeding. Exp. Mol. Pathol. 18:369:379.

Nandy, K. 1972. Brain reactive antibodies in mouse serum as a function of age. J. Gerontol. 27:173-177.

Nandy, K. 1977. Immune reactions in aging brain and senile dementia. Pages 181-196 in K. Nandy and I. Sherwin, eds. The aging brain and senile dementia. Plenum Publishing Corp., New York.

Nandy, K., and V.K. Vijayan. 1979. Cerebellar cell populations, lipofuscin pigment, and acetylcholinesterase activity. Pages 133-142 in D.M. Bowden, ed. Aging in nonhuman primates. Van Nostrand Reinhold, New York.

Napier, J.R., and P.H. Napier. 1967. Handbook of the living primates. Academic Press, London. 456 p.

Nasledova, I.D., and P.A. Silnitsky. 1972. Some age peculiarities of lipid and carbohydate metabolism and the state of the aortic wall in female rabbits. Biull. Eksp. Biol. Med. 73:19-22. (in Russian)

National Cancer Institute (NCI), Biometry Branch. 1971. Preliminary report: Third national cancer survey, 1969 incidence. DHEW Pub. 72-128. U.S. Department of Health, Education, and Welfare, Washington, D.C. 22 p.

National Cancer Institute (NCI). 1973. Workshop on criteria for successful rodent chronic studies. Proceedings of a workshop of the National Cancer Program held April 4-5, 1973 in Bethesda, Maryland. U.S. Department of Health, Education, and Welfare, Washington, D.C. 171 p.

National Center for Health Statistics. 1979. General
    mortality. Section 1, Pages 1-114 - 1-213 in Vital
    Statistics of the United States 1975. Vol. II.
    Mortality. Part A. DHEW Pub. No. (PHS) 79-1114.
    U.S. Department of Health, Education, and Welfare,
    Washington, D.C.
National Commission on Diabetes. 1975. Report of the
    National Commission on Diabetes to the Congress of
    the United States. U.S. DHEW Pub. No. 76-1018. U.S.
    Department of Health, Education, and Welfare, Wash-
    ington, D.C. 4 vol.
National Institute on Aging (NIA). 1977. Our future
    selves. A research plan toward understanding aging.
    DHEW Pub. No. (NIH) 77-1096. U.S. Department of
    Health, Education, and Welfare, Washington, D.C.
    60 p.
National Institute on Aging (NIA) and National Institute
    of General Medical Sciences (NIGMS). 1978. Workshop
    on Pharmacology and Aging. Report on a workshop held
    September 15-16, 1977 in Bethesda, Maryland. DHEW Pub.
    No. (NIH) 78-353. U.S. Dept. of Health, Education, and
    Welfare, Washington, D.C. 28 p.
National Institutes of Health (NIH). 1964. Standard No.
    1. Animal feed processing sanitation. Division of
    Research Resources. National Institutes of Health,
    Bethesda, Maryland. Unpublished.
Navia, J.M. 1977. Experimental periodontal disease.
    Pages 312-337 in Animal models in dental research. The
    University of Alabama Press, University of Alabama,
    Birmingham, Alabama.
Navia, J.M., and C.E. Hunt. 1976. Nutrition, nutrition-
    al diseases and nutrition research applications. Pages
    235-267 in J.E. Wagner and P.J. Manning, eds. The bi-
    ology of the guinea pig. Academic Press, New York.
Neel, J.V. 1962. Diabetes mellitus. A "thrifty" geno-
    type rendered detrimental by "progress"? Am. J. Hum.
    Genet. 14:353-362.
Nelson, J.F., C.F. Holinka, and C.E. Finch. 1976a. Age-
    related changes in estradiol binding capacity of mouse
    uterine cytosol. Page 34 in Program, 29th Annual
    Meeting of The Gerontological Society, held October
    13-17, 1976 in New York. The Gerontological Society,
    Washington, D.C.
Nelson, J.F., C.F. Holinka, K.R. Latham, J.K. Allen, and
    C.E. Finch. 1976b. Corticosterone binding in cysto-
    sols from brain regions of mature and senescent male
    C57BL/6J mice. Brain Res. 115:345-351.

Nelson, J.F., L.S Felicio, and C.E. Finch. In press. Ovarian hormones and the etiology of reproductive aging in mice. Chapter 4 in A.A. Dietz, ed. Aging - its chemistry. American Association for Clinical Chemistry, Washington, D.C.

Nevalainen, T.O., W.J. White, C.M. Lang, and B.L. Munger. 1978. The effect of spontaneous diabetes mellitus on fatty acid oxidation, β-hydroxybutyrate dehydrogenase activity and respiratory coupling of hepatic mitochondria in the guinea pig (Cavia porcellus). Clin. Exp. Pharmacol. Physiol. 5:212-222.

Newberne, J.W., V.B. Robinson, L. Estill, and D.C. Brinkman. 1960. Granular structures in brains of apparently normal dogs. Am. J. Vet. Res. 21:782-786.

Newberne, P.M. 1979. Nutrition of the hamster. Pages 127-138 in F. Homburger, ed. Symposium on the Syrian hamster in toxicology and carcinogenesis research. Proceedings of a symposium held November 30-December 2, 1977 in Boston, Massachusetts. Bio-Research Institute, Cambridge, Massachusetts.

Newell, G.K., and R.E. Beauchene. 1975. Effects of dietary calcium level, acid stress, and age on renal, serum, and bone responses of rats. J. Nutr. 105:1039-1047.

Newman, M.G., S.S. Socransky, E.D. Savitt, D. Propas, and A. Crawford. 1976. Studies of the microbiology of periodontosis. J. Periodontol. 47(7):373-379.

Newman, M.G., M. Sandler, W. Ormerod, L. Angel, and P. Goldhaber. 1977. The effect of dietary Gantrisin® supplements on the flora of periodontal pockets in four Beagle dogs. J. Periodontal Res. 12:129-134.

Newton, C.D., A.J. Lipowitz, R.E. Halliwell, H.L. Allen, D.N. Biery, and H.R. Schumacher. 1975. Rheumatoid arthritis in dogs. J. Am. Vet. Med. Assoc. 68:113-121.

Nielsen, S.W. 1969. Spontaneous hematopoietic neoplasms of the domestic cat. Natl. Cancer Inst. Monogr. 32:73-94.

Nielsen, S.W., L.S. Mackey, and W. Misdorp. 1976. International histologic typing of tumors of domestic animals. XVIII. Tumors of the kidney. Bull. WHO 53:237-245.

Niewoehner, D.E., and J. Kleinerman. 1973. Effects of experimental emphysema and bronchiolitis on lung mechanics and morphometry. J. Appl. Physiol. 35:25-31.

Nissen, H.W., and A.H. Riesen. 1964. The eruption of permanent dentition of chimpanzee. Am. J. Phys. Anthropol. 22:285-294.

Noell, W.K., V.S. Walker, B.S. Kang, and S. Berman. 1966. Retinal damage by light in rats. Invest. Ophthalmol. 5:450-476.

Nolen, G. 1972. Effect of various restricted dietary regimens on the growth, health and longevity of albino rats. J. Nutr. 102:1477-1494.

Nordin, B.E.C. 1973. Metabolic bone and stone disease. Churchill Livingstone, Edinburgh; Williams and Wilkins, Baltimore. 305 p.

Nordmann, J. 1972. Problems in cataract research. Ophthalmic Res. 3: 323-359.

Norris, M.L., and C.E. Adams. 1972a. Aggressive behavior and reproduction in the Mongolian gerbil, Meriones unguiculatus, relative to age and sexual experience at pairing. J. Reprod. Fertil. 31:447-450.

Norris, M.L., and C.E. Adams. 1972b. Mortality from birth to weaning in the Mongolian gerbil, Meriones unguiculatus. Lab Anim. 6:49-53.

Norris, M.L., and C.E. Adams. 1972c. Incidence of cystic ovaries and reproductive performance in the Mongolian gerbil, Meriones unguiculatus. Lab. Anim. 6:337-342.

Norton, W.T., and S.E. Poduslo. 1973. Myelination in rat brain: Changes in myelin composition during brain maturation. J. Neurochem. 21:759-773.

Notkins, A.L. 1978. Virus-induced diabetes mellitus. Arch. Virol. 54:1-17.

Nyman, S., H.E. Schroeder, and J. Lindhe. 1979. Suppression of inflammation and bone resorption by indomethacin during experimental periodontitis in dogs. J. Periodontol. 50:450-461.

Oberling, C., M. Riviere, and F. Haguenae. 1960. Ultrastructure of clear cells in renal carcinomas and its importance for the demonstration of their renal origin. Nature 186:402-403.

Obrist, W.D. 1972. Cerebral physiology of the aged: Influence of circulatory disorders. Pages 117-134 in C.M. Gaitz, ed. Aging and the brain. Plenum Publishing Corp., New York.

O'Dea, K., and S. Koletsky. 1977. Effect of caloric restriction on basal insulin levels and the in vivo lipogenesis and glycogen synthesis from glucose in the Koletsky obese rat. Metabolism 26:763-772.

O'Dell, B.L., K.H. Kilburn, W.N. McKenzie, and R.J.
Thurston. 1978. The lung of the copper-deficient rat.
Am. J. Pathol. 91:413-423.

Oettle, A.G. 1967. The multimammate mouse. Pages 468-
477 in W. Land-Petter, A.N. Worden, B.F. Hill, J.S.
Paterson, and H.G. Vevers, eds. The UFAW Handbook on
the care and management of laboratory animals. 3rd ed.
The Williams and Wilkins Company, Baltimore; E. & S.
Livingston Ltd., Edinburgh.

Ofner, P., R.L. Verra, R.F. Morfin, M.A. Adiapoulios, and
I. Leav. 1974. Pages 111-124 in M. Goland, ed. Nor-
mal and abnormal growth of the prostate. Charles C.
Thomas, Springfield, Illinois.

Ogletree, M.L., and A.M. Lefer. 1976. Influence of non-
steroidal anti-inflammatory agents on myocardial ischemia in the cat. J. Pharmacol. Exp. Ther. 197:582-593.

Ohye, C., and D. Albe-Fessard. 1978. Rhythmic discharges
related to tremor in humans and monkeys. Pages 37-48
in N. Chalazonities and M. Boisson, eds. Abnormal
neuronal discharges. Raven Press, New York.

Oldstone, M.B., and F.J. Dixon. 1974. Aging and chronic
virus infection: Is there a relationship? Fed. Proc.
33:2057-2059.

Olesen, H.P., O.A. Jensen, and M.S. Norn. 1974. Congenital hereditary cataract in Cocker Spaniels. J.
Small Anim. Pract. 15:741-750.

Olson, G.A., and R.P. Shields. 1977. Salmonellosis in
a gerbil colony. J. Am. Vet. Med. Assoc. 171:970-972.

Onodera, T., A.B. Jenson, J-W. Yoon, and A.L. Notkins.
1978. Virus-induced diabetes mellitus: Reovirus in
fection of pancreatic β cells in mice. Science 201:
529-531.

Ordy, J.M. 1975. Neurobiology and aging in nonhuman primates. Adv. Behav. Biol. 16:575-597.

Ordy, J.M. and K.R. Brizzee. 1977. Age-declines in
learning, short-term memory, arousal and aggression in
relation to cell loss from cortex and hippocampus of
the rat. Page 348 in Vol. 3, Abstracts of the 7th
annual meeting of the Society for Neuroscience held
November 6-10, 1977 in Anaheim, California. Society
for Neuroscience, Bethesda, Maryland.

Ordy, J.M., B. Kaack, K.R. Brizzee. 1975. Life span
neurochemical changes in the human and nonhuman primate
brain. Pages 133-189 in H. Brody, D. Harman and J.M.
Ordy, eds. Clinical, morphologic, and neurochemical
aspects in the aging central nervous system. Vol. 1.
Aging series. Raven Press, New York.

Orsini, M.W. 1961. The external vaginal phenomena characterizing the stages of the estrous cycle, pregnancy, and pseudopregnancy, lactation, and the anestrous hamster, Mesocricetus auratus Waterhouse. Proc. Anim. Care Panel 11:193-206.

Osborne, C.A., K.H. Johnson, V. Perman, W.D. Schol. 1968a. Amyloidosis in the dog. J. Am. Vet. Med. Assoc. 153:669-688.

Osborne, C.A., V. Perman, J.H. Sautter, J.B. Stevens, and G.F. Hanlon. 1968b. Multiple myeloma in the dog. J. Am. Vet. Med. Assoc. 153:1300-1319.

Osborne, C.A., D.G. Low, D.R. Finco. 1972. Canine and feline urology. W.B. Saunders Co., Philadelphia. 417 p.

Osetowska, E. 1966. Étude anatomopathologique sur le cerveau de chiens séniles. Pages 497-502 in F. Luthy and A. Bischoff, eds. Proceedings of the 5th International Congress of Neuropathology, held August 31-September 3, 1965 in Zurich, Switzerland. International Congress Series No. 100. Excerpta Medica Foundation, Amsterdam.

O'Steen, W.K. 1970. Retinal and optic nerve serotonin and retinal degeneration as influenced by photoperiod. Exp. Neurol. 27:194-205.

O'Steen, W.K. 1979. Hormonal and dim light effects in retinal photodamage. Photochem. Photobiol. 29:745-753.

O'Steen, W.K., C.R. Shear, and K.V. Anderson. 1972. Retinal damage after prolonged exposure to visible light. A light and electron microscopic study. Am. J. Anat. 134:5-22.

O'Steen, W.K., K.V. Anderson, and C.R. Shear. 1974. Photoreceptor degeneration in albino rats: Dependency of age. Invest. Ophthalmol. 13:334-339.

Outzen, H.C. 1969. Ageing and resistance to infection in germfree C_3Hf mice. Pages 207-217 in E. Mirand and N. Back, eds. Germfree biology. Experimental and clinical aspects. Plenum Publishing Corp., New York.

Outzen, H.C., and H.I. Pilgrim. 1967. Differential mortality of male and female germfree C_3H mice introduced into a conventional colony. Proc. Soc. Exp. Biol. Med. 124:52-56.

Pacific Northwest Laboratory. 1979. Pacific Northwest Laboratory annual report for 1978 to the DOE Assistant Secretary for Environment. Part 1. Biomedical sciences. PNL-2850, Part 1.

Paffenholz, V. 1978. Correlation between DNA repair of embryonic fibroblasts and different life span of 3 inbred mouse strains. Mech. Ageing Dev. 7:131-150.

Page, R.C. 1977. Etiology of peridontal disease. Pages 85-106 in S. Schluger and R. Yuodelir, eds. Periodontal disease. Lea and Febiger, Philadelphia.

Page, R.C., and H.E. Schroeder. 1976. Pathogenesis of inflammatory periodontal disease. Lab. Invest. 33:235-249.

Page, R.C., and H.E. Schroder. In press. Spontaneous chronic periodontitis in adult dogs. A clinical and histopathological survey. J. Periodontol.

Page, R.C., D.M. Simpson, W.F. Ammons, and L.R. Schectman. 1971. Periodontal disease: Are plasma cells and lymphocytes an essential component? Proc. Soc. Exp. Biol. Med. 138:947-951.

Page, R.C., D.M. Simpson, W.F. Ammons, and L.R. Schectman. 1972. Host tissue response in chronic periodontal disease III. Clinical, histologic and ultrastructural features of advanced disease in a colony-maintained marmoset. J. Periodontal Res. 7:283-296.

Page, R.C., D.M. Simpson, and W.F. Ammons. 1975. Host tissue response in chronic inflammatory periodontal disease IV. The periodontal and dental status of a group of aged great apes. J. Periodontol. 46:144-155.

Page, R.C., L.D. Engel, A.S. Narayanan, and J.A. Clagett. 1978. Chronic inflammatory gingival and periodontal disease. J. Am. Med. Assoc. 240:545-550.

Paget, G.E., and P.G. Lemon. 1965. The interpretation of pathology data. Pages 382-405 in W.F. Ribelin and J.R. McCoy, eds. Pathology of laboratory animals. Charles C. Thomas, Springfield, Illinois.

Paget, O., and M. Baumgarter-Gamauf. 1953. Histologische untersuchungen an einer dominant erblichen form einer cataract bein der hausmaus. Osten. Zool. Ztschr. 85:238-244.

Pakes, S.P. 1969. The somatic chromosomes of the Mongolian gerbil (Meriones unguiculatus). Lab. Anim. Care 19:857-861.

Palecek, F., and R. Holusa. 1971. Spontaneous occurrence of lung emphysema in laboratory rats. Physiol. Bohemoslov. 20:335-344.

Panel on Biomedical Research, National Advisory Council on Aging. 1978. Our future selves. A research plan toward understanding aging. Report of the Panel on Biomedical Research, National Advisory Council on

Aging. DHEW Pub. No. (NIH) 78-1445. U.S. Department
of Health, Education, and Welfare, Washington, D.C.
44 p.

Papadaki, L., J.O.W. Beilby, J. Chowaniec, W.F. Coulson,
A.J. Darby, J. Newman, A. O'Shea, and J.R. Wykes.
1979. Hormone replacement therapy in the menopause;
a suitable animal model. J. Endocrinol. 83: 67-77.

Paré, W.P. 1969. Interaction of age and shock intensity
on acquisition of a discriminated conditioned emotional
response. J. Comp. Physiol. Psychol. 68:364-369.

Parfitt, A.M. 1976. The actions of parathyroid hormone
on bone: Relation to bone remodeling and turnover,
calcium homeostasis, and metabolic bone disease. Part
1. Mechanisms of calcium transfer between blood and
bone and their cellular basis: Morphological and
kinetic approaches to bone turnover. Metab. Clin. Exp.
25:809-844.

Parfitt, A.M., and H. Duncan. 1975. Metabolic bone
disease affecting the spine. Pages 599-720 in R.
Rothman and F. Simeone, eds. The spine. W.B. Saunders, Philadelphia.

Park, S.S., Y. Kikkawa, I.P. Goldring, M.M. Daly, M.
Zelefsky, C. Shim, M. Spierer, and T. Morita. 1977.
An animal model of cigarette smoking in Beagle dogs.
Am. Rev. Respir. Dis. 115:971-979.

Parke, D.V., P.J. Sacra, and P.C. Thornton. 1978. Experimental atherosclerosis in the Wistar rat. Br. J.
Pharmacol. 63:346P-347P.

Parkening, T.A. 1976. Retention of ova in oviducts of
senescent mice and hamsters. J. Exp. Zool. 196:307-
314.

Parkening, T.A., and A.L. Soderwall. 1973. Delayed embryonic development and implantation in senescent
golden hamsters. Biol. Reprod. 8:427-434.

Parkening, T.A., and A.L. Soderwall. 1975. Delayed
fertilization and preimplantation loss in senescent
golden hamsters. Biol. Reprod. 12:618-631.

Parkening, T.A., I.-F. Lau, S.K. Saksena, and M.-C. Chang.
1978. Circulating plasma levels of pregnenolone,
progesterone, estrogen, luteinizing hormone, and
follicle stimulating hormone in young and aged C57BL/6J
mice during various stages of pregnancy. J. Gerontol.
33:191-196.

Parker, J.C., M.D. Whiteman, and C.B. Richter. 1978.
Susceptibility of inbred and outbred mouse strains to
Sendai virus and prevalence of infection in laboratory
rats. Infect. Immun. 19:123-130.

Patel, M.S. 1977. Age-dependent changes in the oxidative metabolism in rat brain. J. Gerontol. 32:643-646.

Pathak, S., T.C. Hsu, and F.E. Arrighi. 1973. Chromosomes of Peromyscus (Rodentia, Cricetidae). IV. The role of heterochromatin in karyotypic evolution. Cytogenet. Cell Genet. 12:315-326.

Patnaik, A.K., S.K. Liuand, and G.F. Johnson. 1976. Feline intestinal adenocarcinoma. A clinicopathologic study of 22 cases. Vet. Pathol. 13:1-10.

Patnaik, A.K., A.I. Hurvitz, and G.F. Johnson. 1977. Canine gastrointestinal neoplasms. Vet. Pathol. 14:547-555.

Patnaik, A.K., A.I. Hurvitz, and G.F. Johnson. 1978. Canine gastric adenocarcinoma. Vet. Pathol. 15:600-607.

Patterson, R., and D.B. Sparks. 1962. The passive transfer to normal dogs of skin reactivity, asthma and anaphylaxis from a dog with spontaneous ragweed pollen hypersensitivity. J. Immunol. 88:262-268.

Patterson, R.M., M. Roberts, and J.J. Pruzansky. 1969. Comparisons of reaginic antibodies from three species. J. Immunol. 102(2):466-475.

Patrick, J.M., and A. Howard. 1972. The influence of age, sex, body size and lung size on the control and pattern of breathing during CO_2 inhalation in caucasians. Respir. Physiol. 16:337-350.

Peckham, J.C., J.R. Cole, W.L. Chapman, Jr., J.B. Malone, Jr., J.W. McCall, and P.E. Thompson. 1974. Staphlococcal dermatitis in Mongolian gerbils (Meriones unguiculatus). Lab Anim. Sci. 24:43-47.

Peckham, S.C., C. Entenman, and H.W. Carroll. 1962. The influence of a hypercaloric diet on gross body and adipose tissue composition in the rat. J. Nutr. 77:187-197.

Pedersen, N.C., and R. Pool. 1978. Canine joint disease. Vet. Clin. North Am. 8(3):465-493.

Pederson, N.C., K. Weisner, J.J. Castles, G.V. Ling, G. Weiser. 1976. Non-infectious canine arthritis: The inflammatory, nonerosive arthritides. J. Am. Vet. Med. Assoc. 169:304-310.

Peehl, D.M., and R.G. Ham. 1978. Requirements for growth and differentiation of human keratinocytes. Abstract CU340. J. Cell. Biol. 79(2, Part 2):78a.

Peiffer, R.L. 1978. Cataract resorption in a spider monkey. J. Am. Vet. Med. Assoc. 173:1234-1235.

Peiffer, R.L., and K.N. Gelatt. 1976. Cataract in a woolly monkey. Mod. Vet. Pract. 57:609-610.

Pelkonen, R. 1971. Metabolic aspects of the climacterium. Acta Obstet. Gynecol. Scand. 50(Suppl.):16-23.

Pencharz, R.I., and J.A. Long. 1933. Hypophysectomy in the pregnant rat. Am. J. Anat. 53:117-135.

Peng, M.-T., and H.-O. Huang. 1972. Aging of hypothalamic-pituitary-ovarian function in the rat. Fertil. Steril. 23:535-542.

Peng, M.-T., Y.I. Peng, and F.N. Chen. 1977. Age-dependent changes in the oxygen consumption of the cerebral cortex, hypothalamus, hippocampus, and amygdala in rats. J. Gerontol. 32:517-522.

Penha, P.D., L. Amaral, and S. Werthamer. 1972. Ozone air pollutants and lung damage. Ind. Med. Surg. 41(3):17-20.

Perry, E.K., R.H. Perry, P.H. Gibson, G. Blessed, and B.E. Tomlinson. 1977a. A cholinergic connection between normal aging and senile dementia in the human hippocampus. Neurosci. Lett. 6:85-89.

Perry, E.K., R.H. Perry, G. Blessed, and B.E. Tomlinson. 1977b. Necropsy evidence of central cholinergic deficits in senile dementia. Lancet 1:189.

Perzigian, A.J. 1973. Osteoporotic bone loss in two prehistoric populations. Am. J. Phys. Anthropol. 39: 87-96.

Peters, R.L. 1972. Incidence of spontaneous neoplasms in breeding and retired breeder BALB/c mice throughout the natural life span. Int. J. Cancer 10:273-282.

Pet Food Institute fact sheet. 1978. Pet Food Institute, Washington, D.C.

Pettegrew, R.K., and K.L. Ewing. 1971. Life history study of oxygen utilization in the C57BL/6 mice. J. Gerontol. 26:381-385.

Petty, W.C., and R. Karler. 1965. The influence of aging on the activity of anticonvulsant drugs. J. Pharmacol. Exp. Ther. 150(3):443-448.

Pfeiffer, E., and E.W. Busse. 1973. Mental disorders in later life--affective disorders; paranoid, neurotic, and situational reactions. Pages 107-144 in E.W. Busse and E. Pfeiffer, eds. Mental illness in later life. American Psychiatric Association, Washington, D.C.

Pfingst, B.E., R. Hienz, J. Kimm, and J. Miller. 1975. Reaction-time procedure for measurement of hearing I: Suprathreshold functions. J. Acoust. Soc. Am. 57: 421-430.

Philip, B., and P.A. Kurup. 1977. Cortisol and lysosomal stability in normal and atheromatous rats. Atherosclerosis 27:129-139.

Philipson, B. 1973. Changes in the lens related to the reduction of transparency. Exp. Eye Res. 16:29-39.

Piantanelli, L., R. Brogli, P. Bevilacqua, and N. Fabris. 1978. Age-dependence of isoproterenol-induced DNA synthesis in submandibular glands of BALB/c mice. Mech. Ageing Dev. 7:163-169.

Pick, R., P.J. Johnson, and G. Glick. 1974. Deleterious effects of hypertension on the development of aortic and coronary atherosclerosis in stump-tail macaques (Macaca speciosa) on an atherogenic diet. Circ. Res. 35:427-482.

Pickrell, J.A., S.J. Schluter, J.J. Belasich, E.V. Stewart, J. Meyer, C.H. Hobbs, and R.K. Jones. 1974. Relationship of age of normal dogs to blood serum constituents and reliability of measured single values. Am. J. Vet. Res. 35:897-903.

Pickrell, J.A., D.V. Harris, J.L. Mauderly, and F.F. Hahn. 1976. Altered collogen metabolism in radiation-induced interstitial pulmonary fibrosis. Chest 69(Suppl.): 311-316.

Pilbeam, D. 1972. The ascent of man, an introduction to human evolution. MacMillan, New York. 207 p.

Pincus, T. 1980. Endogenous murine type C viruses. Pages 77-130 in J.R. Stephenson, ed. Molecular biology of RNA tumor viruses. Academic Press, New York.

Pitt, B., and H.W. Strauss. 1976. Myocardial imaging in the noninvasive evaluation of patients with suspected ischemic heart disease. Am. J. Cardiol. 37: 797-806.

Pitts, L.L., L.L. Rudel, B.C. Bullock, and T.B. Clarkson. 1976. Sex differences in the relationship of low density lipoproteins to coronary atherosclerosis in Macaca fascicularis. Abstract No. 487. Fed. Proc. 35:293.

Platt, H. 1970. Canine chronic nephritis. I. Observations on the pathology of the kidney. J. Comp. Pathol. 61:140-149.

Poiley, S.M. 1950. Breeding and care of the Syrian hamster (Cricetus auratus). Pages 118-152 in E.J. Farris, ed. The care and breeding of laboratory animals. Wiley Interscience, New York.

Poiley, S.M. 1960. A systematic method of breeder rotation for noninbred laboratory animal colonies. Proc. Anim. Care Panel 10(4):159-166.

Poirier, L.J. 1960. Experimental and histological study of midbrain dyskinesias. J. Neurophysiol. 23:534-551.

Poirier, L.J. 1975. Dopaminergic agonists in animal models of parkinsonism. Adv. Neurol. 9:327-335.

Poirier, L., M. Filion, P. Langelier, and L. Larochelle. 1975a. Brain nervous mechanisms involved in the so-called extrapyramidal motor and psychomotor disturbances. Prog. Neurobiol. 5:197-243.

Poirier, L.J., J.C. Pechadre, L. Larochelle, J. Dankova, and R. Boucher. 1975b. Stereotaxic lesions and movement disorders in monkeys. Adv. Neurol. 10:5-22.

Poisson, D., A. Marillaud, and G. Galand. 1974. Remarks about stereotaxic atlases of the rabbit brain. Exp. Neurol. 43:474-476.

Pollard, M., and J. Kajima. 1970. Lesions in aged germ-free Wistar rats. Am. J. Pathol. 61:25-32.

Polson, A.M. 1977. Interactions between periodontal trauma and marginal periodontitis. Int. Dent. J. 27:107-113.

Pomerance, A., and J.C. Whitney. 1970. Heart valve changes common to man and dog. A comparative study. Cardiovasc. Res. 4:61-66.

Pontén, J. 1977. Abnormal cell growth (neoplasia) in aging. Pages 536-560 in C.E. Finch and L. Hayflick, eds. Handbook of the biology of aging. Van Nostrand Reinhold, New York.

Ponzio, F., N. Brunello, and S. Algeri. 1978. Catecholamine synthesis in brains of ageing rats. J. Neurochem. 30:1617-1620.

Poppe, E. 1942. Experimental investigations of the effects of roentgen rays on the eye. Norske Videnskaps - Akademie i Oslo Skrifter. Jacob Dybwad, Oslo, Norway. 102 p.

Port, C.D., W.R. Richter, and S.M. Moise. 1970. Tyzzer's disease in the gerbil (Meriones unguiculatus). Lab. Anim. Care 20:109-111.

Port, C.D., K.V. Ketels, D.L. Coffin, and P. Kane. 1977. A comparative study of experimental and spontaneous emphysema. J. Tox. Environ. Health 2:589-640.

Porter, H., D.H. Doty, and C.M. Bloor. 1971. Interaction of age and exercise on tissue lactic dehydrogenase activity in rats. Lab. Invest. 25(6):572-576.

Post, F. 1968. The factor of aging in affective illness. Pages 105-116 in A. Coppen and A. Walk, eds. Recent developments in affective disorders. British Journal of Psychiatry, Special Publication No. 2. Headly Brothers, Ltd., Ashford, Kent.

Post, R.H. 1964. Hearing acuity variation among negroes and whites. Eugen. Q. 11:65-81.

Pour, P., N. Kmoch, E. Greiser, U. Mohr, J. Althoff, and A. Cardesa. 1976a. Spontaneous tumors and common diseases in two colonies of Syrian hamsters. I. Incidence and sites. J. Natl. Cancer Inst. 56:931-936.

Pour, P., U. Mohr, A. Cardesa, J. Althoff, and N. Kmoch. 1976b. Spontaneous tumors and common diseases in two colonies of Syrian hamsters. II. Respiratory tract and digestive system. J. Natl. Cancer Inst. 56:937-948.

Pour, P., U. Mohr, J. Althoff, A. Cardesa, and N. Kmoch. 1976c. Spontaneous tumors and common diseases in two colonies of Syrian hamsters. III. Urogenital system and endocrine glands. J. Natl. Cancer Inst. 56:949-962.

Pour, P., U. Mohr, J. Althoff, A. Cardesa, and N. Kmoch. 1976d. Spontaneous tumors and common diseases in two colonies of Syrian hamsters. IV. Vascular and lymphatic systems and lesions of other sites. J. Natl. Cancer Inst. 56:963-974.

Powell, W.J., Jr., D.R. DiBona, J. Flores, and A. Leaf. 1976. The protective effect of hyperosmotic mannitol in myocardial ischemia and necrosis. Circulation 54:603-615.

Powers, J.M., and S.S. Spicer. 1977. Histochemical similarity of senile plaque amyloid to apudamyloid. Virchows Arch. A. 376:107-115.

Prasse, K.W. 1975. Disorders of the leukocytes. Pages 1627-1663 in S.J. Ettinger, ed. Textbook of veterinary internal medicine. Diseases of the dog and cat. Vol. 2. W.B. Saunders Co., Philadelphia.

Prathap, K. 1973. Spontaneous aortic lesions in wild Malaysian long-tailed monkeys (Macaca irus). J. Pathol. 110:135-143.

Pratt, P.C., and G.A. Klugh. 1967. Chronic expiratory air-flow obstruction-cause or effect of centrilobular emphysema. Dis. Chest 52:342-349.

Price, D. 1963. Comparative aspects of development and structure in the prostate. Natl. Cancer Inst. Monogr. 12:1-27.

Price, G.B., and T. Makinodan. 1972. Immunologic deficiencies in senescence. I. Characterization of intrinsic deficiencies. J. Immunol. 108:403-412.

Price, K.S., I.J. Farley, and O. Hornykiewicz. 1978. Neurochemistry of Parkinson's disease: Relation between striatal and limbic dopamine. Adv. Biochem. Psychopharmacol. 19:293-300.

Prichard, R.W., T.B. Clarkson, H.B. Lofland, and H.O. Goodman. 1964a. Pigeon atherosclerosis. Am. Heart J. 67:715-717.

Prichard, R.W., T.B. Clarkson, H.O. Goodman, and H.B. Lofland. 1964b. Aortic atherosclerosis in pigeons and its complications. Arch. Pathol. 77:244-257.

Prier, J.E., and R.S. Brodey. 1963. Canine neoplasia. A prototype for human cancer study. Bull. WHO 29: 331-344.

Prior, J.T., D.M. Kurtz, and D.D. Ziegler. 1961. The hypercholesteremic rabbit: An aid to understanding arteriosclerosis in man? Arch. Pathol. 71:672-684.

Proshina, L. Ya. 1973. Age-specific peculiarities of uveites and the part played by biogenic amines in their development. Vestn. Oftal'mol. 1:17-22. (in Russian)

Prout, T.E. 1975. The use of screening and diagnostic procedures: The oral glucose tolerance test. Pages 57-67 in K.E. Sussman and R.J.S. Metz, eds. Diabetes mellitus. 4th ed. American Diabetes Association Inc., New York.

Pudel, V.E. 1978. Human feeding in the laboratory. Pages 66-74 in G.A. Bray, ed. Recent advances in obesity research: II. Proceedings of the 2nd International Congress on Obesity, held October 23-26, 1977 in Washington, D.C. Newman Publishing, Ltd., London.

Pugach, B.V. 1975. Age-related peculiarities of the effect of angiotenosin-2 on some hemodynamic indices. Farmakol. Toksikol. 38:427-430. (in Russian)

Pugh, J.E., M.R. Horwitz, and D.J. Anderson. 1974. Cochlear electrical activity in noise-induced hearing loss: Behavioral and electrophysiological studies in primates. Arch. Otolaryngol. 100:36-40.

Pump, K.K. 1974. Fenestrae in the alveolar membrane of the human lung. Chest 65:431-436.

Puri, S.K., and L. Volicer. 1977. Effect of aging on cyclic AMP levels and adenylate cyclase and phosphodiesterase activities in the rat corpus striatum. Mech. Ageing Dev. 6:53-58.

Quadri, S.K., G.S. Kledzik, and J. Meites. 1973. Reinitiation of estrous cycles in old constant-estrous rats by central-acting drugs. Neuroendocrinology 11:248-255.

Quattropani, S.L. 1978. Serous cysts of the aging guinea pig ovary. II. Scanning and transmission electron microscopy. Anat. Rec. 190(2):285-298.

Rabkin, M., M.B. Bellhorn, and R.W. Bellhorn. 1977. Selected molecular weight dextrans for in vivo permeability studies of rat retinal vascular disease. Exp. Eye Res. 24:607-612.

Radcliffe, J.D., and A.J.F. Webster. 1976. Regulation of food intake during growth in fatty and lean female Zucker rats given diets of different protein content. Br. J. Nutr. 36:457-469.

Rampy, L.W., K.D. Nitschke, T.J. Bell, and J.D. Burek. 1979. Interim results of two-year inhalation toxicologic studies of methylene chloride in rats and hamsters. Page A185, Abstract No. 370 in Abstracts of papers presented at the 18th Annual Meeting of the Society of Toxicology, held March 11-15, 1979 in New Orleans, Louisiana. Academic Press, New York.

Randall, P., P. Amaral, and L.S. Ringering. 1978. Effects of chronic neuroleptics on catalepsy and stereotypic behavior in aging mice. Page 114 in Abstracts of the 31st annual meeting of The Gerontological Society, held November 16-20, 1978 in Dallas, Texas. The Gerontological Society, Washington, D.C.

Ranney, R.R., and E.H. Montgomery. 1973. Vascular leakage resulting from topical application of endotoxin to the gingiva of the Beagle dog. Arch. Oral Biol. 18:963-970.

Ranney, R.R., and H.A. Zander. 1970. Allergic periodontal disease in sensitized squirrel monkeys. J. Periodontol. 41:12-21.

Ranson, S.W., C. Fisher, and W.R. Ingram. 1938. Adiposity and diabetes mellitus in a monkey with hypothalamic lesions. Endocrinology 23:175-181.

Rao, G.V.G.K., and H.H. Draper. 1969. Age-related changes in the bones of adult mice. J. Gerontol. 24: 149-151.

Rapport, M.M., and S.E. Karpiak. 1978. Immunological perturbation of neurological functions. Pages 73-88 in K. Nandy, ed. Senile dementia: A biomedical approach. Developments in neuroscience. Vol. 3. Elsevier North-Holland Biomedical Press, New York.

Ratcliffe, H.L., and H. Luginbuhl. 1971. The domestic pig: A model for experimental atherosclerosis. Atherosclerosis 13:133-136.

Rauther, M. 1909. Neue Beitrage zur Kenntnis des Urogenitalsystems der Saugetiere. Denkschr. med.-naturwiss. Ges. Jena 15:417-466.

Rawlins, R.G. 1975. Age changes in the pubic symphysis of Macaca mulatta. Am. J. Phys. Anthropol. 42:477-488.

Raymond, T.L. 1974. Cholesterol metabolism in pig-tailed macaques and squirrel monkeys: Analysis of long-term kinetic studies and identification of body pools.

Doctoral dissertation, Department of Pathology, The Bowman Gray School of Medicine, Wake Forest University, Winston-Salem, North Carolina.

Raynaud, A. 1942. Existence de variations dans l'etat de developpement des tubules glandulaires de la prostate femelle d'*Apodemus sylvaticus* L. C.R. Acad. Sci. 215:382-384.

Rebel, W., and T. Stegmann. 1973. Enzym-histochemische Darstellung (SDH, LDH, Gluc-6-P-DH) von Stoffwechsel-veranderungen im hypertrophischen Myokard der Ratte. Virchows Arch. A 359:361-372.

Redman, H.C. 1980. Survival distribution of Beagle dogs maintained in laboratory colonies. Unpublished paper available from Dr. Hamilton Redman, Lovelace Inhalation Toxicology Reseach Institute, Albuquerque, New Mexico.

Redman, H.C., C.H. Hobbs, and A.H. Rebar. 1979. Survival distribution of Syrian hamsters (*Mesocricetus auratus*, Sch:SYR) used during 1972-1977. Pages 108-117 *in* F. Homburger, ed. The Syrian hamster in toxicology and carcinogenesis research. Progress in experimental tumor research. Vol. 24. S. Karger, Basel.

Reed, J.M., L.J. Schiff, A.M. Shefner, and M.C. Henry. 1974. Antibody levels to murine viruses in Syrian hamsters. Lab. Anim. Sci. 24:33-38.

Reed, O.M. 1973. *Papio cynocephalus* age determination. Am. J. Phys. Anthropol. 38:309-314.

Rehfeld, C.E., J.A. Blomquist, and G.N. Taylor. 1972. The Beagle. Pages 47-57 *in* B.J. Stover and W.S.S. Jee, eds. Radiobiology of plutonium. J.W. Press, University of Utah, Salt Lake City, Utah.

Reichel, W., J. Hollander, J.H. Clark, and B.L. Strehler. 1968. Lipofuscin pigment accumulation as a function 23:71-78.

Reid, L. 1963. An experimental study of hypersecretion of mucus in the bronchial tree. Br. J. Exp. Pathol. 44:437-445.

Reid, L. 1978. The cell biology of mucus secretion in the lung. Pages 138-150 *in* W.M. Thurlbeck and M.R. Abell, eds. The lung. Structure, function and disease. International Academy of Pathology. Monographs in Pathology, No. 19. The Williams and Wilkins Co., Baltimore.

Reid, M.E. 1958. The guinea pig in research. Publication No. 557. Human Factors Research Bureau, Inc., Miami, Florida.

Reif, J.S., and D. Cohen. 1979. Canine pulmonary disease: A spontaneous model for environmental epidemiology. Pages 241-250 in Animals as monitors of environmental pollutants. Proceedings of a symposium cosponsored by the Northeastern Research Center for Wildlife Diseases, Registry of Comparative Pathology, and Institute of Laboratory Animal Resources, held at the University of Connecticut in 1977. National Academy of Sciences, Washington, D.C.

Reif, J.S., and W.H. Rhodes. 1966. The lungs of aged dogs: A radiographic morphomogic correlation. J. Am. Vet. Radiol. Soc. 7:5-11.

Reimer, K.A., and R.B. Jennings. 1979. The changing anatomic reference base of evolving myocardial infarction. Circulation 60:866-876.

Reimer, K.A., M.M. Rasmussen, and R.B. Jennings. 1973. Reduction by propranolol of myocardial necrosis following temporary coronary artery occlusion in dogs. Circ. Res. 33:353-363.

Reis, D.J., R.A. Ross, and T.H. Joh. 1977. Changes in the activity and amounts of enzymes synthesizing catecholamines and acetylcholine in brain, adrenal medulla, and sympathetic ganglia of aged rat and mouse. Brain Res. 136:465-474.

Reisine, T.D., J.Z. Fields, H.I. Yamamura, E.D. Bird, E. Spokes, P.S. Schreiner, and S.J. Enna. 1977. Neurotransmitter receptor alterations in Parkinson's disease. Life Sci. 21:335-344.

Reisine, T.D., H.I. Yamamura, E.D. Bird, E. Spokes, and S.J. Enna. 1978. Pre- and postsynaptic neurochemical alterations in Alzheimer's disease. Brain Res. 159: 477-481.

Renold, A.E. 1968. Spontaneous diabetes and/or obesity in laboratory rodents. Adv. Metab. Disord. 3:49-84.

Renold, A.E., W. Stauffacher, and G.F. Cahill, Jr. 1972. Diabetes mellitus. Pages 83-118 in J.B. Stanbury, J.B. Wyngaarden, and D.S. Fredrickson, eds. The metabolic basis of inherited disease. McGraw-Hill Book Co., New York.

Renshaw, H.W., G.L. VanHooser, and N.K. Amend. 1975. A survey of naturally occurring diseases of the Syrian hamster. Lab. Anim. 9:179-191.

Reyniers, J.A., and M.R. Sacksteder. 1958. Observations on the survival of germfree C_3H mice and their resistance to a contaminated environment. Proc. Anim. Care Panel 8:41-53.

Reynolds, R.D., G.J. Kelliher, D.M. Ritchie, J. Roberts, and A.B. Beasley. 1979. Comparison of the arrhythmogenic effect of myocardial infarction in the cat and dog. Cardiovasc. Res. 13:152-159.

Reznik, G., H. Reznik-Schüller, and A. Emminger. 1975. Comparative studies of blood from hibernating and non-hibernating European hamsters (Cricetus cricetus L.). Lab. Anim. Sci. 25:210-215.

Rheinwald, J.C., and H. Green. 1975. Formation of a keratinizing epithelium in culture by a cloned cell line derived from a teratoma. Cell 6:317-330.

Ribelin, W.E., and J.R. McCoy [eds.] 1965. Pathology of laboratory animals. Charles C. Thomas, Springfield, Illinois. 436 p.

Rich, S.T. 1968. The Mongolian gerbil (Meriones unguiculatus) in research. Lab. Anim. Care 18:235-243.

Richey, D.P., and A.D. Bender. 1977. Pharmacokinetic consequences of aging. Ann. Rev. Pharmacol. Toxicol. 17:49-65.

Richter, C.B. 1970. Application of infectious agents to the study of lung cancer: Studies on the etiology and morphogenesis of metaplastic lung lesions in mice. Pages 365-382 in P. Nettesheim, M.G. Hanna, Jr., and J.W. Deatherage, Jr., eds. Morphology of experimental respiratory carcinogenesis. U.S. Atomic Energy Commission Symposium Series 21. Proceedings of a symposium held May 13-16, 1970 at Gatlinburg, Tennessee. U.S. Department of Energy, Washington, D.C.

Riederer, P., and S. Wuketich. 1976. Time course of nigrostriatal degeneration in Parkinson's disease. J. Neural Transm. 38:277-301.

Riegle, G.D., and J. Meites. 1976. Effects of aging on LH and prolactin after LHRH L-dopa, methyl-dopa, and stress in male rats. Proc. Soc. Exp. Biol. Med. 151:507-511.

Riegle, G.E., J. Meites, A.E. Miller, and S.M. Wood. 1977. Effect of aging on hypothalamic LH-releasing and prolactin inhibiting activities and pituitary responsiveness of LHRH in the male laboratory rat. J. Gerontol. 32:13-18.

Riegle, G.E., and A.E. Miller. 1978. Aging effects on the hypothalamic-hypophyseal-gonadol system in the rat. Pages 159-192 in E.L. Schneider, ed. The aging reproductive system. Vol. 4. Aging series. Raven Press, New York.

Rigaudiere, N., G. Pelardy, A. Robert, and P. Delost. 1976. Changes in the concentrations of testosterone and androstenedione in the plasma and testis of the guinea pig from birth to death. J. Reprod. Fertil. 48(2):291-300.

Riggs, B.L., and J.C. Gallagher. 1977. Evidence for bihormonal deficiency state (estrogen and 1,25 dihydroxy vitamin D) in patients with postmenopausal osteoporosis. Pages 639-648 in A.W. Norman, K. Schaefer, J.W. Coburn, H.F. DeLuca, D. Fraser, H.G. Grigoleit, and D.V. Herrath, eds. Vitamin D: Biochemical, chemical and clinical aspects related to calcium metabolism. DeGruyter, Berlin.

Riggs, B.L., C.D. Arnaud, J. Jowsey, R.S. Goldsmith, and A.J. Kelly. 1973. Parathyroid function in primary osteoporosis. J. Clin. Invest. 52:181-184.

Riley, V., D.H. Spackman, and G.A. Santisteban. 1978. The LDH virus: An interfering biological contaminant. Science 200:124-126.

Rings, R.W., and J.E. Waagner. 1972. Incidence of cardiac and other soft tissue mineralized lesions in DBA/2 mice. Lab. Anim. Sci. 22:344-352.

Ritchie, D.M., G.J. Kelliher, A. MacMillan, W. Fasolak, J. Roberts, and S. Mansukhani. 1979. The cat as a model for myocardial infarction. Cardiovasc. Res. 13:199-206.

Ritchie, J.L., G.B. Trobaugh, G.W. Hamilton, K.L. Gould, K.A. Narahara, J.A. Murray, and D.L. Williams. 1977. Myocardial imaging with thallium-201 at rest and during exercise. Comparison with coronary arteriography and resting and stress electrocardiography. Circulation 56:66-71.

Robbins, S.L. 1974a. Systemic diseases. Pages 259-313 in Pathologic basis of disease. W.B. Saunders Co., Philadelphia.

Robbins, S.L. 1974b. Small intestine. Pages 930-950 in Pathologic basis of disease. W.B. Saunders Co., Philadelphia.

Robbins, S.L. 1974c. The colon. Pages 951-973 in Pathologic basis of disease. W.B. Saunders Co., Philadelphia.

Robbins, S.L. 1974d. The breast. Pages 1265-1296 in Pathologic basis of disease. W.B. Saunders Co., Philadelphia.

Roberts, J.A. 1972. The male reproductive system. Pages 878-888 in R.N.T-W. Fiennes, ed. Pathology of Simian primates. Part I. General Pathology. S. Karger, Basel.

Roberts, J., and P.B. Goldberg. 1975. Changes in cardiac membranes as a function of age, with particular emphasis on reactivity to drugs. Adv. Exp. Med. Biol. 61: 119-148.

Roberts, J., and P.B. Goldberg. 1976. Changes in basic cardiovascular activities during the lifetime of the rat. Exp. Aging Res. 2(6):487-517.

Roberts, R., P.D. Henry, and B.E. Sobel. 1975. An improved basis for enzymatic estimation of infarct size. Circulation 52:743-754.

Roberts, S.R., and L.C. Helper. 1972. Cataracts in Afghan hounds. J. Am. Vet. Med. Assoc. 160:427-432.

Robertson, D.M., and J.P. Creasman. 1972. Effects of topical Thio-TEPA on rat eyes. Am. J. Ophthalmol. 73:73-77.

Robinson, D.G., Jr. 1975. Gerbil care and maintenance. Gerbil Digest 2(2). Available from Tumblebrook Farm, Inc., West Brookfield, Massachusetts. 4 p.

Robinson, F.R. 1976a. Hamster. Pages 253-270 in E.C. Melby, Jr. and N.H. Altman, eds. Handbook of laboratory animal science. Vol. III. CRC Press, Inc., Cleveland, Ohio.

Robinson, F.R. 1976b. Naturally occurring neoplastic disease. V. Guinea pig. Pages 275-278 in E.C. Melby, Jr. and N.H. Altman, eds. Handbook of laboratory animal science. Vol. III. CRC Press, Inc., Cleveland, Ohio.

Robinson, F.R., and F.M. Garner. 1973. Histopathologic survey of 2500 German Shepherd military working dogs. Am. J. Vet. Res. 34:437-442.

Robinson, N.E., and J.R. Gillespie. 1973a. Lung volumes in aging Beagle dogs. J. Appl. Physiol. 35:317-321.

Robinson, N.E., and J.R. Gillespie. 1973b. Morphologic features of the lungs of aging Beagle dogs. Am. Rev. Respir. Dis. 108:1193-1199.

Robinson, N.E., and J.R. Gillespie. 1975. Pulmonary diffusing capacity and capillary blood volume in aging dogs. J. Appl. Physiol. 38:647-650.

Robinson, R. 1973. Acromelanic albinism in mammals. Genetica 44:454-458.

Rodin, J. 1978. Has the distinction between internal versus external control of feeding outlived its usefulness? Pages 75-85 in G.A. Bray, ed. Recent advances in obesity research: II. Proceedings of the 2nd International Congress on Obesity, held October 23-26, 1977 in Washington, D.C. Newman Publishing, Ltd., London.

Rogers, J.B., and H.T. Blumenthal. 1960. Studies on guinea pig tumors. I. Report on fourteen spontaneous guinea pig tumors, with a review of the literature. Cancer Res. 20:191-197.

Rohovsky, M.W., R.A. Griesemer, and L. Wolfe. 1966. The germ-free cat. Lab. Anim. Care 16(1):52-59.

Roldan, A.G., E.J. del Castello, A. Boveris, A.M. Garaza Pereira, and A.O.M. Stoppani. 1971. Decreased activity of 3-hydroxybutyrate dehydrogenase in diabetic liver mitochondria. Proc. Soc. Exp. Biol. Med. 137: 791-793.

Romualdez, A., R.I. Sha'afi, Y. Lange, and A.K. Solomon. 1972. Cation transport in dog red cells. J. Gen. Physiol. 60:46-57.

Rosan, R.C., T.C. Durbridge, M.M. Bieber, and M.C. Cogan. 1970. Oxygen-induced bronchiolar changes in infancy. Arch. Dis. Child. 45:710-717.

Roscoe, H.G., and M.J. Fahrenbach. 1962. Cholesterol metabolism in the gerbil. Proc. Soc. Exp. Biol. Med. 110:51-55.

Rosen, S., and P. Olin. 1965. Hearing loss and coronary heart disease. Arch. Otolaryngol. 82:236-243.

Rosen, S., M. Bergman, D. Plester, A. El-Mofty, and M.H. Satti. 1962. Presbycusis study of a relatively noise-free population in the Sudan. Ann. Otol. Rhinol. Laryngol. 71:727-743.

Rosenberg, H.M., C.E. Rehfeld, and T.E. Emmering. 1966. A method for epidemiologic assessment of periodontal health-disease state in a Beagle hound colony. J. Periodontol. 37:208-213.

Rosenblum, I.Y., H.E. Black, and C.C. Capen. 1979. Diabetes mellitus in the dog. Pages 115-118 in E.J. Andrews, B.C. Ward, and N.H. Altman, eds. Spontaneous animal models of human disease. Vol. I. Academic Press, New York.

Ross, M.D. 1965. A comparison of the normal cochlea with the abnormal of the waltzing mouse. Pages 408-409 in Abstracts of The American Association of Anatomists 78th Annual Meeting, Miami, Florida, April 1965. American Association of Anatomists, Little Rock, Arkansas.

Ross, M.D. 1979. Effects of aging on the otoconia. Pages 163-177 in Special senses in aging. Proceedings of a symposium held October 10-11, 1977 at the University of Michigan, Ann Arbor. Institute of Gerontology, University of Michigan, Ann Arbor, Michigan.

Ross, M.H. 1961. Length of life and nutrition in the rat. J. Nutr. 75:197-210.

Ross, M.H. 1969. Aging, nutrition and hepatic enzyme patterns in the rat. J. Nutr. 97:563-602.

Ross, M.H. 1978. Nutritional regulation of longevity. Pages 173-190 in J.A. Behnke, C.E. Finch, and G.B. Moment, eds. The biology of aging. Plenum Publishing Corp., New York.

Ross, M.H., and G. Bras. 1973. Influence of protein under- and over-nutrition on spontaneous tumor prevalence in the rat. J. Nutr. 103:944-963.

Ross, M.H., and G. Bras. 1975. Food preference and length of life. Science 190:165-167.

Ross, M.H., E. Lustbader, and G. Bras. 1976. Dietary practices and growth responses as predictors of longevity. Nature 262:548-553.

Roth, G.S., and R.C. Adelman. 1975. Age related change in hormone binding by target cells and tissues; possible role in altered adaptive responsiveness. Exp. Gerontol. 10:1-11.

Rothbaum, D.A., D.J. Shaw, C.S. Angeli, and N.W. Shock. 1973. Cardiac performance in the unanesthetized senescent male rat. J. Gerontol. 28:287-292.

Rothfels, K.H., E.B. Kupelwieser, and R.C. Parker. 1963. Effects of x-irradiated feeder layers on mitotic activity and development of aneuploidy in mouse-embryo cells in vitro. Can. Cancer Conf. 5:191-215.

Rothstein, M. 1977. Recent developments in the age-related alteration of enzymes: A review. Mech. Ageing Dev. 6:241-257.

Rotman, M., G.S. Wagner, and A.G. Wallace. 1972. Brady-arrhythmias in acute myocardial infarction. Circulation 45:703-722.

Rouser, G., G. Kritchevsky, A. Yamamoto, and C. Baxter. 1972. Lipids in the nervous system of different species as a function of age. Pages 261-360 in R. Paoletti and G. Kritchevsky, eds. Advances in lipid research. Vol. 10. Academic Press, New York.

Rowe, D.W., E.B. McGoodwin, G.R. Martin, M.D. Sussman, D. Grahn, B. Faris, and C. Franzblau. 1974. A sex-linked defect in the cross-linking of collagen and elastin associated with the mottled locus in mice. J. Exp. Med. 139:180-192.

Rowland, R.E., J.H. Marshall, and J. Jowsey. 1959. Radium in human bone: The microradiographic appearance. Radiat. Res. 10:323-336.

Rowlatt, C., F.C. Chesterman, M.U. Sheriff. 1976. Life-span, age changes and tumor incidence in an aging C57BL mouse colony. Lab. Anim. 10:419-442.

Rowsell, H.C., J.F. Mustard, M.A. Packham, and W.J. Dodds. 1966. The hemostatic mechanism and its role in cardio- vascular disease of swine. Pages 365-376 in L.K. Bus- tad and R.O. McClellan, eds. Swine in biomedical re- search. Proceedings of a symposium held July 19-22, 1965 at the Pacific Northwest Laboratory, Richland, Washington. Batelle Memorial Institute, Pacific North- west Laboratory, Richland, Washington.

Ruben, R.J., G.G. Knickerbocker, J. Sekula, G.T. Nager, and J.E. Bordley. 1959. Cochlear microphonics in man. Laryngoscope 69:665-671.

Rubin, L.F. 1976. Hemeralopia in dogs. Trans. Am. Acad. Ophthalmol. Otolaryngol. 81:OP 677-682.

Rubin, L.F., and R.D. Flowers. 1972. Inherited cataract in a family of Standard Poodles. J. Am. Vet. Med. Assoc. 161:207-208.

Rubin, L.F., S.A. Koch, and R.J. Huber. 1969. Hereditary cataracts in Miniature Schnauzers. J. Am. Vet. Med. Assoc. 154:1456-1458.

Rubin, P., and G.W. Casarett. 1968. Clinical radiation pathology Vol. I. W.B. Saunders Co., Philadelphia. 517 p.

Rudel, L.L., and H.B. Lofland, Jr. 1975. Circulation lipoproteins in nonhuman primates. Primates Med. 9: 224-266.

Ruffin, J.M., W.O. Dobbins, and W.M. Ronfail. 1976. Whipple's disease. Pages 510-517 in H. Bockus, ed. Gastroenterology II. W.B. Saunders Co., Philadelphia.

Ruhren, R. 1965. Normal values for hemoglobin concentra- tion and cellular elements in the blood of Mongolian gerbils. Lab. Anim. Care 15:313-320.

Rumberger, E., and J. Timmermann. 1976. Age-changes of the force-frequency-relationship and the duration of action potential of isolated papillary muscles of guinea pig. Eur. J. Appl. Physiol. 35(4):277-284.

Russell, E.S. 1966. Lifespan and aging patterns. Pages 511-519 in E.L. Green, ed. Biology of the laboratory mouse. McGraw-Hill, New York.

Russell, E.S. 1972. Genetic considerations in the selec- tion of rodent species and strains for research in aging. Pages 33-53 in D.C. Gibson, ed. Development of the rodent as a model system of aging. Book I. DHEW Pub. No. (NIH) 72-121. U.S. Department of Health, Education, and Welfare, Washington, D.C.

Russell, S.W., J.A. Gomey, and J.O. Trowbridge. 1971. Canine histiocytic ulcerative colitis: The early lesion and its progression to ulceration. Lab. Invest. 25:509-515.

Rust, J.H., R.J. Robertson, E.F. Staffeldt, G.A. Sacher, D. Grahn, and R.J.M. Fry. 1966. Effects of lifetime periodic gamma-ray exposure on the survival and pathology of guinea pigs. Pages 217-244 in P.J. Lindop and G.A. Sacher, eds. Radiation and ageing. Proceedings of a colloquium held June 23-24, 1966 in Semmering, Austria. Taylor and Francis, Ltd., London.

Ryan, J.M. 1979. Effect of different fetal bovine serum concentrations on the replicative life span of cultured chick cells. In Vitro 15:895-899.

Ryan, S.F., T.N. Vincent, R.S. Mitchell, G.F. Filley, and G. Dart. 1965. Ductectosia: An asymptomatic pulmonary change related to age. Med. Thorac. 22:181-187.

Sacher, G.A. 1966. The Gompertz transformation in the study of injury-mortality relationship. Application to late radiation effects and ageing. Pages 411-441 in P.J. Lindop and G.A. Sacher, eds. Radiation and ageing. Taylor and Francis, London.

Sacher, G.A. 1976. Evaluation of the entropy and information terms governing mammalian longevity. Interdiscip. Top. Gerontol. 9:69-82.

Sacher, G.A. 1978. Longevity, aging and death: An evolutionary perspective. Gerontologist 18:112-119.

Sacher, G.A., and R.W. Hart. 1978. Longevity, aging and comparative cellular and molecular biology of the house mouse, Mus musculus, and the white-footed mouse, Peromyscus leucopus. Pages 71-96 in D. Bergsma and D.E. Harrison, eds. Genetic effects on aging. Birth defects original article series. Vol. 14, No. 1. A.R. Liss, New York.

Sacksteder, M.R. 1976. Occurrence of spontaneous tumors in the germfree F344 rat. J. Natl. Cancer Inst. 57: 1371-1373.

Sade, D.S., K. Cushing, P. Cushing, J. Dunaif, A. Figueroa, J. Kaplan, C. Taner, D. Rhodes, and J. Schneider. 1977. Population dynamics in relation to social structure of Cayo, Santiago. Yearb. Phys. Anthropol. 20: 253-262.

Saito, S., Y. Kurokawa, and H. Sato. 1977. Effects of various diets on growth, longevity and incidence of spontaneous tumors of Praomys (Mastomys) natalensis. Sci. Rep. Res. Inst. Tohoku Univ. Ser. C 24:33-42.

Salazar, A.E. 1961. Experimental myocardial infarction. Induction of coronary thrombosis in the intact closed-chest dog. Circ. Res. 9:1351-1356.

Salter, R.B., and P. Field. 1960. The effects of continuous compression on living articular cartilage. J.
Bone Joint Surg. 42-A:31-49.

Salzman, C., and R.I. Shader. 1978a. Depression in the
elderly. I. Relationship between depression, psychologic defense mechanisms and physical illness. J. Am.
Geriatr. Soc. 26:253-260.

Salzman, C., and R.I. Shader. 1978b. Depression in the
elderly. II. Possible drug etiologies; differential
diagnostic criteria. J. Am. Geriatr. Soc. 26:303-308.

Sander, C.H., and R.F. Langham. 1968. Canine histiocytic
ulcerative colitis. A condition resembling Whipple's
disease, colonic histiocytosis, and malakopakia in man.
Arch. Pathol. 85:94-100.

Sarich, V.M., and J.E. Cronin. 1976. Molecular systema-
tics of the primates. Pages 141-169 in M. Goodman and
R.E. Tashian, eds. Molecular anthropology. Plenum
Publishing Corp., New York.

Sarks, S.H. 1976. Ageing and degeneration in the macular
region: A clinico-pathologic study. Br. J. Ophthalmol.
60:324-341.

Sass, B., L.S. Rabstein, R. Madison, R.M. Nims, R.C.
Peters, and G. Kelloff. 1975. Incidence of spontaneous neoplasms in F344 rats throughout the natural life
span. J. Natl. Cancer Inst. 54:1449-1456.

Satakopan, V.N., and P.A. Kurup. 1977. Changes in the
proteoglycans of tissues in rats fed atherogenic diet.
Indian J. Biochem. Biophys. 14:172-175.

Saxe, S.R., J.C. Greene, H.M. Bohannan, and J.R. Vermil-
lion. 1967. Oral debris, calculus and periodontal
disease in the Beagle dog. Periodontics 5:217-225.

Scadding, J.G. 1977. Definition and clinical categories
of asthma. Pages 1-10 in T.J.H. Clark and S. Godfrey,
eds. Asthma. W.B. Saunders Co., Philadelphia.

Schacter, S., and J. Rodin. 1974. Obese humans and rats.
Lawrence Erbaum Associates, Potomac, Maryland. 182 p.

Schall, W.D. 1974. Malabsorption-syndromes (malassimilation). Pages 742-747 in R.W. Kirk, ed. Current veterinary therapy. V. Small animal practice. W. B.
Saunders Co., Philadelphia.

Schall, W.D., and V. Perman. 1975. Diseases of the red
blood cells. Pages 1581-1626 in S.J. Ettinger, ed.
Textbook of veterinary internal medicine. Diseases of
the dog and cat. Vol. 2. W.B. Saunders Co., Philadelphia.

Schalm, O.W. 1964. Canine hematology. Vet. Scope 9:2.

Schalm, O.W. 1965. Veterinary hematology. 2nd ed. Lea and Febiger, Philadelphia. 646 p.

Schalm, O.W. 1971. Comments on feline leukemia: Clinical and pathologic features, differential diagnosis. J. Am. Vet. Med. Assoc. 158:1025-1031.

Schardein, J.L., J.E. Fitzgerald, and D.H. Kaump. 1968. Spontaneous tumors in Holtzman-source rats of various ages. Pathol. Vet. 5:238-252.

Schectman, L.R., W.F. Ammons, D.M. Simpson, and R.C. Page. 1972. Host tissue response in chronic periodontal disease II. Histologic features of the normal periodontium and histologic and ultrastructural manifestations of disease in the marmoset. J. Periodontal Res. 7: 195-212.

Schei, O., J. Waerhaug, A. Lovdal, and A. Arno. 1959. Alevolar bone loss as related to oral hygiene and age. J. Periodontol. 30:7-16.

Scheibel, A.B. 1978. Structural aspects of the aging brain. Spine systems and the dendritic arbor. Pages 353-374 in R. Katzman, R.D. Terry, and K.L. Bick, eds. Alzheimer's disease: Senile dementia and related disorders. Vol. 7. Aging series. Raven Press, New York.

Scheibel, M.E., R.D. Lindsay, J. Tomujasu, and A.B. Scheibel. 1975. Progressive dendritic changes in aging human cortex. Exp. Neurol. 47:392-403.

Schemmel, R., O. Mickelsen, and Z. Tolgay. 1969. Dietary obesity in rats: Influence of diet, weight, age, and sex on body composition. Am. J. Physiol. 216:373-379.

Schemmel, R., O. Mickelsen, and J.L. Gill. 1970. Dietary obesity in rats: Body weight and body fat accretion in seven strains of rats. J. Nutr. 100:1041-1048.

Schiff, L.J., A.M. Shefner, P.W. Barbera, and S.M. Poiley. 1973. Microbial flora and viral contact status of Chinese hamsters (Cricetulus griseus). Lab. Anim. Sci. 23:899-902.

Schlettwein-Gsell, D. 1970. Survival curves of an old age rat colony. Gerontologia 16:111-115.

Schlotthauer, C.F. 1932. Observations on the prostate gland of the dog. J. Am. Vet. Med. Assoc. 81:645-650.

Schmidt, M.J. and J.F. Thornberry. 1978. Cyclic AMP and cyclic GMP accumulation in vitro in brain regions of young, old and aged rats. Brain Res. 139:169-177.

Schmidt, R.R. 1971. Ophthalmic lesions in nonhuman primates. Vet. Pathol. 8:28-36.

Schmidt, S.Y., E.L. Berson, and K.C. Hayes. 1976. Retinal degeneration in cats fed casein. I. Taurine deficiency. Invest. Ophthalmol. 15:47-52.

Schneider, E.L., and Y. Mitsui. 1976. The relationship between in vitro cellular aging and in vivo human age. Proc. Natl. Acad. Sci. USA 73:3584-3588.

Schotterer, A. 1928. Beitrag zur Feststellung der Einzahl in verschiedenen Altersperioden vei der Hunden. Anat. Anz. 65(113):177-192.

Schreiner, B.F., S.M. Michaelson and C.L. Yuile. 1968. The effects of thoracic irradiation upon cardiopulmonary function in the dog. Am. Rev. Respir. Dis. 99:205-218.

Schroeder, H.E., and J. Lindhe. 1975. Conversion of stable established gingivitis in the dog into destructive periodontitis. Arch. Oral Biol. 20:775-782.

Schroeder, H.E., and J. Lindhe. 1980. Condition and pathological features of rapidly destructive experimental periodontitis in dog. J. Periodontol. 51:6-20.

Schroeder, H.E., J. Lindhe, A. Hugoson, and S. Münzel-Pedrazzoli. 1973. Structural constituents of clinically normal and slightly inflamed dog gingiva. A morphometric study. Helv. Odontol. Acta 17:70-83.

Schroeder, H., M. Graf de Beer, and R. Attström 1975. Initial gingivitis in dogs. J. Periodontal Res. 10:128-162.

Schuchman, S.M. 1974. Individual care and treatment of mice, rats, guinea pigs, hamsters and gerbils. Pages 558-614 in R.B. Kirk, ed. Current veterinary therapy. V. Small animal practice. W.B. Saunders Co., Philadelphia.

Schuknecht, H.F. 1964. Further observations on the pathology of presbycusis. Arch. Otolaryngol. 80:369-382.

Schuknecht, H.F. 1974. Pathology of the ear. Commonwealth Fund Publication Series. Harvard University Press, Cambridge, Massachusetts. 503 p.

Schultz, A.H. 1969. The life of primates. Universe Books, New York. 281 p.

Schuster, J. Von, G. Lämmler, and J. Thyssen. 1972. Normalwerte verschiedner enzme im serum von Mastomys natalensis (Smith, 1834). Z. Versuchstierk. 14:83-93.

Schwartz, A. (ed.) 1971. Methods in pharmacology. Vol. 1. Appleton-Century-Crofts, New York. 585 p.

Schwartz, J.C., M. Bavdry, M.P. Martres, J. Costenin, and P. Protias. 1978. Increased in vivo binding of ^{3}H-pimozide in mouse striatum following repeated administration of haloperidol. Life Sci. 23:1785-1790.

Schwartz, J.H., I. Tattersall, and N. Eldredge. 1978. Phylogeny and classification of the primates revisited. Yearb. Phys. Anthropol. 21:95-133.

Schwartz, P. 1970. Amyloidosis: Cause and manifestations of senile deterioration. Charles C Thomas, Springfield, Illinois. 395 p.

Schwartz, P.J., H.L. Stone, and A.M. Brown. 1976. Effects of unilateral stellate ganglion blockade on the arrhythmias associated with coronary occlusion. Am. Heart J. 92(5):589-599.

Schwartz, S.M. 1978. Selection and characterization of bovine aortic endothelial cells. In Vitro 14:966-980.

Schwarzbrott, S.S., J.E. Wagner, and C.G. Fisk. 1974. Demodicosis in the Mongolian gerbil (Meriones unguiculatus): A case report. Lab. Anim. Sci. 24:666-668.

Schwartzman, R.M., J.H. Rockey, and R.E. Holliwell. 1971. Canine reaginic antibody characterization of the spontaneous anti-ragweed and induced anti-dinitrophenyl reaginic antibodies of the atopic dog. Clin. Exp. Immunol. 9:549-569.

Schwentker, V. 1963. The gerbil. A new laboratory animal. Ill. Vet. 6:1-15.

Schwentker, V. 1968. Care and maintenance of the Mongolian gerbil. Tumblebrook Farm, Inc., West Brookfield, Massachusetts. 13 p.

Sclafani, A., and D. Springer. 1976. Dietary obesity in adult rats: Similarities to hypothalamic and human obesity syndromes. Physiol. Behav. 17:461-471.

Scott, R.F., E.S. Morrison, J. Jarmolych, S.C. Nam, M. Kroms, and F. Coulston. 1967a. Experimental atherosclerosis in rhesus monkeys. I. Gross and light microscopy features and lipid values in serum and aorta. Exp. Mol. Pathol. 7:11-33.

Scott, R.F., R. Jones, A.S. Daoud, O. Zumbo, F. Coulston, and W.A. Thomas. 1967b. Experimental atherosclerosis in rhesus monkeys. II. Cellular elements of proliferative lesions and possible role of cytoplasmic degeneration in pathogenesis as studied by electron microscopy. Exp. Mol. Pathol. 7:34-57.

Seegal, B.C., M.W. Hasson, E.C. Gaynor, M.S. Rothenberg. 1955. Glomerulonephritis produced in dogs by specific antisera: I. The course of the disease resulting from injection of rabbit antidog-kidney serum. J. Exp. Med. 102:789-805.

Segall, P.E., and P.S. Timiras. 1975. Age-related changes in thermo-regulatory capacity of tryptophan-deficient rats. Fed. Proc. 34:83-85.

Seibold, H.R., and R.H. Wolf. 1973. Neoplasms and proliferative lesions in 1065 nonhuman primate necropsies.
Lab. Anim. Sci. 23:533-539.

Severson, J.A., and C.E. Finch. 1978. Dopamine receptors
in the striatum of C57BL/6J male mice during aging.
Page 121 in Abstracts of the 31st annual meeting of
The Gerontological Society, held November 16-20, 1978
in Dallas, Texas. The Gerontological Society, Washington, D.C.

Shaar, C.J., J.S. Euker, G.D. Riegel, and J. Meites.
1975. The effects of castration and gonadal steroids
on serum luteinizing hormone and prolactin in young
and old rats. J. Endocrinol. 66:45-51.

Shah, B.G., G.V.G. Krishnarao, and H.H. Draper. 1967.
The relationship of Ca and P nutrition during adult
life and osteoporosis in aged mice. J. Nutr. 92:30-
42.

Shah, G.B., S.R. Shah, and H.C. Merchant. 1968. Evolutionary changes in electrocardiographic patterns in
various age groups in Indians. Indian Heart J. 20:
278.

Shain, S.A., and R.W. Boesel. 1978. Androgen receptor
content of the normal and hyperplastic canine prostate.
J. Clin. Invest. 61:654-660.

Shain, S.A., B. McCullough, and W.M. Nitchuk. 1979. Primary and transplantable adenocarcinomas of the A x C
rat ventral prostate gland: Morphologic characterization and examination of C_{19}-steroid metabolism by
early-passage tumors. J. Natl. Cancer Inst. 62:313-
322.

Sharawy, A.M. and S.S. Socransky. 1967. Effect of human
streptococcus strain GS-5 on caries and alveolar bone
loss in conventional mice and rats. J. Dent. Res.
46:1385-1391.

Shatney, C.H., D.J. MacCarter, and R.C. Lillehei. 1976a.
Effects of allopurinol, propranolol and methylprednisolone on infarct size in experimental myocardial infarction. Am. J. Cardiol. 37:572-580.

Shatney, C.H., D.J. MacCarter, and R.C. Lillehei. 1976b.
Temporal factors in the reduction of myocardial infarct
volume by methylprednisolone. Surgery 80:61-69.

Shaw, J.H., and A.M. Auskaps. 1954. Studies on the dentition of the marmoset. Oral Surg. Oral Med. Oral
Pathol. 7:671-677.

Shell, W.E., J.K. Kjekshus, and B.E. Sobel. 1971. Quantitative assessment of the extent of myocardial infarction in the conscious dog by means of analysis of

serial changes in serum creatine phosphokinase activity. J. Clin. Invest. 50:2614-2625.

Shellabarger, C.J., R.D. Brown, A.R. Rao, J.P. Shauley, V.P. Bond, A.M. Kellerer, H.H. Rossi, L.J. Goodman, and R.E. Mills. 1974. Rat mammary carcinogenesis following neutron or x-radiation. Pages 391-401 in Biological effects of neutron irradiation. Unipub, New York.

Sherman, B.M., S.G. Korenman. 1975. Hormonal characteristics of the human menstrual cycle throughout reproductive life. J. Clin. Invest. 55:699-706.

Sherman, B.M., J.H. West, and S.G. Korenman. 1976. The menopausal transition: Analysis of LH, FSH, estradiol and progesterone concentrations during menstrual cycles of older women. J. Clin. Endocrinol. Metab. 42:629-636.

Shevchuk, V.G. 1973. Effect of acetylcholine and catecholamines on hemodynamics at various stages of ontogenesis. Vestn. Akad. Med. Nauk. SSSR 28:52-55. (in Russian)

Shimmins, J., W.R. Lee, D.A. Smith, and N. Lucie. 1971. A study of calcium deposition in the skeleton of a dog using autoradiography. Calcif. Tissue Res. 8:121-132.

Shin, K.S., R.R. Bell, and H.H. Draper. 1976. Effect of estrogen on bone resorption induced by excess dietary P in mature and aged female rats. Abstract No. 1623. Fed. Proc. 35:499.

Shklar, G. 1966. Periodontal disease in experimental animals subjected to chronic cold stress. J. Periodontol. 37:377-383.

Shock, N.W. 1976. Cardiac performance and age. Pages 3-24 in H.I. Russek, ed. Cardiovascular problems. University Park Press, Baltimore.

Shore, B., and V. Shore. 1976. Rabbits as a model for the study of hyperlipoproteinemia and atherosclerosis. Pages 123-141 in C.E. Day, ed. Atherosclerosis drug discovery. Plenum Publishing Corp., New York.

Shreiner, D.P., M.L. Weisfeldt, and N.W. Shock. 1969. Effects of age, sex and breeding status on the rat heart. Am. J. Physiol. 217(1):176-180.

Shumaker, R.C., S.K. Paik, and W.D. Houser. 1974. Tumors in the Gerbil-linae: A literature review and report of a case. Lab. Anim. Sci. 24:688-690.

Sie, T.-L., H.H. Draper, and R.R. Bell. 1974. Hypocalcemia, hyperparathyroidism and bone resorption in rats induced by dietary phosphate. J. Nutr. 104:1195-1201.

Siegel, E.T. 1977. Endocrine diseases of the dog. Lea and Febiger, Philadelphia. 212 p.

Siegel, M.I., and P.W. Sciulli. 1973. Eruption sequence of the deciduous dentition of Papio cynocephalus. J. Med. Primatol. 2:247-248.

Siekert, R.G., Jr., B.A. Dicke, M.T.R. Subbiah, and B.A. Kottke. 1975. Cholesterol balance in atherosclerosis-susceptible and atherosclerosis-resistant pigeons. Res. Commun. Chem. Pathol. Pharmacol. 10:181-184.

Siemers, P.T., C.B. Higgins, W. Schmidt, W. Asburn, and P. Hagan. 1978. Detection, quantitation, and contrast enhancement of myocardial infarction utilizing computerized axial tomography: Comparison with histochemical staining and 99m Tc-pyrophosphate imaging. Invest. Radiol. 13:103-109.

Siiteri, P.K. and J.D. Wilson. 1970. Dihydrotesterone in prostatic hypertrophy. The formation and content of dihydrotesterone in the hypertrophic prostate of man. Clin. Invest. 49:1737-1745.

Silberberg, M., and R. Silberberg. 1945. The influence of sex and breeding on skeletal ageing of mice. Anat. Rec. 91:89-106.

Silberberg, M., and R. Silberberg. 1950. Effects of a high fat diet on the joints of aging mice. Arch. Pathol. 50:828-846.

Silberberg, M., and R. Silberberg. 1960. Osteoarthrosis in mice fed diets enriched with animal and vegetable fat. Arch. Pathol. 70:385-390.

Silberberg, M., and R. Silberberg. 1962. Osteoarthrosis and osteoporosis in senile mice. Gerontologia 6:91-101.

Silberberg, M., and R. Silverberg. 1963a. Modifying action of estrogen on the evolution of osteoarthrosis in mice of different ages. Endocrinology 72:449-451.

Silberberg, M., and R. Silberberg. 1963b. Role of sex hormones in the pathogenesis of osteoarthrosis of mice. Lab. Invest. 12:285-289.

Silberberg, R. 1977. Epiphyseal growth and osteoarthrosis in blotchy mice. Exp. Cell Biol. 45(1-2):1-8.

Silberberg, R., and M. Silberberg. 1950. Growth and articular changes in slowly and rapidly developing mice fed a high-fat diet. Growth 14:213-230.

Silberberg, R., W.G. Stamp, P.A. Lesker, and M. Hasler. 1970. Aging changes in ultrastructure and enzymatic activity of articular cartilage of guinea pigs. J. Gerontol. 25(3):184-198.

Silberberg, R., M. Hasler, and P.A. Lasker. 1973. Aging of the shoulder joint of guinea pigs. Electron microscopic and quantitative histochemical aspects. J. Gerontol. 28(1):18-34.

Silverman, J., and J.-M. Chavannes. 1977. Biological values of the European hamster (Cricetus cricetus). Lab. Anim. Sci. 27:641-645.

Simms, H.S. 1967. Longevity studies in rats. I. Relation between life span and age of onset of specific lesions. Pages 733-747 in E. Cotchin and F.J.C. Roe, eds. Pathology of laboratory rats and mice. Blackwell Scientific Publications, Oxford; F.A. Davis Company, Philadelphia.

Simons, E.L. 1972. Primate evolution, an introduction to man's place in nature. MacMillan, New York. 322 p.

Simpkins, J.W., G.P. Mueller, H.H. Huang, and J. Meites. 1977. Evidence for depressed catecholamine and enhanced serotonin metabolism in aging male rats: Possible relation to gonadotropin secretion. Endocrinology 100:1672-1678.

Simpson, D.M., and B.E. Avery. 1974. Histopathologic and ultrastructural features of inflamed gingiva in the baboon. J. Periodontol. 45:500-510.

Simpson, G.G. 1945. The principles of classification and a classification of mammals. Bulletin of the American Museum of Natural History. Vol. 85. American Museum of Natural History, New York. 350 p.

Simson, M.B., W. Harden, C. Barlow, and A.H. Harken. 1979. Visualization of the distance between perfusion and anoxia along an ischemic border. Circulation 60:1151-1155.

Singh, S.N. 1973. Effect of age on the activity and citrate inhibition of malate dehydrogenase of the brain and heart of rats. Experientia 29:42-43.

Singh, S.N., and M.S. Kanungo. 1968. Alternations in lactate dehydrogenase of the brain, heart, skeletal muscle, and liver of rats of various ages. J. Biol. Chem. 243:4526-4529.

Sisk, D.B. 1976. Physiology. Pages 63-98 in J.E. Wagner and P.J. Manning, eds. The biology of the guinea pig. Academic Press, New York.

Sivam, S.P., and S.D. Seth. 1978. Metoprolol - a new cardioselective beta adrenoceptor antagonist in experimental cardiac arrhythmias. Indian J. Med. Res. 68:176-182.

Skougaard, M.R., and G.S. Beagrie. 1962. The renewal of gingival epithelium in marmosets (Callithrix jacchus) as determined through autoradiography with tritiated thymidine. Acta Odontol. Scand. 20:467-484.

Skougaard, M.R., and B.M. Levy. 1971. Collagen metabolism in periodontal membrane of the marmoset. Influence of peridontal disease. Scand. J. Dent. Res. 79:518-522.

Skow, L.C., R.R. Fox, and J.E. Womack. 1978. Inherited enzyme variation among JAX strains of domestic rabbits. J. Hered. 69:165-168.

Sladek, J.R., T.H. McNeil, P. Walker, and C.D. Sladek. 1979. Monoamine and neurophysin systems. Pages 80-99 in D.M. Bowden, ed. Aging in nonhuman primates. Van Nostrand Reinhold, New York.

Slauson, D.O., D.H. Gribble, and S.W. Russell. 1970. A clinico-pathological study of renal amyloidosis in dogs. J. Comp. Pathol. 80:335-343.

Smelser, G.K., and L. Von Sallman. 1949. Correlation of microscopic and slit lamp examination of developing hereditary cataracts of mice. Am. J. Ophthalmol. 32:1703-1712.

Smith, C.S. 1971. Spontaneous neoplasms in germfree BALB/cPi mice. Proc. Soc. Exp. Biol. Med. 138:542-544.

Smith, D.M., M.R.A. Khairi, and C.C. Johnston. 1975. The loss of bone mineral with aging and its relationship to risk of fracture. J. Clin. Invest. 56:311-318.

Smith, G.S., R.L. Walford, and M.R. Mickey. 1973. Lifespan and the incidence of cancer and other diseases in selected long-lived inbred mice and their F_1 hybrids. J. Natl. Cancer Inst. 50:1195-1213.

Smith, J.R., and K.I. Braunschweiger. 1979. Growth of human embryonic fibroblasts at clonal density: Concordance with results from mass cultures. J. Cell. Physiol. 98:597-602.

Smith, J.R., and L. Hayflick. 1974. Variation in the life-span of clones derived from human diploid cell strains. J. Cell Biol. 62:48-53.

Smith, R.A., E.A. Termer, and C.A. Glomski. 1976. Erythrocyte basophilic stippling in the Mongolian gerbil. Lab. Anim. 10:379-383.

Smith, R.A., and C.A. Glomski. 1977. Embryonic and fetal hemopoiesis in the Mongolian gerbil (Meriones unguiculatus). Anat. Rec. 189:499-517.

Smith, R.S., H. Hoffmann, and C. Cisar. 1969. Congenital cataract in the rat. Arch. Ophthalmol. 81:259-263.

Smith, W.O., M.K. DuVal, W. Joel, W.T. Honska, and S. Wolf. 1960. Gastric astrophy in dogs induced by administration of normal human gastric juice. Gastroenterology 39:55-61.

Snell, K.C. 1967. Renal disease of the rat. Pages 105-148 in E. Cotchin and F.J.C. Roe, eds. Pathology of rats and mice. Blackwell Scientific Publications, Oxford; F.A. Davis Company, Philadelphia.

Snell, K.C., and H.L. Stewart. 1965. Adenocarcinoma and proliferative hyperplasia of the prostate gland in female Rattus (Mastomys) natalensis. J. Natl. Cancer Inst. 35:7-14.

Snell, K.C., and H.L. Stewart. 1975. Spontaneous diseases in a closed colony of Praomys (Mastomys) natalensis. Bull. WHO 52:645-650.

Snyder, W.S., M.J. Cook, E.S. Nasset, L.R. Karhausen, G.P. Howells, and I.H. Tipton. 1975. Report of the task group on reference man. International Committee on Radiation Protection. Pub. No. 23. Pergamon Press, New York. 480 p.

Soames, J.V., and R.M. Davies. 1977. Intracellular collagen fibrils in early gingivitis in the Beagle dog. J. Periodontal Res. 12:378-386.

Socransky, S.S., C. Hubersak, and D. Propas. 1970. Induction of periodontal destruction in gnotobiotic rats by a human oral strain of Actinomyces naeslundii. Arch. Oral Biol. 15:993-995.

Söderholm, G., and R. Attström. 1977. Vascular permeability during initial gingivitis in dogs. J. Periodontal Res. 12:395-401.

Söderholm, G., and J. Egelberg. 1973. Morphological changes in gingival blood vessels during developing gingivitis in dogs. J. Periodontal Res. 8:16-20.

Soga, J. 1977a. Historical background of mastomys research. Pages 1-8 in J. Soga and H. Sato, eds. Praomys (Mastomys) natalensis. The significance of their tumors and diseases for cancer research. The Daiichi Printing Co., Ltd., Niigata, Japan.

Soga, J. 1977b. Maintenance and breeding problems of mastomys. Pages 13-18 in J. Soga and H. Sato, eds. Praomys (Mastomys) natalensis. The significance of their tumors and diseases for cancer research. The Daiichi Printing Co., Ltd., Niigata, Japan.

Soga, J., and H. Sato [eds.] 1977. Praomys (Mastomys) natalensis. The significance of their tumors and diseases for cancer research. The Daiichi Printing Co., Ltd., Niigata, Japan. 201 p.

Soga, J., H. Kanahara, K. Tazawa, and K. Hiraide. 1969. A new experimental animal, Praomys (Mastomys) natalensis, its spontaneous tumor production. Niigata Med. J. 83:372-378. (in Japanese.)

Sokoloff, L. 1956. Natural history of degenerative joint disease in small laboratory animals: 4. Degenerative joint disease in the laboratory rat. Arch. Pathol. 62:140-142.

Sokoloff, L. 1959. Osteoarthritis in laboratory animals. Lab. Invest. 8:1209-1217.

Sokoloff, L. 1960. Comparative pathology of arthritis. Adv. Vet. Sci. 6:193-250.

Sokoloff, L. 1969. The biology of degenerative joint disease. University of Chicago Press, Chicago. 162 p.

Sokoloff, L., and G.E. Jay. 1956. Natural history of degenerative joint disease in small laboratory animals. 2. Epiphyseal maturation and osteoarthritis of the knee of mice of inbred strains. Arch. Pathol. 62: 129-139.

Sokoloff, L., K.C. Snell, and H.L. Stewart. 1967. Degenerative joint diseases in Praomys (Mastomys) natalensis. Ann. Rheum. Dis. 26:146-154.

Sokolovsky, V. 1972. Achalasia and paralysis of the canine esophagus. J. Am. Vet. Med. Assoc. 160:743-755.

Solleveld, H.H. 1978. Types and quality of animals in cancer research. Acta Zool. Pathol. Antverp. 72:5-18.

Sorrentino, R.N., and J.R. Florini. 1976. Variations among individual mice in binding of growth hormone and insulin to membranes from animals of different ages. Exp. Aging Res. 2:191-205.

Sparschu, G.L., and R.J. Christie. 1968. Metastatic calcification in a guinea pig colony: A pathological survey. Lab. Anim. Care 18(5):520-526.

Spath, J.A., Jr., D.L. Lane, and A.M. Lefer. 1974. Protective action of methylprednisolone on the myocardium during experimental myocardial ischemia in the cat. Circ. Res. 35:44-51.

Spencer, J.T. 1973. Hyperlipoproteinemias in the etiology of inner ear disease. Laryngoscope 83:639-678.

Spitz, R.A. 1946. Anaclitic depression. Psychoanal. Study Child Monogr. Ser. 2:313-342.

Spitzer, R.L., J. Endicott, and E. Robins. 1978. Research diagnostic criteria: Rationale and reliability. Arch. Gen. Psychiat. 21:240-248.

Spoerri, P.E., P. Glees, and E. El Ghazzawi. 1974. Accumulation of lipofuscin in the myocardium of senile

guinea pigs: Dissolution and removal of lipofuscin
following dimethylaminoethyl p-chlorophenoxy-acetate
administration. An electron microscopic study. Mech.
Ageing Dev. 3(5-6):311-321.

Sprague, H.B. 1954. The normal senile heart. Pages 359-
371 in E.J. Stieglitz, ed. Geriatric medicine. 3rd
ed. J.B. Lippincott Co., Philadelphia.

Spratto, G.R., and R.E. Dorio. 1978. Effect of age on
acute morphine response in the rat. Res. Commun. Chem.
Pathol. Pharmacol. 19(1):23-36.

Sprott, R.L. 1975. Behavioral characteristics of
C57BL/6J, DBA/2J, and B6D2F$_1$ mice which are potentially
useful to gerontological research. Exp. Aging Res.
1:313-323.

Sprouse, R.F. 1976. Mycoses. Pages 153-161 in J.E.
Wagner and P.J. Manning, eds. The biology of the
guinea pig. Academic Press, New York.

Spurling, N.W. 1977. Haematology of the dog. Pages 365-
440 in R.K. Archer and L.J. Jefscott, eds. Comparative
clinical haematology. Blackwell Scientific Publications, Oxford.

Squire, R.A. 1966. Feline lymphoma. A comparison with
the Burkitt tumor of children. Cancer 19:447-453.

Squire, R.A., M. Bush, E.C. Melby, L.M. Neely, and B.
Yarbrough. 1973. Clinical and pathological study of
canine lymphoma: Clinical staging, cell classification
and therapy. J. Natl. Cancer Inst. 51:565-574.

Staats, J. 1976. Standardized nomenclature for inbred
strains of mice: Sixth listing. Cancer Res. 36:
4333-4377.

Stafford, T.J. 1974. Maculopathy in an elderly subhuman
primate. Mod. Probl. Ophthalmol. 12:214-219.

Stahl, S.S. 1973. Marginal lesion. Pages 94-166 in H.M.
Goldman and D.W. Cohen, eds. Periodontal therapy. 5th
ed. C.V. Mosby Co., St. Louis, Missouri.

Stahl, S.S., and R. Gerstner. 1960. The response of the
oral mucosa and periodontium to simultaneous administration of corisone and somatotropic hormone in young
adult male rats. Arch. Oral Biol. 1:321-324.

Stanley, N.F. 1974. The reovirus murine models. Prog.
Med. Virol. 18:257-272.

Stanley, N.F., and D. Keast. 1967. Murine infection with
reovirus 3 as a model for the virus induction of autoimmune disease and neoplasia. Pages 281-289 in M.
Pollard, ed. Perspectives in virology. Vol. V.
Academic Press, New York.

Stara, J.F., and E. Berman. 1967. Development of an outdoor feline colony for long term studies in radiobiology. Lab. Anim. Care 17:81-92.

Stary, H.C. 1974. Cell proliferation and ultrastructural changes in regressing atherosclerosis lesions after reduction of serum cholesterol. Pages 187-190 in G. Schettler and A. Weizels, eds. Atherosclerosis III, Proceedings of the Third International Symposium. Springer-Verlag, Berlin.

Stebbins, W.C. 1970. Studies of hearing and hearing loss in the monkey. Pages 41-66 in W.C. Stebbins, ed. Animal psychophysics: The design and conduct of sensory experiments. Appleton-Century-Crofts, New York.

Stebbins, W.C. 1973. Hearing of Old World monkeys (Cercopithecinae). Am. J. Phys. Anthropol. 38:357-364.

Steblay, R.W., and M.H. Lepper. 1961. Some immunologic properties of human and dog glomerular basement membrane. II. Nephritis produced in dog by rabbit antihuman glomerular basement membrane sera. J. Immunol. 87:636-646.

Steinberg, R.H., M. Reid, and P.L. Lacey. 1973. The distribution of rods and cones in the retina of the cat (Felis domesticus). J. Comp. Neurol. 148:229-248.

Stemerman, M.D., and R. Ross. 1972. Experimental atherosclerosis. I. Fibrous plaque formation in primates, an electron microscope study. J. Exp. Med. 136:769-789.

Stoltzner, G. 1976. Diet restriction, longevity and immunity in aging mice. Page 43 in Program, 29th Annual Meeting of the Gerontological Society, held October 13-17, 1976 in New York. The Gerontological Society, Washington, D.C.

Stoner, G.D., G. Myers, Y. Katoh, F. Jackson, B.F. Trump, B.R. Brinkley, and C.C. Harris. 1978a. Culture of human bronchial epithelial cells. Abstract No. CU305. J. Cell Biol. 79(2, Part 2):66a.

Stoner, G.D., C.C. Harris, D.G. Bostwick, R.T. Jones, B.F. Trump, E.W. Kingsbury, E. Fineman, and C. Newkirk. 1978b. Isolation and characterization of epithelial cells from bovine pancreatic duct. In Vitro 14:581-590.

Storer, J.B. 1978. Effect of aging and radiation in mice of different genotypes. Pages 55-70 in D. Bergsma and D.E. Harrison, eds. Genetic effects on aging. Birth defects original article series. Vol. 14, No. 1. A.R. Liss, Inc., New York.

Stott, G.G., W.E. Haensley, and R. Getty. 1971. Age changes in the weight of the ovary of the dog. Exp. Gerontol. 6:37-42.

Stover, B.J., and W.S.S. Jee [eds.] 1972. Radiobiology of plutonium. J.W. Press, Salt Lake City, Utah. 552 p.

Strasser, H. 1968. A breeding program for spontaneously diabetic experimental animals: Psammomys obesus (sand rat) and Acomys cahirinus (spiny mouse). Lab. Anim. Care 18(3):328-338.

Strasser, H., and W. Schumacher. 1968. Breeding dogs for experimental purposes. II. Assessment of 8-year breeding records for two Beagle strains. J. Small Anim. Pract. 9:603-612.

Strawbridge, H.T.G. 1960. Chronic pulmonary emphysema (an experimental study). II. Spontaneous pulmonary emphysema in rabbits. Am. J. Pathol. 37:309-331.

Strehler, B.L. 1977. Time, cells, and aging. 2nd ed. Academic Press, New York. 456 p.

Stroganova, N.P. 1975. Peculiarities of cardiac activity in renal form of experimental hypertension with different hemodynamic characteristics. Kardiologiya 15:48-53. (in Russian)

Stromberg, K., J.C. Azizkhan, and K.V. Speeg, Jr. 1978. Isolation of functional human trophoblast cells and their partial characterization in primary cell culture. In Vitro 14:631-638.

Strong, J.P. 1976. Atherosclerosis in primates. Introduction and overview. Primates Med. 9:1-15.

Strong, J.P., and H.C. McGill, Jr. 1967. Diet and experimental atherosclerosis in baboons. Am. J. Pathol. 50:669-690.

Strong, J.P., J. Rosal, R.H. Deupree, and H.C. McGill, Jr. 1966. Diet and serum cholesterol levels in baboons. Exp. Mol. Pathol. 5:82-91.

Strong, J.P., D.A. Eggen, and H.C. Stary. 1976. Reversibility of fatty streaks in rhesus monkeys. Primates Med. 9:300-320.

Stuart, B.P., R.D. Phemister, and R.W. Thomassen. 1975. Glomerular lesions associated with proteinuria in clinically healthy dogs. Vet. Pathol. 12:125-144.

Stuchlikova, E., M. Juricava-Horakova, and Z. Deyl. 1975. New aspects of the dietary effect on life prolongation in rodents. What is the role of obesity in aging? Exp. Gerontol. 10:141-144.

Sturges, J., and L. Reid. 1973. The effect of isoprenaline and pilocarpine on (a) bronchial mucus secreting tissue and (b) pancreas, salivary glands, heart, thymus, liver and spleen. Br. J. Exp. Pathol. 54:388-403.

Subcommittee on Feed Composition, Committee on Animal Nutrition, Agricultural Board, National Research Council, U.S. and Committee on Feed Composition, Research Branch, Department of Agriculture, Canada. 1969. United States—Canadian tables of feed composition. 2nd rev. National Academy of Sciences, Washington, D.C. 92 p.

Sufrin, G., R.Y. Kirdani, A.A. Sandberg, and G.P. Murphy. 1975. Estrogen binding and estrogen receptors in the prostate. Surg. Forum 26:584-586.

Suomi, S.J., and H.F. Harlow. 1978. Production and alleviation of depressive behaviors in monkeys. Pages 131-172 in J.D. Maser and M.E.P. Seligman, eds. Psychopathology: Experimental models. Freeman, San Francisco.

Susini, C., and M. Lavau. 1978. In-vitro and in-vivo responsiveness of muscle and adipose tissue to insulin in rats rendered obese by a high-fat diet. Diabetes 27:114-120.

Suter, P.F., and S.J. Ettinger. 1975. Chronic respiratory disorders. Pages 724-753 in S.J. Ettinger, ed. Textbook of veterinary internal medicine. Diseases of the dog and cat. Vol. 1. W.B. Saunders Co., Philadelphia.

Sweany, S.K., W.T. Moss, and F.J. Haddy. 1959. The effects of chest irradiation on pulmonary function. J. Clin. Invest. 38:587-593.

Sweet, R.D., and F.H. McDowell. 1975. Five years' treatment of Parkinson's disease with levodopa. Therapeutic results and survival of 100 patients. Ann. Intern. Med. 83:456-463.

Sylvia, A.L., and M. Rosenthal. 1979. Effects of age on brain oxidative metabolism in vivo. Brain Res. 165:235-248.

Takaro, T., and S.M. White. 1973. Unilateral severe experimental pulmonary emphysema. Am. Rev. Resp. Dis. 108:334-357.

Taketa, F., M.H. Attermeier, and A.G. Mauk. 1972. Acetylated hemoglobins in feline blood. J. Biol. Chem. 247(1):33-35.

Talbert, G.B. 1971. Effect of maternal age on postimplantation reproductive failure in mice. J. Reprod. Fertil. 24:449-452.

Talbert, G.B. 1977. Aging of the female reproductive system. Pages 318-356 in C.E. Finch and L. Hayflick, eds. Handbook of the biology of aging. Van Nostrand Reinhold, New York.

Tang, L.C., and G.C. Cotzias. 1977. L-3,4-Dihydroxy-phenylalanine-induced hypersensitivity simulating features of denervation. Proc. Natl. Acad. Sci. USA 74: 2126-2129.

Tanimoto, K. 1943. Studies on mammals in relation to bubonic plague in Manchuria. Dobutsugaku Zasshi 55: 117-127.

Tappen, N.C., and A. Severson. 1971. Sequence of eruption of permanent teeth and epiphyseal union in New World monkeys. Folia Primatol. 15:293-312.

Tataryn, I.V., P. Lomax, D.R. Meldrum, J.G. Bajorek, and H.L. Judd. 1980. Postmenopausal hot flashes: A disorder of thermoregulation? Abstract No. 84, Page 52 in Society for Gynecologic Investigation scientific abstracts. Abstracts of the 27th annual meeting held March 19-22, 1980 in Denver, Colorado. Society for Gynecologic Investigation, c/o Dr. W. Anne Reynolds, Office of Academic Affairs, Ohio State University, Columbus, Ohio.

Taylor, C.B., D.E. Patton, and G.E. Cox. 1963. Atherosclerosis in rhesus monkeys. VI. Fatal myocardial infarction in a monkey fed fat and cholesterol. Arch. Pathol. 76:404-412.

Taylor, G.N., L. Shabestari, J. Williams, C.W. May, W. Angus, and S. McFarland. 1976. Mammary neoplasia in a closed Beagle colony. Cancer Res. 36:2740-2743.

Templeton, G.H., J.T. Willerson, M.R. Platt, and M. Weisfeldt. 1978. Contraction duration and diastolic stiffness in aged canine left ventricle. Pages 169-173 in T. Kobayashi, T. Sano, and N.S. Dhalla, eds. Heart function and metabolism. Recent advances in studies on cardiac structure and metabolism. Vol. 11. University Park Press, Baltimore.

Terry, R.D. 1968. Electron microscopic studies of Alzheimer's disease and of experimental neurofibrillary tangles. Pages 213-224 in O.T. Bailey and D.E. Smith, eds. The central nervous system. Williams and Wilkins, Baltimore.

Terry, R.D. 1978. Aging, senile dementia, and Alzheimer's disease. Pages 11-14 in R. Katzman, R.D. Terry, and K.L. Bick, eds. Alzheimer's disease: Senile dementia and related disorders. Vol. 7. Aging series. Raven Press, New York.

Terry, R.D., and H.M. Wisniewski. 1972. Ultrastrucuture of senile dementia and of experimental analogs. Pages 89-116 in C. Gaitz, ed. Aging and the brain. Advances in behavioral biology. Vol. 3. Plenum Publishing Corp., New York.

Terry, R.D., and H. Wisniewski. 1977. Structural aspects of aging in the brain. Pages 3-9 in C. Eisdorfer and R.O. Friedel, eds. The cognitively and emotionally impaired elderly. Yearbook Medical Publishers, Chicago.

Thackray, A.C., and R.B. Lucas. 1974. Atlas of tumor pathology. 2nd series. Fascicle 10. Tumors of the major salivary glands. Armed Forces Institute of Pathology, Washington, D.C. 144 p.

Thakur M.L., A. Gottschalk, and B.L. Zaret. 1979. Imaging experimental myocardial infarction with indium-111-labeled autologous leukocytes: Effects of infarct age and residual regional myocardial blood flow. Circulation 60:297-305.

Thaxter, T.H., R.A. Mann, and C.E. Anderson. 1965. Degeneration of immobilized knee joint in rats. Histological and autoradiographic study. J. Bone Joint Surg. 47-A:567-585.

Thiessen, D.D., K. Owen, and G. Lindzey. 1971. Mechanisms of territorial marking in the male and female Mongolian gerbil (Meriones unguiculatus). J. Comp. Physiol. Psychol. 77:38-47.

Thompson, J.H., C. Su, J.C. Shih, D. Aures, L. Choi, S. Butcher, W.S. Loshota, M. Simon, and D. Silva. 1974. Effects of chronic nicotine administration and age on various neurotransmitters and associated enzymes in male Fischer 344 rats. Toxicol. Appl. Pharmacol. 27:41-59.

Thompson, J.S. 1969. Atheromata in an inbred strain of mice. J. Atheroscler. Res. 10:113-122.

Thompson, L.W., H.J. Michalewski, and R.E. Saul. 1978. Age differences in cortical evoked potentials: A comparison of normal older adults and individuals with CNS disorders. Pages 139-154 in K. Nandy, ed. Senile dementia: A biomedical approach. Elsevier, Amsterdam.

Thompson, S.W., R.A. Huseby, M.A. Fox, C.L. Davis, and R.D. Hunt. 1961. Spontaneous tumors in the Sprague Dawley rat. J. Natl. Cancer Inst. 39:303-309.

Thornback, J. [ed.] 1978. Red Data Book. Vol. 1. Mammalia. Rev. ed. International Union for Conservation of Nature and Natural Resources, Morges, Switzerland.

Thorpe, L.W., and T.J. Connors. 1975. The distribution of uterine glycogen during early pregnancy in the young and senescent golden hamster. J. Gerontol. 30:149-153.

Thung, P.L., L.M. Boot, and O. Muhlbock. 1956. Senile changes in the estrous cycles and in ovarian structure in some inbred strains of mice. Acta Endocrinol. 23:8-23.

Thurlbeck, W.M. 1976. Major problems in pathology. Vol. 5. Chronic airflow obstruction in lung diseases. W.B. Saunders Co., Philadelphia. 456 p.

Thurlbeck, W.M., and G.E. Angus. 1975. Growth and aging of the normal human lung. Chest 67:35-75.

Thurlbeck, W.M., D. Malaka, and K. Murphy. 1975. Goblet cells in the peripheral airways in chronic bronchitis. Am. Rev. Resp. Dis. 112:65-69.

Thurm, D.A., K.W. Samonds, and J.G. Fleagle. 1975. An atlas for the skeletal maturation of the cebus monkey. Harvard University School of Public Health, Boston. 19 p.

Till, J.E., and E.A. McCulloch. 1961. A direct measurement of radiation sensitivity of normal mouse bone marrow cells. Radiat. Res. 14:213-222.

Tilley, L.P., S.K. Liu, R. Gilbertson, D.M. Wagner, and P.F. Lord. 1977. Primary myocardial disease in the cat. A model for human cardiomyopathy. Am. J. Pathol. 87:493-513.

Timiras, P.S. 1972a. Diseases of aging. Pages 469-476 in P.S. Timiras, ed. Developmental physiology and aging. The MacMillan Co., New York.

Timiras, P.S. 1972b. Cardiovascular alterations with age: Atherosclerosis. Pages 477-501 in P.S. Timiras, ed. Developmental physiology and aging. The MacMillan Co., New York.

Timiras, P.S., D.B. Hudson, and S. Oklund. 1973. Changes in central nervous system free amino acids with development and aging. Prog. Brain Res. 40:267-275.

Timms, B.G., J.A. Chandler, and F. Sinowatz. 1976. The ultrastructure of basal cells of rat and dog prostate. Cell Tissue Res. 173:543-554.

Tirgari, M., and L.C. Vaughan. 1975. Arthritis of the canine stifle joint. Vet. Rec. 96:394-399.

Tissot, R.G., and C. Cohen. 1972. A new congenital cataract in the mouse. J. Hered. 63:197-201.

Todaro, G., and H. Green. 1963. Quantitative studies of the growth of mouse embryo cells in culture and their development into established lines. J. Cell Biol. 17:299-313.

Tomanek, R.J. 1970. Effects of age and exercise on the extent of the myocardial capillary bed. Anat. Rec. 167:55-62.

Tomanek, R.J., and U.L. Karlsson. 1973. Myocardial ultrastructure of young and senescent rats. J. Ultrastruct. Res. 42:201-220.

Tomlinson, B.E., and G. Henderson. 1976. Some quantitative cerebral findings in normal and demented old people. Pages 183-204 in R.D. Terry and S. Gershon, eds. Neurobiology of aging. Vol. 3. Aging series. Raven Press, New York.

Tomlinson, B.E., G. Blessed, and M. Roth. 1970. Observations on the brains of demented old people. J. Neurol. Sci. 11:205-242.

Toole, J.R., and N.M. Sulkin. 1974. Changes in cerebral arteries with aging. Pages 133-148 in G.J. Maletta, ed. Survey report on the aging nervous system. DHEW Pub. No. (NIH) 74-296. U.S. Department of Health, Education, and Welfare, Washington, D.C.

Trapp, G.A., G.D. Miner, R.L. Zimmerman, A.R. Mastri, and L.L. Heston. 1978. Aluminum levels in brain in Alzheimer's disease. Biol. Psychiatry 13:709-717.

Travis, D.F., and A. Travis. 1972. Ultrastructural changes in the left ventricle rat myocardial cells with age. J. Ultrastruct. Res. 39:124-148.

Treloar, A.E., R.E. Boynton, B.G. Behn, and B.W. Brown. 1967. Variation of the human menstrual cycle through reproductive life. Int. J. Fertil. 12:77-126.

Trentin, J.J. 1950. Vaginal sensitivity to estrogen as related to mammary tumor incidence in mice. Cancer Res. 10:580-583.

Troup, G.M., G.S. Smith, and R.L. Walford. 1969. Life span, chronologic disease patterns and age-related changes in relative spleen weights for the Mongolian gerbil (Meriones unguiculatus). Exp. Gerontol. 4:139-143.

Turnbull, B.W., and T.J. Mitchell. 1978. Exploratory analysis of disease prevalence data from survival/sacrifice experiments. Biometrics 34:555-570.

Tursov, V.S. [ed.] 1973. Pathology of tumours in laboratory animals. Vol. I, Part 1. Tumours of the rat. IARC Pub. No. 5. International Agency for Research on Cancer, World Health Organization, Lyon, France. 281 p.

Tursov, V.S. [ed.] 1976. Pathology of tumours in laboratory animals. Vol. I, Part 2. Tumours of the rat. IARC Pub. No. 6. International Agency for Research

on Cancer, World Health Organization, Lyon, France.
319 p.

Tust, M. 1958. Cataracta hereditaria mit mikrophthalmus
bei der hausmous. Z. Menschl. Vererb. Konstitutionsl.
34:593-600.

Tuttle, R.S. 1966. Age-related changes in the sensitivity of rat aortic strips to norepinephrine and associated chemical and structural alterations. J. Gerontol. 21(4):510-516.

Uhthoff, H.K., and Z.F.G. Jaworski. 1978. Bone loss in
response to long term immobilization. J. Bone Joint
Surg. 60-B:420-429.

Ullrich, R.L., M.C. Jernigan, and J.B. Storer. 1977.
Neutron carcinogenesis dose and dose-rate effects in
BALB/c mice. Radiat. Res. 72:487-498.

Umbach, R.E., R.C. Lange, J.C. Lee, and B.L. Zaret. 1978.
Temporal changes in sequential quantitative Thallium-
201 imaging following myocardial infarction in dogs:
Comparison of four- and twenty-four-hour infarct images.
Yale J. Biol. Med. 51:597-603.

United States Department of Agriculture (USDA). 1979.
Animal welfare enforcement. FY 1978. Report of the
Secretary of Agriculture to the President of the Senate
and the Speaker of the House of Representatives. U.S.
Department of Agriculture, Washington, D.C. 23 p.

Upton, A.C., A.W. Kimball, J. Furth, K.W. Christenberry,
and W.H. Benedict. 1960. Some delayed effects of
atom-bomb radiations in mice. Cancer Res. 20:1-62.

Urist, M.R. 1960. Observations bearing on the problem
of osteoporosis. Pages 18-45 in K. Rodahl, V.R.
Nicholson, and E.M. Brown, Jr., eds. Bone as a tissue.
McGraw-Hill, New York.

Urist, M.R., M.S. Gurvey, and D.O. Fareed. 1970. Long-
term observations on aged women with pathologic osteoporosis. Pages 3-37 in U.S. Barzel, ed. Osteoporosis.
Grune and Stratton, New York.

Vainisi, S.J., G.A. Fishman, E.D. Wolf, and G.K. Boese.
1976. Cone-rod dystrophy in the Guinea baboon. Trans.
Am. Acad. Ophthalmol. Otolaryngol. 81:OP 725-730.

Valtonen, M.H., and A. Oksanen. 1972. Cardiovascular
disease and nephritis in dogs. J. Small Anim. Pract.
13:687-697.

van der Linden, W., and F. Bergman. 1977. Change in bile
composition during gallstone formation in gerbils. Z.
Ernaehrungswiss. 16:115-119.

van der Schoot, P. 1976. Changing pro-oestrous surges of luteinizing hormone in aging 5-day cyclic rats. J. Endocrinol. 69:287-288.

van der Waaij, D., and C.A. Sturm. 1968. Antibiotic decontamination of the digestive tract of mice. Technical procedures. Lab. Anim. Care 18:1-10.

van der Waaij, D., J.M. Berghuis-de Vries, and J.E.C. Lekkerkerk-van der Wees. 1971. Colonization resistance of the digestive tract in conventional and antibiotic treated mice. J. Hyg. 69:405-411.

Vandevelde, M., C.E. Greene, and D.J. Hoff. 1976. Lower motor neuron disease with accumulation of neurofilaments in a cat. Vet. Pathol. 13:428-435.

Van Heyningen, R. 1971. Galactose cataract: A review. Exp. Eye Res. 11:415-426.

Van Hoosier, G.L., Jr., and L.R. Robinette. 1976. Viral and chlamydial diseases. Pages 137-152 in J.E. Wagner and P.J. Manning, eds. The biology of the guinea pig. Academic Press, New York.

Van Kruiningen, H.J. 1975. The ultrastructure of macrophages in granulomatous colitis of Boxer dogs. Vet. Pathol. 12:446-459.

Van Kruiningen, H.J., R.J. Montali, and J.D. Strandberg. 1965. A granulomatous colitis of dogs with histologic resemblance to Whipple's disease. Vet. Pathol. 2: 521-544.

van Pelt, F.G., and M.J. Blankwater. 1972. Immunological and clinical-chemical investigations on blood, urine, and kidney in aging Praomys (Mastomys) natalensis with spontaneous glomerulonephritis. Gerontologia 18:200-216.

van Steenis, G., and R. Kroes. 1971. Changes in the nervous system and musculature of old rats. Vet. Pathol. 8:320-332.

van Wagenen, G. 1970. Menopause in a subhuman primate. Anat. Rec. 166:392. (Abstract)

van Wagenen, G. 1972. Vital statistics from a breeding colony. J. Med. Prim. 1:3-28.

van Wagenen, G., and M.E. Simpson. 1973. Postnatal development of the ovary in Homo sapiens and Macaca mulatta and induction of ovulation in the macaque. Yale University Press, New Haven, Connecticut. 306 p.

van Zutphen, L.F.M., and R.R. Fox. 1977. Strain differences in response to dietary cholesterol by JAX rabbits: Correlation with esterase patterns. Atherosclerosis 28:435-446.

van Zutphen, L.F.M., M.G.C.W. den Bieman, W.C. Hulsmann, and R.R. Fox. 1980. Genetic and physiological aspects of cholesterol accumulation in hyperresponding and hyporesponding rabbits. Unpublished paper available from Dr. L.F.M. van Zutphen, Vakgroet Zootechniek, Department of Animal Genetics, University of Utrecht, Utrecht, The Netherlands.

Vaughan, D.W. 1977. Age-related deterioration of pyramidal cell basal dendrites in rat auditory cortex. J. Comp. Neurol. 171:501-516.

Vaughan, D.W., and A. Peters. 1974a. Electron microscopic studies of Wallerian degeneration in rat optic nerves. J. Comp. Neurol. 140:207-225.

Vaughan, D.W., and A. Peters. 1974b. Neuroglial cells in the cerebral cortex of rats from young adulthood to old age: An electron microscope study. J. Neurocytol. 3:405-429.

Verkratsky, N.S. 1970. Acetylcholine metabolism peculiarities in aging. Exp. Gerontol. 5(1):49-56.

Vernon, D.F. 1962. Idiopathic sprue in a dog. J. Am. Vet. Med. Assoc. 140:1062-1067.

Verrusio, A.C., and F.C. Fraser. 1966. Identity of mutant genes "shrivelled" and cataracta congenita subcapsularis in the mouse. Genet. Res. 8:377-378.

Verzar, F. 1959. Note on the influence of procain (novocain), para-aminobenzoicacid or diethylethanolamin on the ageing of rats. Gerontologia 3:351-358.

Vessell, E.S., C.M. Lang, W.J. White, G.T. Passananti, R.N. Hill, T.L. Clemmens, D.K. Liu, and D. Johnson. 1976. Environmental and genetic factors affecting the response of laboratory animals to drugs. Fed. Proc. 35:1125-1132.

Vijayan, V.K. 1977. Cholinergic enzymes in the cerebellum and the hippocampus of the senescent mouse. Exp. Gerontol. 12:7-11.

Villa, S., M. Mysliwiec, and G. de Gaetano. 1977. Prostacyclin and atherosclerosis in rats. Lancet 1: 1216-1217.

Vincent, A.L., and L.R. Ash. 1978. Further observations on spontaneous neoplasms in the Mongolian gerbil, Meriones unguiculatus. Lab. Anim. Sci. 28:297-300.

Vincent, A.L., D.D. Porter, and L.R. Ash. 1975. Spontaneous lesions and parasites of the Mongolian gerbil, Meriones unguiculatus. Lab. Anim. Sci. 25:711-722.

Vision research. 1978. A national plan: 1978-1982. Vol. 2. Panel reports. DHEW Pub. No. (NIH) 78-1259.

U.S. Department of Health, Education, and Welfare, Washington, D.C. 484 p.

Vizek, M., and I. Albrecht. 1973. Development of cardiac output in male rats. Physiol. Bohemoslov. 22:573-580.

Vo'ino-Iasenetski'i, V.V., and N.E. Dumbrova. 1974. Age-related changes in Descemet's membrane and Descemet's endothelium according to data of electron microscopy. Oftal'mol. Zh. 29:614-618. (in Russian)

von Hippel, E. 1930. Embryologische untersuchungen uber Vererbung angeborener Katarakte uber Schichtstar des Hundes sowie uber eine besondere Form von Kapselkata-rakt. Arch. f. Ophth. 124:300-324.

von Knorring, J. 1970. Effect of age on the collagen content of the normal rat myocardium. Acta Physiol. Scand. 79:216-225.

Von Voigtlander, P.F., S.J. Boukma, and G.A. Johnson. 1973. Dopaminergic denervation supersensitivity and dopamine stimulated adenyl cyclase activity. Neuropharmacology 12:1081-1086.

Von Voigtlander, P.F., E.G. Losey, and H.J. Triezenberg. 1975. Increased sensitivity to dopaminergic agents after chronic neuroleptic treatment. J. Pharmacol. Exp. Ther. 193:88-94.

Vyskocil, F., and E. Gutmann. 1972. Spontaneous transmitter release from nerve endings and contractile properties in the soleus and diaphragm muscles of senile rats. Experientia 28:280-281.

Wackers, F.J.Th., E.B. Sokole, G. Samson, J.B. v.d. Schoot, K.I. Lie, K.L. Liem, and H.J.J. Wellens. 1976. Value and limitations of thallium-201 scintigraphy in the acute phase of myocardial infarction. N. Eng. J. Med. 295:1-5.

Wagner, W.D. 1978. Risk factors in pigeons genetically selected for increased atherosclerosis susceptibility. Atherosclerosis 31: 453-463.

Wagner, W.D., and T.B. Clarkson. 1975. Comparative primate atherosclerosis. II. A biochemical study of lipids, calcium, and collagen and atherosclerosis. Exp. Mol. Pathol. 23:96-121.

Wagner, W.D., T.B. Clarkson, M.A. Feldner, and R.W. Prichard. 1973. The development of pigeon strains with selected atherosclerotic characteristics. Exp. Mol. Pathol. 19:304-319.

Wagner, W.D., R.W. St. Clair, and T.B. Clarkson. 1978. Angiochemical and tissue cholesterol changes of Macaca fascicularis fed an atherogenic diet for 3 years. Exp. Mol. Pathol. 28:140-153.

Walburg, H.E., Jr., and G.E. Cosgrove. 1967. Ageing in irradiated and unirradiated germfree ICR mice. Exp. Gerontol. 2:143-158.

Walford, R.L. 1969. The immunological theory of aging. Williams and Wilkins, Baltimore; Munksgaard, Copenhagen. 248 p.

Walike, B.C., C.J. Goodner, D.J. Koerker, E.W. Chideckel, and L.W. Kalnasy. 1977. Assessment of obesity in pigtailed monkeys (Macaca nemestrina). J. Med. Primatol. 6:151-162.

Walker, E.P. 1975a. Order: Rodentia. Pages 665-1082 in Mammals of the world. Vol. II. 3rd ed. The Johns Hopkins University Press, Baltimore.

Walker, E.P. 1975b. Rodentia; Caviidae; Genus: Cavia, Pallas, 1766. Page 1016-1017 in Mammals of the world. Vol. II. 3rd ed. The Johns Hopkins University Press, Baltimore.

Walker, E.P. 1975c. Order: Carnivora. Pages 1146-1282 in Mammals of the world. Vol. II. 3rd ed. The Johns Hopkins University Press, Baltimore.

Walker, J.P., and J. Boas-Walker. 1973. Properties of adenyl cyclase from senescent rat brain. Brain Res. 54:391-396.

Wallace, R.B., and J. Altman. 1970. Behavioral effects of neonatal irradiation of the cerebellum. II. Quantitative studies in young-adult and adult rats. Dev. Psychobiol. 2:266-272.

Wallace, R.B., C.E. Daniels, and J. Altman. 1972. Behavioral effects of neonatal irradiation of the cerebellum. III. Qualitative observations in aged rats. Dev. Psychobiol. 5:35-41.

Walsh, P.C., and J.D. Wilson. 1976. The induction of prostate hypertrophy in the dog with androstanediol. J. Clin. Invest. 57:1093-1097.

Walton, M. 1977a. Degenerative joint disease in the mouse knee; radiological and morphological observations. J. Pathol. 123:97-107.

Walton, M. 1977b. Degenerative joint disease in the mouse knee; histological observations. J. Pathol. 123:109-122.

Walton, M. 1977c. Studies of degenerative joint disease in the mouse knee joint; scanning electron microscopy. J. Pathol. 123:211-217.

Ward, A.A., W.S. McCulloch, and H.W. Magoun. 1948. Production of an alternating tremor at rest in monkeys. J. Neurophysiol. 11:317-330.

Ward, B.C., and W. Moore, Jr. 1969. Spontaneous lesions in a colony of Chinese hamsters. Lab. Anim. Care 19: 516-521.

Ward, J.M., C.H. Sodiekoff, and O.W. Schalm. 1969. Myeloproliferative disease and abnormal erythrogenesis in the cat. J. Am. Vet. Med. Assoc. 155:879-888.

Warner, M.R. 1976. Age incidence and site distribution of mammary dysplasias in young Beagle bitches. J. Natl. Cancer Inst. 57:57-61.

Waser, P.M. 1978. Postreproductive survival and behavior in a free-ranging female mangabey. Folia Primatol. 29:142-160.

Watkins, P.J. 1975. The bladder in diabetes. Practioner 214:56-59.

Waxman, S. 1973. Metabolic approach to the diagnosis of megaloblastic anemias. Med. Clin. North Am. 58:315.

Wayner, M.J., Jr., and R. Emmers. 1958. Spinal synaptic delay in young and aged rats. Am. J. Physiol. 194: 403-405.

Webb, S.W., A.A.J. Adgey, and J.F. Pantridge. 1972. Autonomic disturbance at onset of acute myocardial infarction. Br. Med. J. 3:89-92.

Weber, G., P. Fabbrini, L. Resi, R. Jones, D. Vesselinovitch, and R.W. Wissler. 1977. Regression of arteriosclerotic lesions in rhesus monkey aortas after regression diet. Atherosclerosis 26:535-547.

Webster, W.S., T.B. Clarkson, and H.B. Lofland. 1968. Carbon monoxide aggravated atherosclerosis in the squirrel monkey. Exp. Mol. Pathol. 13:36-50.

Wehrmacher, W.H., J.V. Talano, M.P. Kaye, and W.C. Randall. 1979. The unbalanced heart. Animal models of cardiac dysrhythmias. Cardiology 64:65-74.

Weibust, R.S., and G. Schlager. 1968. A genetic study of blood pressure, hematocrit and plasma cholesterol in aged mice. Life Sci. 7:1111-1119.

Weihe, W.H. 1973. Effect of temperature on the action of drugs. Ann. Rev. Pharmacol. 13:409-425.

Weinbaum, G., V. Marco, T. Ikeda, B. Mass, D.R. Meranze, and P. Kimbel. 1974. Enzymatic production of experimental emphysema in the dog. Route of exposure. Am. Rev. Resp. Dis. 109:351-357.

Weir, B.J. 1974. Reproductive characteristics of the hystricomorph rodents. Symp. Zool. Soc. London 34: 265-301.

Weisbroth, S.H. 1972. Pathogen-free substrates for gerontological research: Review, sources, and comparison

of barrier-sustained versus conventional laboratory
rats. Exp. Gerontol. 7:417-426.

Weisbroth, S.H. 1974. Neoplastic diseases. Pages 331-
375 in S.H. Weisbroth, R.E. Flatt, and A.L. Kraus,
eds. The biology of the laboratory rabbit. Academic
Press, New York.

Weisbroth, S.H., R.E. Flatt, and A.L. Kraus [eds.] 1974.
The biology of the laboratory rabbit. Academic Press,
New York. 496 p.

Weisfeldt, M.L. 1975. Function of cardiac muscle in
aging rat. Adv. Exp. Med. Biol. 61:95-118.

Weisfeldt, M.L., W.A. Loeven, and N.W. Shock. 1971.
Resting and active mechanical properties of trabeculae
carneae from aged male rats. Am. J. Physiol. 220:
1921-1927.

Weiss, L., K. Mayeda, and M. Dully. 1970. The karyotype
of the Mongolian gerbil, Meriones unguiculatus. Cy-
tologia 35:102-106.

Weisse, I., H. Stotzer, and R. Seitz. 1974. Age dependent and light dependent changes in the rat eye.
Virch. Arch. A 362:145-156.

Welch, M.H. 1977. Obstructive diseases. Pages 556-677
in C.A. Guenter and M.H. Welch, eds. Pulmonary medicine. J.B. Lippincott, Philadelphia.

Wensinck, F., and J.G.H. Russeler-van Embden. 1971. The
intestinal flora of colonization-resistant mice. J.
Hyg. 69:413-421.

Werboff, J., and J. Havlena. 1962. Effects of aging on
open field behavior. Psychol. Rep. 10:395-398.

Werthamer, S., L.H. Schwarts, J.J. Carr, and L. Sosking.
1970. Ozone induced pulmonary lesions: Severe epithelial changes following sublethal doses. Arch.
Environ. Health. 15:16-21.

Wessler, S. 1976. Introduction: What is a model? Pages
xi-xvi in Animal models of thrombosis and hemorrhagic
diseases. Report of a workshop organized by the Institute of Laboratory Animal Resources (ILAR) Committee
on Animal Models for Thrombosis and Hemorrhagic Diseases, held March 12-13, 1975 at the National Academy
of Sciences, Washington, D.C. DHEW Pub. No. (NIH)
76-982. U.S. Department of Health, Education, and
Welfare, Washington, D.C.

Wesson, L.D., Jr. 1969. Renal hemodynamics in physiological states. Pages 96-108 in Physiology of the
human kidney. Grune and Stratton, New York.

Wever, E.G., J.A. Vernon, and M. Lawrence. 1958. The nature of the cochlear potentials in the monkey. Acta Otolaryngol. 49:38-46.

Wexler, B.C. 1964. Correlation of adrenal cortical histopathology with arteriosclerosis in breeder rats. Acta Endocrinol. 45:613-631.

Wexler, B.C. 1970. Co-existent arteriosclerosis, PAN, and premature dying. J. Gerontol. 25:373-380.

Wexler, B.C. 1975. Metabolic and histopathologic changes in arteriosclerotic versus non-arteriosclerotic rats following isoproterenol-induced myocardial infarction with superimposed diabetes. Metabolism 24:1321-1337.

Wexler, B.C. 1976. Comparative effects of prolactin, perhenazines and reserpine on non-arteriosclerotic (virgin) vs arteriosclerotic (breeder) rats. Atherosclerosis 24:19-36.

Wexler, B.C., and B.P. Greenberg. 1974. Adrenal corticomedullary function in arteriosclerotic (virgin) rats. Atherosclerosis 20:155-172.

Wexler, B.C., and B.P. Greenberg. 1978. Clofibrate retardation of naturally-occurring arteriosclerosis in repeatedly bred male and female rats. Atherosclerosis 29:329-344.

Wexler, B.C., and J.T. Judd. 1970. Acute myocardial histopathology in normal and arteriosclerotic rats during isoproterenol induced infarction. Br. J. Exp. Pathol. 51:646-652.

Wexler, B.C., and G.W. Kittinger. 1963. Myocardial necrosis in rats: Serum enzymes, adrenal steroid and histopathological alterations. Circ. Res. 13:159-171.

Wexler, B.C., K.T. Judd, R.F. Lutmer, and J. Saroff. 1971. Spontaneous arteriosclerosis in female and male gerbils (Meriones unguiculatus). Atherosclerosis 14:107-119.

Wexler, B.C., S.G. Iams, and J.T. Judd. 1976. Arterial lesions in repeatedly bred spontaneously hypertensive rats. Circ. Res. 38:494-501.

Wheeldon, E.B., and H.M. Pirie. 1974. Measurement of bronchial wall components in young dogs, adult normal dogs and adult dogs with chronic bronchitis. Am. Rev. Resp. Dis. 110:609-615.

Wheeldon, E.B., and R.G. Breeze. 1979. Chronic bronchitis. Pages 181-182 in E.J. Andrews, B.C. Ward, and N.H. Altman, eds. Spontaneous animal models of human disease. Vol. II. Academic Press, New York.

Wheeldon, E.B., H.M. Pirie, E.W. Fisher, and R. Lee. 1974. Chronic bronchitis in the dogs. Vet. Rec. 94: 466-471.

Wheeldon, E.B., H.M. Pirie, and R.G. Breeze. 1976. A histochemical study of the tracheobronchial epithelial mucosubstances in normal dogs and dogs with chronic bronchitis. Folia Vet. Lat. 6:45-58.

Whikehart, D.R., and M.B. Lees. 1973. Amino- and carboxyl-terminal amino acids of proteolipid proteins. J. Neurochem. 20:1303-1315.

White, P., M.J. Goodhardt, J.P. Keet, C.R. Hiley, L.H. Carrasco, I.E.I. Williams, and D.M. Bowen. 1977. Neocortical cholinergic neurons in elderly people. Lancet 1:668-671.

Whiting, S.J., and H.H. Draper. 1980. The role of sulfate in the calciuria of high-protein diets in adult rats. J. Nutr. 110:212-222.

Whitney, J.C. 1967. The pathology of the canine genital tract in false pregnancy. J. Small Anim. Pract. 8: 247-263.

Whitney, J.C. 1974. Observations on the effect of age on the severity of heart valve lesions of the dog. J. Small Anim. Pract. 15:511-522.

Wiberg, G.S., H.L. Trenholm, and B.B. Coldwell. 1970. Increased ethanol toxicity in old rats: Changes in LD_{50}, in vivo and in vitro metabolism, and liver alcohol dehydrogenase activity. Toxicol. Appl. Pharmacol. 16(3):718-727.

Wichmann, J., R. Löser, H.P. Diemer, and W. Lochner. 1978. Pharmacological alterations of coronary collateral circulation: Implication to the steal-phenomenon. Pfluegers Arch. 373:219-224.

Wightman, S.R., P.A. Pilitt, and J.E. Wagner. 1978. Dentostomella translucida in the Mongolian gerbil (Meriones unguiculatus). Lab. Anim. Sci. 28:290-296.

Wilde, G., M. Cooper, and R.C. Page. 1977. Host tissue response in chronic periodontal disease. VI. The role of cell-mediated hypersensitivity. J. Periodontal Res. 12:179-196.

Wilhelmi, G., and R. Faust. 1976. Suitability of the C57 Black mouse as an experimental animal for the study of skeletal changes due to ageing, with special reference to osteoarthrosis and its response to tribenoside. Pharmacology 14:289-296.

Will, J.A., and J.M. Kay. 1974. Hypertensive pulmonary vascular disease associated with papain emphysema in rats. Respiration 31:208-220.

Willems, J.L., J. Roelandt, H. De Geest, H. Kesteloot, and J.V. Joosens. 1970. The left ventricular ejection time in elderly subjects. Circulation 42:37-42.

Willerson, J.T., R.W. Parkey, L.M. Buja, and F.J. Bonte. 1979. Technetium-99m stannous pyrophosphate "hot spot" imaging to detect acute myocardial infarcts. Cardiovasc. Clin. 10:139-148.

Williams, J.R., H. Nagasdawa, J.B. Robertson, and J.B. Little. 1979. Patterns of growth in embryonic Syrian hamster cells in vitro. Unpublished paper available from J.A. Williams, Department of Radiology, The George Washington University School of Medicine and Health Sciences, Washington, D.C.

Williams R.H. 1975. Etiologic, pathophysiologic and clinical interrelationships in diabetes. Johns Hopkins Med. J. 136:25-37.

Williams, R.H., and W.J. Thompson. 1973. Effect of age upon guanyl cyclase, adenyl cyclase and cyclic nucleotide phosphodiesterases in rats. Proc. Soc. Exp. Biol. Med. 143:382-387.

Willis, R.A. 1948. Pathology of tumors. Butterworth, London. 992 p.

Wilson, P.D. 1973. Enzyme changes in aging mammals. Gerontologia 19:79-125.

Wilson, R.W. 1973. Cigarette smoking, disability days and respiratory conditions. J. Occup. Med. 15:236.

Wintheiser, J.G., D.A. Clauser, and N.C. Tappen. 1977. Sequence of eruption of permanent teeth and epiphyseal union in three species of African monkeys. Folia Primatol. 27:178-197.

Wisniewski, H.M. 1978. Possible viral etiology of neurofibrillary changes and neuritic plaques. Pages 555-557 in R. Katzman, R.D. Terry, and K.L. Bick, eds. Alzheimer's disease: Senile dementia and related disorders. Vol. 7. Aging series. Raven Press, New York.

Wisniewski, H.M. 1979. The aging brain. Pages 148-152 in E.J. Andrews, B.C. Ward, and N.H. Altman, eds. Spontaneous animal models of human disease. Vol. II. Academic Press, New York.

Wisniewski, H.M., and D. Soiser. 1979. Neurofibrillary pathology: Current status and research perspectives. Mech. Ageing Dev. 9:119-142.

Wisniewski, H.M., and R.D. Terry. 1973. Morphology of the aging brain, human and animal. Prog. Brain Res. 40:167-186.

Wisniewski, H.M., and R.D. Terry. 1976. Neuropathology of the aging brain. Pages 265-280 in R.D. Terry and

S. Gershon, eds. Neurobiology of aging. Vol. 3.
Aging series. Raven Press, New York.

Wisniewski, H.M., R.D. Terry, and A. Hirano. 1970a.
Neurofibrillary pathology. J. Neuropathol. Exp.
Neurol. 29:163-176.

Wisniewski, H.M., A.B. Johnson, C.S. Raine, W.J. Kay, and
R.D. Terry. 1970b. Senile plaques and cerebral amyloidosis in aged dogs. A histochemical and ultrastructural study. Lab. Invest. 23:287-296.

Wisniewski, H.M., B. Ghetti, and R.D. Terry. 1973.
Neuritic (senile) plaques and filamentous changes in
aged rhesus monkeys. J. Neuropathol. Exp. Neurol.
32:566-584.

Wisniewski, H.M., B. Ghett, P.S. Spencer, and R.D. Terry.
1974. Neuritic (senile) plaque--an expression of a
cortical form of axonal dystrophy. J. Neuropathol.
Exp. Neurol. 33:187.

Wisniewski, H.M., M.E. Bruce, and H. Fraser. 1975. Infectious etiology of neuritic (senile) plaques in mice.
Science 190:1108-1110.

Wisniewski, H.M., H.K. Narang, and R.D. Terry. 1976.
Neurofibrillary tangles of paired helical filaments.
J. Neurol. Sci. 27:173-181.

Wissler, R.W., R.H. Hughes, L.E. Frazier, G.S. Getz, and
D. Turner. 1965. Aortic lesions and blood lipids in
rhesus monkeys fed "table prepared" human diets. Circulation 32:220.

Wolf, E.D., S.J. Vainisi, and R. Santos-Anderson. 1978.
Rod-cone dysplasia in the Collie. J. Am. Vet. Med.
Assoc. 173:1331-1333.

Woolcock, A.J., and P.T. Macklem. 1971. Mechanical factors influencing collateral ventilation in human, dog
and pig lungs. J. Appl. Physiol. 30:99-115.

Worgul, B.V., and H. Rothstein. 1975. Radiation cataract
and mitosis. Ophthalmol. Res. 7:21-32.

Wostmann, B.S. 1968. Germ-free versus non-germ-free ani-
mals in gerontological research. Pages 52-61 in The
laboratory animal in gerontological research. Pro-
ceedings of a symposium organized by the Institute of
Laboratory Animal Resources (ILAR) Committee on Animal
Research in Gerontology, held November 10, 1967 in St.
Petersburg, Florida. National Academy of Sciences,
Washington, D.C.

Wostmann, B.S. 1975. Nutrition and metabolism of the
germ-free mammal. World Rev. Nutr. Diet. 22:40-92.

Wostmann, B.S., M. Beaver, K. Bartizal, and D. Madsen. 1978. Gnotobiotic gerbils. Pages 132-135 in Proceedings of the 4th International Symposium on Contamination Control held September 10-13, 1978 in Washington, D.C. For information contact the Department of Microbiology, University of Notre Dame, Notre Dame, Indiana 46556.

Wright, N.G. 1967. The relationship between the virus of infectious canine hepatitis and interstitial nephritis. J. Small Anim. Pract. 8:67-70.

Wright, R.R. 1961. Elastic tissue of normal emphysematous lungs. Am. J. Pathol. 39:355-367.

Wulff, V.J., M. Piekielnick, and M.J. Wayner. 1963. The ribonucleic acid content of tissues of rats of different ages. J. Gerontol. 18:322-325.

Wunder, J.A., W.W. Briner, and G.P. Calkins. 1976. Identification of the cultivable bacteria in dental plaque from the Beagle dog. J. Dent. Res. 55:1097-1102.

Yagil, G. 1976. Are altered glucose-6-phosphate dehydrogenase molecules present in aged liver cells? Exp. Gerontol. 11:73-78.

Yakely, W.L. 1978. A study of heritability of cataracts in the American Cocker Spaniel. J. Am. Vet. Med. Assoc. 172:814-817.

Yakely, W.L., G.A. Hegreberg, and G.A. Padgett. 1971. Familial cataracts in the American Cocker Spaniel. J. Am. Anim. Hosp. Assoc. 7:127-135.

Yamaguchi, N., H. Weisberg, and G.B.J. Glass. 1967. Intestinal vitamin B-12 absorption in the dog: Evidence against an intrinsic factor mechanism. Gastroenterology 52:1145. (Abstract)

Yamamoto, M., and T.H. Ingalls. 1972. Delayed fertilization and chromosome anomalies in the hamster embryo. Science 176:518-521.

Yamamoto, M., T. Shimada, A. Endo, and G. Watanabe. 1973. Effects of low dose x-irradiation of the chromosomal non-disjunction in aged mice. Nature New Biol. 244:206-208.

Yamatake, Y., S. Sasagawa, S. Yanaura, and N. Kobayashi. 1977. Allergy induced asthma with Ascaris suum administration to dogs. Jpn. J. Pharmacol. 27:285-293.

Yanagimachi, R., and M.C. Chang. 1961. Fertilizable life of golden hamster ova and their morphological changes at the time of losing fertilizability. J. Exp. Zool. 148:185-203.

Yang, Y.H. 1965. Polyarteritis nodosa in laboratory rats. Lab. Invest. 14:81-88.

Yerganian, G., J.H. Gagnon, and A. Battaglino. 1978. Angioimmunoblastic lymphadenopathy, immunoblastic sarcoma of B cells. Animal model: Autoimmune-prone inbred Armenian hamster. Am. J. Pathol. 91:209-212.

Yodaikeu, R.E., and V. Pardo. 1975. Diabetic capillaropathy. Hum. Pathol. 6(4):455-465.

Yoon, C.H. 1979. Recent advances in hamster genetics. Pages 157-161 in F. Homburger, ed. Symposium of the Syrian hamster in toxicology and carcinogenesis research. Proceedings of a symposium held November 30-December 2, 1977 in Boston, Massachusetts. Bio-Research Institute, Cambridge, Massachusetts.

Yoon, C.H., and J. Slaney. 1972. Hydrocephalus: A new mutation in the Syrian golden hamster. J. Hered. 63: 344-346.

Young, D.M., A.W. Fetter, and L.C. Johnson. 1979. Osteoarthritis (osteoarthrosis; degenerative joint disease). Pages 257-261 in E.J. Andrews, B.C. Ward, and N.H. Altman, eds. Spontaneous animal models of human disease. Vol. II. Academic Press, New York.

Yu, B.P., H.A. Bertrand, and E.J. Masoro. In press. Nutrition-aging influence of catecholamine-promoted lipolysis. Metabolism.

Zahm, H. 1965. Die Ligamenta decussata im gesunden und arthrotischen Kniegelenk des Hundes. Kleintier-Prax. 10:38-47.

Zahor, Z., and V. Czabanova. 1977. Experimental atherosclerosis of the heart valves in rats following a long-term atherogenic regimen. Atherosclerosis 27:49-57.

Zeman, F.J. 1967. A semipurified diet for the Mongolian gerbil (Meriones unguiculatus). J. Nutr. 91:415-420.

Ziem, M., H. Coper, I. Broermann, and S. Strauss. 1970. Comparative studies of some effects of amphetamine in rats of different ages. Naunyn-Schmiedeberg Arch. Pharmacol. 267(3):208-223.

Zimmerman, E.G., C.W. Kilpatric, and B.J. Hart. 1978. The genetics of speciation in the rodent genus Peromyscus. Evolution 32:565-570.

Zorzoli, A., and J.B. Li. 1967. Gluconeogenesis in mouse kidney cortex. Effect of age and fasting on glucose production and enzyme activities. J. Gerontol. 22: 151-157.

Zs.-Nagy, I., and V. Zs.-Nagy. 1975. Age-dependence of heat-induced strand separation of DNA in situ in post-mitotic cells of rat brain as revealed by acridine orange microfluorimetry. Mech. Ageing Dev. 4:349-360.

Zucker, L.M., and T.F. Zucker. 1961. Fatty, a new mutation in the rat. J. Hered. 52:275-278.

Zwaan, J., and R.M. Williams. 1968a. Morphogenesis of the eye lens in a mouse strain with hereditary cataracts. J. Exp. Zool. 169:407-421.

Zwaan, J., and R.M. Williams. 1968b. Studies on the development of a hereditary cataract in the house mouse. Anat. Rec. 160:456-457. (Abstract)

Zwaan, J., and R.M. Williams. 1969. Cataracts and abnormal proliferation of the lens epithelium in mice carrying the cat[Fr] gene. Exp. Eye Res. 8:161-167.